MANAGEMENT OF ABDOMINAL HERNIAS

CONTENTS

CONTRIBUTORS

H. Brendan Devlin, CBE, MD, FRCS
Fir Tree House
Hilton
Yarm
North Yorkshire

Andrew Kingsnorth, BSc, MS, FRCS
Postgraduate Medical School Hospital
Derriford Hospital
Plymouth

P. J. O'Dwyer, FRCSI
Academic Department of Surgery
Western Infirmary
Glasgow

Karen Bloor, BA, MSc
Department of Health Science and Clinical Evaluation
Alcuin College
University of York

PREFACE TO THE FIRST EDITION

Another book on hernia? Well, not quite! My intention was to produce a neat practical book on hernia, not an exhaustive text. But a book about hernias would be incomplete without mention of the past, hence the 'practical book' has become encrusted with history and anecdote, and conceivably the book is more readable for this.

Almost all the material included has already been published elsewhere – the skeleton is the section on hernia in the current edition of *Rob and Smith's Operative Surgery*, also published by Butterworths, whereas other parts have appeared in the *Lancet*, the *British Journal of Surgery*, the *Annals of the Royal College of Surgeons of England*, *Surgery*, *Surgical Review I* and *Recent Advances*. The work on economics and administration has appeared in the *Lancet*, the *Health and Social Services Journal*, various Department of Health publications and, most importantly, in the *Royal College of Surgeons of England Guidelines for Day Case Surgery* (1985). I am grateful to the respective editors and authorities for permission to reproduce from these articles, and in some cases to expand them.

Hernias, their complications and their management continue to use much surgical resources; repair of a groin hernia is the commonest operation in males and the third commonest operation in British hospitals. Sadly, the results of hernia surgery are still far from ideal. Long hospitalization spells, perioperative complications and, above all, unacceptable recurrence rates disfigure our surgical audit.

Practically every book about hernias reiterates the cliché that too often the repair of a hernia is undertaken by the inexperienced or infrequent operator – the statement does have added cogency in an era of health care cost containment and computerized medical records. It is now easy to compare durations of stay and complication rates and then, using record linkage, to identify the recurrence receiving treatment elsewhere some years later. You no longer need a surgical training to undertake this accounting of results!

The results of hernia repair are improved by specialization. The Shouldice clinic in Toronto dictates the Gold Standard. The anatomical variations and technical difficulties of hernia surgery are sufficient to warrant specialization so that the advisability of specialist hernia units, similar to the regional cardiothoracic units in the National Health Service, merits consideration. Whereas we can debate whether primary hernia repair should remain in the province of the 'general' surgeon, recurrent and incisional hernia repairs demand extra skills and such cases should always be referred to experts.

The prevention of iatrogenic, incisional hernia should be a priority for abdominal surgeons and gynaecologists, yet in all series of incisional hernioplasties surgeon failure at the initial operation is often well documented. The use of inappropriate suture material, sloppy technique, haematoma and sepsis are the all too frequent progenitors of the troublesome incisional hernia.

In setting out my stall, twenty years' experience of hernia surgery, I acknowledge the influence of teachers, particularly the late Frederick Gill, PRCSI, who persuaded me to make myself a surgeon, Austin Marsden, FRCS, who convinced me there is a hernia problem, and Sir Hugh (Lyn) Lockhart-Mummery who taught me so much about surgical technique and its gentleness. To these gentlemen I owe a major debt. Caroline Doig, Allan Kark, Nick Barwell, James Bourke and Frank Glassow have all shared their experience and interest in hernia surgery with me. Percy Payne and Maurice Down have explained all about trusses and demonstrated these appliances to me. Above all, these two gentlemen told me much of the history of British hernia surgery which has corrected my perspective of the recent past.

My colleagues in Stockton-on-Tees and in the North East have referred many of the more complex hernias to me, hernias that have presented technical challenges but afforded me new insights into the anatomy and pathology of hernia. Former junior colleagues have contributed greatly; P. Tiwari, Ranu Singh, A.K. Sahay, Dirk Muller, Denis Quill, Peter Gillen and Bruce Waxman deserve a special mention. Peter Gill and Elizabeth Dillon have undertaken numerous X-ray and ultrasound examinations of hernias for me over the years and both deserve my particular thanks. Angus McNay and Katherine Denham have helped me with statistical problems. I thank Ron Lawler for the photomicrographs (Plates I, II, IIIB).

Permanent members of our department who have a major impact on my perception of hernia surgery include Laurence Rosenberg and Greg Rubin. Mary Fell has undertaken all our socioeconomic interviewing and managed all our research into these fields. Irene Anderson has checked references and done a myriad of secretarial tasks.

Elizabeth Clemo and her staff at North Tees Medical Library have undertaken all the library searches. The libraries of the Royal Society of Medicine and the Royal College of Surgeons of England have tracked down all the more difficult and obscure books I needed. Alexandra MacLean kindly checked and indexed the references for me.

The photographic work has been done by Ken Watson at the Department of Medical Photography at North Tees. The artwork is by Gillian Lee, and it has been a great pleasure to work with her. Surgery books are nothing without artwork; Gillian has put as much into this venture as I have. John Lunn advised me about anaesthesia and persuaded me about other aspects of hernia surgery and surgical audit. Former registrars have assisted me very generously in preparing the various drafts of the text: Simon Raimes, Nigel Fox, Stewart Nicholson, Tom Keane and Paul Stuart deserve my special thanks for their patience and tolerance in that task.

The main burden of turning all this into a book has fallen to Julie Davies. She has painstakingly converted all my handwriting into neat typescript, word processed this and finalized the ultimate manuscript.

Books need publishers and sub-editors; Butterworths have supported and encouraged me throughout the enterprise. My particular thanks go to John Harrison and to Bob Pearson for all the work they have undertaken.

Lastly, and most importantly, my personal secretary, Anne Lindsley, has kept our surgical service on the road despite my involvement in this project.

To all of these colleagues, and to many others, I must express my thanks for their help and enthusiasm.

H. B. D.

Note on terminology. Hernia repair, herniotomy, herniorrhaphy and hernioplasty are terms that are almost but not quite interchangeable. Herniotomy (Gk *temnein*, to cut), herniorrhaphy (Gk *rhaphe*, a seam) and hernioplasty (Gk *plassein*, to mould) connote slightly different meanings. Herniotomy is appropriate to the inguinal operation in children only and I have used it solely in that context. Otherwise, sometimes herniorrhaphy, sometimes hernioplasty is correct, but to switch terms about within the book makes reading difficult. I have, therefore, settled for hernioplasty throughout, perhaps realizing that effective hernia surgery requires all the skills of tissue handling and repair that plastic surgeons so rightly emphasize.

PREFACE TO THE SECOND EDITION

This second edition reflects the rapidly changing world of hernia surgery since 1988. A new, younger, author has participated fully in this new edition.

Three events have precipitated the need for a new edition: the concept of the 'tension free' repair introduced by Irving Lichtenstein, the revolution caused by the laparoscope and the increased role of economics in the contemporary cost-constrained healthcare system.

The realization from the work of Raymond Read, that underlying most, or all, abdominal wall hernias is a defect in the fascia transversalis and that this layer needs replacing, is the seminal advance of replacement by prosthetic mesh introduced by Lichtenstein. This has very important messages for hernia surgeons. Incorporation of this concept into everyday practice is a powerful reason why a new book about hernias is needed.

The new biocompatible plastic meshes and the widespread adoption of mesh replacement repairs in hernia surgery is an important, almost revolutionary, development of contemporary surgery

The laparoscope and its need for a role has captured patients' and surgeons' imaginations and required some overview of the use of this tool in hernia repair. Coupled with this, added cogency has been given to questions of cost and outcomes in evaluation of laparoscopic surgery. The laparoscope makes this new edition inevitable.

There is now a consensus that money will always be limited for surgery and surgeons must perforce adopt cost efficient and effective surgery. These important conclusions are spelt out in the (Revised) *Guidelines for Day Case Surgery* issued by the Royal College of Surgeons of England in 1992.

Above all, this new edition has benefited enormously from the resurgence of interest in the age-old problem of hernia surgery.

The authors' friendship and conversations with many hernia surgeons world-wide is reflected in this new text. European surgeons Kark, Schumpelick, Paul, Nilsson, Stoppa and Kux; Transatlantic surgeons Wantz, Gilbert, Skandalakis, Bendavid, Alexander and Rutkow; Indian surgeons Sahay, Doctor and Rajan, and many others world-wide, have all indirectly participated in this work.

In this Second Edition the artwork is again drawn by Gillian Lee. It has been an enormous pleasure for both of us to work with her.

Elizabeth Clemo and the librarians at North Tees General Hospital, Tina Craig and Michelle Gunning of the Library, Royal College of Surgeons of England have always very willingly helped find different texts for us.

Our secretaries Valerie Peel and Jill Laurence have worked fabulously to put the manuscript into shape.

Our publishers and, especially Nick Dunton, have been a great support throughout the whole venture. Doreen Ramage, our senior production editor, has patiently guided us throughout; we thank her particularly.

Finally, we have written the book together, so whatever its faults and omissions they are our failings alone.

Andrew Kingsnorth
H. Brendan Devlin

A protrusion of any viscus from its proper cavity is denominated a hernia. The protruded parts are generally contained in a bag by the membrane with which the cavity is naturally invested.

Sir Astley Cooper, 1804

Temerity born of ignorance would seem the only judgement to be passed upon one who would offer any further contribution upon the cure of hernia.

Marcy, 1887

It will appear excess of daring to write at the present day of the radical treatment of inguinal hernia.

Bassini, 1890

A surgeon can do more for the community by operating on hernia cases and seeing that his recurrence rate is low than he can be operating on cases of malignant disease.

Sir Cecil Wakeley, 1940

. . . the larger the series, the more valuable are the figures offered; and the percentage of patients returning for follow-up is also of great significance . . .

L. M. Zimmerman, 1971

1 GENERAL INTRODUCTION AND HISTORY OF HERNIA SURGERY

Ancient and renaissance hernia surgery

Hernias are among the oldest surgical challenges. The Egyptians (1500 BC), the Phoenicians (900 BC) and the Ancient Greeks (Hippocrates, 400 BC) diagnosed hernia. The word 'hernia' is derived from the Greek (εθνος), meaning a bud or shoot. The Hippocratic school differentiated between hernia and hydrocele – the former was reducible and the latter transilluminable.[778]

Celsus (AD 40) documented Roman surgical practice: taxis was employed for strangulation, trusses and bandages could control the reducible hernia, and operation was only advised for pain and for small hernias in the young. The sac could be dissected through a scrotal incision, the wound then being allowed to granulate. Scar tissue was perceived as the optimum replacement for the stretched abdominal wall. Galen (AD 200) intro-

duced the concept of 'rupture', with the peritoneum forcing its way through the abdominal wall. The last of the Graeco-Roman medical encyclopaedists, Paul of Aegina (AD D 700), distinguished complete scrotal from incomplete inguinal herniation or bubonocele. For scrotal hernia, he recommended ligation of the sac and the cord with sacrifice of the testicle.

During the long dark conformity of the Middle Ages three important advances in herniology were nevertheless made. Guy de Chauliac, in 1363, distinguished femoral from inguinal hernia. He developed taxis for incarceration, recommending the head-down, Trendelenburg position.[226] In 1556 Franco, an itinerant Swiss barber-surgeon, introduced a grooved director which allowed him to divide the ring of the constriction in strangulated hernia without hazarding the bowel. He recommended reducing the contents and closing the defect with linen suture.[314]

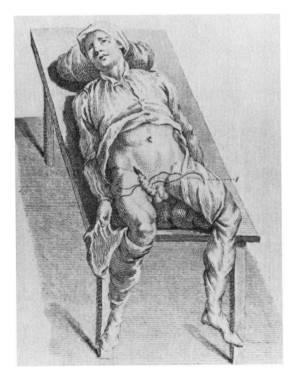

Figure 1.1 Ligation of strangulated omentum in a strangulated right scrotal hernia. The wound then granulated. The patient survived and the hernia did not recur. Operation by Cheselden in 1721[175]

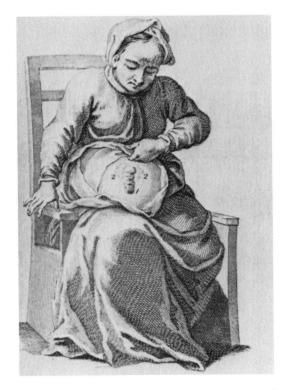

Figure 1.2 Development of a preternatural colon fistula (colostomy) after strangulation of an umbilical hernia. The wound was trimmed. The patient survived many years 'voiding the excrements at the umbilicus'. Operation by Cheselden about 1721[175]

In 1559 Stromayr, a German surgeon from Lindau, published a remarkable contribution to surgery. His book *Practica Copiosa* describes sixteenth-century hernia surgery in great detail and is comprehensively illustrated. Stromayr differentiated direct and indirect inguinal hernia and advised excision of the sac and of the cord and testicle in indirect hernia.[901]

The Renaissance brought burgeoning anatomic knowledge, now based on careful cadaver dissection. William Cheselden successfully operated on a strangulated right inguinal hernia on the Tuesday morning after Easter 1721. The intestines were easily reduced and adherent omentum was ligated and divided. The patient survived and went back to work[175] (Figure 1.1).

Without adequate interventional surgery some patients survived hernia strangulation when spontaneous, preternatural fistula occasionally followed infarction and sloughing of a strangulated hernia. Cheselden's Margaret White survived for many years 'voiding the excrements through the intestine at the navel' after simple local surgery for a strangulated umbilical hernia.[175] The closure of such a fistula in the absence of distal bowel pathology was described by Le Dran, who had noted that it was quite common for poor people with incarcerated hernias to mistake the tender painful groin lump for an abscess and incise it themselves. He found that these painful wounds with faecal fistulas required no more than cleaning and dressing. Often the wound would heal, nature preferring to send the faeces along the natural route to the anus[540] (Figure 1.2).

The anatomical era: Pott and Cooper

Sir Percival Pott described the pathophysiology of strangulation in 1757 and recommended surgical management (Figure 1.3): 'I am perfectly satisfied that the cause of strangulated hernia is most frequently . . . a piece of intestine (in other respects sound and free of disease) being so bound by the said tendon, as to have its peristaltic motion and the circulation through it impeded or stopped.'[757] Fifty years later Astley Cooper implicated venous obstruction as the first cascade in the circulatory failure of strangulation: 'By a stop being put to the return of blood through the veins which produces a great accumulation of this fluid and a change of its colour from the arterial to the venous hue.' Nevertheless ligature, the insertion of setons and castration remained the mainstays of treatment prior to the publication of Astley Cooper's monograph in 1804[193] (Figure 1.4).

Modern surgery commences with Lister's discovery of the nature of sepsis and his introduction of antisepsis about 1870.[570, 810] Halsted introduced gloves in 1896 and when von Mickulicz translated antiseptic surgery to aseptic technique in 1904, the scene was finally set for the techniques of modern hernia surgery to develop.[245]

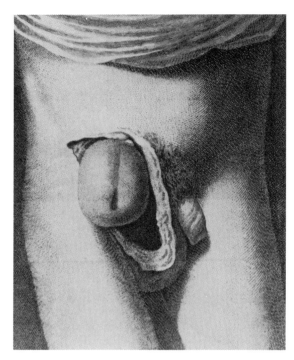

Figure 1.3 Intestine strangulated by the 'tendon' so that the venous circulation through it is stopped, leading to gangrene. Described by Pott in 1757[757]

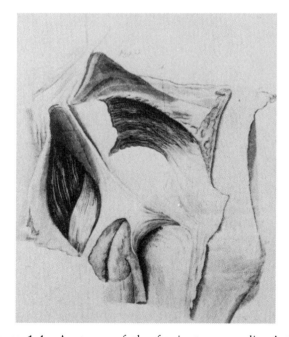

Figure 1.4 Anatomy of the fascia transversalis. Astley Cooper (1804) demonstrated the fascia extending behind the inguinal ligament into the thigh to be the femoral sheath. He first recognized the fascia transversalis and its importance in groin herniation[193]

Initial surgical attempts at hernioplasty were based on static concepts of anatomic repair using natural or modified natural materials for reconstruction. Wood (1863) described subcutaneous division and suture of the sac and fascial separation of the groin from the scrotum. Czerny (1876), in Prague, pulled the sac of an inguinal hernia through the external ring, ligated it, amputated the redundant sac and allowed the neck to spring back to the deep ring.[213] MacEwen (1886), of Glasgow, bundled the sac up on itself and stuffed it back along the canal so that it would act as a cork or tampon and stop up the internal ring[590] (Figure 1.5). Kocher (1907), surgery's first Nobel Prize winner, invaginated the sac on itself and fixed it laterally through the external oblique[508] (Figure 1.6). Suffice to say, none of these operations has stood the test of time.

Marcy, Bassini and Halsted and their disciples

As so often in surgery a new concept was needed before further progress could be made in herniology. Two pioneers – the American Marcy (1871)[608] and the Italian Bassini (1884) – vie for priority for the critical breakthrough.[72-74] Both appreciated the physiology of the inguinal canal and both correctly understood how each anatomic plane, transversalis fascia, transverse and oblique muscles, and the external oblique aponeurosis, contributed to the canal's stability. Read, having carefully surveyed all the evidence, agrees with Halsted[385] that Bassini got there first.[776]

Although both contributed to herniology, Bassini made another seminal advance when he subjected his

technique to the scrutiny of the prospective follow-up. Bassini's 1890 paper is truly a quantum leap in surgery;[74] indeed, if it is read alongside the contribution of Haidenthaller, from Billroth's clinic – reporting a 30%, early recurrence rate – which appears in the same volume

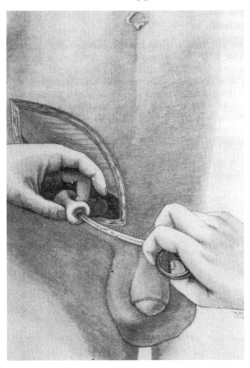

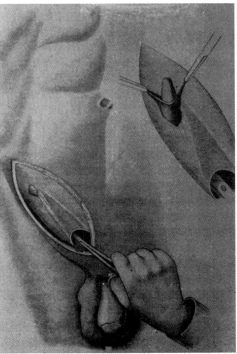

Figure 1.6   Invagination of the sac which is fixed laterally by suturing its stump to the external oblique. No formal dissection or repair of the deep ring was made. Operation by Kocher in 1907[508]

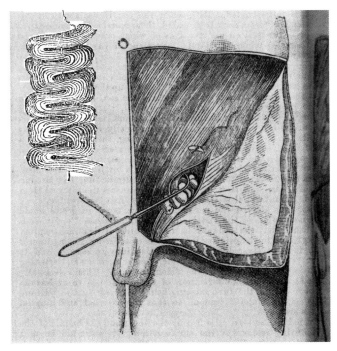

Figure 1.5   The operation of MacEwen 1886. The dissected indirect sac is bundled up and then used as an internal stopper or pad to prevent further herniation along the valved canal[590]

of *Langenbeck's Archiv fur Klinische Chirurgie*, Bassini's stature is further enhanced.[782]

Marcy directed his attention to the deep ring in the fascia transversalis; his operation for indirect inguinal hernia entailed closure of the deep ring with fascia transversalis only, the object being the recreation of a stable and competent deep ring. In 1871 he reported two patients operated on during the previous year 'in which I closed the (deep) ring with the interrupted sutures of carbolized catgut followed by permanent cure'.[608]

Bassini had become interested in the management of inguinal hernia in about 1883, and from 1883 to 1889 he operated on 274 hernias. After trying the operations of Czerny and Wood he modified his approach and attempted a radical cure, so that the patient would not require a truss after surgery. He decided to open the inguinal canal and approach the posterior wall of the canal; gradually he was focusing onto the deep ring and fascia transversalis. Seven times he opened the canal, resected the sac and closed the peritoneum at the internal ring. He then constructed a tampon of the excess sac at the internal ring and sutured this sac stump, or tampon, to the deep surface of the external oblique. One of his seven patients died three months after the operation from an unrelated cause. Post-mortem examination showed the sutured portion of the neck, the 'stopper' or tampon, to be completely reabsorbed. Bassini deduced that although the risk of recurrent herniation was diminished by this technique it did not afford adequate tissue repair, and some external support – a truss – would still be needed to prevent recurrence. He now proceeded to complete anatomical reconstruction of the inguinal canal

> ... this might be achieved through reconstruction of the inguinal canal into the physiological condition, a canal with two openings one abdominal the other subcutaneous and with two walls, one anterior and one posterior through the middle of which the spermatic cord would pass. Through a study of the groin, and with the help of an anatomical knowledge of the inguinal canal and inguinal hernia, it was easy for me to find an operative method which answered the above described requirements, and made possible a radical cure without subsequent wearing of a truss. Using the method exclusively I have, during the year 1884, operated on 262 hernias of which 251 were either reducible or irreducible and 11 strangulated.

His series included 206 men and 10 women; the non-strangulated cases were 115 right, 66 left and 35 bilateral inguinal hernias. The age range was 13 months to 69 years. The operations were performed under general narcosis and there were no operative deaths; however, three patients who each had strangulated hernias died postoperatively – one of sepsis, one of shock and one of a chest infection. Bassini's patients were carefully followed up, some to 4½ years, and seven recurrences were recorded. There were, in fact, eight recurrences; Bassini failed to tabulate case 65, a 54-year-old university

professor in Padua with a strangulated right direct inguinal hernia, with a recurrence at eight months. The wound infection rate was 11 in 206 operations and the time to healing averaged 14 days.[74] These statistics compare favourably with reports made up to the 1950s.

Bassini dissected the indirect sac and closed it off flush with the parietal peritoneum. He then isolated and lifted up the spermatic cord and dissected the posterior wall of the canal, dividing the fascia transversalis down to the pubic tubercle. He then sutured the dissected conjoint tendon consisting of the internal oblique, the transversus muscle and the 'vertical fascia of Cooper', the fascia transversalis, to the posterior rim of Poupart's ligament, including the lower lateral divided margin of the fascia transversalis. Bassini stresses that this suture line must be approximated without difficulty; hence the early dissection separating the external oblique from the internal oblique must be adequate and allow good development and mobilization of the conjoint tendon (Figure 1.7).

The Bassini legacy was popularized by Attilo Catterina, Bassini's assistant in Padua in 1887 who later became professor in Genoa in 1904. Catterina was entrusted by Bassini to teach the exact surgical technique. To do this he wrote an atlas of 'The Operation of Bassini'! This has 20 very fine colour plates by the artist Orazio Gaicher. This book was published in London, Berlin, Paris and Madrid in the 1930s and described in detail the uncorrupted Bassini technique, especially the division of the transversalis fascia, resection of the cremaster muscle and complete anatomical survey of all the relevant anatomy nowadays considered so essential.[159, 160] A foretaste of the Shouldice operation![965]

By contrast, Haidenthaller, from Billroth's Clinic in Vienna, reported 195 operations for inguinal hernia, with 11 operative deaths and a short-term recurrence rate of 30.8%.[382]

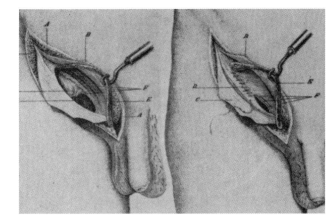

Figure 1.7 Suturing the 'triple layer' (F) (fascia transversalis, transversus tendon and internal oblique) to the upturned edge of the inguinal ligament. An anatomical and physiological repair of the posterior wall of the inguinal canal preserving its obliquity and function. Operation by Bassini in 1890[74]

Although Halsted made important contributions to herniology, his general technical contributions of precise haemostasis, absolute asepsis and the crucial importance of avoiding tissue trauma are easily overlooked. Halsted was always concerned to achieve optimum wound healing, and he not only practised surgery but he experimented and theorized. His observation on closing skin wounds is best repeated verbatim: 'The skin is united by interrupted stitches of very fine silk. These stitches do not penetrate the skin, and when tied they become buried. They are taken from the underside of the skin and made to include only its deeper layers – the layers which are not occupied by sebaceous follicles.[384–386] In today's world haematoma, sepsis and damaged tissue leading to delayed healing mean not only a poor surgical outcome but weigh heavily on the debit side of any economic evaluation. These Halstedian principles should be rigidly applied by any surgeon who undertakes hernia surgery.

Halsted's specific contributions to inguinal hernia surgery do not enjoy the universal assent that his general surgical principles command; indeed, some would suggest that his operations for inguinal hernia are at best meddlesome modifications or corruptions of the major contributions of Marcy and Bassini.

Halsted's first sequence of papers, in 1889, described the operation now known in jargon as Halsted I. In this operation, after high ligation of the sac, Halsted transfixed all the layers of the abdominal wall medial to the sac and sutured them to the lateral structures, carrying his suture medially through both the oblique and transversus muscles, then through the transversalis fascia and laterally through the inguinal ligament and external oblique aponeurosis all in one bite. The sutures were then quilted and tied in a single layer to secure his repair. The cord emerged through the lateral end of this composite wound and was laid subcutaneously. The skin was closed over the cord. Halsted stressed: 'Interrupted strong silk sutures, passed so as to include everything between the skin and the peritoneum are used to close the deeper portion of the wound, which is sewn from the crest of the pubis to the upper outer angle of the incision. The cord now lies superficial to these sutures and emerges through the abdominal muscles about one inch to the inner side of the anterior superior spine of the ileum' (Figure 1.8). Halsted excised 'all but one or two of the veins of the cord'. Subsequently Halsted described complications of his technique: the deep sutures penetrated the bladder and the patient passed urine through the wound, and three cases of testicular atrophy developed.[384] He experimented with silver, copper and brass wire as alternative sutures for wound repair.[385]

Halsted's second sequence of reports, Halsted II, were written in conjunction with his assistant, Bloodgood, who re-investigated and followed up the first 300 patients operated on at Johns Hopkins[103–105] (Figure 1.9).

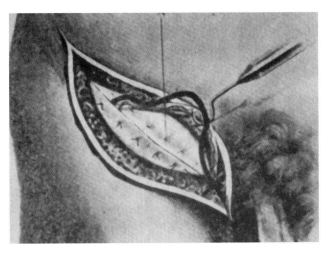

Figure 1.8 The Halsted I operation (1890). Suturing all the medial structures, fascia transversalis, transversus tendon, internal and external oblique, to the lateral structures so that the cord is left subcutaneously. An unanatomical technique which acknowledged the physiological importance of the deep ring[385]

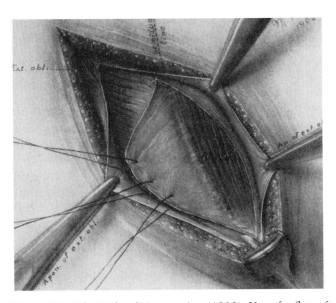

Figure 1.9 The Halsted II operation (1903). Use of a flap of anterior rectus sheath to reinforce the posterior repair[104]

It is difficult to elucidate the exact technique Halsted recommended as definitive at the end of his career. He was a great inventor and evaluator; however, he was convinced of the value of (a) high ligation of the sac, (b) relaxing incisions in the internal oblique aponeurosis to enable the conjoint tendon to be lined up with the inguinal ligament at its medial portion to prevent medial recurrence, and (c) the use of a flap of internal oblique aponeurosis turned down to reinforce the posterior repair. He abandoned subcutaneous transplantation and skeletization of the cord because of the high incidence of hydrocele (25%) and testicular atrophy (10%).

Halsted must be given priority for recognizing the value of an anterior relaxing incision, first described by Wölfler in 1892[994] and subsequently sold in the USA by Rienhoff (1940)[784] and in England by Tanner (1942).[908]

Apart from Halsted, other authors have corrupted or simplified the original Marcy–Bassini concept of a review of the posterior wall of the canal and the correction of any deficits in it, the reconstruction of the patulous deep ring for indirect herniation and the repair of the stretched fascia transversalis in cases of direct herniation. Bull and Coley independently sutured the internal oblique and the aponeurosis over the cord,[131, 188] whereas Ferguson (1899) advised against any mobilization of the cord and, therefore, any review of the posterior wall of the canal:[296] 'Tearing the cord out of its bed is without an anatomic reason to recommend it, a physiologic act to suggest it, an etiological factor in hernia, congenital or acquired, to indicate it, nor brilliant surgical results to justify its continuance ... Leave the cord alone, for it is the sacred highway along which travel vital elements indispensable to the perpetuity of our race.' Ferguson sutured the fascia transversalis **lateral** to the deep ring then, leaving the cord undisturbed, he drew the internal oblique down in front of the cord and sutured it to the inguinal ligament. The external oblique aponeurosis was closed next. Bassini's triple layer – fascia transversalis, transversus muscles and internal oblique – were ignored, Marcy's delineation and closure of the deep ring were forgotten, and the careful exposure of the preperitoneal space or repair of the peritoneum seemed not to be understood.[297]

Ferguson's paper is robust on rhetoric and woefully lacking in outcome measures.[297] Bassini's careful list of patients, complications and recurrences makes a sharp contrast.

Imbrication, or overlapping, of layers was introduced by Wyllys Andrews in 1895. Andrews confessed that his technique was an outgrowth of experience with MacEwan, Bassini, Halsted and similar operations. Andrews laid great stress on careful aseptic technique: '... Finally, I unite the skin itself with a buried suture which does not puncture any of its glands or ducts.' Andrews used collodion only as a dressing. Again the importance of careful surgical technique is emphasized! Andrews stressed the importance of the posterior wall of the canal: 'The posterior wall of the canal ... is narrowed by suturing the conjoined tendon and transversalis fascia firmly to Poupart's ligament.' Andrews recommended the kangaroo tendon introduced by Marcy. Andrews then reinforced the posterior wall with the upper (medial) margin of the external oblique aponeurosis which he drew down behind the cord and sutured to Poupart's ligament. Andrews' intention was to interlock or imbricate the layers. The lower (lateral) flap of the external oblique aponeurosis was then brought up anterior to the cord. Andrews concluded his

article: 'Any successful method of radical cure must be a true plastic operation upon the musculo-aponeurotic layers of the abdominal wall. Cicatricial tissue and peritoneal exudate are of no permanent value.'[24]

The following advantages are claimed for imbrication:

1. A large strong flap of any needed size is available to fill the internal ring.
2. It produces triplicate layers of aponeuroses.
3. The interlocking of layers gives broad surfaces of union.
4. It results in shortening of the anterior as well as the posterior wall of the canal, making them mutually supporting and relieving tension on deep sutures.
5. The cord is amply protected.

Andrews' text is not specific about his management of the fascia transversalis at the deep ring. Did he dissect it and divide it as Bassini recommended or did he just suture it? His text does not clarify the point, but one diagram illustrates the deep ring dissected away from the sac stump with the fascia transversalis of the posterior wall opened (Figure 1.10).

Perhaps we should pause at about 1905 and summarize what empiricism had achieved thus far.

First, all authors agree that division of the neck of the sac and flush closure of the peritoneum is imperative to success.

Second, dissection of the deep ring with exploration of the extraperitoneal space to allow adequate closure of the fascia transversalis anterior to the peritoneum emerges as a cardinal feature. Marcy and Bassini stress the fascia transversalis repair, Halsted emphasized it, Andrews' diagram suggests it. Ferguson did not examine the entire posterior wall, but tightened the internal ring lateral to the emergent cord. All are agreed that the deep ring is patulous in indirect herniation and consequently the fascia transversalis must be repaired. In the English

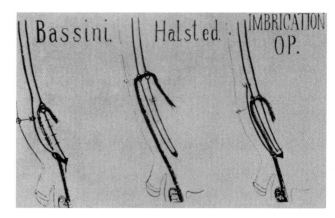

Figure 1.10 Imbrication, lap joint or interlocking of the abdominal layers to effect a sound triplicate repair. The lower (lateral) flap is brought up in front of the cord which is enclosed in a 'new canal'. An attempt to strengthen or buttress the repair. Operation by Andrews in 1895

literature, Lockwood in 1893 clearly emphasized the fascia transversalis and Bassini's 'triple layer'. Lockwood obtained good results by repairing this important layer.[573, 574]

Third, preservation of the obliquity of the canal is suggested by Marcy and Bassini, and by the later Halsted and Bloodgood papers.

Fourth, double breasting (imbrication) of aponeurosis gives improved results and is recommended by Andrews.

Lastly, all the authors stress careful technique. Avoidance of tissue trauma, haematoma and infection leads to impressively better results. Sepsis is an important antecedent of recurrence.

After the nineteenth-century advances of Marcy and Bassini, and the important contribution to surgical technique by Halsted, little of major importance was contributed until the 1920s. Countless modifications of Marcy's and Bassini's operations were made and reported frequently. Except for the contributions of Marcy[609] and Bassini[74] few commentators report any adequate outcome measurements. This literature is vast, opinionated and often pompous. Clearly a new target, and a new rubric to attain it, is required for surgical investigators. At the end of the twentieth century the goal is the measurement of outcomes.[715]

Alternative anatomical approaches to the groin

Alternatives to the anterior (inguinal) approach to the internal ring include the transabdominal (laparotomy)[525, 906] and the extraperitoneal (preperitoneal).[171]

Marcy recognized the advantages of the transabdominal intraperitoneal approach to the ring in 1892:

> It may rarely happen to the operator who has opened the abdomen for some other purpose to find the complication of hernia. When the section has been made considerably large, as in the removal of a large tumour, the internal ring is within reach of the surgeon. Upon reflection, it would naturally occur to any operator that under these conditions it is better to close the internal ring, and reform the smooth internal parietal surface from within by means of suturing. My friend, Dr. N. Bozeman of New York, easily did this at my suggestion in a case of ovariotomy more than 10 years ago.

Marcy attributed the transabdominal technique to the French in 1749.[610] Lawson Tait recommended midline abdominal section for umbilical and groin hernia in 1891.[906]

LaRoque, in 1919, recommended transabdominal repair of inguinal hernias through a muscle-splitting incision about 1 inch (2.5 cm) above the ring. The peritoneum was opened, the sac dissected and then inverted into the peritoneal cavity by grasping its fundus and pulling it back into the peritoneal cavity. The sac was

excised and a repair of the deep ring effected[525] (Figure 1.11).

Battle, a surgeon at St Thomas' Hospital, London, described his approach to repair of a femoral hernia in 1900. Battle pointed out the difficulties of diagnosing femoral hernia and the difficulties, principally the age, sex and comorbidity, of managing patients with femoral hernia. He approached the hernia sac from above through an incision splitting the external oblique above the inguinal ligament. After coping with the peritoneal sac, Battle repaired the femoral canal, constructing a 'shutter' of the aponeurosis of external oblique which he sutured to the pectineus fascia and the pectineal ligament across the abdominal opening of the femoral canal.[76]

The extraperitoneal–preperitoneal approach owes its origin to Cheatle (1920) who initially used a midline incision but subsequently (1921) changed to a Pfannenstiel incision.[171, 172] Cheatle explored both sides, and inguinal and femoral protrusions were reduced and amputated. If needed, for strangulation or adhesions, the peritoneum could easily be opened. The fascia transversalis was visible and easily repaired. Cheatle advised against this approach for direct hernia because the direct region was usually obscured and distorted by the retraction of the rectus muscles.

A.K. Henry, a master anatomist, rediscovered and popularized the extraperitoneal approach in 1936.[418]

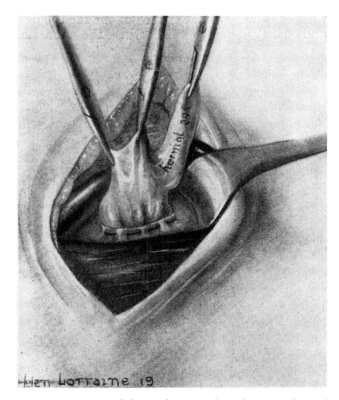

Figure 1.11 Transabdominal approach to the groin through a muscle-splitting incision above the inguinal canal with subsequent closure of the peritoneal sac away from the canal[525]

McEvedy (1950), 10 years after Henry's description, adopted a unilateral oblique incision, retracting the rectus medially, to approach a femoral hernia.[634] In the USA, Musgrove and McCready (1949) adopted the Henry approach to femoral hernia.[685] Mikkelsen and Berne (1954) reported inguinal and femoral hernias repaired by this technique and commended the excellent access obtained even in the obese. Furthermore femoral, inguinal and obturator hernias were all repairable through this 'extended suprapubic approach'.[650]

Two Europeans – Lytle and Fruchaud

In the immediate aftermath of the Second World War two European Surgeon Anatomists, Lytle and Fruchaud, are important contributors.

Lytle was principally concerned with the anatomy and shutter mechanism of the deep inguinal ring. He dissected the deep ring and in a remarkable film demonstrated its prophylactic mechanism in indirect herniation. He was concerned to preserve the mechanism of the ring and at the same time to reinforce its patulous medial margin in indirect herniation. He emphasized that manoeuvres which damaged the lateral 'pillars of the ring' inevitably compromised the physiological shutter mechanism.[585] In a subsequent study he

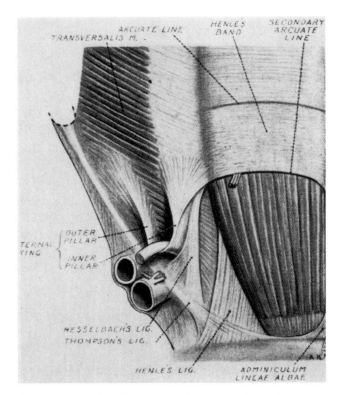

Figure 1.12 The 'shutter mechanism' of canal and the internal anatomy of the deep ring, demonstrating the sling of fascia transversalis which pulls the deep ring up and laterally when the patient strains[587]

clearly described the embryological anatomy of the ring and how it could be repaired, in the fascia transversalis layer, without losing its function[587] (Figure 1.12).

A remarkable Frenchman, Henri Fruchaud, published two books in Paris in 1956: *L'Anatomie Chirurgicale de la Region de l'Aine (Surgical Anatomy of the Groin Region)*[317] and *Le Traitement Chirurgical des Hernies de l'Aine (Surgical Treatment of Groin Hernias)*.[318] Fruchaud combined traditional anatomical studies of the groin, the work of Cooper, Bogros and Madden, with his own extensive anatomical and surgical experience. He invented an entirely new concept – 'the myopectineal orifice' – which combined the traditionally separate inguinal and femoral canals to form a unified highway from the abdomen to the thigh. The abdominocrural tunnel of fascia transversalis extended through this myopectineal orifice, through which all inguinal and femoral hernias pass, as do the iliofemoral vessels. Based on this anatomical concept Fruchaud recommended complete reconstruction of the endo-fascial wall (fascia transversalis) of the myopectineal orifice. This unifying concept forms the basis for all extraperitoneal mesh repairs, open or laparoscopic, of groin hernias (Figure 1.13).

The concept of Fruchaud has been expanded by Stoppa in France and Wantz in the USA into the 'giant reinforcement of the peritoneal sac' repairs of inguinal hernias.[896, 966, 967]

Laparoscopy

Laparoscopic management of inguinal hernias has caught the imagination of surgeons and patients. Ger first reported the laparoscopic closure of the neck of a sac with a Michel clip introduced laparoscopically in 1982.[335] The first patient to be treated by laparoscopic closure of the neck of the sac was under the care of Dr P. Fletcher of the University of the West Indies, operated on the 24th November 1979.[335] Initial techniques of simple closure of the peritoneal neck[336] have gradually given way to transperitoneal plugging of hernia orifices with prosthetics[304] then to transperitoneal patching techniques[199] and now to extraperitoneal patch operations.[199] The requirement for transperitoneal insufflation in the laparoscopic approach to the hernia, with the consequent requirement for general anaesthesia, has lead to questioning of these newer operations. Furthermore, the long-term results of laparoscopic hernia surgery are awaited with interest.[305] The development of better local anaesthetic techniques and the rise of day surgery somewhat dampens the enthusiasm for laparoscopic operations. A rigorous economic evaluation of laparoscopic hernia surgery questions its cost effectiveness and appropriateness in some circumstances[655] (See Chapters 5 and 14).

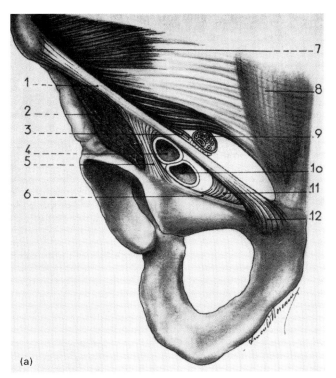
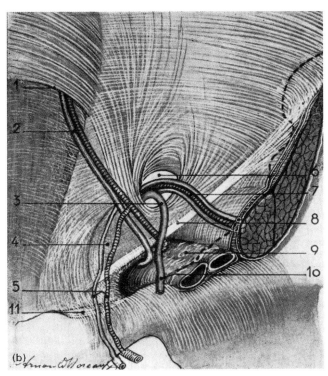

Figure 1.13 (a) Fruchaud's concept of the myopectineal orifice ('l'orifice crural classique') incorporating the inguinal and the femoral canals. An external view showing the two canals separated by the inguinal ligament and internal dissection (b) demonstrating how the muscles of the groin form a tunnel down to the myopectineal orifice[318]

Sutures and prostheses

Suture materials and prosthetics have accumulated another literature. Marcy and Bassini initially favoured carbolized catgut, whereas Halsted settled on silk. Marcy was the first surgeon to use animal sinew, recommending kangaroo tendon in 1881.[609] He also experimented with ox, whale and deer tendon. Interestingly, he performed animal experiments to supplement his understanding of fascial healing, especially when animal tendon was used as a suture.

Kirschner (1910)[503] introduced fascial patches or strips from the thigh into the repair of groin hernias. Then in 1921 Gallie and Le Mesurier[323] introduced the autologous fascia grafts either as overlays or as strip sutures. Somehow the work of the Canadians Gallie and Le Mesurier caught the surgical imagination. Sir Geoffrey Keynes championed these techniques in the UK; he recommended the fascia strip operation for inguinal hernia and a flap of anterior rectus aponeurosis sutured to Cooper's ligament for femoral hernia[491] (Figure 1.14).

Burdick and co-workers, in 1937, researched the fate of implanted fascia and they stressed the disadvantages – sepsis, dissolution of the graft and recurrence of the hernia – when ox fascia and heterologous fascia were used, compared with the good results obtained with autologous fascia.[134]

From these beginnings a large combative literature developed in the 1930s and 1940s, reporting the use of various natural organic prostheses. The dust of these controversies has now largely settled, but we can nevertheless draw conclusions. Homologous and heterologous fascia have no value in hernioplasty; they are, after all, implanted foreign organic matter and undergo complete phagocytic digestion after a time.

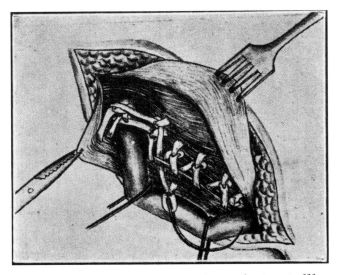

Figure 1.14 Gallie repair using autologous fascia strips[323]

The work on fascia as an adjunct to hernioplasty prompted one of the most bizarre recommendations in the literature. After quoting the data of Burdick, Edwards (1943) dismisses them and continues: 'It is quite safe to implant fascia lata from one individual into the hernial region of a second – a convenient practice when one is dealing with several hernias on the same operation list'.[277]

Smith (1971) reviews his experience with autologous fascia lata grafts; he concludes that the technique has merit, the fascia lata survives and it provides for adequate repair. He reports 32 hernias repaired in this fashion between 1963 and 1970, with only one recurrence. However, he reports that pain and herniation at the donor site in the thigh can be a problem.[874]

McNealy and Classman have the last word: 'Old fascia from an old thigh placed in an old hole in an old man . . . does not aid rejuvenation.'[638] They recommended vitallium plates as an alternative to fascia.

Mair pioneered the use of skin and split skin (cutis) as a repair material. These can now be forgotten; they were abandoned largely because of the persistence of epidermal components which develop cysts of sebum and hair.[604, 605]

Prosthetic metal meshes have been around since Bartlett (1903) described the construction of a silver wire mesh for repair of large defects in the abdominal wall and McGavin of the Dreadnought Seamen's Hospital, Greenwich, introduced the 'silver filigree repair' in 1909 (Figure 1.15).[68, 635] As recently as 1958, 500 patients having a silver filigree operation for an inguinal hernia were reported from Melbourne by Ball.[61] Silver filigree and tantalum gauze can nowadays be ruled out as prosthetics because the metalwork hardens and then fatigue fractures. The fragmentation that ensues is followed by erosion of adjacent musculo-aponeurotic tissue and a worse recurrent hernia or multiple sinuses. The newer steel prostheses may not have this physical disadvantage in the short term. Such an improved stainless steel mesh, Toilinox, has been reported from France in a series of 150 incisional hernia repairs; none of the meshes had to be removed for sepsis. More than 95% of the patients

have an excellent long-term result with neither pain nor recurrence.[918] However, metallic meshes as prostheses for hernia repair have been overtaken by the advent of bio-inert plastics.

Polyvinyl alcohol sponge, introduced by Schofield in 1955, proved difficult to handle in the abdominal wall (as opposed to its excellence in the Wells operation for rectal prolapse[831, 975]) and along with nylon tricot, a lady's garment fabric used by Horwich (1958), is prone to sepsis.[437] Nylon net was subjected to an elegant study by Doran and colleagues in 1961.[264] These prostheses have nowadays disappeared from the repertoire, along with polyethylene plates[919] and vitallium plates.[638]

Polymer meshes, polypropylene (introduced in 1958) and Dacron (1974) have optimum value in hernia prosthetic repair.[34, 940] Flexible carbon fibre (Grafil AS Fibre, Courtaulds Ltd), a satisfactory repair material used in orthopaedic surgery, has been used experimentally in hernia repair recently by Johnson-Nurse and Jenkins.[470] Polytetrafluoride has been employed both in its woven form Teflon[477] mesh and as an expanded soft tissue patch, GoreTex.[389]

Floss silk, a once popular British repair material introduced by Maingot in 1941,[599] produced a very dense fibrous response but was often compromised by infection and sinus formation, leading to its abandonment. Its synthetic analogue, floss nylon, anticipated to be more inert and, therefore, more easily incorporated into fibrous tissue, had similar untoward characteristics in longer term follow-up[132, 602] (Figure 1.16).

Nylon tape, as an alternative to fascial strips, was also employed in a darn operation, with a recurrence rate of 3.7%, and no sinuses.[361] In the same tradition of darn repair, Sames recommended the vas deferens as a suture in hernia repair in 1975.[824]

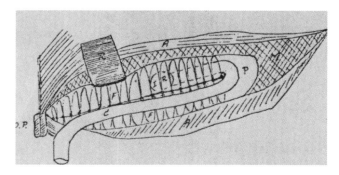

Figure 1.15   McGavin double silver filigree repair (1909);[622] A, aponeurosis; c, cord; F, filigree; M, internal oblique muscle; R, retractor; O.P., os pubis; p, peritoneum; I.R., internal ring

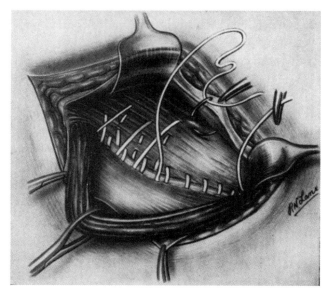

Figure 1.16   Maingot repair using a floss silk darn

Tensionless hernia repair

Irving Lichtenstein is the seminal thinker who introduced tensionless prosthetic repair of groin hernias into everyday, commonplace, outpatient practices. As well as being an office procedure under local anaesthetic, Lichtenstein's technique has pioneered the idea that hernia surgery is special, that it must be performed by an experienced surgeon and cannot be relegated to the unsupervised trainee doing 'minor' surgery. The key feature of Lichtenstein's technique is the 'tensionless' operation. With his co-workers Shulman and Amid, he has developed a simple prosthetic operation which can be performed on outpatients.[18, 564]

Against the simplicity and success of Lichtenstein operations, other techniques – Shouldice and above all laparoscopic methods – have real problems of competition. Harking back to Doran in 1960 the problems of evaluation are now much more complex.[263]

Sutures today

Modern research, following Douglas' pioneer investigation of healing tissue strength in 1952,[266] has elucidated the dynamics of wound healing and clarified our understanding of the functions of sutures.[266] The choice of suture should now reflect scientific fact. This is reviewed in Chapter 6.

Aetiology of hernia

Sir Astley Cooper (1827) first attempted an overview of the aetiology of hernia.[194] He proposed 'predispositions' to hernia including: obesity, repeated pregnancy, general wasting of the body, difficulty of micturition, injury and horse-riding, violent exercise, and food difficult of digestion and habitual costiveness. Bailey (1957) suggested the list should be completed by adding chronic cough and ascites.[56]

Fruchaud's work on the anatomic development of groin hernia stresses the role of the erect human posture and the force of gravity as possible determinants of groin hernia disease. Gravity at the level of the groin results in a constitutional tendency to herniation. 'Every healthy man is a self unknown hernia bearer' according to Fruchaud.[319]

Controversial theories of the aetiology of hernia have been re-evaluated and even restated in the past 100 years – Russell's (1906) 'saccular theory'[808] being restated by the development of indirect inguinal hernia in adult males undergoing peritoneal dialysis, and Sir Arthur Keith's (1924)[487] 'acquired theory' being bolstered by the recent discovery of an elastic collagen deficit in adult male smokers with direct hernias.[955]

European epidemiology

Quite distinct from inherent tissue defects or anatomical variation, the environment and occupation of hernia sufferers also has an influence on hernia development. 'Risk factors': straining at work, heavy lifting, are all implicated. Recent European epidemiology research stresses environmental factors in hernia development.[153, 308]

No history of hernia surgery would be complete without mention of the contribution of Earle Shouldice and his colleagues in Toronto, who have collected and evaluated many thousands of hernia patients.[978] Likewise, in the USA the Veterans Administration hospitals have striven to manage hernias effectively and economically, and in pursuit of these goals have added immensely to our knowledge.

New era of evidence-based medicine

Today any new technique must be based on a careful evaluation of its benefits and costs; benefits must be measured in clinical, social and economic terms. Similarly, benefits are accounted across the whole patient environment and across the whole healthcare system. It is no longer adequate to demonstrate that something 'works'; it must be tested in proper trials to eliminate confounding variables. Patients own their hernias and they must consent to participate in what are becoming increasingly complex trials to evaluate the new techniques. Certainly in the UK all new techniques and technologies should be introduced in the context of properly devised trials.[801]

Chronology of hernia surgery

ANCIENT

1500 BC   Inguinal hernia described in an Egyptian papyrus. An inguinal hernia is depicted on a Greek statuette from this period.[778]

900 BC   Tightly fitting bandages are used to treat an inguinal hernia by physicians in Alexandria. A Phoenician statue depicts this.[778]

400 BC   Hippocrates distinguished hernia and hydrocele by transillumination.[778]

AD 40   Celsus described the older Greek operations for hernia.[162]

AD 200   Galen introduced the concept of 'rupture' of the peritoneum allowed by failure of the belly wall tissues.[778]

AD 700   Paul of Aegina distinguished complete and incomplete hernia. He recommended amputation of the testicle in repair.[778]

MEDIEVAL

1363   Guy de Chauliac distinguished inguinal and femoral hernia.[226]

1556   Franco recommended dividing the constriction at the neck of a strangulated hernial sac.[314]

1559   Stromayr published *Practica Copiosa*, differentiating direct and indirect hernia and advocating excision of the sac in indirect hernia.[810]

RENAISSANCE

1700   Littré reported a Meckel's diverticulum in a hernial sac.[571]

1731   De Garengeot described the appendix in a hernial sac.[227]

1724   Heister distinguished direct and indirect hernia.[415]

1757   Pott described the anatomy of hernia and of strangulation.[757]

1756   Cheselden described successful operation for an inguinal hernia.[175]

1785   Richter described a partial enterocele.[785]

1790   John Hunter speculated about the congenital nature of complete indirect inguinal hernia.[444]

1793   De Gimbernat described his ligament and advocated medial rather than upward division of the constriction in strangulated femoral hernia. This avoided damage to the inguinal ligament and the serious bleeding which sometimes followed.[228]

1804   Cooper published his three-part book on hernia – The plates are a *tour de force*; they are almost life sized and depict anatomy as never before. Cooper defined the fascia transversalis; he distinguished this layer from the peritoneum and demonstrated that it was the main barrier to herniation. He carefully delineated the extension of the fascia transversalis behind the inguinal ligament into the thigh as the femoral sheath and the pectineal part of the inguinal ligament – Cooper's ligament.[193–195]

1811   Colles, who had worked as a dissector for Cooper, described the reflected inguinal ligament.[189]

1816   Hesselbach described the anatomy of his triangle.[424]

1816   Cloquet described the processus vaginalis and observed it was rarely closed at birth. He also described his 'gland', so important in the differential diagnosis of lumps in the groin.[182]

1846   Anaesthesia discovered.[612]

LISTERIAN

1870   Lister introduced antiseptic surgery and carbolized catgut.[570]

1871   Marcy, who had been a pupil of Lister, described his operation.[609]

1874   Steele described a radical operation for hernia.[888]

1875   Annandale successfully used an extraperitoneal groin approach to treat a direct and an indirect inguinal and a femoral hernia on the same side in a 46-year-old man. Annandale plugged the femoral canal with the redundant inguinal hernial sacs.[27]

1876   Czerny pulled the sac down through the external ring, ligated it at its neck, excised it and allowed it to retract back into the canal.[213]

1881   Lucas-Championniere opened the canal and reconstructed it by imbrication of its anterior wall.[581]

1886   MacEwan operated through the external ring; he rolled up the sac and used it to plug the canal.[590]

1887   Bassini published the first description of his operation.[72]

1889   Halsted I operation described.[384]

1890   Coley's operation – placing the internal oblique anterior to the cord which emerged at the pubic end of the repair. This was the most pernicious and least effective corruption of Bassini's operation.[188]

1891   Tait advocated median abdominal section for hernia.[906]

1892   Wölfler designed the anterior relaxing incision in the rectus sheath to relieve tension on the pubic end repair and prevent recurrence at that site.[994]

1893   Lockwood emphasized the importance of adequate repair of the fascia transversalis.[573]

1895   W.J. Mayo – a radical cure for umbilical hernia.[626]

1895   Andrews introduced imbrication or 'double-breasting' of the layers.[24]

1898   Lotheissen used Cooper's ligament in repair of femoral hernia.[579]

1898   Brenner described 'reinforcing' the repair by suturing the cremaster between the internal oblique arch and the inguinal ligament. The fascia transversalis is not inspected. A serious corruption of the Marcy–Bassini strategy.[116]

1899   Ferguson advised leaving the cord undisturbed – a more serious corruption of Bassini.[296]

1901   McArthur darned his inguinal repair with a pedicled strip of external oblique aponeurosis.[628]

1902   Berger turned down a rectus flap to repair inguinal hernia.[89]

MODERN ASEPTIC

1903   Halsted II operation. Halsted abandoned cord skeletonization to avoid hydrocele and testicular atrophy, and adopted Andrews' imbrication and the Wölfler–Berger technique of a relaxation incision and a rectus sheath flap.[385]

1906   Russell – the 'saccular theory' of hernias, postulating that all indirect inguinal hernias are congenital.[808]

1907   Kocher – revised operation for indirect hernia without opening the canal. The sac was dissected, invaginated and transposed laterally.[508]

1909   McGavin used silver filigree to repair inguinal hernias.[635]

1909   Nicol reported paediatric day-case inguinal herniotomy in Glasgow.[698]

1910   Kirschner used a free transplant of fascia lata from the thigh to reinforce the external oblique.[503]

1918   Handley reconstructed the canal using a darn/lattice technique.[394]

1919   LaRoque – transperitoneal repair of inguinal hernia through grid iron (muscle splitting) incision.[525]

1920   Cheatle – extraperitoneal approach to the groin through a midline incision.[171]

1921   Gallie used strips of autologous fascia lata to repair inguinal hernia.[323]

1923   Keith – classic review of the causation of inguinal hernia. He remarked that aponeuroses and fascia are living structures and speculated that a tissue defect could be responsible for the onset of hernias in middle age.[487]

1927   Keynes – surgeon to the London Truss Society – advocated elective operation using fascial graft techniques.[491]

1936   Henry – extraperitoneal approach to groin hernia.[418]

1940   Wakeley – a personal series of 2020 hernias.[958]

1942   Tanner popularized rectus sheath 'slide'.[908]

1945   Lytle reinterpreted the importance of the internal ring.[585]

1945   Mair introduced the technique of using buried skin to repair an inguinal hernia.[604]

1952   Douglas – first experimental studies of the dynamics of healing (aponeurosis) showed that aponeurotic strength was slow to recover and only reached an optimum at 120 days.[266]

1953   Shouldice – a series of 8317 hernia repairs with overall recurrence rate to 10 years of 0.8%. Emphasis on anatomic repair and early ambulation.[851]

1955   Farquharson – an experience of 485 adults who had their hernias repaired as day cases.[292]

1956   Fruchaud – the concept of the myopectineal orifice and fascia transversalis tunnel for all groin hernias.[317]

1958   Marsden – a 3-year follow-up of inguinal hernioplasties. An important contribution to the evaluation of results.[615]

1958   Usher – the use of knitted polypropylene mesh in hernia repair.[940]

1960   Anson and McVay – classic dissections and evaluation of musculoaponeurotic layers based on a study of 500 body halves.[28]

1962   Doran described the pitfalls of hernia follow-up and set out criteria for adequate evaluation.[263]

1970   Lichtenstein showed the interdependence of suture strength and absorption characteristics with wound healing. Demonstrated experimentally the critical role of non-absorbable or very slowly absorbable sutures in aponeurotic healing.[559]

1972   Doran – critical review of short-stay surgery for inguinal hernia in Birmingham.[260]

1973   Glasgow reported 18 400 repairs of indirect hernia with a recurrence rate less than 1%.[354]

1979   Laparoscopic hernia repair first attempted.[335]

1981   Read demonstrated a tissue defect, metastatic emphysema, in smokers with direct herniation.[147]

1981   Chan described patients developing hernia while undergoing continuous ambulatory peritoneal dialysis.[166]

1983   Schurgers demonstrated an open processus vaginalis in a man 5 months after commencement on peritoneal dialysis.[836]

1984   Read postulated an aetiological relationship between smoking, inguinal herniation and aortic aneurysm.[150]

1993   Environmental factors in hernia causation redefined.[153]

2 ESSENTIAL ANATOMY OF THE ABDOMINAL WALL

A detailed knowledge of the normal anatomy and the functions of each structure is necessary to the surgeon treating hernias. The undergraduate student learning anatomy from the cadaver regards anatomical description as unchanging and invariably accurate, the postgraduate student learning more detailed anatomy or revising for an examination in applied surgical anatomy tends to repeat this error. The surgeon who treats groin and abdominal wall hernias knows that the anatomy is not constant; indeed sometimes he is operating on anatomic variants of the normal rather than for pathological processes disorganizing the normal. Philosophically the surgeon who seeks to make a success of hernia repairs should optimize anatomic variations. Today the surgeon should particularize his operation for the anatomy encountered.

The anatomy of the abdominal wall has undergone a major revision in the past 50 years. The work of Anson and McVay on the inguinal canal appeared in 1938, and since then they and their associate Zimmerman have published extensively. Other notable contributors include Askar, Condon, Fruchaud, Griffith, Harkins, Kark, Lytle, Madden, Mizrachy, Nyhus, Ruge, Skandalakis and Van Mameren.

External anatomy – the surface markings

The abdominal wall, bounded by the lower margin of the thorax above, and by the pubes, the iliac crests and the inguinal ligaments below, is easily recognized in the upright man. Vertically down the centre of the abdomen the depression of the linea alba is obvious. The umbilicus lies at the junction of the upper three-fifths and lower two-fifths of the linea alba. In the healthy young adult the rectus muscle is prominent on either side of the linea alba. The rectus muscle is particularly prominent inferolaterally to the umbilicus: this infra-umbilical rectus mound is of surgical importance. With ageing and obesity the lower abdomen sags but the infra-umbilical rectus mound remains obvious and visible to the subject, even into old age.

The outer margin of each rectus is indicated by a convex vertically directed furrow, the semilunar line (linea semilunaris), which is most distinct in the upper abdomen where it commences at the tip of the ninth costal cartilage. At first it descends almost vertically, but inferior to the umbilicus it gently curves medially to terminate at the pubic tubercle. It is along this line that the internal oblique aponeurosis bands and splits to enclose the rectus muscle in the upper two-thirds of the abdomen. The broad furrow of the inferior semilunar line is also described as the Spigelian fascia and is the site of herniation (Chapter 21). In the lower abdomen the configuration varies, a wider pelvis and greater pubic prominence being important female characteristics (Figure 2.1).

The surgeon must be aware of the elastic and connective tissue lines in the skin (Langer's lines) if optimum

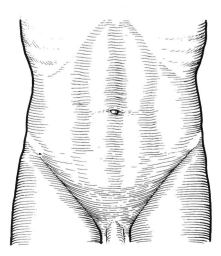 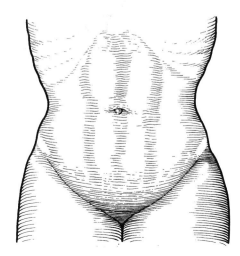

Figure 2.1 Topographical anatomy of the abdomen – the distinctly different male and female characteristics are important in hernia surgery. The boundaries of the abdomen, the costal cartilages above and the crests of the iliac and pubic bones and the inguinal ligament inferiorly are illustrated. The umbilicus, the rectus muscle and the semilunar lines are important surface landmarks

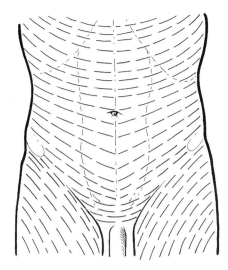

Figure 2.2   Tension lines of the skin (Langer's lines). Incisions at right angles tend to splay and lead to unsightly scars. This adverse phenomenon is enhanced if the incision also crosses a joint crease. Vertical incisions in the groin for hernia repair are particularly unsightly

healing is to be obtained. Incisions made at right angles to Langer's lines gape and tend to splay out when they heal. The longitudinal contraction of the healing wound, particularly when the wound crosses a skin delve or body crease, can make healing very unsightly with contracture and for these reasons vertical incisions over the groin are particularly condemned. However, abdominal access requires adequate vertical incisions and they continue to remain in everyday general surgical and gynaecological practice (Figure 2.2).

The subcutaneous layer

Beneath the skin there is the subcutaneous areolar tissue and fascia. Superiorly over the lower chest and epigastrium this layer is generally thin and less organized than in the lower abdomen where it becomes bilaminar – a superficial fatty stratum (Camper's fascia) and a deeper, stronger and more elastic layer (Scarpa's fascia). Scarpa's fascia is well developed in infancy, forming a distinct layer which must be separately incised when the superficial inguinal ring is approached in childhood herniotomy.

In the lower abdomen the deeper fascia (Scarpa's) is more membranous with much elastic tissue and almost devoid of fat. This fascia does not pass down uninterrupted to the thigh and perineum as the superficial fatty fascia does; instead, the deep fascia is attached to the inner half of the inguinal ligament, to the anterior fascia lata of the thigh and to the iliac crest laterally. Medially it forms a distinct structure containing much elastic tissue and descends, almost as a band, from the pubis to

envelop the penis as the suspensory ligament. Internally it can be traced as a thin layer over the penis and scrotum. Behind the scrotum it becomes continuous with the deep layer of the superficial fascia of the perineum (Colles' fascia) (Figure 2.3).

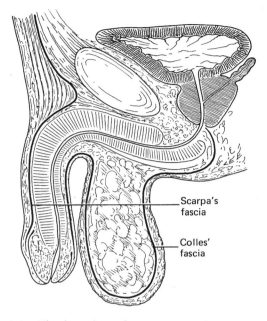

Figure 2.3   The deep elastic fascia (Scarpa's fascia) is stronger over the lower abdomen where it forms a distinct layer that requires division in groin hernia operations

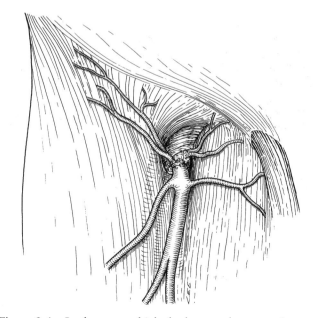

Figure 2.4   In the upper thigh the long saphenous vein goes from superficial to deep to join the femoral vein which is contained in the femoral sheath, an extension of the abdominal fascia transversalis. The femoral sheath is deficient anteriorly where the saphenous vein penetrates it. This weak part of the femoral sheath is the sieve-like cribriform fascia

The superficial fascia in the upper medial thigh has important anatomic features for the hernia surgeon. It is interrupted by the passage, from superficial to deep, of the saphenous vein and other structures, at the saphenous opening or fossa ovalis. Attenuated connective tissue, the cribriform fascia, packs and 'closes' the saphenous opening. Although the cribriform fascia lies in the same plane as the deep fascia, it has many of the structural characteristics of the superficial fascia: it is loose and fatty in texture and is easily distorted by the dilatation of any of the structures in its neighbourhood, a varicose saphenous vein, enlarged lymph nodes and lymphatics, and a femoral hernia. The cribriform fascia is the anterior boundary of the femoral canal at this site (Figure 2.4).

The vessels of the abdominal wall are constant and the experienced operator is used to encountering them in sequence. Superficially they anastomose to make a network in the subcutaneous tissue. The lower intercostal arteries, the musculophrenic and the right and left superior epigastric arteries (continuations of the internal thoracic from the subclavian) supply the abdominal wall cephalad to the umbilicus. Caudal to the umbilicus the superior epigastric vessels are continuous with the inferior epigastric vessels lying deep to the rectus muscle; the inferior epigastric artery arises from the external iliac artery just proximal to the inguinal ligament, The inferior epigastric artery forms the lateral margin of Hasselbach's triangle;[424] the neck of an indirect inguinal hernia is lateral and a direct inguinal hernia medial to this artery.

In addition to the serially arranged vessels, there are three small superficial branches of the femoral artery in the upper thigh (and accompanying veins draining to the saphenous vein) which spread out from the groin over the lower abdomen. These vessels are the superficial circumflex iliac passing laterally and upwards over the inguinal canal, the superficial epigastric coursing upward and medially and the superficial external pudendal making its way medially to supply the skin of the penis and scrotum and, importantly, to anastomose with the spermatic cord vessels to the scrotal contents. All these arteries are encountered in inguinal and femoral hernioplasty; all anastomose adequately both with the serial intercostal and lumbar arteries and across the midline. In most instances they can be divided with impunity, but sometimes they are an important auxiliary blood supply to the testicle (see page 273) (Figure 2.5).

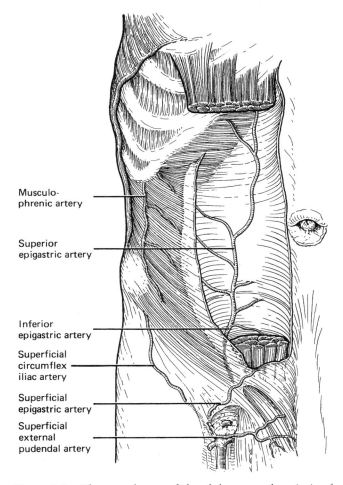

Musculo-
phrenic artery

Superior
epigastric artery

Inferior
epigastric artery

Superficial
circumflex
iliac artery

Superficial
epigastric artery

Superficial
external
pudendal artery

Figure 2.5   The vasculature of the abdomen and groin is of particular interest to the surgeon. Fortunately the vessels all anastomose freely, so surgery does not need to be locked into vascular anatomy, except for the anastomosis of the pudendal with the cord vessels over the pubis. Care should be taken not to dissect the superficial tissues medial to the pubic tubercle to avoid threat to the pudendal anastomosis and the testicle

Superficial nerves

The cutaneous nerves are arranged segmentally, similarly to the intercostal nerves in the thorax. The lower five or six nerves sweep around obliquely to supply the abdominal parietes, giving a lateral cutaneous branch which passes between the digitations of the external oblique muscle; this branch divides into a small posterior nerve which extends back over the latissimus dorsi and a larger anterior nerve which supplies the external oblique and the overlying subcutaneous tissue and skin. The main stem of the intercostal nerve continues forwards and gains the surface by passing through the rectus muscle and emerging through the anterior rectus sheath a centimetre or so from the midline (Figure 2.6).

The most caudal of the abdominal wall nerves are derived from the first lumbar nerve; they are the iliohypogastric and ilio-inguinal nerves. The ilio-inguinal nerve is generally smaller than the iliohypogastric nerve – if one is large the other is smaller and vice versa. Occasionally the ilio-inguinal nerve is very small and may be absent. The anterior cutaneous branch of the iliohypogastric nerve emerges through the aponeurosis of the external oblique just above the superficial

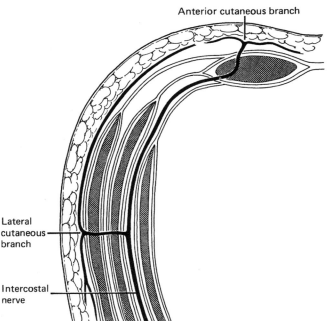

Figure 2.6 The lower abdomen is segmentally supplied by the intercostal nerves. Each nerve has a lateral cutaneous branch which gives anterior and posterior divisions in the subcutaneous tissue. When a local anaesthetic is administered it is important to block the anterior division of the lateral cutaneous branch of these nerves

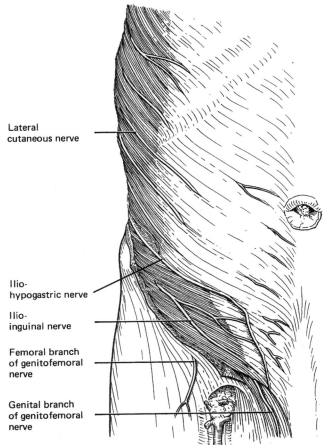

Figure 2.7 The groin area is innervated principally by branches of the first lumbar nerve – the iliohypogastric and ilio-inguinal nerves. These nerves innervate the skin area over the iliac crest (the lateral branch of the iliohypogastric nerve), the suprapubic region (the anterior iliohypogastric nerve) and the side of the scrotum and upper medial thigh (the ilio-inguinal nerve after it emerges from the inguinal canal)

inguinal ring and innervates the skin in the suprapubic region. The ilio-inguinal nerve passes through the lower inguinal canal and becomes superficial by emerging from the superficial inguinal ring to supply the skin of the scrotum and a small area of the medial upper thigh (Figure 2.7).

The genitofemoral nerve arises from the first and second lumbar nerves and completes the innervation of the abdominal wall and groin areas. At first it passes obliquely forwards and downwards through the substance of the psoas major. It emerges from the muscle and crosses its anterior surface deep to the peritoneum, going behind, posterior to, the ureter. It divides a variable distance from the deep inguinal ring into a genital and a femoral branch.

The posterior two-thirds of the scrotum are supplied by S2 and S3 through the perineal and posterior femoral cutaneous nerves. The anterior scrotal cutaneous supply is frequently disrupted in inguinal hernioplasty (Figure 2.8).

The sensory nerve supply of the upper anterior thigh is from the lateral cutaneous nerve of the thigh, the femoral branch of the genitofemoral nerve, the ilio-inguinal nerve and the genital branch of the genito-femoral nerve (Figure 2.9). There is overlap between the territories of these nerves and their pathways also show considerable variation.

The lateral cutaneous nerve of the thigh arises from the dorsal branches of the ventral rami of the second and

third lumbar nerves. It emerges from the lateral border of the psoas major and crosses the iliacus obliquely, running towards the anterior superior spine. It lies in the adipose tissue between the iliopsoas muscle fascia and the peritoneum.

Usually the lateral cutaneous nerve of the thigh forms one single trunk but it may divide into two branches a variable distance proximal to the inguinal ligament (Figure 2.10).[806] The nerve then penetrates the anterior surface of the body by passing deep to the lateral portion of the inguinal ligament; it may lie superficial to the sartorius muscle here or may pass through the sartorius before it becomes superficial to supply the skin of the lateral side of the thigh. The variability of the course of the nerve in the abdomen is considerable and the distance between nerve and the deep inguinal ring also variable.[435] The nerve may traverse the anterior abdominal wall cranial to the inguinal ligament or through the attachment of the ligament to the anterior superior iliac spine.

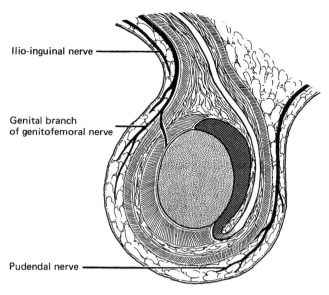

Figure 2.8 The skin of the anterior scrotum is supplied by the ilio-inguinal nerve, L1, and the genital branch of the genitofemoral nerve, L1. These nerves are often disrupted in hernioplasty

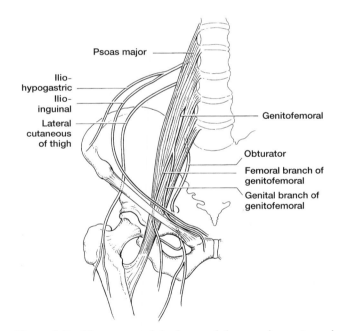

Figure 2.9 The nerves of the lower abdomen, the groin and upper thigh. The lateral cutaneous nerve of the thigh and the femoral branch of the genitofemoral nerve are at special risk in extraperitoneal operations on groin hernia.

The genital branch, a mixed motor and sensory nerve, crosses the femoral vessels and enters the inguinal canal at or just medial to the deep ring. The nerve penetrates the fascia transversalis of the posterior wall of the inguinal ligament either through the deep ring or separately medially to the deep ring. The nerve traverses the inguinal canal lying between the spermatic cord above

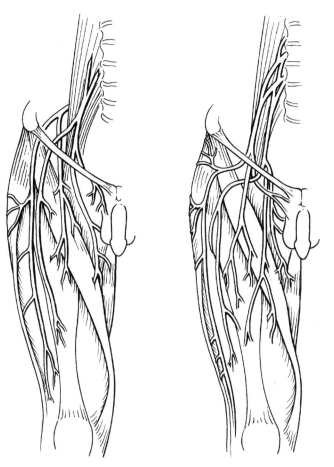

Figure 2.10 The variable anatomy of the lateral cutaneous nerve of the thigh and the femoral branch of the genitofemoral nerve. Both these nerves are in close proximity to the inguinal ligament as they progress to the thigh (After Ruge 1908 – from Van Mameren and Go, 1995[946])

and the upturned edge of the inguinal ligament inferiorly; the nerve is vulnerable to surgical trauma as it progresses along the floor of the canal (the gutter produced by the upturned internal edge of the inguinal ligament). The genital nerve supplies the motor function to the cremaster muscle and the sensory function to the skin of the scrotum.

The femoral branch enters the femoral sheath lying lateral to the femoral artery and supplies the skin of the upper part of the femoral triangle (Figure 2.11).

The scrotal nerve supply is complex.[1000] The autonomic supply of the testis is from T10 to T12, via nerves which accompany the spermatic vessels. These autonomic nerves are motor to the vasculature and to the smooth muscle of the tunica albuginea. However, they also have free, sensory, endings in the interstitial spaces of the testis and convey noxious stimuli which give referred pain in the lower abdomen (T10–T12 segments). The autonomic supply of the vas and epididymis are distinct from those of the testis; pain from these

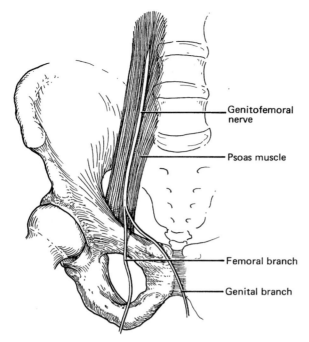

Figure 2.11   The genitofemoral nerve, from L1 and L2, inner-vates the femoral sheath and the skin over it. It needs blocking when a femoral hernia is to be operated under local anaesthetic

structures is felt in the L1 segment, lower than testicular pain, in the distributions of the genitofemoral nerve.

The somatic nerve supply is the genitofemoral nerve, L1 and L2, and the sacral nerve, S2 and S3. The genital branch of the genitofemoral nerve supplies the cord, the cremaster, the tunica vaginalis and, along with the L1 component of the ilio-inguinal nerve, the anterior third of the scrotal skin.

The area lateral to the cord vessels and above the inguinal ligament where the femoral branch of genito-femoral nerve and lateral cutaneous nerve of the thigh lie

has been dubbed the 'triangle of pain' by laparoscopic surgeons because of the hazard of nerve injury by entrap-ment with staples. In this area thick globular adipose tissue can surround and conceal the nerves. On a deeper plane the femoral nerve crosses this triangle with the genitofemoral and lateral cutaneous nerve superficial to it (Figure 2.12).

The external oblique muscle

The external oblique muscle arises by eight digitations from the external surfaces of the lower eight ribs; the upper three digitations alternate with the origins of the serratus anterior and the lower four with those of the latissimus dorsi muscle. The fibres pass downwards and forwards from their origins; the posterior fibres are nearly vertical and are inserted into the anterior external lip of the iliac crest: in contrast, the uppermost fibres run almost horizontally towards the contralateral side. The intervening fibres pursue an intermediate oblique course. All the superior and intermediate fibres end in the strong external oblique aponeurosis.

Superiorly the aponeurosis is relatively thin and passes medially to be attached to the xiphoid process. Inferiorly the aponeurosis is very strong. Along its lower margin the aponeurosis forms the inguinal ligament, which is attached superolaterally to the anterior superior iliac spine and inferomedially to the pubic tubercle. The aponeurosis of the muscle forms the anterior rectus sheath and is inserted, along with its fellow of the oppo-site side, into the linea alba and the front of the pubis. The aponeurosis is broadest inferiorly, narrowest at the umbilicus and broad again in the epigastrium.

The aponeurosis of the external oblique muscle fuses with the aponeurosis of the internal oblique in the anterior rectus sheath. This line of fusion is considerably

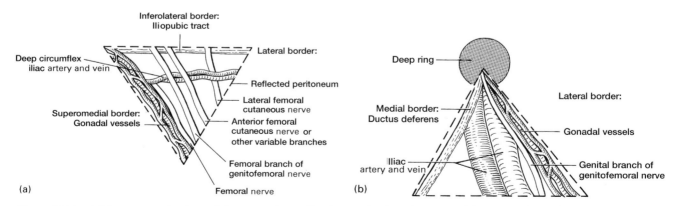

Figure 2.12   (a) Laparoscopic view of the nerves immediately proximal to the inguinal ligament after reflection of the parietal peritoneum. These nerves lie in the adipose tissue just deep to the peritoneum and superficial to the iliopsoas muscle: the 'trian-gle of pain'. (b) Laparoscopic view of the deep inguinal ring and adjacent structures, the 'triangle of doom'. (After Skandalakis *et al.* 1996[866])

medial to the semilunar line – the fusion line is oblique and somewhat semilunar, being more lateral above and more medial below. In fact, the external oblique aponeurosis contributes very little to the lower portion of the anterior rectus sheath. This latter point is of considerable importance in inguinal hernioplasty (Figure 2.13).[640]

There is a defect in the external–oblique aponeurosis just above the pubis. This aperture – the superficial inguinal ring – is triangular in shape and in the male allows passage of the spermatic cord from the abdomen to the scrotum. In the female the round ligament of the uterus passes through this opening. The superficial inguinal ring is not a 'ring'; it is a triangular cleft with its long axis oblique in the same direction but not quite parallel to the inguinal ligament. The base of the triangle is formed by the crest of the pubis and the apex is lateral towards the anterior superior iliac spine. The superficial inguinal ring represents that interval between the aponeurosis of the external oblique which inserts into the pubic bone superiorly and, as the inguinal ligament, inserts into the pubic tubercle inferiorly. The aponeurotic margins of the ring are described as the superior and inferior crura. The spermatic cord, as it comes through the superficial ring, rests on the inferior crus which is a continuation of the floor of the inguinal

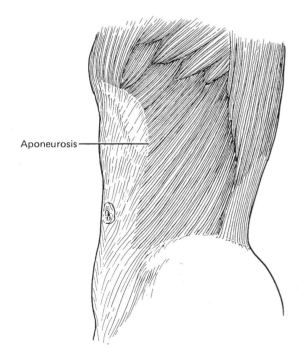

Aponeurosis

Figure 2.13   The external oblique muscle and its aponeurosis invests the abdomen. The aponeurosis of this muscle forms the anterior rectus sheath by fusion to the underlying aponeurosis of the internal oblique. However, this line of fusion, in the lower abdomen especially, is considerably medial to the semilunar line, a point of great importance in inguinal hernioplasty, allowing a 'slide operation' on the internal oblique without compromising the anterior rectus sheath (see page 165)

canal (the upturned internal margin of the inguinal ligament).

The dimensions of the superficial inguinal ring, or aponeurotic cleft, are of surgical importance. Far from being of standard size and predictable extent it may sometimes be snug around the cord and occasionally extend upward and laterally beyond the anterior superior iliac spine. In 80% of cases the cleft is confined to the lower half of the area between the midline and the anterior superior spine, but in the remaining 20% it extends more laterally. In about 2% of cases there are one or more accessory clefts, usually superolaterally to the main cleft; the accessory cleft may transmit the iliohypogastric nerve (Figure 2.14).[28]

The relationship between the apex of the cleft and the deep epigastric vessels (indicating the lateral margin of Hesselbach's triangle) is of crucial importance in closing the inguinal canal anteriorly and containing a potential direct inguinal hernia. Whereas the canal is usually described as closed anteriorly by the external oblique aponeurosis, in only 11% of cases does the apex of the cleft lie less than halfway along a line from the pubic tubercle to the inferior epigastric artery; in 52% the cleft extends to the level of the epigastric vessels and, most importantly, in 37% the apex of the cleft is lateral to the epigastric vessels (Figure 2.15).[28]

The crura of the superficial ring are joined together by intercrural fibres derived from the outer investing fascia of the external oblique aponeurosis. The size and strength of these intercrural fibres vary. In 27% of specimens these fibres do not cross from crus to crus and, therefore, do not reinforce the margins of the cleft[28] (Figure 2.16).

The inguinal ligament is simply the lower margin of the aponeurosis of the external oblique; it is not a condensed thickened ligamentous structure. The ligament presents a rounded surface towards the thigh where the aponeurosis is rolled inwards back on itself to make a groove on its deep surface. Laterally the ligament is attached to the anterior superior iliac spine and medially to the pubic tubercle and via the lacunar and reflected inguinal ligaments to the iliopectineal line on the superior ramus of the pubis. The inguinal ligament is not straight; it is concave, with the concavity directed medially and upward towards the abdomen (Figure 2.17).

The medial attachment, or continuation, of the inguinal ligament as the lacunar (Gimbernat's) and the pectineal (Cooper's) ligament gives a fan-like expansion of the inguinal ligament at its medial end. This expansion has important surgical implications.

The lacunar ligament is a triangular continuation of the medial end of the inguinal ligament. Its apex is at the pubic tubercle, its superior margin continuous with the inguinal ligament, and its medial margin is attached to the iliopectineal line on the superior ramus of the pubis.

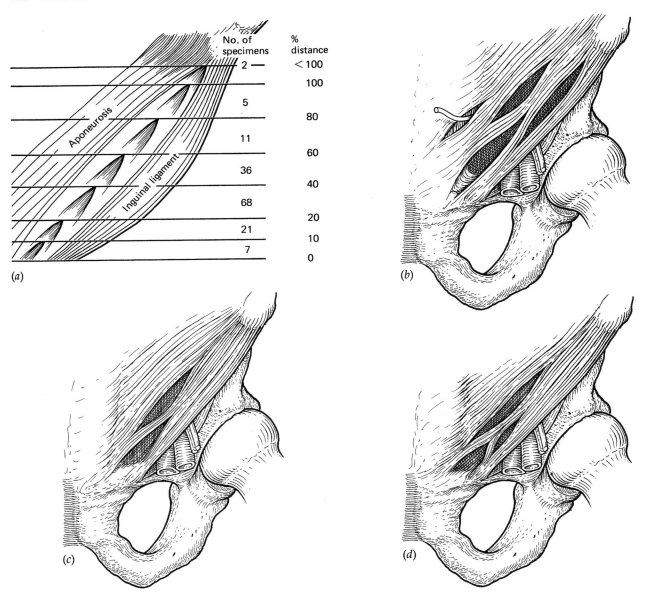

Figure 2.14 The anatomy and dimensions of the superficial inguinal ring are very variable. The 'ring' is a triangular cleft separating the insertions of the external oblique muscles into the pubic crest and the pubic tubercle. Its base is medial and inferior and its apex superior and lateral. In 80% of subjects the apex lies in the medial half of the lower abdomen, but in the remaining 20% the apex approaches the anterior superior iliac spine (**a**). In 2% of subjects, there are accessory clefts superior to the main cleft (**b,c,d**). One of these clefts may transmit the iliohypogastric nerve (**b**) (From Anson, Morgan and McVay, 1960[28])

Its lateral crescentic edge is free and directed laterally, where it is an important rigid structure in the medial margin of the femoral canal. The ligament lies in an oblique plane, with its upper (abdominal) surface facing superomedially and being crossed by the spermatic cord, and its lower (femoral) surface looking anterolaterally. With the external oblique aponeurosis and the inguinal ligament, the superior surface forms a groove for the cord as it emerges from the inguinal canal (Figure 2.18).

The reflected part of the inguinal ligament (Colles') is a broad band of rather thin fibres which arise from the crest of the pubis and the medial end of the iliopectineal line and pass anterosuperiorly behind the superior crus of the subcutaneous inguinal ring to the linea alba. The reflected part of the inguinal ligament is very variable in its extent but it is an important structure closing the potential space in the posterior wall of the inguinal canal between the iliopectineal line and the lateral margin of the rectus muscle (Figure 2.19).

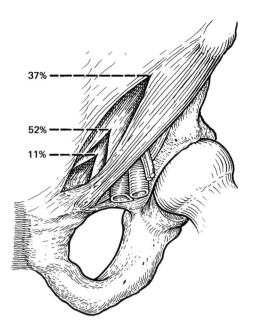

Figure 2.15   The size of the superficial inguinal ring, the cleft in the external oblique, is crucial in closing the inguinal canal anteriorly. In 11% of subjects the cleft extends less than 50% of the length of the inguinal canal, in 52% it extends as far as the deep epigastric vessels, and in 37% the cleft extends lateral to the deep epigastric vessels (From Anson, Morgan and McVay, 1960[28])

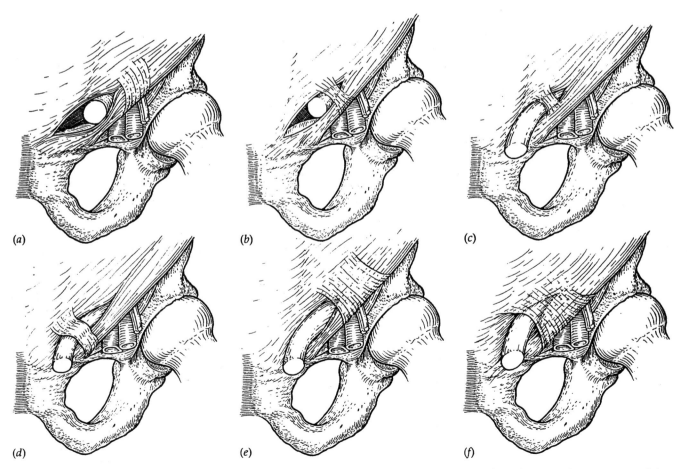

Figure 2.16 (a–l)   Variations in the structure of the superficial inguinal ring. The intercrural fibres between the two crura of the ring are very variable; in 27% of subjects these intercrural fibres do not cross from one crus to the other (From Anson, Morgan and McVay, 1960[28])

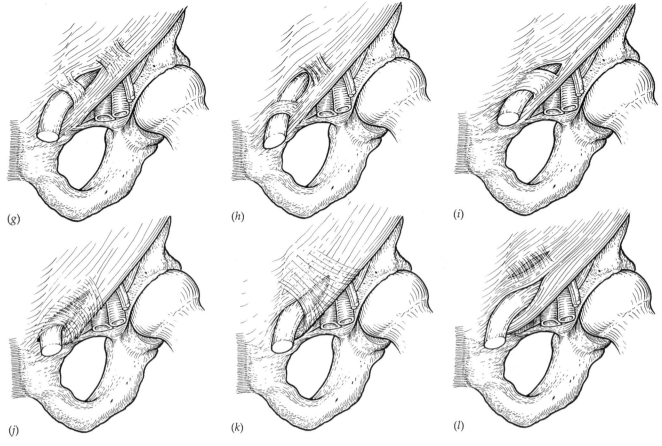

(g)

(h)

(i)

(j)

(k)

(l)

Fig. 2.16 (cont.)

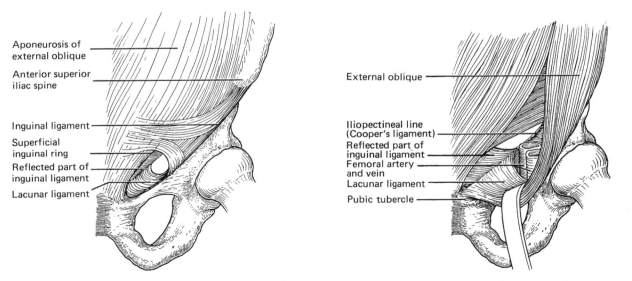

Aponeurosis of
external oblique

Anterior superior
iliac spine

Inguinal ligament

Superficial
inguinal ring

Reflected part of
inguinal ligament

Lacunar ligament

External oblique

Iliopectineal line
(Cooper's ligament)
Reflected part of
inguinal ligament
Femoral artery
and vein
Lacunar ligament

Pubic tubercle

Figure 2.17 The inguinal ligament is the lower margin of the external oblique muscle. Medially it is attached like a fan to the iliopectineal line (Cooper's ligament) and the tubercle of the pubis

Figure 2.18 The upper abdominal surface of the attachment of the inguinal ligament to the pubic tubercle is the floor of the inguinal canal which the cord rests on as it emerges from the canal

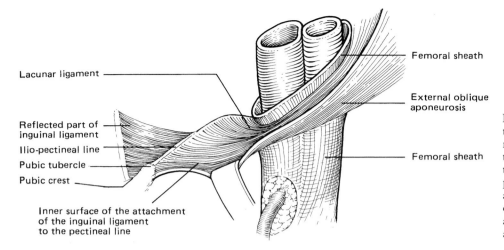

Lacunar ligament

Reflected part of inguinal ligament
Ilio-pectineal line
Pubic tubercle
Pubic crest

Inner surface of the attachment of the inguinal ligament to the pectineal line

Femoral sheath

External oblique aponeurosis

Femoral sheath

Figure 2.19 Medially the posterior wall of the inguinal canal is reinforced by the reflected part of the inguinal ligament, a strong triangular fascia arising from the pubic crest anteriorly to the attachments of the internal oblique and transversus muscles and passing medially to the linea alba into which it is inserted

The internal oblique muscle

The internal oblique muscle arises from the lateral half of the abdominal surface of the inguinal ligament, the intermediate line on the anterior two-thirds of the iliac crest and the lumbodorsal fascia. The general direction of the fibres is upward and medial. The posterior fibres are inserted into the inferior borders of the cartilages of the lower four ribs. The intermediate fibres pass upward and medially and end in a strong aponeurosis which extends from the inferior borders of the seventh and eighth ribs and the xiphoid process to the linea alba throughout its length. The lower fibres, from their origin

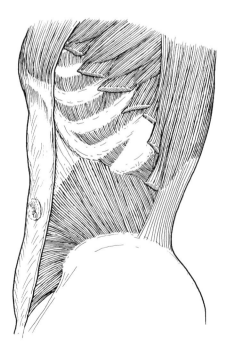

Figure 2.20 The internal oblique muscle arising from the lateral half of the inguinal ligament and the iliac crest to be inserted into the lower costal cartilage and, via its aponeurosis, continuous with its fellow muscle contralaterally

at the inguinal ligament, arch downward and medially: with the lowest fibres of the transversus muscle they pass in front of the rectus muscle, to form the anterior rectus sheath, and insert on the pubic crest and the iliopectineal line behind the lacunar ligament and reflected part of the inguinal ligament (Figure 2.20).

The internal oblique is not invariable in its anatomy in the inguinal region. Its origin may commence at the internal ring or at a variable distance lateral to the ring. The muscle may then insert either into the pubic crest and tubercle or into the lateral margin of the rectus sheath a variable distance above the pubis. There are thus four common combinations of origin and insertion of the internal oblique in the groin. The contribution of the internal oblique to groin anatomy and in particular to the 'defences' of the inguinal canal is very variable. There are racial differences in the anatomy of the internal oblique in the groin (see page 46) (Figure 2.21).

The detailed anatomy of the semilunar line and rectus sheath, and that of the insertion of the lowermost fibres of the internal oblique into the pubic bone, are of surgical significance and warrant more detailed consideration.

At the lateral margin of the rectus muscle the aponeurosis of the internal oblique splits into two lamellae – the superficial lamella passes anterior to the rectus and the deep lamella goes posterior to the rectus. The anterior lamella fuses with the aponeurosis of the external oblique to form the anterior rectus sheath; likewise the posterior lamella becomes fused with the aponeurosis of the underlying transversus muscle. The detailed anatomy varies but has importance in the causation of umbilical and epigastric hernias (see page 218). In the lower part of the abdomen, in an area inferior to a point about midway between the umbilicus and the pubis, the aponeurosis does not split into lamella but courses entirely in front of the rectus to fuse with the overlying aponeurosis of the external oblique (Figure 2.22).

The internal oblique muscle in its lateral fleshy part is not uniform in structure; it is segmented or banded. The

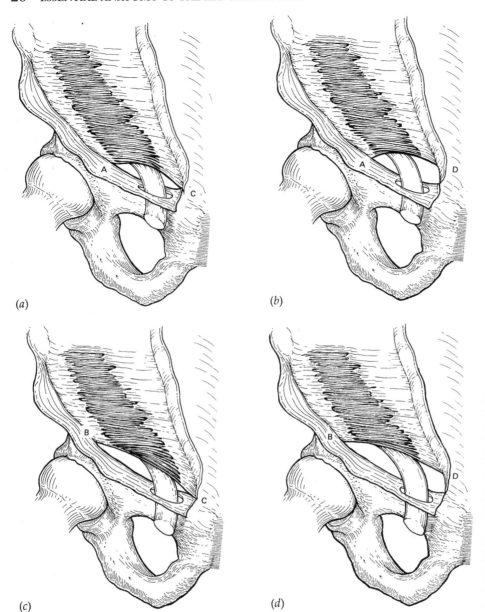

(a)

(b)

(c)

(d)

Figure 2.21 The origin and insertions of the internal oblique muscle and aponeurosis in the inguinal region are variable. The origin of the red muscle fibres is from the lateral inguinal ligament; this origin may extend as far medially as the deep ring (**a**), or the muscle may arise more laterally (**b**). The insertion of the aponeurosis is also variable; it may be inserted into the pubic crest and pubic tubercle (**c**) or solely into the rectus sheath (**d**). This gives four variants of the lower margin of the internal oblique in the inguinal canal: A–C, A–D, B–C, B–D

muscular bands terminate just lateral to the border of the rectus muscle and are most marked in the inguinal and lower abdominal region. The bands are generally

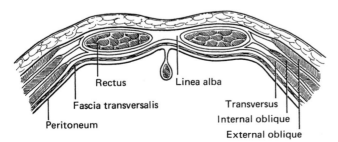

Figure 2.22 Structure of the posterior rectus sheath in the upper abdomen. The internal oblique divides into two lamellae which enclose the rectus. The line of the fascia transversalis is deliberately emphasized

arranged like 'the blades of a fan with the interspaces increasing as the medial extremities are reached.'[878, 1005] The bands may easily be separable up to the point where they fuse with the aponeurosis lateral to the rectus muscle. In a fifth of cases there are potential parietal deficits between these bands. Spigelian hernias occur through these defects of the semilunar line, which are more pronounced in the lower abdomen (see page 233).

At the lowermost part of the internal oblique muscle, adjacent to its origin from the inguinal ligament, the spermatic cord passes through or adjacent to the medial margin of the muscle. Laterally the cord lies deep to the fleshy muscular fibres, then as it emerges alongside the muscle it acquires a coat of cremaster muscle from the muscle.

The fascicles of the lower internal oblique muscle

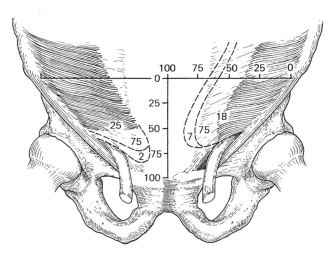

Figure 2.23 Extent of the muscular fibres of the internal oblique. In only 2% of subjects the muscle extends inferiorly to the inguinal canal (left of diagram). Similarly the medial extent of the fleshy muscle fibres varies (right of diagram). The contribution of the internal oblique to the 'defences' of the inguinal canal is very variable (From Anson, Morgan and McVay, 1960,[28] by permission of *Surgery, Gynecology and Obstetrics*)

follow a transverse or oblique direction. Medial to the cord they convert to an aponeurosis which continues to the insertion of the muscle. There is variation in both the medial and the inferior extent of the muscle fibres of the internal oblique.

The fleshy muscle extends to the inferior margin in

only 2% of cases; in 75% the extent is a centimetre or so above the margin, and in 20% there is a broad aponeurotic leaf superior to the spermatic cord. Likewise the fleshy muscle extends as far as the emergent cord in 20%, medial to the cord but not as far medially to the rectus margin in 75%, and medial to the lateral margin of the rectus in 2%.

In clinical practice a direct inguinal hernia is never encountered when the lower margin of the internal oblique is fleshy **and** when the fleshy fibres extend medial to the superficial ring. Direct herniation is most frequently found at operation when the internal oblique muscle is replaced with flimsy aponeurosis in the roof of the inguinal canal (Figure 2.23).[28]

In 52% of cases the lowermost arching fibres of the internal oblique are continuous above with the remainder of the internal oblique muscles but in the remainder a variety of spaces between banding occur. In the medial and lower musculo-aponeurotic plate, defects superior to the spermatic cord may compromise the shutter mechanism of the canal and lead to direct inguinal herniation. Similarly, Spigelian hernia defects can develop between the muscle bands, enter the inguinal canal and present as direct inguinal hernia[935] (Figure 2.24).

Rarely (0.15% of hernia cases), the spermatic cord comes through the fleshy part of the lower muscle belly so that the muscle had an origin from the inguinal ligament medial to emergent cord. In these cases there is prominent banding of the muscle in the lower abdomen so that effectively there is a band caudal to the cord (Figure 2.25).

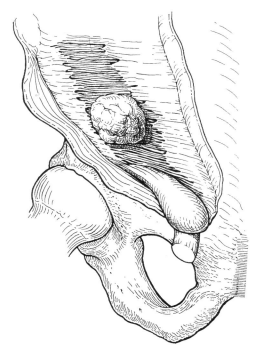

Figure 2.24 A hernia can occur between the banding of the lower internal oblique muscle. Although this hernia is truly a variant Spigelian hernia, it presents as a direct hernia into the inguinal canal

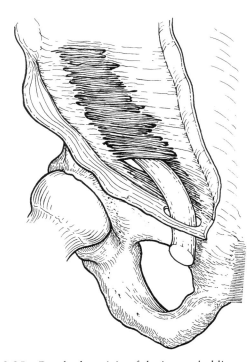

Figure 2.25 Rarely the origin of the internal oblique extends medially to the deep ring so that the cord passes between bands of the muscle

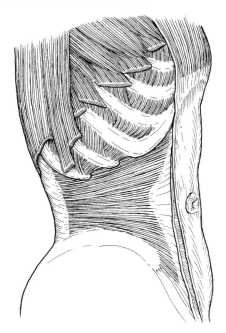

Figure 2.26 The transversus muscle is the deepest of the parietal muscles; it arises from the iliopsoas fascia and the iliac crest in its anterior two-thirds. The muscle extends to the lowest six costal cartilages and to the linea alba and its contralateral fellow

The transverse abdominal muscle

The transversus abdominis is the third and deepest of the three abdominal muscle layers. The muscle arises from the iliopsoas fascia along the internal lip of the anterior two-thirds of the iliac crest. The iliopsoas fascia is continuous with the thoracolumbar fascia (which is effectively the posterior aponeurosis of the muscle extending its origin to the vertebral column), and the costal cartilages of the lower six ribs interdigitating with the origin of the diaphragm (Figure 2.26).

Anteriorly, the muscle fibres end in a strong aponeurosis which is inserted into the linea alba, the pubic crest and the iliopectineal line. For the most part the fibres run transversely, but in the lower abdomen they take on a downward and medial curve so that the lower margin of the muscle forms an arch over the inguinal canal. The lower fibres give way to the aponeurosis which gains insertion into the pubic crest and the iliopectineal line. The insertion of the transverse muscle is broader than that of the internal oblique and consequently its aponeurosis extends further along the iliopectineal line (Figure 2.27).

In the epigastrium and in the lower abdomen, down to a point midway between the umbilicus and the pubis, the transverse aponeurosis fuses with the posterior lamella of the aponeurosis of the internal oblique to form the posterior rectus sheath. In the lowermost abdomen the aponeurosis passes in front of the rectus muscle and fuses with the aponeurosis of the external oblique and internal oblique muscles to form the anterior rectus sheath (Figure 2.28).

The muscle consists of more aponeurosis and much less muscle fibres than either the external or internal oblique muscles. In 67% of cases fleshy muscle covers only the upper part of the inguinal region. In only 14% of cases are any fleshy fibres found in the lowermost fibres arching over the inguinal canal. Similarly, in 71% of subjects the red fibres do not extend medially to the deep epigastric vessels. The aponeurotic portion of the muscle shows its greatest anatomical variation in the inguinal region, where it is most important in hernia repair.

The lower border of the transversus abdominis aponeurosis is called the 'arch'. Above the arch the transversus aponeurosis forms a continuous strong sheet, with no spaces between its fibres. Below the arch the posterior wall of the inguinal canal is closed by transversalis

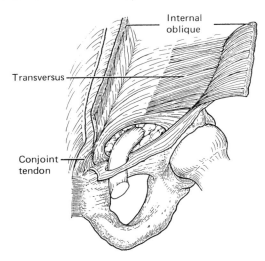

Figure 2.27 The transversus muscle fibres run transversely, except in the lower abdomen where they form a strong aponeurosis (tendon) which is inserted to the pubic crest and the iliopectineal line. The insertion of the transversus tendon is broader than that of the internal oblique. The extent to which this tendon extends along the iliopectineal line determines its contribution to reinforcing the posterior wall of the inguinal canal. In surgical jargon the lowest fibres of the transversus aponeurosis cross over the cord to form the 'roof' of the canal. These white aponeurotic fibres are referred to as the 'arch' by some surgeons (see page 153)

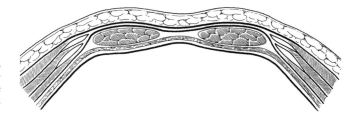

Figure 2.28 Composition of the posterior rectus sheath in the lower abdomen. In the lower abdomen, inferior to the arcuate line of Douglas, the rectus sheath becomes deficient posteriorly. This is related to the variable anatomy of the internal oblique muscle. The fascia transversalis is stronger in the lower abdomen

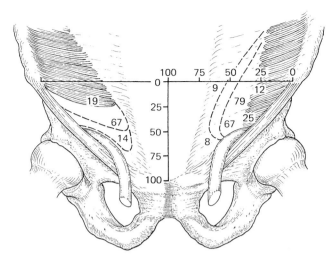

Figure 2.29 The extent of fleshy red muscle in the transversus muscle is much less than in the internal oblique. Only in 14% of subjects is the lower margin of this muscle in the roof of the inguinal canal composed of red muscle (left of diagram). The medial extent of red fibres is similarly restricted; in 71% of subjects muscle fibres do not extent medially to the inferior epigastric vessels (right of diagram)(From Anson, Morgan and McVay, 1960,[28] by permission of *Surgery, Gynecology and Obstetrics*)

fascia only. This is a weak area through which direct herniation can occur. The aponeurotic arch is easily identifiable as a 'white line' of aponeurosis at operation (Figures 2.27 and 2.29).

The conjoint tendon

The transverse fibres of the transversus muscle proceed horizontally to their insertion in the rectus sheath and the linea alba, while the lower fibres course downward, medially and caudally – sometimes to fuse with fibres of the internal oblique as they insert into the anterior pubis and the iliopectineal line.

Only when the aponeuroses of the transversus and the internal oblique are fused some distance lateral to the rectus sheath may the term conjoint tendon be correctly used. Thus the conjoint tendon is the fused aponeuroses of the internal oblique and transversus muscles which is inserted into the anterior 2 cm of the iliopectineal line. The transversus muscle contributes 80% of the conjoint tendon. The conjoint tendon is lateral to the rectus muscle and lies immediately deep to the superficial inguinal ring. It passes down to its insertion deep to the inguinal and lacunar ligaments. The spermatic cord, or round ligament, lies anterior to it as it passes through the superficial inguinal ring.

The conjoint tendon has a very variable structure and in 20% of subjects it does not exist as a discrete anatomic structure. It may be absent or only slightly developed, it may be replaced by a lateral extension of the tendon of

origin of the rectus muscle, or it may extend laterally to the deep inguinal ring so that no interval is present between the lower border of the transversus and the inguinal ligament. A shutter mechanism for the conjoint tendon can only be demonstrated when the lateral side of the tendon, that is the transversus and internal oblique muscles, extend onto and are attached to the iliopectineal line.[976] The extent of this insertion is very variable. In 8% of cases this attachment does not extend lateral to the rectus muscle, leaving the posterior wall of the inguinal canal (fascia transversalis) unsupported; in 31% the attachment extends to the midpoint of the posterior wall between the pubic spine medially and the deep epigastric vessels laterally; in 40% it extends as far as the deep epigastric vessels. In a minority of cases bands of aponeurosis wind off the main aponeurotic arch and are inserted independently into the iliopectineal line. Sometimes, therefore, the lateral margin of the rectus sheath is formed only from the lowermost fibres of the transversus aponeurosis which curve inferiorly to become attached to the pubis – this is called the falx inguinalis.

A few fibres of the lowermost lateral margin of the rectus tendon may be fused with the fascia transversalis in their attachment to the iliopubic ligament – this has been called Henle's ligament (Figure 2.30).

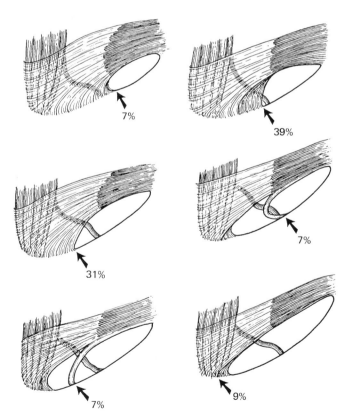

Figure 2.30 The extent of the tendon of transversus abdominis contributes to the posterior wall of the inguinal canal. The arrows indicate the lateralmost extension in the percentages of subjects (From Anson, Morgan and McVay, 1960[28])

To understand the importance of the attachment of the internal oblique and transversus aponeuroses to the iliopectineal line, the posterior aspect of the inguinal canal must be visualized from inside the abdomen. If there is full attachment of the conjoint tendon to the iliopectineal line, the posterior wall of the inguinal canal is completely reinforced by aponeurosis. Absence of this attachment removes this reinforcement and there is then the potential to develop a direct or large indirect hernia.

Of all the anatomic layers the external oblique is the least variable; in the inguinal region it is invariably aponeurotic. The internal oblique and transversus layers are very variable; they may be fleshy almost to the midline, aponeurotic or banded fan-like with the space between the musculo-aponeurotic bands occupied only by the flimsiest fascia. If these local weaknesses are superimposed, herniation is facilitated.

Zimmerman and colleagues have drawn attention to the frequency with which defects occur in the internal oblique and transversus muscles in this area. In 45% of their dissections there was a defect in one or other layer and in 6% these defects, of the lower linea semilunaris, were superimposed. These defects predispose to spontaneous ventral hernias either of preperitoneal fat or more extensive hernias with peritoneal sacs.[1006]

The linea alba, and the rectus sheath and its contents

The linea alba is formed in the midline by the decussation of the fibres of the three aponeuroses. The linea alba is a dense fibrous band which extends from the xiphoid process to the pubic symphysis. The linea is broad in the epigastrium, then broadest at the umbilicus, and below the umbilicus it narrows down to become little more than a line between the two rectus muscles at the pubis. The linea alba is pierced by several small blood vessels and by the umbilical vessels in the fetus.

The anterior rectus muscle sheath forms the most important portion of the abdominal wall aponeuroses. When the anterior sheath is gently dissected, during a paramedian incision for example, it is shown to be made of three lamina. The most superficial fibres are directed downward and laterally; these form the external oblique of the opposite side. The next layer, derived from the external oblique of the same side, has fibres at right angles to the first layer, that is they run downwards and medially. Finally, the third component of the anterior rectus sheath is formed from the anterior lamina of the internal oblique muscle of the same side whose fibres generally run in the same direction as, and parallel to, the fibres of the external oblique of the opposite side. This gives the anterior rectus sheath a triple criss-cross pattern similar to plywood.[41] In the lower abdomen the

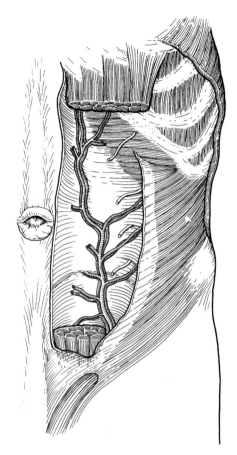

Figure 2.31   Rectus sheath and linea alba. The contents of the rectus sheath are the rectus and pyramidalis muscles, the superior and inferior epigastric vessels and the terminal branches of the lower six thoracic nerves

fusion of the external oblique aponeurosis to the internal oblique aponeurosis is very medial, an important anatomical arrangement that allows a tendon slide to be used to release the tension of the internal oblique in direct inguinal hernia repair without compromising the integrity of the anterior rectus sheath[41] (for further description, see page 165).

The most important feature from a surgical perspective is that the fibres of the rectus sheath run from side to side. Vertical incisions divide fibres while horizontal incisions down closure with sutures encircling fibres rather than between fibres.

The posterior rectus sheath has a similar trilaminar criss-cross pattern above the umbilicus, where it is composed of the posterior lamina of the internal oblique and the aponeurosis of the transversus abdominis muscle from either side.

Within the rectus sheath are the rectus muscles, the pyramidalis muscle, the terminal portions of the lower six thoracic nerves and the superior and inferior epigastric vessels (Figure 2.31).

The rectus muscle is flat and strap-like and extends from the pubis to the thorax. Each muscle is separated

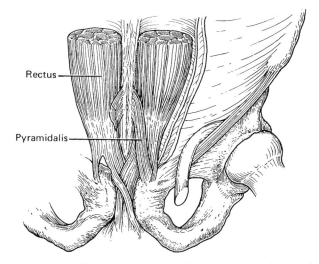

Figure 2.32 The rectus muscle arises by two tendons – the larger and lateral from the crest of the pubis and the smaller and medial from the pubis of the opposite side and from the ligamentous fibres of the symphysis. The pyramidalis is variable; it arises from the ligamentous fibres of the symphysis and adjacent pubis and is inserted into the linea alba

from its fellow of the opposite side by the linea alba. The muscle arises by two tendons; the larger and lateral is attached to the crest of the pubis and the smaller and medial mingles with fibres from the opposite side and arises from the ligamentous fibres over the symphysis pubis. The muscle is inserted by broad bundles into the fifth, sixth and seventh costal cartilages and into the xiphoid by a small medial slip. The rectus muscle has three tendinous intersections – one at the xiphoid, one at the umbilicus and one midway between these two. Sometimes a further incomplete intersection is present below the umbilicus. The intersections extend a variable distance across the muscle mass and are intimately adherent to the anterior lamina of the sheath of the muscle, but have no attachment to the posterior sheath.

The pyramidalis muscle is triangular in shape, arising by its base from the ligaments on the anterior surface of the symphysis pubis and being inserted into the lower linea alba. The muscle is absent in 10% of cases (Figure 2.32).

Function of the anterior abdominal wall

Although the anterior abdominal wall is composed of two halves, right and left, it functions in a co-ordinated fashion. The individual muscles cannot work separately. The upper part is the actively mobile respiratory zone, where the rectus sheath – the flank muscles and the rectus muscle through its tendinous attachments to the rectus sheath – functions as an accessory respiratory muscle. The lower part has no tendinous intersections and is a relatively fixed lower belly support zone. This

anatomical and physiological configuration has been demonstrated using a transillumination silhouette technique by Askar.[41]

The fascia transversalis – the space of Bogros

The fascia transversalis lies deep to the transverse abdominal muscle plane. It is continuous from side to side and extends from the rib cage above to the pelvis inferiorly.

In the upper abdominal wall the fascia transversalis is thin, but in the lower abdomen and especially in the inguinofemoral region the fascia is thicker and has specialized bands and folds within it. In the groin region, where the fascia transversalis is an important constituent of the posterior wall of the inguinal canal and where it forms the femoral sheath inferiorly to the inguinal ligament, the anatomy and function of the fascia transversalis is of particular importance to the surgeon. As originally described by Sir Astley Cooper in 1807 the fascia transversalis, in the groin, consists of two layers.[193] The anterior strong layer covers the internal aspect of the transversalis muscle where it is intimately blended with the tendon of the transversus muscle. It then extends across the posterior wall of the inguinal canal medial to the deep ring aperture and is attached to the inner margin of the inguinal ligament. The deeper layer of fascia transversalis, a membranous layer, lies between the anterior substantial layer of fascia transversalis and the peritoneum. The extraperitoneal fat lies behind this layer between it and the peritoneum (Figure 2.33). The deep epigastric vessels run between the two layers of fascia transversalis.

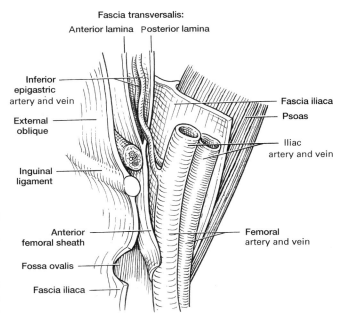

Figure 2.33 The bilaminar fascia transversalis in the groin. (After Read, 1992, Skandalakis *et al.*, 1996[866])

These two distinct layers of fascia transversalis are readily identified laparoscopically and must be opened separately to allow access to the avascular preperitoneal space (of Bogros) when undertaking an extraperitoneal repair of a groin hernia either laparoscopically or by open surgery. The deeper layer extends down behind the inguinal canal and fuses with the pectineal ligament (of Cooper) before continuing downward into the pelvis. The deeper layer fuses with the spermatic cord at the deep ring and continues into the cord as the internal spermatic fascia.[86, 193, 780] The existence of the bilaminar structure of the fascia transversalis at the deep ring was confirmed by Lytle[587] and by Cleland,[181] but its nature disputed by the later anatomists Anson and McVay,[28] and its relevance and importance questioned by experienced surgeons.[191]

The dissection of both layers of fascia transversalis from the cord structures at the deep inguinal ring is an important component of hernioplasty; it allows dissection of an indirect peritoneal sac and the divided peritoneal stump to retract at the deep ring in a classic Bassini and Shouldice operation for indirect hernias.

In the lower abdomen it is attached laterally to the internal lip of the iliac crest, along which line it becomes continuous with the fascia over the iliacus and psoas muscles. From these lateral attachments the fascia extends medially as a continuous curtain, which is interrupted only by the transit of the spermatic cord at the deep inguinal ring. The fascia transversalis invests the cord structures as they pass through it with a thin layer of fascia, the deep spermatic fascia. On the medial margin of the deep ring the fascia transversalis is condensed into

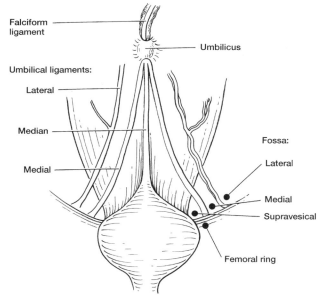

Figure 2.34 Diagram of the posterior aspect of the lower abdominal wall. This area is divided up by the folds produced by the umbilical structures. The median fold is produced by the obliterated urachus, the medial folds by the obliterated umbilical arteries and the lateral umbilical fold thrown up by the inferior deep epigastric vessels.

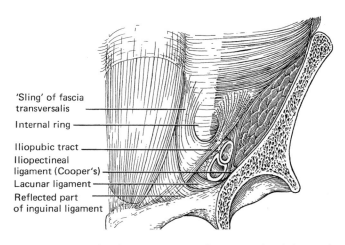

Figure 2.35 The fascia transversalis, or endo-abdominal fascia, is continuous with the fascia on the deep surface of the transversus muscle. In the upper abdomen this fascia is thin and featureless; however, in the lower abdomen and pelvis the fascia transversalis has an important role. It is thickened and includes specialized bands and folds. It forms the posterior wall of the inguinal canal, and at the deep ring it has a condensation medial to the cord. This condensation is part of a U-shaped sling through which the cord passes. This sling hitches the cord up laterally when the transversus muscle contracts. Just above the inguinal ligament the fascia transversalis is thickened as the iliopubic tract. (After Lytle, 1945)

a U-shaped sling, with the cord supported in the concavity of the ring and the two limbs extending superiorly and laterally to be suspended from the posterior aspect of the transversus muscle. The curve of the 'U' lies at or just above the lower border 'arch' of the aponeurosis of the transverse muscle.

This U-shaped fold, the fascia transversalis sling, is the functional basis of the inguinal 'shutter' mechanism; as the transverse muscle contracts during coughing or straining, the column/pillars of the ring are pulled together and the entire sling drawn upwards and laterally. This motion increases the obliquity of exit of the spermatic cord structures through the ring and provides protection from forces tending to cause an indirect hernia (Figure 2.35).[587] The reconstruction of this sling medially with preservation of the function of the ring laterally is the rationale of anterior inguinal hernioplasty. In front of the ring lies the lower border of the transverse muscle and the internal oblique muscle. Each of these structures supports the internal ring and together they provide a very effective valve when the intra-abdominal pressure rises.

The 'shutter' action of the internal ring, the fascia transversalis sling, can be demonstrated readily at operation under local anaesthetic. If the patient is asked to cough, the ring is suddenly pulled upwards and laterally behind the lower margin of the transverse muscle. In the adult with an obliterated processus vaginalis, a flat lid of peritoneum covers the ring internally for the spermatic

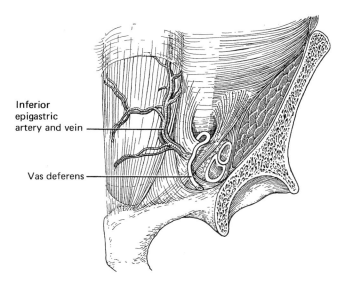

Inferior
epigastric
artery and vein

Vas deferens

Figure 2.36 Seen from behind, the view from within the abdomen, the inferior epigastric vessels are deep, on the abdominal side, of this curtain of fascia transversalis. The vas deferens and cord structures ascend to and hook over the sling of fascia transversalis at the deep ring

vessels and the vas deferens lie extraperitoneally. The spermatic vessels pass down almost vertically retroperitoneally on the psoas muscle. As they enter the narrow gutter of the groin they are joined by the vas deferens: the spermatic cord thus formed turns obligingly upwards and then hooks around the fascia transversalis sling to enter the deep ring, acquiring an investment of internal spermatic fascia as it traverses the ring (Figure 2.36).

The inferior border of the internal ring abuts on a condensation of the fascia transversalis, the iliopubic tract

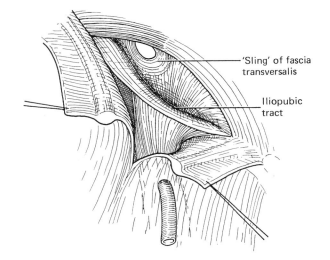

'Sling' of fascia
transversalis

Iliopubic
tract

Figure 2.37 Dissected further anteriorly, if the inguinal ligament is divided, the fascia transversalis can be seen to be continuous with the femoral sheath. The thickening at the junction of fascia transversalis with the femoral sheath is the iliopubic tract. The internal oblique muscle, which arises from the lateral inguinal ligament, acts as a shutter or 'lid' on the deep inguinal ring

or bandelette iliopubienne of Thomson. This small fascial band extends from the anterior superior iliac spine laterally to the pubis medially. The band is a condensation of and integral part of the fascia transversalis; it lies on a plane somewhat deeper than the inguinal ligament which can be readily demonstrated as distinct from it at operation. The iliopubic tract bridges the femoral canal medially and then curves inferiorly and posteriorly to spread out fan-wise to its attachment to a broad area of the superior ramus of the pubis along the iliopectineal line (Cooper's ligament). The iliopubic tract thus forms the inferior margin of the defect in the fascia transversalis in an indirect inguinal hernia and in a direct hernia: it is anterior to the peritoneal sac of a femoral hernia (Figure 2.37).

The fascia transversalis superior to the iliopubic tract extends over the posterior wall of the inguinal canal up to and posterior to the arch of the transverse muscle. Medially the fascia transversalis merges into the rectus sheath and aponeurosis of the transverse muscle or conjoint tendon. The fascia transversalis in the posterior wall of the inguinal canal is supported to a variable extent by the aponeurosis of the transverse muscle as it arches down to its attachment to the pubis and iliopectineal line. Medial to the deep inguinal ring and deep to the fascia transversalis, lying in the extraperitoneal fat between the peritoneum and the fascia, the deep epigastric vessels follow an oblique course upward and medially to the deep aspect of the rectus muscle. This triangular area, bounded by the deep epigastric vessels laterally, the lateral margin of the rectus muscle medially and the inguinal ligament below, is known to surgeons as Hesselbach's triangle; this is the area through which a direct inguinal hernia protrudes.

More exactly, a direct hernia explodes through the fascia transversalis in the area bounded by the iliopubic tract inferiorly, the medial limb of the fascia transversalis sling laterally and the lower margin of the arch of the transversus aponeurosis superiorly.

Condon (1971) has investigated the anatomy of the fascia transversalis using a technique of transillumination of fresh tissue. He clearly shows these anatomic details and defines the margins of the aponeurotic deficiency in the posterior inguinal canal wall through which direct hernia protrudes. This area of fascia transversalis is buttressed anteriorly to a greater or lesser degree by the aponeurosis of the transverse muscle as it inserts to the iliopectineal line. At operation these features – the iliopubic tract, the deep ring and the 'line' of the arch of the transverse aponeurosis – are easily identifiable if the fascia transversalis is adequately dissected. Indeed, the identification of all these features is an essential prerequisite for adequate inguinal hernioplasty[190] (Figure 2.38).

The fascia transversalis in the groin is but a segment of the endo-abdominal fascia. This fascia is distinct in

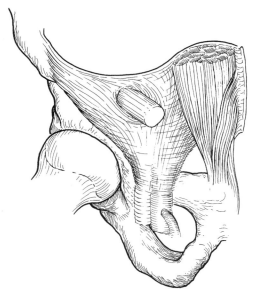

Figure 2.38 From the front, as the surgeon visualizes the subject, the fascia transversalis in the groin resembles a funnel with a valved side vent. The femoral vessels come out of the funnel below and the cord structures out of the 'side vent' which is 'valved' by the sling of the fascia transversalis at the deep ring

the lower abdomen, but is fused into the fascia on the deep surface of the transverse abdominal muscle superiorly. This composite layer, the transverse muscle and its fascia (the fascia transversalis), is the most important of

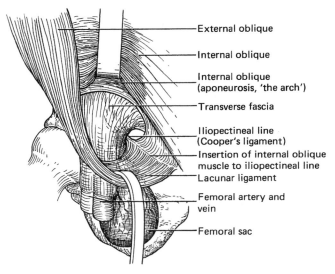

- External oblique
- Internal oblique
- Internal oblique (aponeurosis, 'the arch')
- Transverse fascia
- Iliopectineal line (Cooper's ligament)
- Insertion of internal oblique muscle to iliopectineal line
- Lacunar ligament
- Femoral artery and vein
- Femoral sac

Figure 2.39 A dissection to demonstrate the anatomy of a femoral hernia. The femoral cone of fascia transversalis is stretched on its medial aspect; the hernial sac extends within this cone of fascia transversalis medial to the femoral vein and lateral to the lacunar ligament

the abdominal wall strata in solving the problem of inguinofemoral hernia, as the integrity of this layer prevents herniation. Defects in it, congenital or acquired, are the aetiology of all groin hernias.

The fascia transversalis descends behind the inguinal ligament into the thigh as the sheath of the femoral

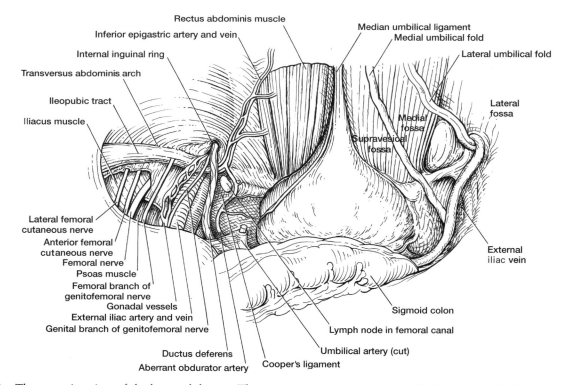

Rectus abdominis muscle
Inferior epigastric artery and vein
Internal inguinal ring
Transversus abdominis arch
Ileopubic tract
Iliacus muscle
Median umbilical ligament
Medial umbilical fold
Lateral umbilical fold
Lateral fossa
Medial fossa
Supravesical fossa
External iliac vein
Lateral femoral cutaneous nerve
Anterior femoral cutaneous nerve
Femoral nerve
Psoas muscle
Femoral branch of genitofemoral nerve
Gonadal vessels
External iliac artery and vein
Genital branch of genitofemoral nerve
Ductus deferens
Aberrant obdurator artery
Cooper's ligament
Lymph node in femoral canal
Umbilical artery (cut)
Sigmoid colon

Figure 2.40 The posterior view of the lower abdomen. The peritoneum is intact on one side, illustrating the fossae projected by the umbilical ligaments. On the contralateral side the peritoneum is reflected to allow visualization of the extraperitoneal structures, the vessels and nerves. (After Van Mameren and Go, 1994[946])

vessels – this is a funnel-like sheath. Inferior to the inguinal ligament the fascia transversalis attaches to the iliopectineal line medially and posteriorly to the femoral vessels. This funnel of fascia transversalis extends into the thigh as far as the fossa ovalis in the deep fascia. This anatomic arrangement allows for a small 'space' medial to the femoral vein through which some lymphatics pass. When a femoral hernia develops, this 'space' is expanded (Figure 2.39).

What, then, is the anatomy of the peritoneum relative to the layering of the abdominal wall we have considered previously? In the lower abdomen the peritoneum is thrown up into five folds which converge as they pass upwards to the umbilicus. The median umbilical fold extends from the apex of the bladder to the umbilicus and contains the remnant urachus. To either lateral side the medial umbilical fold contains the obliterated umbilical artery and more laterally the inferior epigastric vessels raise the lateral umbilical fold. These folds create depressions or fossae in the anterior abdominal peritoneum: the supravesical fossae right and left, and the medial and the lateral inguinal fossae right and left. A further depression on either side is below and medial to the lateral inguinal fossa and separated from it by the inguinal ligament. This overlies the femoral ring and is called the femoral fossa (Figure 2.34).

Hernias egress through these fossae – the femoral through the femoral fossa, the indirect inguinal through the lateral inguinal fossa and the direct through the medial fossa. Internal supravesical hernias can occur in the supravesical fossa (Figure 2.40).

The landmarks are the peritoneal folds, particularly the medial umbilical ligament (containing the obliterated umbilical artery) and the lateral umbilical fold (containing the inferior epigastric vessels). The peritoneum overlying the deep inguinal ring is identified with the testicular vessels and vas deferens clearly visible beneath the peritoneum. The peritoneum is separated from the underlying fascia transversalis by adipose tissue except medial to the deep ring where the peritoneum is more firmly fixed to the subjacent fascia transversalis. Below, posterior to, the inguinal ligament the genital branch of the genitofemoral nerve is seen joining the cord structures at the deep ring.

The lateral cutaneous nerve of the thigh and the femoral branch of the genitofemoral nerve lie rather deeper in the fatty tissue overlying the iliopsoas muscle. Blood vessels are also found in the adipose tissue beneath the peritoneum, in the extraperitoneal plane branches of the deep circumflex iliac vessels laterally and of the ob-turator vessels inferiorly and medially. There is an extensive venous circulation (anastomosis) in the extraperitoneal tissues between the inferior epigastric vein and obturator veins. This venous anastomosis lies between the two lamina of the fascia transversalis in the space of Bogros.[86] This space is

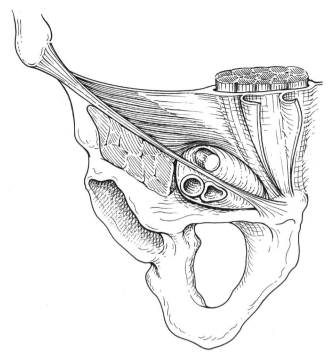

Figure 2.41 The 'myopectineal orifice of Fruchaud': the area of the groin closed by fascia transversalis with the inguinal canal above and femoral canal below the rigid inguinal ligament. (After Wantz, 1991[967])

continuous from side to side and with the pelvic space, the cave of Retzius. The space of Bogros is important for extraperitoneal repair of hernia and is the repository of bleeding in pelvic trauma.

The peritoneum – the view from within

Hernia sacs are composed of peritoneum and they may contain intra-abdominal viscera. From within they consist of the peritoneum, then a loose layer of extraperitoneal fat, then the deep membranous lamina of fascia transversalis, then the vessels such as the epigastric vessels in the space of Bogros, then the stout anterior lamina of fascia transversalis, then the muscles and aponeuroses of the abdominal wall. In the groin these muscles and aponeuroses are variously absent over the inguinal and crural canals. The myopectineal orifice of Fruchaud, which is divided into two parts by the inguinal ligament[319, 967] (Figure 2.41). This concept of one groin aperture is relevant for mesh occlusion repairs, whether anterior open operation or posterior laparoscopic operation. The boundaries of the myopectineal orifice of Fruchaud are superiorly the 'arch' of the transversus muscle, laterally the iliopsoas muscle, medially the rectus muscle and inferiorly the pecten of the pubis.[37]

Between the peritoneum and the fascia transversalis there is a loose layer of extraperitoneal fat, used as an

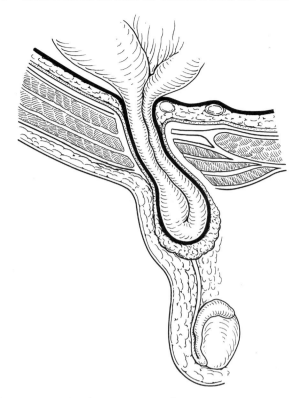

Figure 2.42 As the peritoneum forms an indirect inguinal hernia it carries with it a covering of extraperitoneal fat. This extraperitoneal fat is given the misnomer 'lipoma of the cord' by many surgeons[293]

important landmark in many surgical operations. Hernial protrusions progress from within outward through deficiencies in the musculo-aponeurotic lamina of the abdominal wall; they carry this extraperitoneal fat with them along the track of the hernia sac. Abundance of this fat at the fundus of an indirect inguinal hernia gives rise to the surgical misnomer a 'lipoma of the cord' – in reality this no more than extraperitoneal fat around the fundus of a peritoneal hernia sac (Figure 2.42).

The umbilicus

Between the sixth and tenth week of gestation the abdominal viscera enlarge rapidly so that they cannot be contained within the more slowly enlarging coelom.

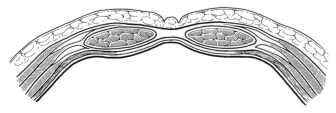

Figure 2.43 Cross-section through the umbilicus. The aponeuroses of all three laminae are fused in the umbilical cicatrix

Viscera are extruded through the broad umbilical deficit into a peritoneal cavity, the exocoelom, which occupies the base of the umbilical cord. At about the tenth week the abdominal cavity has enlarged so much that it can now contain all the extruded viscera, and by the time of birth all the intestines are reduced inside the abdominal cavity proper. At birth the abdominal wall is complete except for the space occupied by the umbilical cord. Running in the cord are the urachus and the umbilical arteries coursing up from the pelvis, and the umbilical vein to the liver. After the cord is ligated the stump sloughs off and the resultant granulating surface cicatrizes and epithelializes from its periphery.

In the normal umbilicus there is a single layer of fused fibrous tissue consisting of the superficial fascia, the rectus sheath and linea alba, and the fascia transversalis. The peritoneum is adherent to the deep aspect of this (Figure 2.43).

The spermatic cord

The spermatic cord is composed of: (a) the arteries – the testicular artery, the cremaster artery and the artery of the vas deferens; (b) the veins – the testicular veins form the pampiniform plexus of veins within the spermatic cord; (c) the lymphatics; (d) the nerves – the genital branch of the genitofemoral nerve and autonomic nerves; (e) the vas deferens; and (f) the processus vaginalis.

The spermatic cord, as it emerges through the abdominal wall from the deep inguinal ring, receives investments of fascia. The fascia transversalis forms a thin, funicular coat called the internal spermatic fascia: the internal oblique invests it with a tracing of muscle fibres, the cremaster muscle, and most superficially it is coated with external spermatic fascia derived from the external oblique aponeurosis at the subcutaneous inguinal ring. Each of these fascial layers requires opening to identify the processus vaginalis or sac of an indirect hernia. Until birth the processus vaginalis, although minute, remains as an uninterrupted diverticulum from the abdominal peritoneum through the length of the cord to the testis, where it opens out to become the tunica vaginalis of the testis. The processus vaginalis closes in most males soon after birth. More recently the persistence of the processus vaginalis into adult life has been confirmed when hydrocele or hernia has complicated peritoneal dialysis in renal failure patients. The theories and mechanism of testicular descent and the development of the processus vaginalis are described in detail in Chapter 9 (Figure 2.44).

An indirect inguinal hernial sac is a similar peritoneal diverticulum which extends into the spermatic cord and occupies the same position as the primitive processus vaginalis. Often indirect hernias also have extraperitoneal fat at their fundus.

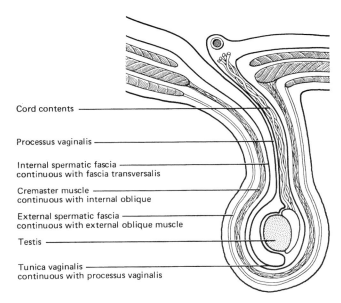

Cord contents

Processus vaginalis

Internal spermatic fascia
continuous with fascia transversalis

Cremaster muscle
continuous with internal oblique

External spermatic fascia
continuous with external oblique muscle

Testis

Tunica vaginalis
continuous with processus vaginalis

Figure 2.44 Section through the spermatic cord and testis. The importance of the layers is demonstrated. The external spermatic fascia is derived from the fascia over the external oblique muscle at the superficial ring, the cremaster arises from the internal oblique muscle and the internal spermatic fascia is the continuation of the fascia transversalis over the cord structures. Each of these layers needs division in inguinal hernia repair

Comparative anatomy

A cool environment for spermatogenesis is a necessity in warm-blooded birds and mammals. Birds, which have high blood temperatures and are invariably cryptorchid, keep their testes cool by an air stream around the abdomen. In some sea-living mammals – whales and sea cows – the testes remain intra-abdominal, but presumably the constant contact with cold water is effective in keeping them cool.

The necessity to have the testes reside in a colder scrotum leads to problems, not only in humans but in domestic and farm animals; the topic of hernia and undescended testicles appears in veterinary textbooks where it has a practical and economic importance of its own. Inguinal hernias are fairly common in pigs and horses, but less common in bovines. The economic consequence of an inguinal hernia in a stallion is considerable; it may incarcerate during mating and forestall full consummation. A similar problem is known in stud bulls. Hernias are relatively common in dogs, but are rather rare in cats. Both male and female dogs are likely to develop inguinal hernias, but the males are more likely to have intestine caught within the hernial sac. When a female dog develops a hernia the usual content is one of the uterine horns and the broad ligament; this can present the danger of strangulation if the bitch becomes pregnant (the content of a congenital hernia in a girl is most likely an ovary and a fallopian tube). In the dog, most veterinary surgeons treat the hernia by orchidectomy (a proposition which is sometimes put forward for the handling of the same situation in the elderly human).

Bats have testicles which are normally intra-abdominal and descend into the scrotum only at the time of mating. In these animals there is a low incidence of hernia and of a patent processus vaginalis. The testicles in bats descend to the scrotum and ascend to the abdomen, although there is no patent processus vaginalis. In small boys with rectractile testicles which disappear up to the external inguinal ring, a hernia is rarely present.[663]

3 EPIDEMIOLOGY AND AETIOLOGY OF PRIMARY GROIN HERNIAS IN ADULTS

In everyday general surgical practice, all varieties of hernia form a substantial workload. Representative figures from the UK are given in Tables 3.1–3.3.[240] The population prevalence and incidence are inextricably linked to surgical operation rates for the procedure.

Epidemiology

Prevalence and incidence data give no indication about the actual or potential demand for hernia surgery. Although incomplete and subject to many pitfalls in interpretation, UK data sources which relate to the need for hernia surgery include: the English Hospital In-Patient Enquiry (HIPE) Data, 1975–1985, the English Hospital Episodes System (HES) Data, 1989/90 and Data on Surgical Activity in Independent Hospitals in the National Health Service (NHS) from local and national surveys.[987]

There have been no true population or community-based studies of the incidence of groin hernia. The closest estimates for the true incidence of inguinal and femoral hernia can be obtained from the 1981/82 *Morbidity Statistics from General Practice (Third National Study).*[798] These figures are probably an underestimate because a proportion of patients will fail to seek medical advice. However, based on these figures the annual incidence of inguinal hernia in England will be of the order of 113 000 per year. The 95% confidence intervals are approximately 80 000–160 000.

The published evidence comes from three main sources. Firstly, population prevalence and incidence: there have been few community-based estimates of the prevalence of groin hernias. None have estimated the incidence. Each has been performed in communities where access to surgery was limited, e.g. African populations. Further research defining the population

Table 3.1 Operations undertaken for groin hernias at North Tees General Hospital, 1969–85 (After Quill *et al.* 1983[765])*

Year	Inguinal in children (<14 years)		Inguinal in adults (>14 years)		Femoral in adults	
	Elective	Emergency	Elective	Emergency	Elective	Emergency
1969	66	10	172	16	13	6
1970	56	8	123	18	15	7
1971	57	7	147	12	17	5
1972	62	11	151	14	9	7
1973	54	9	131	13	8	5
1974	49	7	162	11	11	8
1975	67	6	139	12	12	8
1976	64	6	135	13	9	12
1977	54	8	168	8	8	11
1978	41	5	189	13	7	4
1979	58	5	178	11	7	4
1980	60	7	214	13	14	8
1981	70	1	196	12	14	7
1982	80	2	152	7	17	10
1983	39	4	198	5	12	7
1984	70	7	229	12	8	6
1985	54	1	180	8	24	11

* The incidence of elective inguinal hernioplasty in adults is 90.5 per 100 000 population and for emergency hernioplasty in adults 7.2 per 100 000 population; for elective femoral hernioplasty in adults 6.1 per 100 000 population and for emergency femoral hernioplasty 3.8 per 100 000 population. Over these 17 years no significant trends are demonstrated.

Table 3.2 Incidence of various hernia operations (Cleveland, England; population 568 000; 9 years, mid-1970 to mid-1979) (From Devlin, 1982,[240] with permission)

Inguinal	Male children	1702
	Female children	210
Inguinal	Male adults	5080
	Female adults	416
Femoral	Male adults	195
	Female adults	491
Incisional	Male adults	551
	Female adults	398
Umbilical	Male children	142
	Female children	151
Umbilical	Male adults	142
	Female adults	147

Table 3.3 Distribution of type of hernia in 1000 consecutive cases presenting to an English district hospital[240]

	Hernia type	Male	Female
Children under 14 years	Inguinal	177	20
	Femoral	1	0
	Umbilical	15	16
		193	36
Adults	Inguinal		
	indirect	343	39
	direct	164	1
	pantaloon	21	0
		528	40
	Femoral	20	51
	Umbilical	15	15
	Incisional	57	40
	Obturator	0	1
	Spigelian	2	2
	Grand total:	815	185

incidence of subjects with groin hernias is required. Prevalence estimates are of local value only; they reflect not only the distribution and morbidity in the community but also the success of past local activity. Secondly, 'demand' incidence rates are based on the number of people who seek medical advice for their problem. However, numerous factors may influence this decision and the data must therefore be treated with caution. Estimates of the incidence of inguinal and femoral hernias (Table 3.4) comes from the 1981/82 *Morbidity Statistics from General Practice (Third National Study)* based on consultations with 143 volunteer general practice principals caring for 332 000 patients.[798] Figures 3.1 and 3.2 show incidence rates for inguinal and femoral hernia, each of which denotes a consultation where the patient was seeking medical advice concerning a groin hernia for the first time during the study year. Again, these data

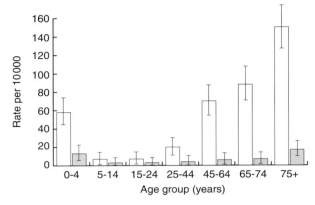

Figure 3.1 Incidence rates of inguinal hernia per 10 000 persons at risk (1981/82 morbidity statistics from general practice, third national study[798]). □= Males; ■ = Females

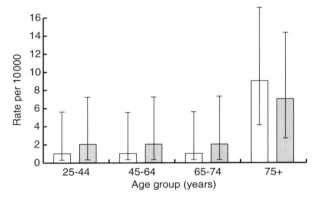

Figure 3.2 Incidence rates of femoral hernia per 10 000 persons at risk (1981/82 morbidity statistics from general practice, third national study[798]). □ = Males; ■ = Females

Table 3.4 Incidence rates (95% confidence limits) of inguinal and femoral hernia per 10 000 persons at risk (1981/82 morbidity statistics from general practice, third national study[798])

Age (years)	Males		Females	
Inguinal hernias				
0–4	58	(44.9,74.8)	13	(6.9,22.2)
5–14	7	(2.8,14.4)	3	(0.6,8.8)
15–24	7	(2.8,14.4)	3	(0.6,8.8)
25–44	20	(12.2,30.9)	4	(1.1,10.2)
45–64	70	(55.5,88.2)	6	(2.2,13.1)
65–74	88	(71.5,108.2)	7	(2.8,14.4)
75+	150	(128.2,175.5)	17	(9.9,27.2)
Femoral hernias				
0–4				
5–14				
15–24				
25–44	1	(0.02,5.6)	2	(0.2,7.2)
45–64	1	(0.02,5.6)	2	(0.2,7.2)
65–74	1	(0.02,5.6)	2	(0.2,7.2)
75+	9	(4.1,17.1)	7	(2.8,14.4)

From ref 967, with permission

must be interpreted with caution because neither the doctors nor the patients may be representative of the general population, and the diagnoses were not validated. The age-specific incidence rates are given with 95% confidence intervals.

Demand for groin hernia surgery in adults

The overall rates for inguinal hernia repair (primary and recurrent) performed in NHS hospitals in England did not change between 1975 and 1990 (Figure 3.3). The total numbers for 1989/90 were 64 998 primary inguinal hernia repairs and 3480 recurrent inguinal hernia repairs (Table 3.5). Age-specific hernia rates have altered considerably since 1975 with a significant increase in the surgical rates for older men. For instance, the age-specific inguinal repair rate for the 65–74-year age group rose

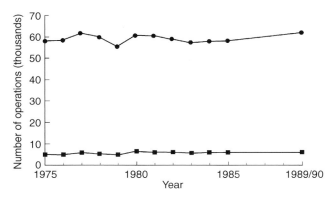

Figure 3.3   Trends in number of inguinal hernia repairs, NHS hospitals in England, 1975–1989/90[989]. ●–● Males; ■–■ Females (From Williams *et al.*, 1992)

from 40 per 10 000 in 1975 to 70 per 100 000 in 1990. This probably reflects improvements in anaesthetic delivery and postoperative recovery in high dependency or

Table 3.5   Number and % of single procedure inguinal hernia operations performed in NHS hospitals, England, 1989/90

Inguinal hernia	Total no. of operations	No. (%) done as single procedure
Primary	64 998	54 090 (83)
Recurrent	3 480	2 790 (80)

From ref. 989, with permission

intensive care units. A more detailed analysis of age-specific inguinal hernia repair rates for males and females is shown in Figure 3.4, which indicates the high rates in infants and men over the age of 55.

Of the approximately 65 000 inguinal and 6000 femoral hernia repairs performed in NHS hospitals in England each year, 10% are emergency operations; these have remained constant for two decades. There has been an expansion in the private sector, which now accounts for 14% of all elective groin operations. Referring to the data in Figures 3.4 and 3.5, it cannot be assumed that these repair rates approximate to the population incidence of inguinal and femoral hernias, because only 60% of groin hernias are referred to specialists for operation.[798] The implications for the English population will be 112 700 new cases per annum for inguinal hernias, and 6900 for femoral hernias. Because a considerable proportion of patients are not undergoing groin hernia surgery, this may account for the 40 000 trusses sold annually.[174, 533] There is considerable variation in surgical rates for populations of health districts in England, and the weak correlations between these rates and supply factors (e.g. consultants per 1000 population) and demand factors (e.g. waiting lists), suggest that a considerable proportion of the variation is accounted for by differences in medical decision making.[989]

Demand incidence is based on surgical procedures. In a stable catchment population, the number of people who

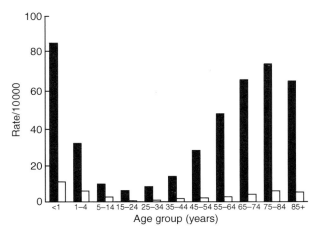

Figure 3.4   Age-specific primary inguinal hernia repair rates, NHS hospitals, England 1989/90[989]. ■ Males; ☐ females (From Williams *et al.*, 1992)

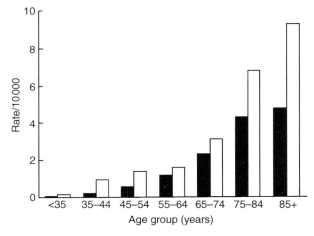

Figure 3.5   Age-specific surgery rates for femoral hernia per 10 000 for males and females, NHS hospitals, England, 1989/90. ■ Males; ☐ females (From Williams *et al.*, 1992[989])

seek surgery during a defined period can be established. At North Tees General Hospital, for example (Table 3.1), the incidence of elective inguinal hernioplasty in adults is 90.5 per 100 000 population, and for emergency hernioplasty 7.2 per 100 000. For elective femoral hernioplasty in adults the incidence is 6.1 per 100 000 population, and for emergency femoral hernioplasty 3.8. Again, there is difficulty in extrapolating these figures for the general population because the catchment population is difficult to define, being influenced by GP referral practices. Of more importance is the demographic structure of the population being studied, which may vary widely between regional populations. The demand for emergency treatment of strangulated inguinal hernia is better defined, being estimated at 3.25–7.16 per 100 000 per annum, in Western Europe.[25, 200] However, deficiencies of available data arise from three facts: firstly, they are based on Health Service use rather than healthcare needs; secondly, patterns of morbidity have an uncertain relationship to indications for treatment; and thirdly patients will seek treatment only if they are aware of the significance of underlying morbidity and the consequences of treatment.

Inguinal hernias are more common than femoral hernias, occurring in ratios of 8:1 or 20:1 depending on the surgical series, and are more common in males, where the inguinal to femoral ratio may be up to 35:1. Seventy per cent of inguinal hernias are indirect and 30% direct. Inguinal and femoral hernias may coexist: 2% of males with inguinal hernias also have a femoral hernia and 50% of those with femoral hernias have a coexisting inguinal hernia. This distribution of groin hernias is illustrated graphically in a large series of 4173 hernias operated on in Truro, south-west England by Barwell 1974–1992[834] (Figure 3.6). Similar figures are reported by Nilsson et al. from Sweden.[703]

Age-standardized hernia surgery rates vary considerably world-wide. For instance, the hernia surgery rate per 100 000 population per year in England and Wales is 100, Norway 200, the USA 280 and Australia 180. The actual approximate number of operations performed per year in respective countries is 80 000 in the UK, 25 000 in Belgium, 100 000 in France and 180 000 in Germany.[835] In the USA, where 550 000 inguinal hernia operations are carried out per year, the annual costs estimated in 1987 were 2.8 billion dollars, or 3% of the total healthcare budget. These figures are obtained from The National Center For Health Statistics (NCHS) through its National Hospital Discharge Survey, which has compiled data on the number of operations performed annually in the USA, from a 5–8% sample of patient records.[811] In the UK hernia surgery rates peak in the 55–85-year age group, at 600 operations per 100 000 population per year, and the incidence of strangulated hernia is 13 per 100 000 population, with a peak in the 80-year-old age group.

In the USA the high rates of hernia surgery may have contributed to the reduction in mortality associated with strangulation. For instance, the mortality for hernia and intestinal obstruction obtained by analysis of statistics data from the NCHS shows a fall in the number of deaths per year per 100 000 population in patients over the age of 15 years, from 5 in 1968 to 3.1 in 1978, and stabilizing at 3.0 in 1988. This was in spite of the fact that hernia patients with intestinal obstruction were on average 15 years older in 1988 than in 1968. In 1971 Medicare discharges for inguinal hernia without intestinal obstruction showed 94% of patients having surgery, with a probability of death at 0.005 (5 per 100 000 population).[651]

Inguinal hernias in adults

Inguinal hernias are more common in males than females, in a ratio of 8:1 or 20:1 in different series. However, there is considerable incidence of underreporting of inguinal hernia, as illustrated by two validity checks in the US National Health Surveys. In both studies half the hernias recorded during the previous year were unreported on interview, and in another study in Baltimore positive reports were received from only 21% of men found to have hernias on clinical examination.

In the literature the incidence varies depending on the source of the count. Approximately 94% of hernias among males are estimated to be in the inguinal region. Ninety-five per cent of inguinal hernia operations are on males. Three times more females undergo femoral hernia operations than males. By the age of 75 years 10–15% of males have already received inguinal hernia surgery. In the period 1975–1990 mortality from inguinal hernia surgery in the UK fell by 22% and for femoral hernia by 55%. In the USA, for inguinal hernia with obstruction,

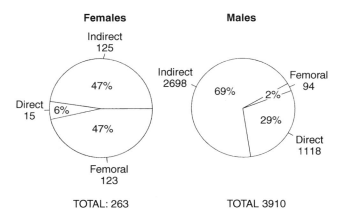

Figure 3.6 Groin hernia diagnoses in males and females, Truro 1974–1992 (From Williams et al., 1992[989])

88% underwent surgery with a mortality rate of 0.05%.[651]

Incidence estimates vary widely. A study of World War I British recruits between the ages of 18 and 41 years shows these variations: in Scotland 31 per 1000 were found, whereas in London and south-east England it was 17–56 per 1000; in men aged 16–30 years the rate was 6 per 1000, whereas in men of 40–50 years it was 24 per 1000. In contradistinction, the rate in Stockport and Manchester was 125 per 1000. Sir Arthur Keith, in 1924, estimated the prevalence at 25 per 1000 males.[487]

The figures from recruits in World War II are equally confusing: the prevalence was generally about 26 per 1000, but a range from 6 to 79.6 per 1000 recruits is given – these are in young males so, bearing in mind that most inguinal hernias occur in the later decades, the overall incidence is probably higher.[1005]

Sixty-five per cent of inguinal hernias in adult European males are indirect in type. Right-sided inguinal hernias in adult males are slightly more frequent than left-sided; 55% occurring on the right, regardless of whether the hernia is indirect or direct. Bilateral hernias are four times more often direct than indirect. In Western series the peak incidence of groin hernias is in the sixth decade.[449]

In Negroid peoples the prevalence of inguinal hernia is higher than in Europeans: in Southern Ghana 7.7% of the adult male population have inguinal hernias,[83] in Rhodesian miners 9%,[287] in Tanzanians 16%,[40] and of the male population of the Island of Pemba, off the Zanzibar coast, 30% have inguinal hernias.[1002] There are tribal differences; for instance, in Ghanaian tribes the prevalence is 7.8% in Gas, 13.5% in Ewes and 3.4% in Akan.[83] In Ghana the male to female inguinal hernia ratio is 31:1, in Gabon it is reported as 3:1, and in East Africa it is 7.65:1. Further geographic differences are reported in Africa: in Badoe's series from Accra 11% of inguinal hernias in adult males are direct,[54] in Hausa from Northern Nigeria 22% are direct,[714] in Lambarene 57% are direct, and in Kampala 42% are direct.[40, 393]

A possible genetic link has been postulated in the Inuit living in the Western Arctic of Greenland. Hernia is common in males and thought to be due to a high prevalence of disorders associated with instability of mesenchymal tissues, such as spondylolisthesis, arthritis and heart block. The Inuit have been living in almost complete genetic isolation for 150–200 generations and have a high incidence and frequency of the HLA-B27 allele. Such polymorphism could result in the frequency of hernia in these peoples.[407]

The difference between the ratio of indirect to direct inguinal hernia in different African locations and the tribal differences in Ghana support a polygenic predisposition. In Japan hernias are twice as frequent in twins,

in Ghana one in every five live births is a twin, twice the rate found in non-Africans – which may account for the higher incidence recorded.[83]

Comparing the age structure of the patients with inguinal hernia operated in Accra with the age structure found in the field study in Ghana shows that all age groups are equally represented in the Accra hospital population, whereas in rural Ghana the prevalence of groin hernia rises with increasing age.[53, 83]

It is impossible to compare these findings. The large-scale surveys of uncomplaining males are drawn from recruits into British and American forces in two world wars and are not, therefore, representative samples of the population. The only field study is from southern Ghana and confirms that inguinal hernias are at least three times more common in Africans than Europeans.

The true prevalence of inguinal hernias can be estimated only by community-based epidemiological studies, the validity of which will depend on the diagnostic criteria used. The presence of a visible, palpable lump may be supplemented by such diagnostic criteria as cough impulse at the internal or external ring and the presence of an incision in the groin. The latter, of course, may represent another form of surgery, such as orchidopexy, rather than hernia. Moreover, recurrent inguinal hernias may not be adequately diagnosed or sub-categorized. These pitfalls are well illustrated by the two studies alluded to above, carried out on British Army recruits in the first and second world wars. The prevalence was 1.6% for groin hernias in recruits aged 30–40 years in World War I and 11% in World War II.[487, 989]

Perhaps the most rigorous epidemiological study carried out was that of Abramson in Western Jerusalem between 1969 and 1971.[2] Males from differing ethnic and social backgrounds were studied, although young males were largely excluded because of national service. The study was performed by interviewing subjects in their homes, where the response rate was high (over 86%). Of these, 91% participated in the second stage of physical examination. Interviewers and examiners had been trained in the use of questionnaires and diagnostic criteria. The results are shown in Table 3.8. The prevalence increased with age in all cohorts studied, and the majority were diagnosed on the basis of a visible swelling. An important finding from the Abramson study was the concordance between interview and examination findings: only 50% of men reported a swelling in the groin on interview, which is in close agreement with the 50% under-reporting revealed from validity checks by the US National Health Surveys.[691] It is obvious from these studies that questionnaire-based data must be supplemented by clinical examination if the true prevalence is to be ascertained, although this may be confounded by problems with diagnostic criteria.

Table 3.6 Percentage of age group with inguinal hernia[2]

| | Age (years) | | | | | | |
	25–34	35–44	45–54	55–64	65–74	75+	Total
No. examined	620	438	300	322	156	47	1883
Current prevalence (excluding successful repairs)	11.9	15.1	19.7	26.1	29.5	34.1	18.3
'Obvious' hernias*	1.0	4.8	9.0	14.3	19.2	29.8	7.6
Unoperated swellings	0.7	3.7	5.7	10.9	13.5	23.4	5.5
Recurrences	0.3	1.4	3.7	3.4	5.8	6.4	2.2
Palpable impulse only	11.0	10.3	10.7	11.8	10.3	4.3	10.7
Lifetime prevalence (including successful repairs)	15.2	19.4	28.0	34.5	39.7	46.8	24.3
'Obvious' hernias*	4.7	9.6	18.3	24.2	30.8	44.7	14.5

From ref. 999, with permission
* 'Obvious' hernias included swellings and repaired hernias and excluded those presenting with a palpable impulse only. The current prevalence of obvious hernias may be less than the combined prevalences of unoperated swellings and recurrences, since a person may have for example an unoperated swelling in one groin and a recurrence in the other.

Femoral hernias in adults

The prevalence and incidence of femoral hernias in the population cannot be determined accurately due to lack of investigation. However, the demand incidence can be estimated as for femoral hernia from the General Practitioner Morbidity Survey of 1981/82, which is summarized in Table 3.4. An incidence figure for England derived from these data is approximately 7000 per year, but the 95% confidence intervals range from approximately 1500 to 24 000.

Femoral hernias are less common than inguinal and account for only 10% of all groin hernias. They are more frequent in females than males in a ratio of 2.5:1 (Table 3.2). Maingot gives femoral hernias in females as eight times more common than in males.[602] Glassow, from Toronto, reports more males than females in his series, in a ratio of 5:3.[352] Glassow's series is of patients undergoing elective operation for inguinal hernia and many of his cases were found as concomitant femoral hernias in men undergoing elective inguinal hernioplasty. Clearly the Toronto series is not representative of wider general surgical practice. In British practice 40% of femoral hernias are admitted as emergency cases with strangulation or incarceration.[765] Females undergo three times as many inguinal hernia as femoral hernia repairs. Femoral hernia is rare in those under 35, is most common in multiparous women and is as common in men as in multiparous women. The ratio of inguinal to femoral hernias is between 10:1 and 8:1. In Accra femoral hernias are rare, accounting for only 1.2%, with an inguinal to femoral ratio of 77:1; in Kampala the ratio is 21.6:1. It is interesting to observe that indirect inguinal hernias outnumber direct inguinal hernias in Accra and in Zaria, Nigeria, whereas in Kampala direct hernias are more frequent. In Kampala there are nine women with

femoral hernias to one man, whereas in West African Hausa the male to female ratio of femoral hernias is 1.2:1.[40, 54, 516, 714, 1002]

The surgical volume for rates of femoral hernia repair in NHS hospitals in England has remained stable between 1975 and 1990, with 5083 primary femoral hernia repairs and 299 recurrent femoral hernia repairs being performed in 1989/90 (Table 3.3). The age-specific data indicate an increasing rate of repair through the decades with a peak in those over 85 years (Figure 3.5).

There is considerable variation in surgical rates for both inguinal and femoral hernia for each district in English Regional Health Authorities. The range for primary inguinal hernia repair is 0.57–24 per 10 000 and for primary femoral hernia repair 0.16–2.3 per 10 000. Such wide variations reflect diversity in clinical practice, demand for and supply of treatment.[989]

Aetiology of primary groin hernia

The pathogenesis of groin hernia is multifactorial. Sir Astley Cooper's 'predispositions' to hernia, in 1827, and the subsequent addition of chronic cough and ascites are now only of historic interest.

Because indirect inguinal hernias are so common in infancy the first surgical speculation was that they were due to a developmental defect. Indirect inguinal hernia arises from incomplete obliteration of the processus vaginalis, the embryological outpocketing of peritoneum that precedes testicular descent into the scrotum. The testes originate along the urogenital line in the retroperitoneum and migrate cordially during the second trimester of pregnancy to arrive at the internal inguinal ring at about six months of intrauterine life. During the last trimester they proceed through the abdominal wall via the inguinal canal and descend into the scrotum, the right slightly later than the left. The processus vaginalis then normally obliterates postnatally except for the portion surrounding and serving as a covering for the testes. Failure of this obliterative process results in congenital indirect inguinal hernia. The modern epidemiological support for this hypothesis has already been reviewed, while the differing familial and tribal incidences, and the coincidence of hernias in twins, are supportive.

John Hunter, in the late eighteenth century, researched the development and descent of the testis in men and domestic animals. He showed that in some inguinal hernias the sac was continuous with the processus vaginalis.[444] Cloquet (1817) observed that the processus vaginalis was frequently not closed at birth.[182] The complete (scrotal) indirect hernia of adult men has the same anatomy as that of the neonate – it is invested by all the layers of the spermatic cord as it transverses the inguinal canal and its sac is continuous with the tunica vaginalis of the testis. Additional support for the congenital theory of indirect inguinal herniation is the finding at autopsy that 15–30% of adult males without clinically apparent inguinal hernias have a patent processus vaginalis at death.[441]

Review of the contralateral side in infantile inguinal hernias reveals a patent processus vaginalis in 60% of neonates and a contralateral hernia in 10–20%. During 20 years of follow-up after infantile hernia repair, 22% of men will develop a contralateral inguinal hernia, of which 41% occur if the initial hernia was on the left and 14% if the initial hernia was on the right.

The introduction of continuous ambulatory peritoneal dialysis for renal failure has demonstrated that the persistent processus vaginalis, if subjected to intra-abdominal pressure, will dilate to give a hydrocele or hernia.[166, 284, 836] This has been reported as late as 2 years in a 61–year-old man recently commenced on continuous ambulatory peritoneal dialysis (CAPD). The development of inguinal hernia in female CAPD patients adds further force to this argument.[196, 419, 836]

Russell, an Australian paediatric surgeon, in 1906 advanced the 'saccular theory' of the formation of hernia, a theory that 'rejects the view that any hernia can ever be "acquired" in the pathological sense and maintains that the presence of a developmental peritoneal diverticulum is a necessary antecedent condition in every case . . . We may have an open funicular peritoneum and we may have them separately or together in infinitely variable gradations.'[808]

It would be apparent from the above that the problem of indirect inguinal hernia is not simply one of a congenital defect, i.e. a persistent patent processus vaginalis. The high frequency of indirect inguinal hernia in middle-aged and older people suggests a pathological change in connective tissue of the abdominal wall to be a contributory factor. Indeed, simple removal of the sac in adults results

in an unacceptably high recurrence rate. Thus the susceptibility to herniation is based on both the presence of a congenital sac and failure of the trans-versalis fascia. In direct inguinal hernia there is no peritoneal sac and the prevalence parallels ageing and other factors including smoking.[276, 774] The absence of an adequate musculo-aponeurotic support for the fascia transversalis and the medial half of the inguinal canal occurs in about a quarter of individuals.[1005] In these men there is deficiency of the lower aponeurotic fibres of the internal oblique muscle, coupled with a narrow insertion of the transversus abdominis onto the superior pubic ramus.[641, 642] Because such a congenital anomaly would be symmetric, this explanation is congruent with the clinical finding that direct hernias are frequently bilateral.

The anatomic disposition of the pelvis, and particularly the height of the pubic arch, may be a significant ethnic characteristic predisposing to inguinal hernia. The height of the pubic arch is measured as the distance of the pubic tubercle from the bispinous line between the innermost parts of the two anterior superior iliac spines. African (Negro) peoples have lower pubic arches than Europeans and a higher incidence of inguinal hernia. In West and East Africa the 'lowness' of the pubic arch is greater than 7.5 cm in 65% of males; in Europeans and in Arabs the arch is less low, 65% of males having a height of between 5 and 7.5 cm (Figure 3.7). In European females 80% have an arch between 5 and 7.5 cm, and they have the lowest incidence of groin hernias.[271, 1002, 1008]

The low arch is associated with a narrower pelvis and with a narrower origin of the external oblique muscle from the lateral inguinal ligament. With these anatomic variations there is a shorter inguinal canal, the deep inguinal ring may be unclosed by the internal oblique. The canal may then be so short that no muscular 'shutter mechanism' is operative[271] (Figure 3.8).

There is another much rarer form of direct hernia where a narrow peritoneal diverticulum comes directly through the conjoint tendon lateral to the rectus and pyramidalis to project at the superficial inguinal ring.

It must be concluded that there are congenital and genetic factors and anatomic variations that render individuals more likely to manifest direct and indirect inguinal hernias.

Sir Arthur Keith (1924)[487] observed: 'There is one other matter which requires further observation. We are so apt to look on tendons, fascial structures and connective tissues as dead passive structures. They are certainly alive, and the fact that hernias are so often multiple in middle aged and old people leads one to suspect that a pathological change in the connective tissues of the belly wall may render certain individuals particularly liable to hernia.' He concluded his argument with a statement regarding 'the importance of a right understanding of the aetiology of hernia . . . If they occur only in those who have hernial sacs already formed during fetal life then we

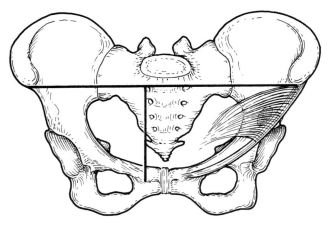

Figure 3.7   The European pelvis is relatively wide with a less deep arch than the Negro pelvis. This ensures that the internal oblique muscle origin from the lateral inguinal ligament is broad, so that the internal oblique muscle 'protects' the deep ring

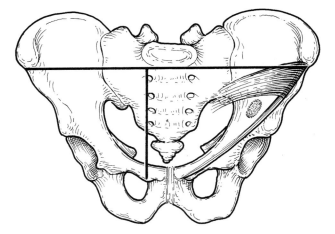

Figure 3.8   The Negro pelvis is narrower than the European, which means that the lowness of the arch of the pelvis is greater in the Negro and the origin of the internal oblique relatively narrower. Hence the internal oblique will not cover the deep ring during straining and the 'shutter mechanism' of the inguinal canal is deficient. Negroes have a 10 times greater incidence of indirect inguinal hernia than Europeans

must either excise the sacs at birth or stand by and do nothing but trust to luck. But if ... the occurrence of hernia is due to circumstances over which we have control then the prevention of hernia is a matter worthy of our serious study.'[487]

Read made the crucial clinical observation which next advanced our understanding of the aetiology of inguinal hernia. In 1970 he noted, when using the preperitoneal approach to the inguinal region, that the rectus sheath is thinner and has a 'greasy' feel in those patients who turned out to have direct defects. This observation was confirmed by weighing samples of constant area; specimens from controls weighed significantly more than those from patients with indirect, pantaloon and direct hernias (in that order). Bilateral hernias were associated with more severe atrophy. Adjustment for age and muscle mass confirmed the validity of the primary observation.[774]

Further evidence in support of a collagen derangement in the transversalis fascia has been presented by Peacock and Madden (1974), who observe that satisfactory repair of adult inguinal hernia depends on the local extent of any collagen deficiency. And, if surgical technical failure can be excluded, the logical treatment of recurrent herniation is a fascial graft or prosthetic repair.[728] This concept has been enthusiastically promulgated by Irving Lichtenstein, one of the earliest protagonists of prosthetic repair for primary inguinal hernia.[563] Hydroxyproline, which comprises 80% of the dry weight of collagen, is strikingly decreased in the rectus sheath of hernia patients.[955] Extraction of the collagen reveals an altered precipitability and a reduced hydroxyproline: proline ratio. Intermolecular cross-linking is unaffected, but synthesis of hydroxyproline is inhibited and there is variability in the diameter of the collagen fibrils in hernia patients.[984] Similar electron microscopic findings are present in pericardial and skin biopsies from these patients[984] and have also been

described in connective tissue tumours,[11] pulmonary emphysema[149] and in scurvy.[556]

These observations led Read, in 1978, to the postulate that inguinal herniation is not a localized defect of the groin fascia, but is a manifestation of a generalized connective tissue disorder similar to emphysema, α_1–antitrypsin deficiency, osteogenesis imperfecta, scurvy, varicose veins and experimental nicotine deficiency.[149] There is both a difference in collagen ultrastructure when it is examined under an electron microscope and in its physicochemical properties as observed by altered precipitability and deficiency in hydroxyproline content. It appears that a fundamental problem in the aponeurosis of men with direct inguinal herniation is a failure of hydroxylation of the collagen molecule.

Berliner in 1984 confirmed these findings by studying biopsies from three sites in patients with inguinal hernia.[92] Degenerative changes in the musculo-aponeurotic fibres were found not only in the transversalis fascia/transversus abdominis of patients with direct inguinal hernias, but also in the transversalis fascia at the superior aspect of the internal ring in patients with indirect inguinal hernia and also distant from the hernia site in grossly abnormal transversus abdominis aponeurosis. The main changes observed were reduction in elastic tissue with a paucity and fragmentation of elastic fibre similar to that seen in Marfan and Ehlers–Danlos syndrome. The implication from these findings is that collagen malsynthesis and enzymolysis play a major role in the aetiology of both direct and indirect inguinal hernia. Indeed, the *in-vitro* synthesis of type I and III collagens and their procollagen mRNAs was determined in a study of isolated skin fibroblasts from patients with inguinal hernia. Fibroblasts incubated with radiolabelled tritiated proline secreted increased amounts of type III procollagen, which suggested that an altered fibroblast phenotype in patients with inguinal hernia could result in reduced collagen fibril assembly and defective connective tissue formation.[316]

Could an uninhibited elastolytic enzyme system cause groin herniation – a similar mechanism to low serum levels of the protease inhibitor α_1–antitrypsin globulin allowing endogenous enzymes to destroy alveoli?[531]

Experimental evidence supports the biochemical hypothesis that the pulmonary connective tissue disorder in emphysema is an imbalance between proteolytic enzyme levels and their inhibitors. Evidence of raised elastolytic enzyme has been found in smokers, and in smokers with inguinal herniation there is a close association between raised elastolytic levels and raised white counts. Leukocytes carry proteolytic and elastolytic enzymes and are actively involved in the lung inflammatory response to cigarette smoke. Could they not also deliver the same proteolytic insult to the fascia transversalis? An association between direct inguinal herniation and aortic aneurysm (as opposed to aortic atherosclerotic occlusive vascular disease) also exists. The prevalence of inguinal hernia (41%) in 119 patients with infrarenal aortic aneurysms was significantly elevated compared with 81 patients with aortic occlusive disease (18.5%) and 293 patients with coronary artery disease (18.1%). Additionally, the number of patients with recent hernia repair (16%) or still awaiting repair (19%) was very high.[548] These findings indicate that up to 66% of patients with non-occlusive infrarenal aortic aneurysm suffer from inguinal hernia. The smoking habits of the three groups were not different, and again the findings support a systemic fibre degeneration.[150] Although the enzymatic elastase content of the wall of abdominal aortic aneurysms is known to be increased, the concept of high levels of circulating elastase has not been confirmed. The term 'metastatic emphysema' has been coined by Cannon and Read (1981) for this generalized connective tissue disorder.[149] We must be cautious in interpreting the experimental data about a proteolytic defect in inguinal hernia patients and then relating it to the proven association with abdominal aortic aneurysm. It is tempting to relate the metastatic emphysema theory of inguinal herniation to Hunt's and Tilson's ideas that aortic aneurysm is a copper transport collagen disorder enhanced by cigarette smoking.[443, 923]

The genetics of inheritance of indirect inguinal hernia

Although there is considerable evidence suggesting the role of genetic factors in the aetiology of inguinal hernia, its mode of inheritance remains controversial.[980] Hypotheses proposed include:

1. Autosomal dominant inheritance with incomplete penetrance.[873]
2. Autosomal dominant inheritance with sex influence.[671, 975]
3. X-linked dominant inheritance.[661]
4. Polygenic inheritance.[212, 827]

A study of 280 families with congenital indirect inguinal hernia in the Shandong province of China has indicated that the mode of transmission in these families is autosomal dominant with incomplete penetrance and sex influence. There is preferential paternal transmission of the gene, which suggests genomic imprinting in its aetiology.[360] In this study the probands had all been operated on by five years of age, the hernia occurring on the right side in 138 probands, and on the left side in 84. This is consistent with the known embryological facts that the right testis descends later than the left, and that the processus vaginalis is therefore obliterated later on the right side than on the left side; hence hernia is more frequent on the right than on the left side.

Indirect inguinal hernia arises from incomplete obliteration of the processus vaginalis, the embryological protrusion of peritoneum that precedes testicular descent into the scrotum. The testes originate along the urogenital line in the retroperitoneum and migrate cordially during the second trimester of pregnancy to arrive at the internal inguinal ring at about six months of intrauterine life. During the last trimester they proceed through the abdominal wall via the inguinal canal and descend into the scrotum, the right slightly later than the left. The processus vaginalis then normally obliterates postnatally except for the portion surrounding and serving as a covering for the testes. Failure of this obliterative process results in congenital indirect inguinal hernia.

It is plausible to speculate that morphogenesis may be determined by single genes and complicated by environmental factors. In the case of indirect inguinal hernia, an autosomally dominantly inherited gene with reduced penetrance and sex influence would therefore be susceptible to environmental factors influencing its expression as a clinical inguinal hernia. In most families, however, a monogenic mode of inheritance is not apparent. Therefore the maternal allele may protect against failure of closure of the patent processus vaginalis. Abdominal hernias are associated with autosomal dominant polycystic kidney disease.[661]

In conclusion, the fact that most affected males have inherited an indirect inguinal hernia gene from their father implicates a role of genomic imprinting in the aetiology of the indirect inguinal hernia phenotype.

Intra-abdominal disease causing hernias

Ascites due to abdominal carcinomatosis, liver or heart disease can present as recent onset herniation. The mechanism is similar to that already described in CAPD patients, with hydrostatic pressure dilating a pre-existing sac and abdominal contents prolapsing into this enlarged space. The sudden onset of a hernia in middle-aged or elderly patients should arouse diagnostic suspicion. It is a sound policy to subject hernial sacs to histological examination, especially in older patients, where ascites is found or when the sac is thickened. Routine histological examination of 'normal appearance' hernial sacs is not recommended; indeed the chance of an unexpected find of pathology in a 'normal' sac is estimated to be 0.00098%.[484] Routine histology is certainly not economically sensible.

Thickening of the sac is not necessarily due to cancer; peritoneum is active tissue and particularly in children and young adults can exhibit over-exuberant tumour-like reaction to mechanical injury to the sac. This mesothelial hyperplasia may follow wearing a truss or occur simply after incarceration. Microscopically there are atypical mesothelial cells; these may be either free or attached to the wall. Mitoses and multinucleated cells are frequently seen. Mesothelial hyperplasia is reactive and not neoplastic in origin.[793]

The development of an abdominal wall hernia may be the initial symptom of decompensated heart or liver disease. Whereas good surgical practice is to repair an uncomplicated hernia, the question of repair in cirrhotics raises other issues. Leonetti *et al.* (1984) report that repair of umbilical hernias in uncontrolled unshunted cirrhotics gave a mortality of 8.3%, a morbidity of 16.6% and a recurrence rate of 16.6%. Umbilical herniorrhaphy in patients with a functioning peritoneovenous shunt was associated with minimal morbidity (7%). These authors suggest that peritoneovenous shunting should be a prerequisite to hernia repair.[551]

Pus can also distend an empty hernial sac, as with any peritoneal recess, during or after general peritonitis. In a review of 32 examples of this phenomenon, 19 were right inguinal, five right femoral, three left inguinal, one epigastric and one umbilical. Acute appendicitis accounted for 16 examples, perforated peptic ulcers for three, one followed pneumococcal peritonitis in a 2-week-old male child, one an acute pyosalpinx and one followed a biliary leak after removal of a common bile duct drain.[205] Every patient with this complication was originally diagnosed as having a strangulated hernia, which is not surprising. If pus is found in a hernial sac, abdominal exploration is mandatory with acute appendicitis being the commonest initial diagnosis, especially in right-sided hernias.[917]

Inguinal hernia and appendicectomy

Hoguet, in 1911, first described the development of inguinal hernia in patients who had undergone previous appendicectomy.[431] He found eight right inguinal hernias in a series of 190 patients who had undergone appendicectomy; he suggested a causal relationship. Other authors have supported this contention.[36, 373]

Right inguinal hernias are more frequent when appendicectomy is performed through a lower, 'more cosmetic' incision which is placed below the anterior superior iliac spine and in which the iliohypogastric nerve is injured. Electromyographic studies have shown conflicting results. While some investigators[35] have shown that denervation of the transversus abdominis muscle in the groin occurs, and could therefore interfere with the shutter mechanism of the deep ring and be a factor in the subsequent development of inguinal hernia, other investigators have failed to detect any abnormality signifying partial or complete denervation of the musculature in and around the right groin.[346]

Using the standard McBurney appendicectomy incision (at right angles to a line from the umbilicus to the anterior superior iliac spine, at a point at the junction of its lateral third and medial two-thirds and parallel to the iliohypogastric nerve which is rarely hazarded if the flank muscles are opened by splitting in their fibre line), there is no evidence that inguinal herniation is a consequence of appendicectomy. In a series of 549 patients who had undergone inguinal hernia repair, the percentage incidence of previous appendicectomy in right-sided hernias was 8.9% ± 1.7% and in left-sided inguinal hernias 11.2% ± 2.1%.[545]

It is the lower, 'more cosmetic' incisions which carry a particular hazard to the iliohypogastric nerve and a propensity to subsequent inguinal herniation. The introduction of effective antibiotics and the reduction of wound complications after appendicectomy have also contributed to the lower incidence of inguinal herniation after appendicectomy nowadays.

Hernias related to trauma and pelvic fracture

Abdominal hernias related to trauma and blunt injury are rare and are only reported following lower abdominal and pelvic injuries. To diagnose a traumatic hernia there must be immediate signs of local soft-tissue injury, bruising, haematoma, etc., and then there must be the early presentation of the symptoms of the hernia. The aponeuroses close to their pelvic attachments are most at risk.

Disruption of the inguinal canal and complete ruptures of the conjoint tendon are recorded.[179] Ryan, from the Shouldice clinic, reports five hernias related to pelvic fractures in 8000 hernia repairs.[818]

Figure 3.9 illustrates an extremely rare case of a patient whose hernia was related to a pelvic fracture: a 40-year-old man developed a 'pantaloon' hernia after fracture of both rami of the pubis in a road traffic

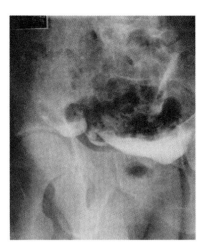

Figure 3.9 Herniography on a 40-year-old man who had sustained a fracture of both pubic rami. The patient developed a 'pantaloon' inguinal hernia

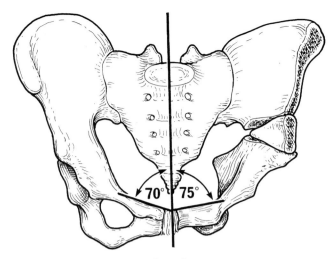

Figure 3.10 Diagram to show how innominate osteotomy predisposes to inguinal herniation

accident. Hernias related to iatrogenic pelvic fractures, for example osteotomy for congenital dislocation of the hip, are of course well known in the literature. Ryan classifies these fracture-related hernias according to the mechanism of the fracture.[818]

1. Due to acute anteroposterior forces acting on the pelvis. In these instances there is tearing of the rectus abdominis origin from the pubic crest. The tearing is maximal on the side opposite to that on which maximum bony displacement had occurred. The damage to the muscle is usually more severe medially than laterally, leading to the development of a broadnecked sac just suprapubically from the midline extending laterally across the attachment of the rectus to the pubic crest.
2. Due to lateral or lateral/vertical forces. These fractures involve the superior pubic ramus with consequent tearing of the fascial and aponeurotic attachments of the inguinofemoral region. In these circumstances a direct inguinal hernia develops through the fascia transversalis immediately above the bony fracture line. A repair of the direct hernia corrects the situation.
3. Due to surgical innominate osteotomy. This hernia occurs in children with congenital dislocated hips. The hernia following innominate osteotomy is either a direct inguinal hernia, a prevascular femoral (Narath's) hernia or a combination of the two.[690]

During innominate (Salter's) osteotomy there is a downward lateral and forward displacement of the lower fragment of the pelvis produced by a combination of hinging and rotation at the symphysis pubis.[823] This procedure leads to an increase in the distance between the edge of the rectus abdominis muscle and the inguinal and pectineal ligaments. There is a consequent weakening in the posterior wall of the inguinal canal. The angle

between the midline (and, therefore, the lateral edge of the rectus muscle) and the superior ramus of the pubis is increased by a minimum of 5 degrees when compared to the opposite side, there is also an increase in the distance from the pubic tubercle to the anterior superior iliac spine. These changes alter the anatomy of the inguinofemoral region predisposing to hernia. It must be stressed that a consequent hernia is rare, and undoubtedly compensatory remodelling of the soft tissues occurs as the child develops after the osteotomy operation (Figure 3.10).

After the removal of autologous bone grafts from the iliac crest, when full thickness grafts are taken from the posterior iliac crest, the inferior lumbar triangle is enlarged predisposing to herniation. These lumbar hernias cause backache and can be complicated by irreducibility and strangulation.[157]

Exertion and herniation

There is no evidence that strong muscular or athletic exertion causes inguinal hernia in the absence of a fascial and/or muscular abnormality – either acquired connective tissue disease or congenital anomaly of the abdominal wall. Indeed, inguinal hernia is rare in weight-lifters.[224] At the moment the relative importance of genetic, anatomic and environmental (smoking and heavy manual work) factors cannot be construed in each case. Manual work or strain is never, or very rarely, the sole cause of inguinal hernia.

Recent research suggests that persistent straining and heavy work is relevant to the development of groin hernia. The environment and occupation have an influence on hernia development. Recent European research has stressed these environmental factors rather than congenital defects in hernia development.[153, 308]

The aetiology of groin hernia has an importance in terms of prevention; smoking is a causal agent.

In medicolegal terms, the situation is confused – an accident or heavy strain at work is generally construed as a causal factor in the onset of a hernia and in the English courts damages are usually awarded. Our current understanding of the aetiology of inguinal hernias casts doubt on judicial reasoning in many of these instances. The legal foundation for compensating a workman who develops a hernia after an accident at his workplace is the commission of a tort or breach of contract by his employer. The heads of damages awarded are for pain or suffering, loss of amenities (usually sex life), pecuniary loss, medical expenses and loss of earning capacity. The role of a pre-existing disability, patent processus vaginalis or metastatic emphysema, will need offsetting against the damages. This is definitely a task for the judiciary, being largely unrelated to the observations of natural science.[488]

Conclusions

The incidence of primary groin hernia varies in different communities. The exact incidence in adult males in the UK is very difficult to estimate, but 16% of adult males will undergo operation for the condition.

The incidence of inguinal hernia is higher in African people, who tend to have a narrower male pelvis than Europeans. The incidence varies considerably between different African tribes.

Genetic and acquired factors each interact to allow a hernia to develop; however, we are forced to the conclusion that a failure of the fascia transversalis to withstand the stresses and strains of life is crucial to the development of inguinal hernia.

A preformed, congenital, peritoneal processus or sac is an important prerequisite of the indirect hernia of childhood or of the indirect sac which is manifest in CAPD patients or in patients with ascites due to cirrhosis or peritoneal malignancy.

A tissue defect is demonstrated in adult males with inguinal herniation. This tissue defect is causally related to smoking. Persistent heavy labouring work is associated with hernia development.

4 LOGISTICS OF HERNIA REPAIR

Trends in surgical care

Before the Victorian economic miracle in the 1860s allowed extensive hospital construction in the British Isles and simultaneously created the urban deprivation which required hospitals as a haven from a hostile unhygienic environment for the working masses when they were ill, most patients recuperated at home after surgical operations. Only the indigent and members of the armed forces were automatically hospitalized if they required surgery or were wounded. Patients with financial means avoided hospital care. This pattern of surgery was usual in the USA and Europe. The tradition of home surgery lingered on in England where, in the spring of 1951, King George VI had a left pneumonectomy for carcinoma of the lung in a Buckingham Palace room which had been turned into an operating theatre.[282]

The regimentation of wartime and the prejudices of officer surgeons on the management of hernias influenced postoperative care in the early days of the National Health Service (NHS). The average time between operation and return to depot in the World War II British Army was 12 weeks: three weeks in bed, with exercises commencing on the twelfth day; three to four weeks in a convalescent hospital, with exercises conducted under instruction; four weeks in a convalescent depot; then a few days' leave. At the end of this time the patient was able to carry out full duties as a 'fighting man'.[277] These orders persisted into peacetime and contributed to conservative surgical practice until they were challenged in the 1960s by Hugh Dudley.[147]

The NHS, from its inception in 1948, also encouraged hospitalization for surgery; the 1962 Hospital Plan envisaged all surgery concentrated in one hospital in each district. The 1969 update of that report, like the earlier report, recommended concentrating surgical services but did not recognize the value of day-case or short-stay facilities. Up to the early 1970s the trend to institutional surgery and recuperation as an in-patient continued remorselessly.[236]

Three forces predicated this – the professionalization of the hospital nursing service, the improvements in surgical technology, requiring more and more sophisticated equipment for even the simplest procedure, and the drive by third-party paymasters (in England the

State) to control costs. Costs are most easily controlled in an institution owned by the paymasters, so surgery in hospital becomes normative. Until the 1990s the concept of the NHS contracting out work to an independent day-care facility was unthinkable. By the 1950s it was accepted that for clinical, social and economic reasons surgery and postoperative recovery should take place in hospital, notwithstanding the example of King Emperors and the whimsy of their surgeon knights!

Administrative and governmental influences were not the only conservative forces; the attitudes of the distinguished 'fathers' of modern surgery were conservative too. Billroth believed that rest and protection were essential for the proper repair of coapted tissues.[97] Halsted, writing on the radical cure of hernia in 1889, stated:

> Our patients are kept on their backs for 21 days. Wounds healed thoroughly throughout are not strong in 21 days . . . are certainly stronger on the fourteenth day than the seventh and certainly stronger on the twenty-first day than on the fourteenth. Just how long wounds of skin and muscle which have healed by first intention . . . in strength we do not know . . . I sometimes question the propriety of allowing, as I do, my patients to walk about on the twenty-first day.[384]

Four years later (1893) Emil Ries, Professor of Gynaecology in Chicago, a man who is truly the English-speaking father of early postoperative ambulation, instituted early rising and rapid convalescence in his unit. In 1893 Ries had visited Morisani's clinic in Naples and while there he was shown a patient who had risen from her bed and walked across the ward during the evening of the day of symphysiotomy, without detriment to herself or her wound. Not only was early ambulation possible, but Ries soon found that recovery was faster too; these patients commenced on a full diet sooner and they had fewer bowel problems. He concluded that with good asepsis and careful surgery there should be no problems. Reis concluded: 'It means a great deal for the business man or labourer or their wives to be put on their own feet in a short time and to be able to return to their work two or three weeks after an abdominal operation.'[787]

Powers investigated the effect of early ambulation on postoperative complications and return to work following hernioplasty in a New York rural community from

1933 to 1953. He clearly demonstrated that the duration of hospital stay could be safely lowered from an average of 14 postoperative days to one day, and this allowed a sixfold increase in the number of operations undertaken. Early ambulation was associated with a dramatic lowering of the hernia recurrence rate.[761] This latter improvement in the recurrence rate should not be ascribed to early ambulation alone; the increased experience of the operating surgeon must have improved his technique too.

Surgery, social mores and economics are not static. Advances in anaesthesia, newer surgical techniques, lower sepsis rates, a healthier and better nourished population, improved home conditions, co-ordinated home nursing and family doctor services, and inexorable cost containment programmes have made us review our indications for in-patient hospital care. High complication rates no longer bedevil anaesthesia and surgery. Furthermore, the benefits of self-help and early mobilization are now appreciated.

Today's *weltschmerz* is cost containment with consumerism, combined with increased longevity, vastly improved medical technology and a quite correct emphasis on efficiency and 'value for money'. Paradoxically, home recuperation after surgery is now the norm often for reasons of patient choice and satisfaction.

Variation in duration of stay of adult hernia patients

Variations in the length of hospital stay were demonstrated by routine hospital statistics in about 1960. These differences in clinical practice soon began to attract interest. The work of Farquharson and of Stephens and Dudley had alerted managers to the benefits of efficient hospital practice, so it is not surprising that non-clinicians should be attracted to investigate the seemingly inexplicable variations in clinical practice.

Farquharson in Edinburgh (1955) reported 458 outpatient hernioplasties. All his patients were operated under local anaesthetic, only 11 developing complications which required admission. He emphasized the therapeutic advantages of early mobilization and the benefit such rapid turnover brought to others awaiting operation. Farquharson found the system clinically satisfying and continued the practice for the rest of his working life.[292]

Stephens and Dudley (1961) reported a study of outpatient varicose veins and hernia operations, emphasizing that for day-case patients and in-patients the same standards of care must be delivered. They stressed the importance of anaesthetic assessment and the organizational rigour that must be instituted.[889]

Davies and Barr (1965) researched the management of uncomplicated inguinal hernias in adults between 16 and 60 years old by 17 consultant surgical teams in three NHS regions – Birmingham, Liverpool and Oxford. Each team provided records of 100 recent patients; in all, 1678 patients were analysed. In the series 80% of the patients were aged between 30 and 59 years of age and 121 (7.2%) were females. One-third were engaged on heavy work, the remainder having light industrial or sedentary occupations. The mean time on the waiting list varied widely; in Birmingham 3.1 months were spent on a waiting list, in Liverpool 3.9 months and in Oxford 6.9 months.[223]

The duration of hospital stay also varied, being shortest in the Oxford region where the waiting list was longest. In Oxford 86% of patients were operated on within a day of admission; in the other two regions there were significantly longer preoperative in-patient stays. In Liverpool, for instance, 27.6% of patients spent two days in hospital prior to operation. The greatest degree of correlation was found between the time spent on the waiting list and the duration of in-patient stay: where the waiting list time was short the in-patient duration was long and vice versa. The study also reviewed operative techniques and suture choice and demonstrated that little had changed despite the classic contributions on these topics by Marsden who had reviewed hernia practice in Liverpool in 1958 and 1962.[614, 615]

This three-region study, at a time when earlier studies of ambulant or short-stay inguinal hernia repair had already been published, demonstrates the innately conservative behaviour of clinicians. The authors, epidemiologists, concluded that a prospective evaluation of techniques and suture materials was needed and an evaluation of the effect of different lengths of stay was urgently required!

Another study, by epidemiologists, of the duration of stay of men undergoing unilateral inguinal hernioplasty in eight Wessex hospitals from 1970 to 1971, showed that the duration of postoperative hospital stay was related to the hospital, more importantly its size and organization, rather than to other factors. Small hospitals had longer durations of stay. Surgeons operating in two hospitals adopted the normative duration of stay of the hospital rather than vice versa. Pressure of work at larger hospitals may compel shorter stays and modify hospital organization.[367]

These studies do show how helpless the surgeon often is when it comes to implementing good clinical policies which challenge the accepted practice for the institution. Clinicians, like their patients, can suffer from the institutionalism that stalks hospital corridors!

Clinically oriented studies of short-stay surgery for hernias include those of Morris (1968),[666] Russell et al. (1977)[807] and Ruckley et al. (1978).[805]

Morris and colleagues randomized patients from the hernia waiting list in Mansfield, Leicestershire, to either in- or out-patient surgery. The only problems they reported were postoperative chest infections and some patients' preference for 48 h postoperative in-patient care.[666]

Russell and colleagues in Stockton-on-Tees conducted a prospective randomized controlled study of day-case operation for hernias or haemorrhoids. No surgical adverse effects were seen when day-case hernioplasties were compared with longer stay hernia operations, but in complications with day-case haemorrhoid operations increased two-fold. He also found, like Morris and co-workers, that some patients preferred an overnight or 24 h stay.[807]

Ruckley and colleagues reviewed the duration of stay of patients requiring surgery for varicose veins; the patients were preselected for suitability and then randomized to care patterns. One hundred and twenty-one were allocated to a 48 h stay in an acute ward, 121 were managed in a convalescent hospital after operation and 117 were discharged directly home to the care of the general practitioner and the community nursing service. Anaesthetic and/or surgical problems necessitated keeping five patients (three convalescent and two day-case) in hospital on the day of operation. Two acute ward patients and one convalescent ward patient required readmission for complications; two of these patients had minor pulmonary emboli and one had undiagnosed chest pain. None of the day cases required readmission for any reason.[805]

Day care involved an average of only eight minutes more working time, including travelling for general practitioners in the three weeks after operation. Forty per cent of patients had no contact whatsoever with their general practitioners during the postoperative period. The average contact times with the community nurse in the three weeks postoperatively were 186 min (for acute ward patients), 204 min (for convalescent ward patients) and 325 min (for day-care patients). The saving in day care compared with seven-day care was £100 (based on Scottish Hospital Statistics, 1975).[838]

Customer reaction was tested and day care was the most acceptable of the three options. Women with children at home preferred day care. The average hospital ward compares unfavourably with most home environments in terms of comfort, menu, personal attention, privacy, hygiene and cross-infection risks. It is not surprising that patients undergoing simple surgery, not subject to postoperative risks of a life-threatening nature, should prefer home care.

The development of 'one-day' out-patient surgery for adults with groin hernias has been slow. Enthusiasts in both North America[329] and the UK have published accounts of such surgery, but universal adoption of these policies is perhaps too adventurous for most surgeons. Although Farquharson, in 1955, reported day-case herniorrhaphy in 485 patients treated over a five-year period in Edinburgh, there can be no doubt that his example did not spread too far afield. In Scotland, in 1967, the median postoperative stay after inguinal herniorrhaphy was eight days, with a range of 2–12 days.[412, 804] In 1974 this remained unchanged at eight days, with 10% of the patients occupying an in-patient hospital bed for three or more days prior to operation. Indeed, in some hospitals 30% of patients rested in hospital for three or more days before surgery.[838] In the Northern Region of the NHS in England, in 1981, 18 528 male adults with inguinal hernia underwent operation. The average duration of stay was 6.9 days and 45% were in hospital for longer than 10 days.

Morgan and her colleagues (1987) have analysed the duration of hospital stay for inguinal hernia repair in adults in the Northern and South East Thames regions of the NHS.[665] In the Northern Region 18% of operations on the under 25–year-old group were performed as day cases; in those 25 years old and over, only 0.6% of inguinal hernia repairs were done as day cases. The mean length of stay for adult inguinal hernia repair in the Northern Region in 1984 was 4.9 days (SD ± 4.5) and in South East Thames Region in 1982 5.4 days (SD ± 4.1). There is a noticeably wide variation. Quite clearly durations of stay, particularly preoperative stay, could be reduced without clinical detriment to the patients. The wide differences between hospitals revealed in this study suggest that organizational as well as clinical inertia contributes to the problem.[665]

Motives other than clinical excellence are likely to encourage short-stay surgery; changing patterns of female behaviour and work, with more nursing falling to male nurses and married women, will dictate the requirement for flexible and no-weekend shift systems. The high cost of institutional overheads will optimize single short-stay facilities which can be closed down completely at weekends. The development of ambulant surgery should reduce the requirement for in-patient facilities. Costs of medical care will continue to remain high and containment of these costs will increasingly become a surgical priority. To date there have been few good prospective studies of short-stay surgery. Such studies need to be adequately controlled to give real comparative data about all the variables, including patient satisfaction. Everyone knows it is possible to remove the appendix on the kitchen table, but is this necessarily a good thing?

To resolve this question a carefully controlled study comparing the social, economic and clinical outcome of the treatment is required. The DHSS commissioned such a study in the early 1970s; however, like so many studies commissioned to bolster administrative policy, it was 'quick and dirty' and did not adequately answer the questions clinicians and their patients find most relevant.[6] The study did not measure the quality of surgical care, although a subsequent report suggests that the 'acid test' of hernia surgery, the recurrence rate of the patients included, was much higher than the best surgery available at the time. Other surgical complications appear to have been above average too. The authors of this study concluded that short-stay hospital care for these conditions saved the hospital and community medical services about £25 per case – this difference is largely accounted for by the difference in the 'hotel costs' of the shorter stay.[6] Herein is the dilemma: any economic or organizational conclusions drawn from a sample in which the clinical and social outcomes are less than optimal are regarded as dubious by both consumers and clinicians.

Day surgery and high quality hernia surgery have been promoted by enthusiasts rather than by administrative decree, day surgery must be of higher quality and safe. Such attributes evolved at North Tees Hospital in the 1970s. In a prospective series of series of inguinal hernioplasties in male adults (16 years old and above) from 1970 to 1982, 718 operations were performed, the mean duration of stay was 4.3 days, 28% were day cases (in-hospital stay up to 8 h), 31% overnight stay (< 24 h) and 41% greater than 24 h. The recurrence rate, the 'acid test', was under 1%. The problem is how to generalize such results.

In recent years the average duration of stay of inguinal hernia patients has fallen consistently and the proportion of patients being treated on an ambulant day-case basis has increased (Table 4.1).

Overall the development of day-case surgery for adults with groin hernias has been slower in the UK than in the USA, where most inguinal hernioplasties are performed on an ambulant basis. Interestingly, the Shouldice Hospital in Toronto, possibly the owners of the 'gold standard' hernioplasty operation, have not endorsed day surgery for groin hernia. They continue with their four-day regime for hernioplasty with progressive supervised postoperative ambulation and rehabilitative exercises.[10, 978]

The impact of contemporary socioeconomic pressures on surgical practice in the UK is well demonstrated by inguinal hernioplasty. There are socioeconomic and age-related variations in the uptake of inguinal hernioplasty,[200] and probably related to these there is an increasing uptake of private practice options.[639] Nichol has estimated that repair of hernias in private practice increased by 77% from 1981 to 1986.[699] Private hernia patients in independent hospitals have the longest stay recorded;[987] this longer stay occurs in all age groups in 1980. We have no more recent data about the duration of stay on the utilization of private facilities in the UK for groin hernia surgery.

The relentless drive of cost constraint has clearly not been as potent in the private sector in the UK as it has in the USA and the NHS.

Hospital-based or independent day-care (ambulatory) surgery facility?

Early day-case surgery was undertaken from traditional wards, but gradually the concept of a special free-standing unit appeared, the first one in the UK being at the Royal Postgraduate Medical School, Hammersmith, London. Short-stay or ambulatory surgery can be accommodated in three separate settings, each of which has its own advantages and disadvantages. First, patients can be admitted into traditional surgical wards. Secondly, a designated unit can be set up as part of an existing surgical general hospital organization. Lastly, a custom-built, free-standing, independent ambulatory care facility can be built.[238, 255, 758]

Each of these settings has advantages. Utilization of main in-patient facilities imposes no extra capital cost because facilities are already on site, but the space occupied by short-stay cases will be vacant and wasted at weekends. A designated unit in a general hospital allows for multidisciplinary utilization; it keeps staff on location and also allows weekend closure, thus cutting expensive nursing costs and allowing staffing by married nurses. An additional advantage that has been claimed is that married nurses develop greater empathy and understanding of the special domestic requirements of day-case patients.

Hospital-based dedicated units are the usual model for day-case surgery; they require less capital and they use existing staff, equipment and support services. They allow for flexibility of staffing and can draw on the parent hospital in times of shortage. Furthermore, if complications arise the patients can be handled within the same institution. The disadvantages include surgeons being called away to more pressing emergencies, so that the day-case plan is 'bumped'. Also, patients' morale may be disadvantaged by having to witness other patients receiving critical care or major surgery. As these dedicated units are part of a larger whole their overheads may be unduly high because they have to carry their share of services required in a major hospital but which are not essential to their more restricted role.

It is the problems of capital provision and overhead costs which have led, particularly in the USA, and more recently in Europe, to free-standing Ambulatory Care Centres. American reviews of surgical care provision now seem to give this type of unit, the Surgicenter, more marks than day care located in traditional medical institutions. Separate registration, standardized preoperative and postoperative regimens and an absence of seriously ill

Table 4.1 Mean duration of stay for inguinal hernioplasty in England and Wales

Year	1975	1980	1985	1990	1995
Duration of stay (days)	7.3	5.7	4.9	3.1	2.1

incumbents make these units more acceptable to the community. Disadvantages may include the lack of in-house medical staff to deal with the infrequent complication.[311]

Patient management policies

Day-case and short-stay surgery depend critically on the administrative and nursing, as well as the surgical, protocol. There must be an easy flow from first patient contact through operation to home, convalescence and return to employment. If this flow is to be effortless the entire programme must be formalized, repeatable and understood by all concerned – including the patient. It is advisable to have standard printed documentation including details of pre-admission (Table 4.2), operation

Table 4.2   Preoperative documentation for management of the day-case patient

Name:	Hospital number:
Date of birth:	Address:
Ward:	
Name of ward sister:	
Ward doctor:	

Date of admission/completion of this
   form:
Reason for admission:
Occupation of patient:
Past medical history:
Previous operations:
Complications of previous operations:
Current drug therapy:
Is there any history of allergies?
Is the patient taking anticoagulants?
Alcohol intake:
Smoking habits:
Does the patient take any other social
   drugs?

Female patients:
   Are you pregnant?
   Date of last menstrual period?
   Are you taking oral contraceptives?
   If 'yes', what DVT prophylaxis has
   been ordered?

Systematic enquiries:
   Cardiovascular system
   Respiratory system
   Other

Active intercurrent illnesses:
Physical examination

Height:	Weight:
Pulse rate:	Blood pressure:
Temperature:	Urinalysis:

Chest examination:
Cardiovascular examination:
ASA grade:

and postoperative care, nursing and consent all on one form. Details of the organization, management and patient selection are extensively reviewed and protocols set out in the *Royal College of Surgeons of England Guidelines for Day Surgery* revised edition 1992.[799, 800]

At the first consultation a diagnosis should be made and a decision to operate (or not) taken. The patient's physical and emotional health and suitability or not for general or local anaesthesia are reviewed, as are home and other relevant social conditions and operation day transportation. Important facts to record include age, weight and height for pharmacological reasons, active intercurrent medical conditions, current drug therapy and social drug composition.

In females, day-case surgery could be inadvisable during pregnancy. The use of oral contraceptives and the requirement for deep vein thrombosis (DVT) prophylaxis will need assessing. Preoperative cessation of oral contraceptives may be advised; however, a six-months off dry period is required if the risk of DVT is to be reduced. The possibility of pregnancy may be a greater risk to the patient. This will require a decision at the initial consultation.

The American Society of Anesthesiologists' (ASA) grade should be recorded. Only patients of ASA classes 1 and 2 can ordinarily be considered suitable for day-case surgery (Table 4.3).[16]

The date and time of operation, and the date and time of discharge, are set at this initial consultation. All medical and nursing process documentation including the consent form, which can be repetitive, time consuming and wearying for the patient, is rolled up into one document to be filled in at the initial consultation. Completed, this checklist is passport, visa, ticket and boarding pass to surgery. When giving consent the patient must clearly understand that he is to be discharged postoperatively with a newly created surgical wound. Failure to obtain this consent and explain its consequences may lead to difficulties later. Patients need to know what to expect and who to contact if they are concerned when they return home.

A very worthwhile and effective preoperative routine can be a nurse assessment clinic. Such a clinic can undertake much of the routine preoperative check of physical status and additionally verify the social context and suitability of the patient for day surgery.[397]

The patient needs instructions that he can review at home; these may be written or as a tape or video (Table 4.4). 'Going home' is the crucial moment for the patient. The emphasis must be on accurately timed discharge. Planned discharge imposes constraints on all the actors; the commitment to predictable discharge is more demanding than the commitment to admission – hence the term 'planned early discharge'.

In order that arrangements and the patient's status remain unchanged, as short an interval as possible

Table 4.3   ASA classification of physical status for surgical patients[16]

Class 1   The patient has no organic, physiological, biochemical or psychiatric disturbance. The pathological process for which operation is to be performed is localized and does not entail a systemic disturbance. Examples: a fit patient with inguinal hernia; fibroid uterus in an otherwise healthy woman.

Class 2   Mild to moderate systemic disturbance caused either by the condition to be treated surgically or by other pathophysiological processes. Examples: non- or only slightly limiting organic heart disease; mild diabetes; essential hypertension; or anaemia. Some might choose to list the extremes of age here, either the neonate or the octogenarian, even though no discernible systemic disease is present. Extreme obesity and chronic bronchitis may be included in this category.

Class 3   Severe systemic disturbance or disease from whatever cause, even though it may not be possible to define the degree of disability with finality. Examples: severely limiting organic heart disease; severe diabetes with vascular complications; moderate to severe degrees of pulmonary insufficiency; angina pectoris or healed myocardial infarction.

Class 4   Severe systemic disorders that are already life threatening, not always correctable by operation. Examples: patients with organic heart disease showing marked signs of cardiac insufficiency, persistent angina, or active myocarditis; advanced degrees of pulmonary, hepatic, renal or endocrine insufficiency.

Class 5   The moribund patient who has little chance of survival but is submitted to operation in desperation. Examples: the burst abdominal aneurysm with profound shock; major cerebral trauma with rapidly increasing intracranial pressure; massive pulmonary embolus. Most of these patients require operation as a resuscitative measure, with little if any anaesthesia.

should occur between the various phases. For example, a groin hernia in a child or adult should be processed within three weeks.

On admission the patient's identity and medical status must be re-checked. It is convenient to use a structured form for this. The site of the operation is checked for cleanliness and freedom from sepsis. It should be indelibly marked, with the patient conscious when this is done.

In the operating room the patient's identity should be checked. Identifying the patient can be most hazardous in children and a fail-safe double-check procedure, with surgeon and anaesthetist separately doing the check, is advised.

An excellent booklet containing details for the patient has been published by the British Association for Day Surgery entitled *Day Surgery* and one on hernia repair

Table 4.4   Instructions to day-case hernia patients

This letter relates to your admission to hospital for repair of your hernia.

In the morning, before you come into hospital, would you please shave your lower abdomen, groin and pubic/scrotal area completely.

It is expected that you will be discharged about 5 p.m. but would you please advise your family to contact Sister on the ward if you have not arrived home by 7 p.m.

You will be given 20 tablets for pain. You should not have any pain, but if you do one of these tablets should be quite sufficient to relieve it.

You should be fit to get up and about as soon as you get home. We strongly advise you to exercise. If possible, you should go out for a walk each day after your operation. At all costs you must keep fully mobile about the house.

Your hernia has been repaired with modern suture material which is very strong, at least as strong as your tissues; this means you can walk and exercise as much as you want. The only restriction may be imposed by pain in the first few days after surgery.

We do *not* advise heavy lifting for about three weeks after surgery.

You must not drive yourself in a car for seven days after surgery; your groin will be stiff and this could interfere with your movement of the pedals.

The skin wound has been stitched internally and then the surface closed with spray-on plastic and a dressing. Keep the wound dry during the first four days. On the fifth day have a warm bath or shower, and when the wound is well wetted remove the dressing and discard it. The would may appear a little red and proud at first, but just keep it clean, washing it each day and drying it carefully. It will heal up to give you a neat red scar in two weeks and an almost invisible white scar in three months.

You will be fit to resume office work in three to seven days.

You will be fit to resume heavy work – labouring, gardening, scaffolding, coalmining, etc. – eight weeks after operation. Swimming can be resumed four weeks after operation; violent sports, rugby, soccer or squash, can be resumed gradually after four weeks to full activity at twelve weeks. Sexual activity is best resumed gently from two to four weeks after operation. Any activity that does not cause pain is good for you. Early resumption of work enhances would healing and will reduce the chance of recurrence of your hernia.

If you have any complications you can either contact your own doctor or the ward here.

Hernia Repair Operation, Questions and Answers published by the Royal College of Surgeons of England. In the USA a similar patient booklet, *Hernias of the Groin*, by Professor George Wantz of New York, can be recommended. It must be stressed again that patient information is vital to successful modern hernia short-stay surgery.[800, 802]

Pre-discharge criteria

Patients need to be fully conscious prior to discharge. They also must be mobile and able to care for themselves. They must be taking fluids by mouth, not nauseated and 'happy' on oral analgesics and be able to medicate themselves adequately when they arrive home. Voiding urine may be difficult after a hernia repair, especially for the male. Micturition must be accomplished prior to departure from hospital. The patients must understand their care plan, the management of the wound and the management of pain and discomfort.

The patient needs to take home with him full details of his operation, whatever medication he has been advised and what postoperative regimen is planned. These should be given to him so that if something goes awry he can hand all this information to the doctor or nurse who attends in an emergency.

Simultaneously the patient's family doctor and nursing staff should be advised that the patient has undergone the operation, that he has been discharged, what has been done and what postoperative care is advised. It must again be stressed that postoperative care is properly the responsibility of the operating surgeon.

Cannon and colleagues at the Middlesex Hospital, London, have reviewed the reasons for delayed discharge in a consecutive series of 104 unselected patients undergoing planned repair of an inguinal hernia. It was intended to discharge all of them from hospital within 48 h after operation; however, taking into account social and clinical factors only 54 patients were proposed for 48 h discharge and of these 24 (44%) were discharged on time. Of the 104 patients, 62 (60%) were discharged on the planned day, but only 24 (23%) left hospital 48 h after surgery. The most frequent reason for delaying discharge was a persistent postoperative pyrexia, which occurred in 24 patients. In retrospect, Cannon and co-workers report that a raised postoperative temperature did not foreshadow any more important clinical complications and should not therefore be a criterion for delaying discharge from hospital.[82, 151]

Inner city deprivation is sometimes advanced as an argument against planned early discharge. However, although adverse social circumstances may preclude the inclusion of some patients in such a scheme, the reality is that a well-constructed system can function in most communities.

Postoperative care

The aim should be minimal care, if possible without professional input. Postoperative pain control should be demand-led and self-prescribed by the patient. Wounds should be doctor and nurse non-dependent. Sutures or clips that need skilled removal should not be used and dressings should easily be undertaken by the patient. Techniques used should not impose an additional burden on family doctors. It is possible to construct a surgical system that is free-standing and not transferring its workload onto other carers.

Postoperative care should not impose costs above expected in-patient costs on the patient or his family. Research has confirmed that the trousseau effect of admission to traditional hospital care, plus the costs of spouses visiting, is at least as expensive as the cost of additional meals, spouse attention and other incidentals of home convalescence.[807]

Day-case surgery is only advantageous if it is well co-ordinated and free of problems; it is not an excuse to divest oneself of responsibility for postoperative care.[800]

Sleep

Even relatively minor surgical interventions can cause major, though temporary, disruptions of sleep in otherwise healthy individuals. Preoperative sleep is often forgotten, most patients admitted to hospital showing diminished preoperative sleep on the night before surgery. Anxiety, a new environment and clock-fixed nursing routines are important determinants of this. Admitting the patient on the day of operation overcomes many of these difficulties.

For the first two nights postoperatively, sleep is characterized by restlessness, lightness and the almost complete absence of rapid eye movement and delta sleep.[486] The consequences of these postoperative sleep disturbances are uncertain, but there is evidence that sleep deprivation causes psychological instability and may also be a precursor of poor wound healing.

The adverse effect of the hostile ward environment on sleep is again a strong argument for day-care surgery. However, in both day-care and hospital-care surgery the case for adequate analgesics and hypnotics in the perioperative phase must be emphasized.

Day-case surgery for children

As early as 1909 the Royal Glasgow Hospital for Children reported that out-patient surgery was satisfactory for children with inguinal hernias, but 25 years later surgeons were still keeping children in bed for three weeks after hernia repairs.[698] This has mostly changed and out-patient herniotomy in paediatric practice is now well established.[50]

The experience, in Brighton, Sussex, of treating children with hernias, hydroceles and other minor conditions as day cases demonstrates all the advantages of the system. One hundred children were studied; each child was initially diagnosed and recommended for day-case surgery in the surgical clinic. The children were then reviewed in a special anaesthetic clinic and finally the parents and the family doctors were asked to complete a questionnaire about the patient care incident.[32]

Of the 100 patients, there were 72 boys and 28 girls, and 64 of them were aged under 5 years old. Four patients were deemed unfit for day-case anaesthesia and a further two patients developed respiratory infections just prior to operation, necessitating a rescheduling. One child was detained in hospital with a haematoma, but no child required readmission or intervention by the family doctor for complications.

The family doctors were enthusiastic about the scheme – two even included their own children in the subsequent day-care programme! Ninety-two per cent of the parents replying to the questionnaire approved. The low duration of child–parent separation, the involvement of the parents in the day-care admission and the devolution of postoperative nursing to the parents were all considered advantages.

The economic aspects were not quantified, but the programme did relieve the pressure on beds, reduced the night nurse workload and reduced the waiting list. All of these were economic positives. However economically advantageous a day-case programme may be, unless it appeals to patients (and parents) it cannot be regarded as successful. This study illustrates clinical, social and economic success.[672] The organization of day care for children needs to be exact; an outstanding system has been developed in Southampton by Atwell.[50] This topic is further explored in Chapter 9.

Convalescence and return to work

In general, the philosophy of day-case and short-stay surgery should encourage early mobility and a rapid return to work. The rate of healing of fascial wounds dictates how soon the patient can walk and how soon the patient can return to work. Fascial wounds sutured with non-absorbable suture material have 70% of their final strength immediately on completion of the operation (see page 70); in comparison, fascial wounds sutured with catgut lose all the tensile strength imparted by the catgut within one month, at a time when wound healing has only contributed 30% of normal tissue integrity.

These researches provide the experimental basis for permitting early unrestricted physical exertion after surgery. Blodgett and Beattie, in 1947, demonstrated no adverse effects consequent on early mobilization after hernia repair.[102] In a series of over 2000 patients undergoing inguinal hernia repair, Lichtenstein and co-workers demonstrated that the recurrence rate was 0.9%, despite immediate postoperative resumption of normal activity.[561] At the Shouldice clinic the patients get up off the operating table and walk back to their rooms, and their recurrence rate is the best in the world.[978]

Baumber (1971) reviewed the time of return to work in 54 adult males with inguinal hernia: the range of time off was from 3 to 91 days, with a mean of 45 days for indirect and 56 days for direct hernia. He records that occupational physical stress did not influence the recurrence rate.[77]

Glassow (1976) has pointed out that 12.5% of all surgical admissions to general hospitals in Britain are for hernia repairs. In England and Wales 80 000 hernioplasties are performed each year, nine out of ten of these are for inguinal hernias. Thus if the practice of early return to work at about eight weeks after operation were adopted, 3212 working man-years per year could be gained.[354]

Palumbo has suggested that the loss of defensive reflexes in the immediate postoperative period may predispose to damage if the patient is encouraged to take too much activity before the anaesthetic effects have completely worn off. Our experience in undertaking hernia repairs under general anaesthetic has not suggested to us that early activity should be contraindicated. All our patients have been mobilized as soon as they have regained consciousness and, indeed, one patient got up immediately following surgery and went for a walk in the hospital precincts.[721]

Ross reviewed retrospectively 260 adult males who had undergone inguinal hernia repair and found that there was no evidence that a prolonged convalescent period reduces the subsequent hernia recurrence rate. However, he does conclude that many patients restrict their postoperative activities after inguinal hernia repair for much longer than is necessary. He recommends that the patients should be advised to resume their normal activities immediately after discharge and should remain off work for up to four weeks only if they are engaged in occupations which are physically very strenuous. He suggests that this advice should be given to the patient by the surgeon prior to the patient's discharge from hospital.[796]

In the only controlled study of the effect of early return to work after elective repair of inguinal hernias, Bourke and co-workers compared early return to work at 48 days after operation with standard return to work 65 days after operation. They note that there is considerable monetary benefit for the workers to return to work at the earlier date. They found no evidence of a higher recurrence rate in patients who resumed even strenuous activities at the earlier date. The self-employed in Bourke's study returned to work 31 days after operation. Their financial incentive to return to work was great. Seventy per cent of the self-employed in their study were heavy workers. The most compelling reason to attempt to change attitudes to return to work after hernioplasty is that the workers themselves lose money by prolonged convalescence. This was estimated to be £19.86 per week (at 1978 prices).[111]

Attitudes of management in industry need to alter too: the most depressing fact to emerge from the studies in Nottingham is the negative attitude of a major industry to early re-employment after hernioplasty. The more realistic economic climate prevailing since 1984 may modify this atavism.

In the armed forces the surgeon can control the date of resumption of full duties. An experiment to test the safety of early return to work in the Royal Navy and Royal Marines concluded there was no contraindication or increased recurrence rate to servicemen resuming full physical duty three weeks after repair of an uncomplicated unilateral inguinal hernia.[910]

The Middlesex Hospital, in 1982, published a report of a series of inguinal hernias repaired on a short-stay basis. They advised early return to work after operation and achieved an average time off work of 52 days. In 1985 they published a further series of results, the difference being explicit advice to return to work 28 days after surgery. In this latter series they achieved a mean duration of absence from work of 37 days. An additional one week of work beyond that advised by the surgeon was the norm.[84, 151]

Return to work is most often dictated by other factors than the rate of wound healing. Barwell, in a study of 399 hernia repairs using the Shouldice technique, observes that the self-employed returned to work far sooner than those whose employers allowed them generous insurance coverage (this confirms the earlier observation of Bourke and co-workers). He further observes that provided a non-absorbable suture is used for the repair, the likelihood of recurrence is independent of the time off work.[70] Barwell's insight into the economic drive of self-employment and its association with early return to work has, perhaps, more cogency than all the exhortations of doctors![69]

Semmence and Kynch, reviewing the return to work of patients in Oxford, were unable to account for the different durations of time off work. Age, social class, type of operation and amount and duration of sick pay only accounted for part of the variance in time off work. The type of occupation and the amount of duration of sick pay were the only statistically significant contributions. The heavier the job the longer the employee took to return to work. Paradoxically, the more the sick pay and the longer it lasted the less time the men took off work.[842]

General practitioner attitudes to return to work after hernioplasty have been studied. Questionnaires were sent to 50 family doctors and 38 (76%) were returned. Thirty-one respondents were of the opinion that a period of inactivity after hernia repair helps to reduce the chances of a recurrence of the hernia, five disagreed and one 'did not know'. The mean recommended time off work after operation was 53 days (range 28 days to 26 weeks). All the respondents agreed that a distinction should be made according to the occupation of the patient, a person doing light work and a retired person being advised a shorter convalescence than a heavy worker. The average time off work in the UK after repair of a unilateral inguinal hernia is 70 days.[842] The observations that general practitioners encourage longer periods off work than the operating surgeons are confirmed by Cannon and colleagues from the Middlesex Hospital, London.[151]

In 1993 the Royal College of Surgeons of England Clinical Guidelines on the Management of Groin Hernias in Adults recommended patients should be fit to return to office work after two weeks following an inguinal hernioplasty and back to heavy work after four weeks.[801] There are, however, no published randomized studies to support these recommendations. Shulman has challenged this advice, stating that there is no reason for any caution following mesh repair.[858] Proponents of the mesh repair in the UK have suggested that return to work is quicker after 'their operation'.[483] Rider et al. have shown that return to work correlates closely with the patient's preconceived idea.[786] Education preoperatively by the surgeon would surely be of crucial importance in influencing a patient's decision but this needs to be consistent and evidence-based. Jarrett has undertaken an important study of consultants and general practitioners' attitudes to return to work after surgery. He has demonstrated that the mean time off work recommended by general practitioners is about twice that recommended by surgeons.[464] The most recent surgical literature only adds to confusion about return to work; surgeons continue to advise early return to work while GPs, perhaps for social reasons, delay return to work.[789, 801] The only randomized study of laparoscopic hernia surgery in England also found that general practitioners' fears were an important factor in delaying return to work.[113]

The key to early return to work after surgery probably rests with the surgeon: his explanation has more impact than an explanation from the general practitioner. The economic advantages of early return to employment clearly have an important role in resuming work after surgery.

Driving should be prohibited for seven days or so after hernia repair, not for reasons of recurrence but because the foot reaction time does not return to normal before then.

Further research on return to work and social activity is summarized on page 193.

Conclusions

Day-case surgery is clinically feasible for most children with hernias and for at least 30% of adults with primary hernias.

Day-case surgery requires technical and organizational excellence if the long-term results are going to be worthwhile and if complications are to be avoided.

After surgery, early return to work should be encouraged. We all need educating in the benefits of modern surgical technology.

Despite the clear demonstration of the feasibility and clinical excellence of day-case and short-stay surgery for inguinal hernias, the average duration of stay in most hospitals remains above the 3.7 days reported from the Middlesex Hospital in 1985 and the 4.3 days reported from North Tees General Hospital in 1986. Both of these units are in areas of urban deprivation, suggesting that the behavioural attitudes of the surgeons rather than the social circumstances of the population served need modification.

5 ECONOMICS OF HERNIA REPAIR

with Karen Bloor

Introduction

> It is now recognised that resources will never be adequate to support all that surgery has to offer, and that we must all be conscious of the need to make the most efficient use of what resources there are (Royal College of Surgeons 1992).[800]

Economic evaluations of new and existing healthcare interventions are an essential input into decision making. Healthcare systems around the world face steady increases in expenditure resulting from demographic change and improvements in medical technology. Increasingly, funders must choose which interventions will be provided and which will not be reimbursed from limited public funds. This creates difficult choices, as systems are no longer limited by what is technically possible to improve the health of patients but by what is practically possible given resource constraints. In a situation where resources are scarce, all choices about who will be treated have an opportunity cost – the value of the benefit foregone. Health economics and the techniques of economic evaluation aim to maximize the amount of health which is produced within the scarce resources available.

It is no longer sufficient to consider the clinical or therapeutic effects of healthcare interventions: purchasing choices will be predicated on studies which identify, measure and value what is given up when an intervention is used (the cost) and what is gained (improved patient health outcomes). This requires explicit economic evaluation of healthcare interventions. This requirement is likely to increase, particularly in the UK National Health Service, as purchasers (District Health Authorities and GP fundholders) develop their role within the internal market. Purchasers have a fixed budget and are aware of the opportunity costs of interventions. Increasingly they are likely to require evidence of effectiveness and cost effectiveness, and they will develop contracts and enforce protocols to ensure this.

Economic evaluation values both inputs (costs) and outcomes (consequences) of an intervention, comparing more than one alternative. This builds upon clinical evaluations which assess efficacy (can an intervention work, in experimental circumstances?) and effectiveness (does it work, in normal clinical practice?) to assess efficiency (does it provide the greatest benefit at least cost to society?). The type of economic evaluation depends upon the outcome measure chosen:

1. Cost minimization analysis is appropriate only when the outcomes of two or more interventions have been demonstrated to be equivalent, in which case the least costly alternative is the most efficient, and only cost analysis is required.
2. Cost effectiveness analysis includes both costs and outcomes using a single outcome measure, usually a natural unit. This allows comparisons between treatments in a particular therapeutic area where effectiveness is unequal, but not between therapeutic areas where natural outcome measures differ.
3. Cost utility analysis combines multiple outcomes into a single measure of utility (e.g. a quality adjusted life year, or QALY). This allows comparisons between alternatives in different therapeutic categories with different natural outcomes.
4. Cost benefit analysis links costs and outcomes by expressing both in monetary units, forcing an explicit decision about whether an intervention is worth its cost. Various techniques have been used to attach monetary values to health outcomes, but the technique remains rare in health economics.

Technological innovation in surgery and in other areas (for example diagnostic innovation) is not regulated in the same way as innovative pharmaceutical therapies. A new pharmaceutical product is subjected to rigorous clinical trials to identify evidence of safety and efficacy, before licensing for public use by the Committee on the Safety of Medicines. Increasingly, new and existing pharmaceutical products are also subjected to well defined economic evaluation, to show evidence of effectiveness and efficiency. Guidelines issued by the Department of Health state that 'the economic evaluation of pharmaceuticals should become part of taking decisions about treatment', and set out clear guidelines regarding how a high-quality economic evaluation should be carried out.[234]

The careful procedures that control the introduction of innovative pharmaceutical products are essential for innovative surgical and diagnostic therapies. How, then, should technological innovations such as laparoscopic surgery be introduced? All such pioneering innovations should be evaluated in well designed trials. There are difficulties in implementing randomized controlled trials of surgical techniques due to the difficulties of blinding, but a carefully designed trial can mitigate these problems. Clinical trials protect the safety of patients and ensure that new technologies produce effective healthcare. Economic evaluations ensure that such health gains are purchased at least cost. The guidelines applied to pharmaceutical products, intended to protect society's health and scarce resources, should also be applied to surgical innovations.

The principle of evaluating innovative surgical interventions was accepted by the Department of Health in a press release in 1995, which announced that major innovations were to be 'scrutinised, evaluated and then, if approved, fast tracked throughout the health service'.[235] A major advance should, under a new system, be subjected to clinical trials and a central register would give information on approved operations. The register could then be consulted by purchasers as a measure of the effectiveness of various operations and procedures. This register, the Safety and Efficacy Register of New Interventional Procedures (SERNIP), is managed by the Academy of Medical Royal Colleges, and funded by the Department of Health. Doctors are asked to register new techniques which they intend to pilot, and to check the register to discover the current status of new invasive procedures.[112] An advisory committee convened by SERNIP will then assess all known data and assign the procedure to one of four categories:

1. Safety and efficacy unsatisfactory – procedure must not be used.
2. Safety and efficacy established – procedure can be used.
3. The procedure is sufficiently similar to one of established safety and efficacy to raise no reasonable doubts and can be used.
4. Safety and efficacy is not established. Controlled evaluation is needed.

The proposed system is voluntary and clinically controlled and in time economic evaluation of innovative invasive procedures will be required, as is the case for pharmaceutical products.

Economics of hernia repair

Hernia repair is an established and effective procedure, and its relatively low cost amongst surgical procedures means that economic evaluation of the procedure itself is no longer a priority. Hernias create pain and discomfort for patients and limit ability to work or carry out other productive activities. While the increased risk of

Table 5.1 Health status yield per £ for three selected treatments provided by the NHS, at November 1981 prices (From Hurst, 1984, with permission of the Controller of Her Majesty's Stationery Office)[446]

Treatment	Health status yield	Cost of treatment (£)	Health status yield per £'000 cost
Home haemodialysis	191.25	160 000	1.2
Successful renal transplant and subsequent maintenance	197.30	35 000	5.6
Uncomplicated hernia repair	5.53	420	13.2

surgical procedures in elderly people means that repair of some small direct hernias may not be mandatory, there would seem to be clear clinical and economic arguments in favour of carrying out hernia repairs amongst the majority of the working population.[801]

Hurst, a health economist, has compared the benefits and costs of hernia repair with the benefits and costs of home dialysis for renal failure, and with the benefits and costs of a successful renal transplant. Drawing on a measure of health status which measures two dimensions of health (disability and distress), and using DHSS cost data, Hurst calculates the health status yield per pound sterling for the three selected treatments. Using this cost-benefit equation, uncomplicated hernia repair comes out better than a successful renal transplant and a renal transplant is better value than continuous home haemodialysis.[446] Memories of Cecil Wakeley's (1940)[958] aphorism crowd in to confirm that refined clinical judgement may well be as valuable in evaluating the benefits of clinical care as the statistical gymnastics of contemporary health economists!

Innovations in the procedure of hernia repair and the management of patients should, however, be subject to economic evaluation, ideally based upon a randomized controlled trial. Recent developments in hernia repair include the expansion of day-case surgery and the introduction of laparoscopic hernia repair. These developments require a clinical and economic evidence base.

Economics of day-case surgery

Reductions in length of stay for many surgical and other in-patient procedures result from improvements in surgical procedures reducing recovery time, changing preferences of patients, and financial and political pressures on hospitals to reduce costs, increase activity and reduce waiting times. Day-case surgery is often preferred by patients, and it may encourage early mobilization and reduce the risk of hospital-acquired infection.[805]

Day-case treatment for hernia repair may result in good outcomes for lower costs than other organizational forms of care.[120, 804] The Royal College of Surgeons recommends that at least 30% of elective hernioplasties should be performed on a day-case basis.[800]

Length of in-patient stay generally has a positive relationship with the costs of a hospital episode, and so reducing length of stay should reduce average costs per hospital episode.[241] However, this may not translate into overall cost savings for a healthcare purchaser, for the following reasons:

1. Costs may be shifted from hospitals to primary and community care, with more GP visits and higher use of community nursing services, particularly for elderly patients. This was illustrated by Russell *et al.*, with day-case patients receiving slightly more GP consultations and considerably more district nurse visits than long-stay patients (5.96 compared with 1.79).[807] Economic evaluations should therefore consider a patient episode longer than just in-patient stay, by including costs of readmission and costs and benefits elsewhere in the healthcare system.
2. For a surgical in-patient episode, the most resource-intensive period is at the beginning of the stay, when surgery and initial recovery takes place. This means that reducing length of stay may create fewer cost savings than anticipated – reducing in-patient stay from ten days to five will not halve costs.
3. A reduction in the demand for hospital beds may not result in cash savings, unless it allows ward closures. In most cases, reducing length of stay enables more activity, from faster throughput of patients, which is likely to increase overall financial costs.[241]
4. More patients may become eligible for surgery if social and domestic barriers are removed, and less invasive procedures reduce the threshold for services.[120]

Economic appraisal is unlike surgical decision-making. Economists analyse the results of their interventions by comparing them within different scenarios: as the scenarios change – employment prospects, labour relations – the economics change too! Surgeons are used to evaluating their outcomes over time with the scenario held constant. For instance, with day-case surgery and a constant surgeon-related scenario, one impact of shortening the patients' stay will be empty beds – which the surgeon will perceive as the currency of an 'efficiency saving'. The economist would not call this a 'saving'; the concept of 'opportunity cost' means that no 'benefit' has accrued until the empty beds (resources) are put to some alternative use. 'Benefit' is thus not necessarily the same to the surgeon as to the economist.

Any economic appraisal of day-case surgery must, therefore, first address the crucial issue of 'benefit'. Are the benefits to be:

1. More surgery – using the freed resources to undertake a greater volume of surgery or more complex innovative surgery?
2. A redeployment of the freed resources towards a different client group, for example elderly or mentally ill people?
3. A reduction in overall health service expenditure by the amount saved?

A day-case surgery policy will need to be appraised in the 'short run' and the 'long run'. Short-run benefits may be very difficult to gain; for instance, a reduction in surgical bed requirements by 15 may confer no benefit since you cannot knock down half a 30-bed ward and reduce staff costs by 50% overnight! While there may be no short-run gains, the long-run gains could be substantial and allow explicit alterations to existing surgical and nursing practice. Consequently new hospital provision could include less traditional in-patient surgical wards and instead have dedicated day-case units.

Stepping through the looking-glass, more day-case surgery will need less capital expenditure on surgical in-patient facilities, and fewer nursing staff will need employing for the same volume of work in the long term.

The quantification of savings accruing from a day-case policy is difficult; four approaches have been advanced:

1. Comparing the bills paid by patients in private practice (Rockwell, 1982).[791]
2. The analytical device of holding the level of service constant and estimating the benefits that could be bought with the now unused resources (Russell *et al.*, 1977).[807]
3. The technique of comparing average *per diem* in-patient and out-patient costs.[136] Farquharson (1955) produced the seminal paper advocating this type of economic evaluation.[292]
4. Comparing and computing the one-year costs of a day-care facility with the one-year costs of a traditional in-patient unit.[799]

In the North American literature, where direct patient billing on an item for service basis is the norm, it is possible to compare the charges which patients pay for different durations of stay. Flanagan and Bascom (1981),[307] Coe (1981)[184] and Rockwell (1982)[791] compared costings of day-case inguinal hernia repair with in-patient repair and reported substantial savings ranging to 70%. Rockwell reported the financial benefits of out-patient surgery for hernia in the Deaconess Hospital, Spokane, Washington, USA. In a series of 50 men operated between 1977 and 1981, 42 were returned home the evening of operation. General, spinal and local anaesthesia were used and patients were not discharged unless they were drinking and voiding satisfactorily. The best results were in middle-aged males with unilateral indirect hernia repair. Only one patient with a bilateral repair returned home the same evening. The average hospital bill for the last 10 patients in the series was $617, compared with an average cost of $1119 for a control group having traditional in-patient care. This represents savings of $502 per patient (at 1981 prices). Rockwell now employs out-patient management for all his inguinal hernia repairs in adults (Table 5.2).

This approach has economic cogency if viewed from the perspective of the paying patient, but the price paid may in part reflect the economic stance of the institution, profit making or not, as well as being influenced by outside regulatory bodies – Medicare in the USA and a provident association in the UK.

Russell et al. (1977) conducted a randomized prospective study of day-case versus in-patient care for inguinal hernia repair and haemorrhoidectomy.[807] They included in their analysis the costs to the hospital and the community medical and nursing services, and the direct and indirect costs to the patients (of extra amenities for home convalescence, spouse off-work support, transportation to visit in-patients, etc.). Holding the level of service constant, if day-case surgery allowed closure of a ward, each four days of convalescence in hospital forgone would save £24 per patient. Alternatively, if day-case avoided the construction of a new ward, four days of postoperative care would be worth £33. They estimated the costs of additional community medical and nursing support at £4; thus savings to the NHS would be between £20 and £29 per patient (all at 1974 prices). Furthermore, the tangible and intangible costs to the patients were similar whether they were given day-care or traditional in-patient care. The duration of time off work was not related to duration of hospitalization. In overall terms their results suggest that day-case surgery for the conditions studied may lead to cost reductions of the order of 40–50%.

Burn (1983), using NHS per diem average costings, estimated the 7488 minor surgical cases treated in Southampton as 48 h in-patients at a cost of £1 686 148, whereas if they had been treated as day cases the overall cost would be £409 893, a saving of £1 276 255. A day case costing £54.74 compared with a 48 h in-patient costing of £225.18, a net gain of 75%. Although this approach can be challenged on methodological grounds,

particularly because the various components of the hospital budget are too many and too diverse and the differences in service intensity on different in-patient days too great to allow an average per diem calculation to adequately reflect an individual patient cost profile, there is no doubt that immense savings would follow a transfer of minor surgery from in-patient to day-case status. Burn correctly estimates that 50% of district general hospital surgery could be done on a day-case basis, with staggering savings on a national scale.[136]

In a quasi-controlled study of paediatric surgical day care, Evans and Robinson (1980), in Vancouver, found a resource saving of 60% when compared with more traditional surgical practice.[288] Their technique of attributing costs is similar to disease costing recently introduced in the UK and should enable different operative strategies to be compared. The problem of the different tangible and intangible costs borne by patients which were measured directly by Russell and co-workers is bypassed by the 'revealed preference' argument: the patients preferred day care when given the option; therefore it must economically be at least as good as in-patient care.

Direct comparison of the personnel costs (in 1985 prices) of an operating suite open 24 hours a day, 365 days a year, with an operating suite open 8 a.m. to 5 p.m. five days a week shows that the unit open 45 hours per week saves £121 178 (£160 961 – £39 783) (75% of costs). Similarly, comparing a five-day ward with a traditional always-open ward gives nursing cost savings of 65%. The argument for day-case 30 min operations from a dedicated five-day ward and theatre has sound financial support.[242]

Bailey, an economist from the Audit Commission in the UK, has proposed an alternative strategy to determine the resources that might be released as a result of a change from in-patient to day-case while treating an equivalent patient. He states that the costs of day surgery are substantially less than in-patient care but it is misleading to interpret such measures as 'savings'. The resource implications of more day surgery should be estimated directly by looking at precisely what changes are planned to take place.[57]

In conclusion, there is evidence that the unit costs of day-case surgery are much lower than in-patient care of the order of 40–75% per treatment episode, however calculated. These lower unit costs will free resources to do more surgery or for alternative uses. Day-case surgery has been found to be superior to in-patient surgery in terms of wound infection and return to work, although this finding is not statistically significant.[174] Day-case surgery is also becoming increasingly acceptable to patients. A dedicated five-day care unit allows more resources to be saved compared with day cases in a traditional theatre suite and ward where all the resources cannot easily be redeployed, particularly in the short run. This is consistent with the conclusions of a US

Table 5.2 Cost comparison of out-patient vs. in-patient repair of inguinal hernia (From Devlin, 1985, by courtesy of the Royal College of Surgeons of England)[242]

Reference	Out-patient costs ($)	In-patient costs ($)	Savings ($)
Rockwell (1982)[789]	617	1119	502
Coe (1981)[179]	398	1168	770
Flanagan and Bascom (1981)[301]	300	1000	700

review of cost effectiveness of management of hernia by Millikan and Deziel (1996).[655] These authors concluded that the most cost effective approach to hernia repair would use an ambulatory surgical centre with open mesh repair for primary inguinal hernia and failed primary suture repair.[655]

INCENTIVES AND DAY-CASE HERNIOPLASTY

To date, resource savings from day-case surgery in the NHS have largely been used to expand surgical services either quantitatively or qualitatively. Every hospital experienced this phenomenon in the 1970s. It has been quantified and shown that as resources are liberated by day-case work they are used up in other surgical endeavours. This extra work sucks in further resources and the overall surgical budget becomes larger.

Increasing the proportion of day cases in the surgical unit mix will lead to a fall in the average cost of each patient treated. This may enable more cases to be operated upon, and even though the marginal costs of doing each extra case within normal working hours are low the aggregated cost to the hospital will be higher, although greater demand will initially be met and the queue reduced. If there is no queue and no excess demand, reducing the costs should allow premises to be closed and staff made redundant, with considerable reduction in fixed and estate costs and in wages. The cost of doing an extra case after-hours in a day-case unit, when staff must be paid overtime, is a very high marginal price – a fact to be remembered when case scheduling is considered.

If day-case surgery is used to cut unit costs and increase the overall volume of surgery, this extra burden of rising productivity will fall on the surgeons and nurses. There are reports of the proportion of day cases

Table 5.3 Theatre and ward costs (From Devlin, 1985, by courtesy of the Royal College of Surgeons of England)[242]

Theatre	Open 24h per day 365 days per year, 168h per week (£)	Open 8 a.m.–5 p.m. Monday to Friday 45h per week (£)
Cost per year		
Medical staff	25 594	10 923
Nursing staff	131 367	28 860
Total	160 961	39 783
Cost of 30 min operation	17472 per year[a]	9.21
Cost of 30 min operation (4160 per year[b])	38.69	9.57

[a] The cost of a 30 min operation is similar if the theatres are 100% used for a 'night shift' in addition to 100% occupancy of the daytime. The staffing assumptions of these calculations may be obtained from the author.
[b] Low utilization of fully staffed operating theatres dramatically increases the unit costs of each operation episode.

rising to close to 40%, in some units, with consequent increases in surgical throughputs. Ultimately the increased output may demand an alteration on the supply side of the equation, and more doctors and nurses may then need to be employed to cope with increased demand.[242] While the relation between demand and output of a surgical service is elastic in the short term, in the longer term supply inevitably must be increased to allow greater output.

It must be apparent that there is no economic incentive for surgeons and other hospital employees to expand day-case surgery. Substantial savings can only be achieved by maintaining constant the quantity of surgery done, not allowing day cases to increase the output, and by closing premises and dismissing redundant staff. Such a policy is unlikely to make surgeons who take up day-case surgery popular!

Economics of laparoscopic surgery

The introduction and rapid diffusion of laparoscopic surgical techniques since the pioneering laparoscopic removal of a gall bladder by the French surgeon Phillippe Mouret in 1987 has been accepted with 'unbridled enthusiasm' and often without question by surgeons, the media and the general public. 'Keyhole surgery' techniques continue to be developed, and laparoscopic hernia repair is gaining acceptance in surgical practice, without adequate clinical and economic evaluation.

Laparoscopic surgery has spread rapidly through many surgical specialties, and there are major knowledge gaps about its clinical and economic attributes. Searches of clinical literature reveal a large number of papers about laparoscopic surgery, but many of these studies are of small numbers of patients, with insufficient follow-up, very narrow clinical endpoints and little measurement of the cost consequences of these techniques. There have been few large-scale multicentre pragmatic trials involving a broad range of clinicians in different environments. Making policy decisions which result in the transfer of substantial amounts of resources on the basis of small studies carried out by enthusiasts in the field is likely to be inefficient and inappropriate.[655] One of the consequences of this unevaluated adoption of laparoscopic cholecystectomy as 'the gold standard'[877] has been an unprecedented rise in cholecystectomy rate and thus increased cost.[547]

Some 'economic' arguments have been used to support the rapid diffusion of laparoscopic surgery. Studies often quote reductions in the length of in-patient hospital stay in comparison with standard surgical procedures and imply that this will necessarily save hospitals money. This is, however, not necessarily the case, and hospital managers are increasingly questioning the appropriateness of procedures which involve purchase of sophisticated and expensive capital equipment and considerably increased theatre time, resulting in lower patient throughput for surgical procedures. Available time in the operating theatre is a scarce resource, and although operating time in laparoscopic surgery declines as experience increases, Cuschieri (1994) estimates that on average it will continue to take about one-third longer than the corresponding conventional operation, with the excess of time over open surgery the higher the more complicated the basic operation.[208]

The effect of length of in-patient stay on health service resource use is an important issue in many studies. Cuschieri (1994) estimates that discharge may on average be expected to be less than 48 h.[208] This is thought to result in cost savings from earlier discharge and earlier return to normal activities including work; however, economists such as Sculpher (1993) note that this may not always be the case.[840] Firstly, a reduction in the demand for hospital beds may not result in cash savings, unless it allows ward closures. This is unlikely as laparoscopic surgery represents a small proportion of all hospital procedures and as conventional surgical backup facilities are need for procedures that result in complications. In addition, laparoscopy does not release other resources used for surgical procedures, particularly theatre time, and some laparoscopic procedures replace non-invasive therapies rather than open surgery. Also, many studies concentrate on initial hospitalizations, ignoring readmission rates. It is important to remember that lengths of in-patient stay have been falling for many years, and the additional savings from laparoscopic surgery may be lower than anticipated.

Complication rates are an important determinant of the overall costs of any surgical procedure. Complications with laparoscopic surgery procedures, such as bile duct injuries with laparoscopic cholecystectomy, have been well documented (4–10, see Table 1 from Soper et al. (1994)[877]). Most bile duct injuries have also occurred early in a surgeon's experience, highlighting the need for careful training and accreditation of surgeons, and clinical practice guidelines.[841] The rate of

conversions from laparoscopic operations to open operations ranges from 1.8 to 8.5%, and tends to be highest early in a surgeon's experience.[877] The cost implications of complication rates include increased operating time, increased length of in-patient stay, increased care burden on families or other carers and increased time for the patient to return to work or normal activities.

A recent systematic review of the effectiveness and safety of laparoscopic cholecystectomy showed that effectiveness of this procedure is similar to that of open and mini-cholecystectomy.[269] Complete alleviation of symptoms was achieved in 60–70% of patients. However, safety profiles differ, with more technical support and specialized surgical equipment required for the laparoscopic procedure. Differences in complication rates were difficult to assess because of methodological problems and differences between studies. In particular, studies often do not have sufficient statistical power to identify clinically important differences in outcomes, particularly bile duct injury, because the rate of adverse events is low.

Sculpher (1993)[840] argues that laparoscopic surgery has a different 'production function' to conventional surgical techniques – i.e. it requires a different mix of inputs to the production process – more inputs of theatre and medical staff time, more sophisticated equipment, and less inputs of inpatient bed days (see Figure 5.1). The overall effect on hospital costs and on overall costs to society is unclear, and requires economic evaluation. Evaluation should be long term, in order to include any effects of different readmission rates, and should include not only hospital costs and effects but also the burden on community based services, patients and carers, which may change due to earlier discharge.[840]

The 'production function' description of surgery is useful in considering other issues. The appropriate level of individual and centre specialization should be determined by evidence of economies of scale. If a centre specializes in laparoscopic surgery, this may influence costs per patient, as theatre time may be reduced as familiarity with the procedure increases. In addition,

Table 5.4   Results of laparoscopic cholecystectomy[840]

Study	Year of study	No. of patients	Procedures converted to open operations	Mortality	Major complications*	Common bile-duct injury
Larson et al.[528]	1992	1963	4.5	0.1	2.1	0.3
Southern Surgeons Club[913]	1991	1518	4.7	0.07	1.5	0.5
Cuschieri et al.[209]	1991	1236	3.6	0	1.6	0.3
Soper et al.[877]	1992	618	2.9	0	1.6	0.2
Spaw et al.[884]	1991	500	1.8	0	1.0	0
Lillemoe et al.[569]	1992	400	4.0	0	5.0	0.5
Wolfe et al.[993]	1991	381	3.0	0.9	3.4	0

* These include myocardial and cerebrovascular events, pneumonia, haemorrhage, bile leakage and iatrogenic injury to the bile duct or bowel.

Inputs   **Outcomes**

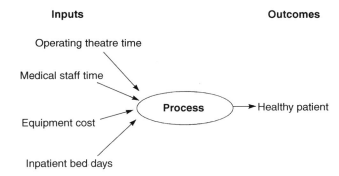

Figure 5.1   A surgical production function (source: Sculpher, 1993[840])

outcomes may be improved, particularly by reduced complication rates. However, the appropriate level of individual and centre specialization requires careful evaluation: could the alleged benefits of centralization be matched by careful training and treatment protocols at local levels? Identification of the conditions necessary for the production of efficient laparoscopic procedures is absent but inhibits neither unsubstantiated assertions by policy makers nor significant investments in new facilities.

Laparoscopic hernia repair

Laparoscopic hernia repair is currently being adopted in many centres, although its potential clinical and economic benefits are particularly unclear.[535] Soper *et al.* (1994) describe laparoscopic inguinal hernia repair as an 'operation gaining acceptance'.[877] Several techniques for laparoscopic hernia repair have been used, including closure or plugging of the hernia and various types of patch repairs, most commonly a tension-free mesh. Laparoscopic repair of inguinal hernias, unlike other laparoscopic procedures that duplicate traditional open surgical approaches, represents a departure from standard hernia repair. It requires the use of general anaesthesia, with its associated risks, whereas the conventional procedure can be done under local anaesthetic. There is also a small risk of serious injury to intra-abdominal organs that is not associated with the open procedure.[855] This shows parallels with laparoscopic cholecystectomy, and the associated risk of bile duct injury; therefore learning curve effects are likely to apply. During the learning process the procedures take longer, and there may be an increased risk to the patient. Complication rates are generally higher for surgeons less familiar with the technique of laparoscopic surgery, and this applies across specialties. See *et al.*[841] have evaluated the relationship between complication rates and surgeon-dependent variables following a laparoscopic training course, finding a significant inverse correlation between complication rates of individual surgeons and the number of laparoscopic procedures performed,

concluding that the rate of complications associated with the clinical learning curve can be reduced by additional education following an initial course in laparoscopy.[841]

A number of studies have investigated the effectiveness of laparoscopic versus open inguinal hernia repair, but only a minority of these studies used randomized controlled trials. Stoker *et al.* (1994)[895] randomized 150 UK patients to laparoscopic or open hernia repair. The laparoscopic procedure took significantly longer for unilateral repairs (50 min compared with 35 min for the open procedure). There was a downward trend in operating times as experience was gained with the new technique. The study reported reduced pain in laparoscopic repair (less self-administered analgesia and better pain analogue scores), earlier return to normal activity (3 days vs. 7 days) and earlier return to work (7 days vs. 14 days).[535]

These positive outcomes are not supported by an Australian randomized study of 86 day case patients by Maddern *et al.* (1994).[596] Operative time was similar for both procedures (30 min for the open group and 35 for the laparoscopic group), but open patients were discharged after a significantly shorter time than laparoscopic patients (135 min vs. 225 min). During the follow-up period there were two recurrent hernias and one small bowel obstruction in the laparoscopic group. Pain scores, activity levels, analgesia requirements and time to return to work were not significantly different following surgery in either group, leading the authors to conclude that 'the added cost of laparoscopic hernia repair at this stage does not warrant its widespread use in unilateral hernia repairs.'[596]

Payne *et al.* (1994)[726] randomized 100 patients to laparoscopic or open inguinal herniorrhaphy, finding similar operative and hospitalization times, but faster return to work for laparoscopic patients (9 vs. 17 days). Again, laparoscopic repair was considerably more expensive than open repair (US$3093 (£2062) vs. US$2494 (£1663)).

Barkun *et al.* (1995) reported results of 92 patients randomized at two Canadian hospitals.[63] Time in the operating theatre was reported to be similar, but the duration of time for which the anaesthetist was responsible for the patient was longer for the laparoscopic group (132 min vs. 109 min). There was no detectable statistical difference between groups with respect to duration of hospitalization and convalescence. The laparoscopic group may have had slightly less pain after operation, but similar percentages of patients complained of discomfort at seven-day follow-up, and there was no significant difference in the perioperative change in quality of life at seven days. After one month, improvement in quality of life was shown to be greater in the laparoscopic group using the Nottingham Health Profile, but this was not observed using a visual analogue scale. Total direct costs were found to be on average CN$1223.84 (around £612) for the open group and CN$1718.12 (£860) for the laparoscopic group.

Finally, Lawrence et al. (1996) used a UK randomized controlled trial as the basis of an economic evaluation of laparoscopic versus open inguinal hernia repair, on data collected from 104 day-case patients.[535] The mean total health service cost of laparoscopic repair was £1074 vs. £489 for open repair. Linking this additional cost with the additional pain-free days in the laparoscopic group showed an additional cost per pain free day of £109 (95% CI £41–393). The authors concluded that there were strong arguments against the introduction of laparoscopic hernia repair until evidence on long-term outcomes becomes available.

A literature review and survey questionnaire carried out by the American Medical Association also investigated the appropriateness of laparoscopic herniorrhaphy for inguinal hernias. Reviewing evidence and presenting this to 75 panellists with a special interest in laparoscopic surgery or hernias, the procedure was rated as 'promising' in terms of safety and 'investigational' in terms of effectiveness for repair of primary inguinal and bilateral inguinal hernias. The repair of recurrent inguinal hernias was rated as investigational in terms of safety and effectiveness. Nine per cent of the responders (4/47) said that they would prefer the laparoscopic technique (with mesh) for repair of their own small unilateral inguinal hernia, while the remaining 91% (43/47) would prefer repair by inguinal incision (with or without mesh). These percentages were similar, whether or not the respondents had ever performed a herniorrhaphy using a laparoscopic technique.[460]

These clinical and economic studies do not support the rapid diffusion of laparoscopic techniques which has occurred in other procedures. Clinical benefits are uncertain, particularly given the additional risk of general anaesthesia compared to local anaesthetic, and the potential for injury to intra-abdominal organs. Both these risks are small, and the possible serious adverse events are only likely to be shown in large sample randomized trials, or meta-analysis of such trials. In a review of laparoscopic cholecystectomy, Downs et al. revealed the problem of small studies with insufficient statistical power to identify small but clinically important differences in the rate of adverse events. This problem applies equally in the area of laparoscopic hernia repair.[269]

The economic arguments which may be weak for other laparoscopic procedures are almost non-existent for laparoscopic hernia repair. There is no potential for reducing in-patient stay, as the open procedure can be carried out on a day-case basis. Time in the operating theatre appears to be longer, and the only real economic benefit is a possibility of slightly faster return to work and normal activities. This benefit may offset some of the additional costs, but only if a perspective broader than that of the NHS is adopted.

Mistakes made in the rapid diffusion of laparoscopic techniques with inadequate evaluation in other specialties should not be repeated in hernia repair. Surgical innovations should be based on evidence rather than enthusiasm, and managed into practice only in ways which ensure the safe, effective and efficient treatment of patients. If surgeons fail to manage innovations into practice efficiently, central regulators and local purchasers are likely to impose surgical protocols to do so.

Conclusions

It is no longer sufficient to consider only the clinical and therapeutic effects of healthcare: purchasing choices require explicit economic evaluation to identify, measure and value costs and patient health outcomes. Surgical interventions are no exception to this.

Hernia repair is an established and effective procedure for most patient groups, and its relatively low cost amongst surgical procedures means that economic evaluation of the procedure itself is not a priority. However, innovations in the procedure of hernia repair and the management of patients, such as day case and laparoscopic hernia repair, should be subject to economic evaluation.

The unit costs of day-case surgery are lower than those of traditional in-hospital care. Any money saved will enable more operations to be done and more patients to be treated. Alternatively, savings generated could be used to develop other services.

Laparoscopic surgery has spread rapidly through many surgical specialties but there are still major knowledge gaps about its clinical and economic attributes. The potential clinical and economic benefits of laparoscopic hernia repair are particularly unclear given the need for general anaesthesia and the possibility of rare but serious injuries to intra-abdominal organs. This procedure should not be adopted widely without large-scale clinical trials and economic evaluations.

6 PRINCIPLES IN HERNIA SURGERY

General principles

There are three principles which dictate the management of all abdominal wall hernia patients.

1. The patient must be resuscitated. The continued mortality from hernia operations, particularly the mortality and morbidity of strangulated femoral hernias in older women, is almost entirely due to operating when the patient is in a less than optimal physiological condition. Hernias never require emergency surgery, although they may require urgent surgery as soon as the patient is rendered fit. To operate before adequate rehydration and renal function is restored, or before the cardiorespiratory status is assessed and stabilized, is to court disaster.[9,15] Four or five hours of careful resuscitation may be needed in the most ill patients.[128] Even in the very elderly mortality can be reduced to a minimum; death is usually a result of complications of the strangulated hernia rather than associated diseases which should have been adequately treated before the urgent operation.[327] For elective hernia repair the same golden principle applies – do not operate until the patient has been fully assessed and is in an optimum physiological state. An analysis of 175 patients with ages greater than 66 years, of whom 58% were ASA grade III or higher, revealed that elective or urgent operation can be carried out with zero mortality, provided prompt diagnosis and treatment of primary systemic diseases is performed. Appropriate anaesthesia, such as local anaesthetic or epidural anaesthesia, should be given careful consideration in those not fit for general anaesthesia. Thus, severe systemic disease that limits activity but is not incapacitating is not a contraindication for elective groin hernia repair.[340] *Temporis medicina fere est*: 'The art of medicine is a question of timeliness': Ovid.
2. The contents must be reduced after inspection at open operation and following careful inspection for viability. If strangulation has occurred infarcted contents resected. The dangers of forcible reduction of contents into an inadequate cavity when there is 'lack of storage capacity of the abdominal cavity' or when organs have lost the right of domain must be appreciated (see pages 243, 244).
3. The defect must be repaired. In all abdominal wall hernias the principle is to repair each layer of the defect discreetly or reinforce weak layers with mesh to restore the patient's anatomy so that it resembles the normal unoperated condition. The process of repair in aponeurosis is slow. Only tendinous/aponeurotic/fascial structures can be successfully sutured together: suturing red fleshy muscle to tendon or fascia will not contribute to permanent union of these structures. Nor will it reconstruct anything resembling the normal anatomy!

Haemostasis

Careful haemostasis and tissue handling is most important if haematoma formation and sepsis are to be avoided. Larger vessels, especially the veins in the subcutaneous fat, should be carefully ligated, taking care not to leave large stumps of tissue to undergo absorption. For ligatures, metric 3.5 braided polyglycolic acid (Dexon) or metric 3.5 braided polyglactin 910 (Vicryl) are used. Chromic catgut is not recommended because of its adverse effect on wound healing (see below). Diathermy is employed for haemostasis in small vessels.

Haematomas are more likely to occur if local anaesthesia with adrenaline is used, and extra care with haemostasis is then advised. Closed suction drains are strongly recommended whenever there is extensive dissection, particularly if there is 'dead space' in which haematoma or serum may collect. The use of closed suction drains can significantly improve wound healing and convalescence.[79] When large incisional hernias are repaired, suction drains are mandatory.

Sepsis

Sepsis is the great hazard to hernioplasty, particularly when non-absorbable suture material is used. Scrupulous surgical technique is vital if infection is to be avoided. The skin may be covered at the site of operation with sterile adherent film, which is not removed until the wound is closed.[274] Sutures should not be used to close the skin, for by their very nature they have potential for introducing bacteria into the subcutaneous tissue along their tracks.[26] Postoperative wound infection increases the rate of hernia recurrence by a factor of four.[248, 348]

Wound healing

Important variables in hernia repair are the rate at which the aponeurosis regains strength and the stability of the healing process. Many of the factors that regulate wound healing are under the control of the surgeon, and an appreciation of their effects and their clinical significance can aid in the proper care of the patient.

Much of the data on wound healing have been gathered by animal experimentation; there are, however, important species differences in animals and care must be exercised in translating all animal research directly into clinical practice. For example, catgut skin closure in dogs is characterized by a rapid gain in wound strength with little cellular reaction, whereas in rats and rabbits there is a slow gain in strength and a most intense cellular reaction to catgut skin sutures.[950]

The pioneering work on the maturation and development of tensile strength in wounds was reported by Howes and his group in 1933. They reported the healing of experimental skin, fascial, muscle and gastric wounds in dogs. They observed a lag phase extending from wounding until the fifth or sixth day. During the lag phase the wound appeared quiescent, the wound strength did not increase and wound apposition was maintained by the sutures only (Figure 6.1).[438, 439]

Next there was a phase of fibroplasia, during which wound strength increased rapidly, reaching a maximum around the fourteenth to sixteenth day.

Howes mentioned a third phase – the maturation phase – which he did not study longitudinally. He attributed much of the restoration of mechanical strength to the fibroblastic phase. In this he was mistaken: had he studied the maturation phase he would have discovered that this late phase, rather than the fibroblastic phase, was critical in the healing of aponeurotic wounds.

Douglas (1952) studied the rate of tensile strength gain of incisions in the lumbodorsal aponeurosis of rabbits. He found that the rate of tensile strength was slow, much slower than earlier reports suggested – about 50% of the original strength was gained at 50 days and only 80% regained at one year postoperatively.[266, 267] Mason and Allen (1941) had made similar observations on the healing of tendons. They observed that if the tendon was rested the rate of gain in strength during the maturation phase was slower than if active motion was permitted,[620] this observation providing a sound experimental basis for advocating early ambulation in hernia surgery.

The lag (or latent) phase extends from the time of wounding until the fourth to sixth day in humans. During this phase the inflammatory reaction prepares the wound for subsequent healing by removing debris, necrotic tissue and bacteria. At the same time there is mobilization and migration of fibroblasts and epithelial cells and accumulation of non-collagenous proteins and glycoproteins. During the lag phase only the gluing of the fibrin holds the wound edges together This point needs stressing. At this stage, wound security is a property of the suture material not the tissue.

At about the fourth to sixth post-wounding day, proliferating fibroblasts begin to synthesize collagen, mucopolysaccharides and glycoproteins. This is the fibroblastic stage of repair. The collagen quickly aggregates into fibres. Once this production of collagen commences there is the most rapid increase in the tensile strength of the wound.

As the fibroblastic phase runs down, the phase of maturation begins. During this, further wound strength gain is due to intra- and intermolecular collagen remodelling and cross-linking. This remodelling takes six months to a year for completion. Probably it is the failure of this remodelling that accounts for the late appearance of incisional hernias in healed laparotomy wounds.[283, 392, 950]

To obtain optimal repair in hernia wounds it is necessary to incise the aponeurosis or fascia prior to suturing it. Incised fascial and aponeurotic wounds heal faster and are ultimately considerably stronger than invaginated or infolded aponeurotic or fascial wounds. This is because incision of tissues initiates the normal cascade healing mechanisms which ultimately lead to formation of organized collagen and mature strong connective tissue. Invagination with interrupted or running suture causes areas of local ischaemia with disorganized healing and defects of collagen formation which can become apparent as areas of weakness with potential for recurrence of hernia. Continuous suturing of aponeurosis by spreading tension gives better ultimate healing than interrupted sutures. Aponeurotic wound healing is accelerated if there has been previous recent wounding.

The rate of wound healing and the ultimate tensile strength of wounds is adversely affected by severe

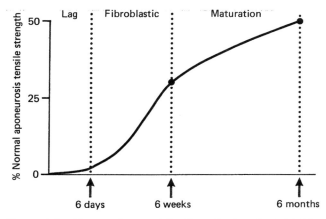

Figure 6.1 Phases of wound healing. During the initial lag phase the wound is quiescent and during the fibroplastic phase wound strength increases rapidly over a few days; however, it is in the third, maturation, phase that significant and permanent strength gain occurs

protein deficiency, vitamin C deficiency, prolonged hypo-volaemia, increased blood viscosity, intravascular coagulation, cold vasoconstriction and chronic stress. Hypoxia, some drugs, irradiation and other factors can be critical in wound healing. For the surgeon, the most important variables are suture strength to maintain wound apposition until collagen synthesis is well advanced and exercise of the healing tendon or aponeurosis which speeds the entire process.[312, 620, 825, 830]

Sutures

'The material used for sutures is probably not very important' observed Aird, in 1957 (Figure 6.2).[8] Forty years have now passed since Aird summarized in one sentence the choice of a suture for hernia repair.[8] During these years the dynamics of wound healing have been defined and a revolution has overtaken sutures.[38] The modern surgeon should choose a suture according to objective biological data and marry biological science to surgical craft. Naturally occurring sutures – silk, linen and catgut – are obsolete; synthetic fibres are today's choice.[899]

Prior to this revolution a wide variety of materials were used for surgical sutures and ligatures. Silk was Halsted's favourite suture in the 1880s and subsequently. Marcy recommended catgut and kangaroo tendon for repairing the aponeurotic and fascial layers of hernias. Linen and cotton sutures, floss silk, strips of aponeurosis and fascia lata, even the vas deferens, have all been tried and found wanting. Halsted experimented with brass and copper wire. Silver wire and stainless steel wire have all been used at some time for hernia repair.[187]

In the past the choice of suture material was based on availability and experience. And most importantly the *obiter dicta* of a former chief decided the acolyte's initial behaviour or, as Charles Mayo has stated, experience

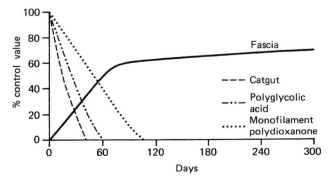

Figure 6.2 Relationship of wound strength gain to the rate of wound healing in aponeurotic wounds. Absorbable sutures do not survive long enough to ensure wound stability. Polydioxanone occupies an intermediate position between the traditional catgut and the absorbable polymers on the one hand and the non-absorbables on the other

can consist of doing the same thing wrongly over and over again. Until recently surgeons have concentrated on the mechanical properties of the suture and often paid scant attention to the interaction of the host tissue and the suture. Three postulates summarize the mechanical and biological relations of suture and tissue.[949]

1. Sutures should at least be as strong as the normal tissue through which they are placed.
2. If the tissue reduces suture strength with time, the relative rates at which the suture loses strength and the wound gains strength are important.
3. If the suture alters the biology of wound healing, the impact of this alteration is important.

If these postulates are accepted, and then applied to the healing wound, the surgeon requires information about the normal strength of the tissue, the rate of gain of strength in the wounded tissue, the strength of the suture, the rate at which the suture loses strength when embedded in tissue, and about the interaction of suture and tissue. Only after considering these factors can the surgeon proceed to account for the handling and knotting properties, the 'memory', ease of sterilization and shelf life of the suture.

The least helpful surgeon-dependent variables are tissue trauma and sepsis epitomized by Marcy in 1900: 'a wound made and maintained aseptic in well vitalized structures held at rest in easy co-option by buried sutures will be followed by a non-inflammatory primary union.'[609]

Sir Berkeley Moynihan, at the inaugural meeting of the Association of Surgeons in 1920, set out the essential conditions for sutures and ligatures which must remain within the wound.[678] Such material should ideally: (a) achieve its purpose – be sufficient to hold parts together, close a vessel, etc.; (b) disappear as soon as its work is accomplished; (c) be free from infection; (d) be non-irritant.

Sutures are either absorbable or non-absorbable and made from natural or synthetic products, distinctions that are increasingly blurred by modern polymer chemistry.

Tissues that are mainly formed of collagen/fascia/aponeurosis tend to heal slowly, so that only about 50% of their original tensile strength has been recovered at three months; thus absorbable sutures, whether natural or synthetic, do not generally persist long enough for adequate structural integrity to be restored. However, the healing curve of these tissues, a curve that reflects the laying down of collagen, is initially steep, so that fascia aponeurotic wounds of the abdominal wall closed with absorbable sutures or, more particularly, the modern synthetics, may just have enough strength to withstand disruption unless there are major forces, such as coughing, applied to them. In contrast, tissues which do not contain much structural collagen heal and gain their initial tensile strength much more rapidly, the gut being a particular example of this.[947]

The suture material must retain its strength for long enough to maintain tissue apposition and allow sound union of tissues to occur. In aponeurotic wounds a non-absorbable or very slowly absorbable suture material must therefore be employed. The inherent disadvantageous properties of non-absorbable suture materials – proneness to sepsis, adverse tissue reaction and sinus formation – have led surgeons to seek compromises for hernia repair. The unpredictability inherent in the manufacture of biological absorbable materials such as catgut and their considerable tissue reactivity in the body suggest that the use of standardized synthetic materials is preferable in modern surgical practice.[948]

Catgut was mentioned by Galen nearly 2000 years ago. It is made from the submucosa of herbivore intestine and although it is still in use today it has all the disadvantages of a natural product. Lister, in 1908, championed the use of catgut which had been soaked in chromic acid, because of its antimicrobial properties and its absorption into the body.[570] Catgut has remained in surgical use until recently and its properties in wound healing have been studied extensively. Plain catgut evokes a severe pyogenic response in tissue, which leads to a rapid loss of its tensile strength. Large plain catgut sizes are absorbed almost as fast as fine gauges, but the added intensity of reaction when thicker catgut is used delays healing, so that although thicker catgut is initially stronger the adverse effects outweigh the advantages and wounds heal less well. Chromic catgut initially provokes a slow inflammatory response, but this increases to about 10 days when foreign body giant cells appear. Once the giant cell attack commences, the chromic catgut rapidly loses strength, again before the wound has gained adequate intrinsic strength. Although catgut has good knot security in the dry state, the knots in catgut become very insecure when exposed to body tissues.[537, 538] Extruded collagen sutures have the same characteristics as catgut and do not offer any marked advantages.[478]

Clinical observations confirm the high incidence of abdominal aponeurotic wound failure when catgut alone is used, and for this reason catgut alone should never be used for abdominal wound closure or for hernia repair.[905]

Catgut is of historic interest only and has no place in modern hernia surgery.

Table 6.1 lists the properties of natural and synthetic suture material.

SYNTHETIC ABSORBABLE SUTURES

The first polymer possessing reasonable physical and biological properties was synthesized in the 1960s by Du Pont Research Laboratories. It was a braided polyester suture made of poly-L-lactide. The first commercially available absorbable synthetic suture was also a braided polyester, polyglycolic acid (PGA, Dexon), introduced in 1971. In 1974 another braided polyester suture, polyglactin 910 (Vicryl), a copolymer of lactide and glycolide, was introduced.[905]

The basic ingredients of these polymers and their eventual breakdown products are lactic acid, glycolic acid or a combination of the two. Compared with catgut and collagen these biodegradable polymer sutures have some interesting properties. Catgut and collagen are digested by cellular enzymes and, therefore, excite an intense cellular reaction which prolongs the lag phase in wound healing. The new polyester sutures degrade by hydrolysis and do not excite cellular activity; indeed they will hydrolyse similarly in vitro if placed in buffer solution at body temperature. Consequently they do not delay wound healing. Because they are synthetic materials produced under tight manufacturing controls they are also much more uniform and predictable in their dimensions and tensile strength than the biologically made natural fibres formerly used.

There are disadvantages. The polymer sutures, while they possess greater and more predictable strength than catgut or collagen, are also much harsher and stiffer fibres. These sutures have to be braided to provide good handling characteristics and carefully tied to avoid slippage on the first throw when tied. Because of their stiffness only extremely fine monofilaments can be used in surgery, their usefulness being confined to microsurgery and ophthalmology.

In order to overcome the abrasive quality of these fibres and to improve tying, coated polymer sutures have been introduced. The coating decreases the 'drag' through tissues and allows sliding of knots for better control.

Polydioxanone (PDS) is a newer more flexible polyester suture, introduced in 1981. Its greater flexibility, compared with PGA and polyglactin 910, allows it to be used as a monofilament. Like all the polyesters it degrades by hydrolysis and excites little tissue reaction; however, its rate of degradation is much slower than that of PGA or polyglactin 910. Polydioxanone suture was completely absorbed from rat muscle by 180 days versus 60–90 days for polyglactin 910 and 120 days for PGA suture. In vivo polydioxanone retains its strength for longer than other synthetic absorbable sutures: 58% versus 1–5% at four weeks and 14% versus 0% at eight weeks.[552, 773]

The place of synthetic absorbable sutures in hernioplasty is unclear. There were early favourable reports of the use of PGA sutures (Dexon) for laparotomy closure. Irvin et al. (1976) compared PGA, polyglactin and polypropylene in a randomized clinical trial. They reached the conclusion that there was little to choose between these sutures. The trial was small: 161 cases

Table 6.1 Properties of common suture materials (From Kapadia, 1983,[478] with permission)

Material	Nature	Type	Tissue response	Retention of tensile strength in vivo	Handleability	Potential advantages/ disadvantages
Catgut	Sheep submucosa	Absorbable	Inflammation more marked with plain catgut than chromic	Plain, $\frac{2}{3}$ lost in 5–6 days; chromic, $\frac{2}{3}$ lost in 10–15 days	Moderate	Unpredictable loss of tensile strength; potentiation of sepsis, although this is limited by absorption, variability of natural product
Reconstituted collagen	Sheep mucosa	Absorbable	Inflammation as with catgut	As for chromic catgut	Moderate	As for catgut but more reliable product
Polyglycolic and polyglactin 910	Synthetic polymer	Absorbable	Slight; absorbed with variable but muted inflammatory reaction	Variable; $\frac{1}{2}$ lost in 15 days	Good	Predictable loss of tensile strength; less potentiation of sepsis than catgut
Polydioxanone	Synthetic polymer	Absorbable	Slight	$\frac{1}{2}$ lost in 28 days	Moderate	As above
GTMC	Synthetic polymer	Absorbable	Minimal mononuclear response; no inflammatory activity	20% lost in 14 days; 60% lost in 3 months	Very good	Predictable; stronger *in vitro* than nylon or polypropylene
Linen	Vegetable	Non-absorbable	Moderate inflammation	$\frac{1}{3}$–$\frac{1}{2}$ strength lost in 3–6 months	Very good	Cheap; variable supply and performance
Silk	From silk worm	Non-absorbable	Mild to moderate inflammation	$\frac{1}{2}$ strength lost in 2–12 months	Very good	Fairly cheap; cost likely to rise; variable supply
Nylon	Synthetic polyamide	Non-absorbable	Minimal	$\frac{2}{3}$ strength retained up to 6 months	Poor in monofilament; good in braid	Knot slippage in monofilament
Polypropylene	Synthetic	Non-absorbable	Minimal	As for nylon	Superior to monofilament nylon	Elastic; knot slippage; can fracture, e.g. artery
Coated polyester	Synthetic (PTFE-coated braid)	Non-absorbable	Minimal to moderate	As for nylon	Good (braid + monofilament coat)	Knot slippage; coat fracture leads to increased inflammatory response
Polytetrafluoro-ethylene	Synthetic (expanded PTFE)	Non-absorbable	Minimal	As for nylon	Good	Expanded microstructure allows incorporation into tissues; minimal suture line bleeding (artery)
Polybutester	Synthetic	Non-absorbable	Minimal	As for nylon	Good but more elastic than nylon or polypropylene	Size for size it is straight; pull strength greater than nylon
Stainless steel	Synthetic	Non-absorbable	Virtually nil	Monofilament shows fatigue fractures at 1 year	Poor in monofilament; moderate in practice	Inert; troublesome knots and wound pain

randomized equally to each suture, a layered closure was used – the wound failure rate was 5.8% for polyglactin, 9.6% for PGA and 8.8% for polypropylene. Wound failure was closely related to wound infection.[454] When PGA was compared with nylon mass closure the rate of wound failure was 12.5% in the PGA group, compared with 4.7% in the nylon group. It was concluded that closure of abdominal wounds with absorbable sutures does not appear to be justified.[129] Polyglactin and polydioxanone sutures have prolonged tissue integrity compared with PGA and may therefore be more satisfactory for laparotomy. Polydioxanone is as good as a non-absorbable.[544] It does need stressing that it takes years to assess the final outcome of a wound closure technique and until this assessment is made by enthusiastic clinical researchers, ordinary regular surgeons should continue to use tested and proven suture techniques.[542, 543]

NON-ABSORBABLE SUTURES

For closure of aponeurosis a non-absorbable monofilament flexible material with good knotting properties is at present the ideal. Of the suture materials available, stainless steel wire provides the greatest strength and knot security by a wide margin. However, the poor handling characteristics of wire limits its usefulness, despite its additional advantage of minimal tissue reaction. Silk has long been considered the standard non-absorbable suture material and has enjoyed widest use. Silk was recommended by Halsted and by Whipple.[384, 983] In terms of strength and knot security silk is distinctly inferior to many other materials, and the tissue reaction to silk correlates with the incidence of granuloma and sinuses in clinical use. Cotton was introduced in 1940 during World War II when silk was relatively unobtainable. Its strength is similar to silk, but its handling characteristics are inferior – again it has a high incidence of granuloma and sinus formation. Cotton is similar to linen in many properties.

Nylon was developed by the Du Pont Company and introduced as an alternative to silk in 1943.[646] Compared with silk, nylon has distinct advantages: it can be used as a monofilament, it loses less strength when wet (15% versus 25%), it is stronger, it causes much less tissue reaction. However, it is not as flexible, it is difficult to handle and to knot, and the knots have a tendency to slip. Monofilament nylon undergoes both plastic (irreversible) and elastic (reversible) elongation when subjected to tension. When 1 BPC nylon is stretched using a force of 5 kg, the total elongation produced is 22.5%, of which 6.9% is irreversible. When aponeurotic wounds are closed with nylon and then the sutures are tightened to 5 kg to produce 'compression' of the wound, the suture stretches by 27.7%.[625] This plastic irreversible elongation has an importance in closing fascial wounds: unless the nylon is tightened adequately, its elongation

when the patient breathes and moves will lead to loss of apposition of the wound edges and ultimately to wound failure.

Monofilament polypropylene is an alternative to nylon. The advantages of polypropylene are greater flexibility and easier handling characteristics. It knots better than nylon.[420, 422]

Braided non-absorbable sutures have distinctly better handling and knotting characteristics than monofilaments, but they give the least good results for suturing aponeurosis and repairing hernias. The particular problems are infection and the persistent sinuses and so braids should be abandoned. If infection occurs in a wound repaired with a non-absorbable braid, there is no alternative to removing the suture. With monofilaments, infection can be controlled and suture removal is not needed. Others have confirmed the unsuitability of braided non-absorbable sutures in hernia repair.[471]

Mechanical factors in abdominal wound closure

Wounds are not set in their dimensions, but undergo change as they heal. Not only do the wounds themselves change, but the cavities or tissues they contain alter, and these alterations critically vary the dimensions of the wound.

The events of wound healing lead to oedema of the wound and then to the development of a healing ridge and fibroblast proliferation as collagen placement gets under way. Oedema of the wound by increasing wound bulk increases the tension in each suture bite. If suture bites are initially tight this increase in tension may lead to (a) suture breakage, (b) knot failure or (c) cutting out. These same three consequences develop from changes in body compartments beneath suture lines. In the abdomen, extreme examples of this phenomenon occur. In voluntary inspiration, pregnancy and abdominal distension, mean alterations of girth of 6%, 18% and 27% have been measured, while simultaneously the mean xiphoid to pubis distance increases by 12%, 15% and 37%, respectively (Table 6.2). In these circumstances an abdominal wound will increase in length by an estimated 30% overall.

The alterations in wound length that occur during healing have a critical impact on the technique of suturing an abdominal wound. Jenkins has analysed this geometrically[467] and concluded that the ratio of suture length (SL) to wound length (WL) is critical to aponeurosis repair.

An SL:WL ratio of 4:1 or more is optimum; if the SL:WL ratio decreases below 2.5:1 the risk of wound disruption increases geometrically. Wound disruption is inevitable as the SL:WL ratio approaches 1:1. This mathematical analysis (Jenkins' rule) is confirmed when tested in clinical practice.

Table 6.2 Increases in girth and xiphoid–pubis distance caused by abdominal distension (From Jenkins, 1976,[466] with permission)

Abdominal distension associated with:	Type of measurement	Percentage increase in distension	
		Mean value	Extreme value
Voluntary inspiration (n = 18)	Girth	6	11
	Xiphoid–pubis	12	18
Caesarean section (n = 27)	Girth	18	94
	Xiphoid–pubis	15	36
Gut obstruction or paralytic ileus (n = 5)	Girth	27	53
	Xiphoid–pubis	37	67

In hernia repair it is important to take deep bites of aponeurosis, to place the sutures close together, observing Jenkins' rule, to make the suture bites irregular to avoid splitting between the strands of aponeurosis and to tighten the sutures to allow for plastic elongation of the polymer in the postoperative period.

SUTURE LENGTH

The healing of midline laparotomy incisions was observed in a prospective clinical study by Israelsson and Jonsson.[456, 457] A total of 1023 patients were included from August 1989 to June 1993. Wound dehiscence occurred in five patients (0.5%) and was associated with wound infection and suture technique. Wound infection occurred in 97 (9%) and was associated with suture technique. Incisional hernia occurred in 118 of 808 patients (15%) at one year and was associated with suture technique. Overweight was not associated with an increased rate of incisional hernia when the SL:WL ratio was 4.0–4.9. The rate of wound problems, infection and incisional hernia is lower when the SL:WL ratio is greater than 4.0. This clinical confirmation of Jenkins' rule is an important confirmation of the mathematical concept postulated in 1976.

KNOTS

The knot is the weakest part of a suture and knot efficiency is a crucial component of the suture technique. Conventional knots cause a 40% decrease in the strength of most suture materials except for nylon (and probably polypropylene). Self-locking knots permit the end of a continuous suture to slide inside the knot, thus absorbing some of the energy which would otherwise be transmitted to the knot and cause it to break.[724] Additionally, self-locking knots are less bulky than more conventional knots, thus diminishing the risk of infection and sinus formation.[734, 930]

Skin closure

Sutures, penetrating the skin and then tied on the surface, are the traditional closure method for wounds. Alternatives include subcuticular sutures, skin clips which do not penetrate the full skin thickness and most recently plastic tape adherent to the skin.

The requirements for adequate skin closure are that the skin edges should be held together in apposition for sufficient time to allow the skin to grow together. To promote rapid healing, the edges should not move in relation to each other and tension should be minimal to prevent necrosis. Careful suturing should prevent the introduction of sepsis. Lastly, but perhaps of overriding importance to the patient, a good cosmetic result is needed.

Clean or contaminated surgery demands different regimens for wound management. One of the oldest surgical principles is that a frankly contaminated wound should be left open. The wound which is expected to be compromised by early (reactionary) haemorrhage is managed by delayed primary suture. If localized infection is anticipated, interrupted sutures may allow early drainage. These are the traditions of wound care. Hernia operations nowadays are clean operations – we are searching for quick uncomplicated healing with the best functional and cosmetic results. Hence we should review our methods of skin closure and optimize skin healing as far as possible.

Conventional (traditional) skin suturing techniques do have certain disadvantages – the needle passing through the skin on either side carries fragments of both epidermis and skin organisms down its track and into the depths of the subcutaneous tissue. This causes an increased wound infection rate than when skin closure by a sutureless technique is used. The complications of suture track infection are greater when a multi-strand suture is used and when the tension upon the wound edges is too great. Poor technique in inserting the sutures and subsequent oedema after suturing lead to localized ischaemia and a poor cosmetic result.

Clips avoid the problem of introducing deep infection into the wound. Michel-type clips may produce localized tension and cause local pressure necrosis. Unless they are removed within 24–48 h, this local ischaemia can cause tissue necrosis and a permanently poor cosmetic result. Currently available disposable applicators for the introduction of wire skin clips with a rectangular configuration of the closed clip give excellent results, although cost may be a factor in discouraging their use. Closure with adherent tape gives excellent healing.[274, 732, 909]

A randomized controlled clinical trial comparing skin closure using vertical mattress sutures of monofilament nylon and steel clips in laparotomy incisions has confirmed the significant advantage of avoiding skin sutures. In a consecutive series of 341 wounds (182 skin sutured and 159 closed with clips), the infection rate in the sutured wounds was 17.0% versus 6.3% in those closed with clips (χ^2 = 9.26; $P<$ 0.01).[745]

Subcutaneous absorbable sutures may be the favourite method with surgeons, nurses and patients. In a randomized trial four different methods of thigh wound closure after removal of the saphenous vein for coronary artery bypass grafting were used.[26] Continuous nylon vertical mattress sutures, continuous subcuticular absorbable PGA sutures, metal skin clips and adhesive sutureless closure (Opsite) were compared. Assessment of the healing showed subcuticular PGA to be more effective than skin clips or vertical mattress nylon sutures. The final cosmetic result showed subcuticular PGA to be superior to sutures or skin clips and as effective as sutureless adherent closure. Subcuticular absorbable sutures do not require removal; this is an economic saving and is a considerable advantage in day-case surgery.[770] For skin closure in hernia wounds from 1970 to 1978 we used Michel clips, from 1978 to 1984 skin tapes only and since 1984 we have used subcuticular clear polydioxanone. The results of the polydioxanone have been excellent. The suture does not require removing and the wounds are non-nurse dependent. Wound healing is quick and neat and, most importantly, the lack of through-skin sutures has removed much of the postoperative pain.

Prostheses in hernia repair

McArthur (1901) recommended using fascia lata to repair hernias.[628] Kirschner (1910) used a free graft of fascia lata to repair the defect[503] and Gallie, in 1921, used strips of autologous fascia lata to darn the muscular structures together.[323] Hamilton reported 47 large hernias repaired with an onlay fascia lata graft in the University of Louisville over a 21-year period. No patches sloughed but the hernia recurred in five cases.[390] Mair introduced buried whole thickness skin for hernioplasty in 1945.[604]

Bartlett, in 1903, used an 'improved filigree' of silver wire to repair incisional hernias[68] and McGavin, in a classic 1909 article on the radical cure of inguinal hernia, advocated the use of a filigree of silver wire to maintain and reinforce the approximation of muscular structures to Poupart's ligament.[635] Throckmorton and Koontz independently, in 1947, introduced tantalum gauze.[511, 922] As recently as 1958 Ball, from Melbourne, reported 500 cases repaired with a silver wire filigree and having good results.[61]

Thompson recommended a semi-rigid plastic insert in 1948.[919] Schofield, in 1955, used polyvinyl alcohol sponge[631] and Usher introduced polypropylene mesh in 1959.[937] Doran et al. (1961) investigated the use of nylon net in inguinal hernia repair.[264]

Over these years what have we learned about the ideal properties of prostheses, the indications for prostheses and their fixation at operation?

The ideal properties of an implantable soft-tissue prosthesis are: (a) it should remain inert and stable; (b) it should not be modified by the body after implantation; (c) it should not excite a chemical reaction; (d) it should not excite a biological reaction (inflammatory, granulomatous, carcinogenic or allergenic); (e) it should not itself undergo physical change after implantation and should remain perpetually flexible.[523]

Each of the biological prostheses has disadvantages and enthusiasm for them has evaporated. Heterologous fascia lata or pericardium is a foreign tissue which undergoes necrosis after insertion and does not survive to provide any long-term support. Homologous fascia lata does survive, but there is only a limited quantity of it available and there are reports of troublesome complications at the donor site.[134] Buried skin survives; indeed it survives so well that the dermal appendages continue to function, producing dermoid cysts. Squamous carcinoma has developed in some buried skin grafts.[874]

The technique of buried skin graft repair of a primary inguinal hernia was compared to 'Bassini's repair' by Piper (1969).[746] In the 'skin graft' technique the whole thickness graft was taken as an ellipse from the wound during initial exploration. The skin was sutured under tension between the conjoint tendon and the inguinal ligament. Linen thread was used to hold the graft in position. In the series of 189 buried skin repairs, the recurrence rate at two years was 15.3% for direct and 10.8% for indirect hernias. The sepsis rate was 7% and discharge continued for up to 30 months, with an average of 8.8 months in wounds that became infected. There was an incidence of dermoid cysts of 3.2%.

In summary, fascia lata is an acceptable repair tissue but is not nowadays recommended. Buried skin should never be used – the complications of sepsis, cysts and malignancy outweigh any usefulness it may have appeared to have in the past.

Metallic prostheses include stainless steel mesh, tantalum gauze and Toilinox stainless steel mesh. The original stainless steel used prior to 1940 and tantalum gauze used up to the 1960s were both inert and easy to insert.[52, 265, 656, 921] However, work hardening with fatigue fracture made both of them inadequate in the long term. When they fractured, parts of the mesh would wander or even erode into body cavities, causing bowel fistulas, or out through the skin with ulceration. Patients found these metallic implants very painful and uncomfortable. For these reasons most surgeons abandoned them. Toilinox*, a new metal prosthesis manufactured in France, appears not to have these undesirable properties. It is a prosthesis of stainless steel made of strands 76 μm in diameter, woven to 20 strands/cm, with spaces between the strands 0.424 mm square. These characteristics provide resistance to infection and a good fibrous ingrowth into the mesh. The material is manufactured in pieces 15 cm × 30 cm. It is easily cut to size. Fines (1972) reports its use in ventral hernias and in recurrent groin hernias. He recommends placing it deeply, if possible in the preperitoneal layer.[300] It is reported to be safe even when placed in contact with omentum and small intestine. It is fixed in position with nylon.

Further experiences with this prosthesis are reported by Thomeret *et al.* (1960),[918] Verges and Jaupitre (1973)[951] (who performed simultaneous open prostatectomy) and Validire *et al.* (1986).[943] The mesh can be used preperitoneally or fastened to the anterior rectus sheath after linea alba repair. The mesh is tolerant of sepsis which will resolve without the mesh being removed. Fixation of the mesh with nylon or PGA is reported.

Synthetic plastic meshes must be the first choice today. They are in infinite supply, relatively cheap to produce and can be readily cut to whatever size is required.

Polyvinyl alcohol sponge was the first synthetic prosthesis used to repair large aponeurotic defects in Newcastle upon Tyne in 1955. In Liverpool, Charles Wells used this prosthesis in his ingenious operation for rectal prolapse. Sepsis and sinus formation were early on recognized as complications; the sponge had to be removed for these reasons in the first patient treated. However, if the sponge was placed deeply with peritoneum behind it to separate it from gut and fascia and a layer of subcutaneous fat anteriorly, so that it was exposed to a good blood bath, healing by fibrous tissue investment occurred and infection and sinus formation was then less of a problem.[831] In the long term ongoing sepsis with sinus formation has been prominent. The mesh is very difficult to remove to control the sepsis and is strongly not recommended.

Non-absorbable synthetics were introduced in the 1940s and pioneered for the repair of hernia by Usher in 1958, with the first generation of Marlex mesh made of polyethylene (a Philips petroleum product).[937] Initial problems arose because of difficulties with sterilization and the suture material used for fixation. The original woven product was modified in 1962 with the construction of a knitted mesh with greater flexibility which could be stretched in both its axes, eliminating the problem of unravelling after cutting.[938] Polypropylene mesh (Marlex and Prolene) produced by closely controlled polymerization of Prolene, a derivative of propane gas, is the most widely used prosthetic material in repair of hernias. It has a burst strength of more than 172.5 kPa, which is in excess of the estimated intra-abdominal pressure generated in the inguinal wall by a cough, estimated to be 20–30 kPa. Its flexibility is indicated by an extensibility of 60% (warp) and 20% (weft). Marlex is composed of a monofilament, knitted woven mesh with large pore sizes of about 620 μm. It is argued that pore size is of paramount importance.[20] Pore size is estimated by measuring the smallest and largest of the two longest perpendicular axes of the pore. Biomaterials that contain pores of 10 μm in diameter or less may increase the risk of infection because bacteria can shelter in such spaces, where they are inaccessible to polymorphonuclear granulocytes, which average 10–15 μm in diameter. Similarly, the largest pore size should be greater than 90 μm, which is the optimal size for the rapid ingrowth of vascularized connective tissue and the laying down of collagen and fibrous tissue. A smaller pore size does not allow fibrocytic and collagen infiltration of the host tissue into the mesh which should occur in the first month after implantation. Non-absorbable synthetic materials that contain pore sizes of less than 90 μm tend to be infiltrated with macrophages and histiocytes, which form granulomas with young, loose granulation tissue in and around the mesh. Biomaterials available today include monofilamented polypropylene mesh (Marlex and Prolene) (Figures 6.3 and 6.4), multifilamented polypropylene mesh (Surgipro) (Figure 6.5), multifilamented polyester mesh (Mersilene†) (Figure 6.6), multifilamented polytetrafluoroethylene (PTFE) mesh (Teflon) (Figure 6.7), and expanded PTFE soft tissue patch (GoreTex‡). Except for the monofilamented polypropylene meshes, namely Marlex and Prolene, the other synthetic non-absorbable meshes are based on a pore size of less than 90 μm in all dimensions, such as expanded PTFE soft-tissue patch, or contain one dimension of the weave or weft which is microporous, such as polyester mesh (Mersilene) and multifilamented polypropylene mesh (Surgipro). Because of this element of microporosity, these meshes excite a weak fibrous, granulomatous and histiocytic reaction rather than the ingrowth of strong collagen tissue and fixation to neighbouring tissues.[17]

The choice of non-absorbable synthetic mesh for laparoscopic hernioplasty should be given special

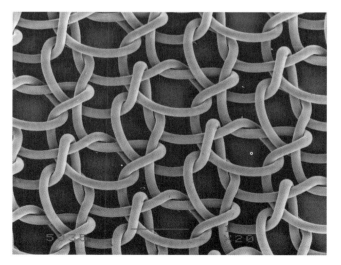

Figure 6.3 Scanning electron micrograph of monofilamented polypropylene mesh (Marlex). (Reproduced with permission from Brenner, 1995[117])

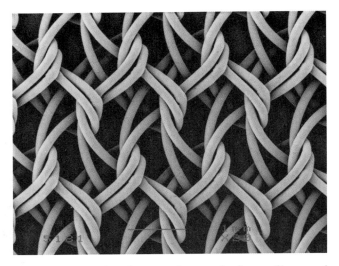

Figure 6.4   Scanning electron micrograph of monofilamented polypropylene mesh (Prolene). (Reproduced with permission from Brenner, 1995[117])

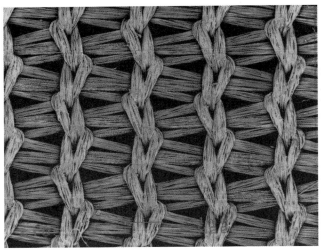

Figure 6.6   Scanning electron micrograph of multifilamented polyester mesh (Mersilene). (Reproduced with permission from Brenner, 1995[117])

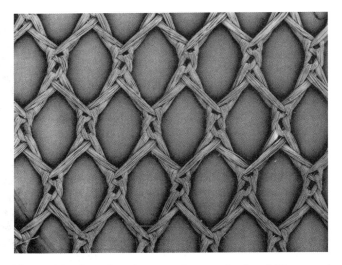

Figure 6.5   Scanning electron micrograph of multifilamented polypropylene mesh (Surgipro). (Reproduced with permission from Brenner, 1995[117])

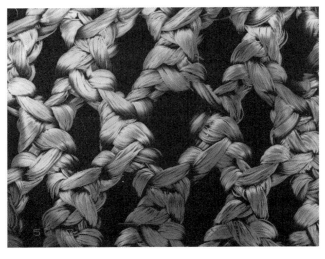

Figure 6.7   Scanning electron micrograph of expanded multi-filamented polytetrafluoroethylene soft tissue patch (GoreTex) mesh. (Reproduced with permission from Brenner, 1995[117])

consideration because the endoscopic surgeon has special requirements. These include an additional element of stiffness so that the material does not curl up and wrinkle during staple or suture fixation in a vertical position. The material must also be net-like so that the laparoscopic surgeon may view the posterior aspect and ensure the staples or sutures are not penetrating vital structures or nerves. Finally, in any intraperitoneal or intra-abdominal approach there is a risk of adhesion formation in and around the opened and resutured peritoneum, which may lead to adherence of bowel with the risk of intestinal obstruction or fistulation. Thus the development of a composite mesh made of a layer of macroporous monofilamented polypropylene on the

parietal side and a layer of absorbable synthetic material, such as the polyglycolic acid polymers (Dexon and Vicryl), on the intestinal side. This would allow infiltration of the host connective tissue into the polypropylene mesh, yet prevent adhesions on the intestinal aspect. Such composites might also have an application in the repair of chest wall and diaphragmatic defects.

Mersilene, a multifilamented Dacron polyester mesh, is readily available: the 40-denier fabric is used in groin hernia repair and the heavier gauge 70-denier in incisional hernia repair. Like the monofilament polypropylene meshes Marlex and Prolene and the multifilamented PTFE mesh, Mersilene is knitted. This provides advantages for the incorporation of fibrous and collagen tissues when compared with the woven meshes. However, Mersilene is a multifilamented polyester and as such will exclude polymorphonuclear leukocytes but not bacteria, so the risk of infection, granuloma formation and sinus tract formation is increased. A special property of Mersilene as a braided Dacron polyester is that it lacks a plastic memory allowing it to conform to structures in the preperitoneal space. For this reason it has proven to be especially attractive to French surgeons for use in the GPRVS preperitoneal hernia repair. It has given excellent results in both British and French experience.[896, 897] When placed deep to the muscles in the extraperitoneal layer (see page 174), sepsis rates of under 3% are recorded. However, because of its multifilament nature it is less well tolerated by the body than polypropylene and excites a more intense inflammatory response. Because of its flexibility and pliability, Mersilene has been advocated for repair of incisional hernias, but here again the potential for infection and exposure of any small part of the mesh to the peritoneal cavity or bowel increases the likelihood of adhesion formation and intestinal obstruction. Nevertheless, this thin widely meshed net allows early fixation to the surrounding tissues as a result of the rapid ingrowth of fibrous and connective tissue.

Multifilamented polytetrafluoroethylene (PTFE) mesh (Teflon) and expanded PTFE (ePTFE) soft tissue patch (GoreTex) have long been available as vascular prostheses and, more recently, become available as a sheet to replace abdominal wall or inguinal defects and as a suture. The ePTFE soft tissue patch is purely microporous (pore size less than 10–70 μm). Matching PTFE expanded sutures are also available. The suture is composed of a single strand of PTFE expanded to produce a microstructure that is greater than 50% air by volume; as a result the suture has a greater diameter (volume) than other available sutures for the same strength. The suture is swaged to a same diameter needle which makes the suture fill the needle track after insertion. PTFE excites minimal reaction and the equal size of suture to needle hole prevents haemorrhage after its insertion. The use of Teflon mesh in incisional hernia repair is reported by Kalsbeek.[477] This material has not been widely used and is not recommended as a first-choice prosthesis. Because of its microporous nature ePTFE soft tissue patch encourages an inadequate host tissue incorporation when used for groin hernia repair by either the anterior or preperitoneal open approach. Early experience with PTFE with the porous weave mesh was not favourable because of infection and rejection. The introduction by Gore and Associates in 1975 of a microporous expanded PTFE (ePTFE) material has overcome these problems.[684, 945] Because of the minimal cellular infiltration into ePTFE, it is used extensively in cardiovascular surgery as a pericardial membrane substitute and material for vascular grafts. Experimental studies in

animals have confirmed that, compared with monofilament polypropylene materials, ePTFE causes an insufficient fibrous response and becomes infiltrated with fine fibrils rather than dense, organized collagen. However, there is an almost total lack of adhesion formation and ePTFE may be the preferred prosthesis when there is a possibility that mesh and viscera are in close proximity.[523, 532] Only one series reports the use of ePTFE as an onlay mesh for open inguinal hernia repair and the results were good.[94]

Marlex mesh has been useful for the repair of giant inguinoscrotal inguinal hernias. After reduction of the hernia the defect is repaired with Marlex mesh followed by creation of a midline anterior wall defect to increase intra-abdominal capacity; this defect is covered with Marlex mesh and closure of this midline defect is completed by rotation of a flap of inguinoscrotal skin.[649]

For recurrent, complex and bilateral groin hernias a midline preperitoneal approach has been used in 672 patients with placement of the ePTFE patch by anchorage to the ligament of Cooper, suture around the cord and finally anchorage of the upper part to the posterior surface of the rectus. A respectable recurrence rate of 2.7% in these difficult hernias was achieved.[719] A smaller series in which 81 patients with difficult inguinal hernias were treated with a tension-free ePTFE patch achieved excellent results at four-year follow-up, no complications due to adhesions, bowel erosion or bowel obstruction, and the formation of only one seroma and one wound infection.[489] For routine use as a prosthetic material in primary inguinal hernia, multifilamented PTFE cannot be recommended. For complex hernias, where there is a risk of contact of the mesh with bowel or for preperitoneal prosthetic mesh repair, ePTFE is an option, albeit an expensive one. It is certainly on the list of options for materials to be used by laparoscopic surgeons. However, because it is floppy and opaque there is increased difficulty with fixation with staples or sutures. A more rigid material with memory is easier to handle.

Multifilamented polypropylene mesh (Surgipro) is a microporous biomaterial recently introduced (USS Surgical Corporation). It has gained popularity as a result of its promotion by the laparoscopic instrument manufacturers. However, objective evaluation or follow-up of a large series of patients using this biomaterial has not been performed.

The use of absorbable biomaterials, such as the polyglycolic acid polymers (Dexon and Vicryl), is limited. These meshes rapidly lose strength due to fragmentation and hydrolysis, losing bursting strength after three weeks. They are unsatisfactory, therefore, for use in permanent wall replacement.[523] Absorbable prosthetic material may be used for temporary abdominal closure in contaminated cases, or as a buffer between exposed bowel and a non-absorbable prosthetic mesh. Although absorbable polyglactin mesh is replaced by mature collagenous tissue, it is not strong enough to resist intra-abdominal pressure and prevent recurrent hernia formation.[20] Implantation of polyglactin (Vicryl) mesh or polyglycolic acid (Dexon) mesh is therefore unsatisfactory for safe and successful hernia repair. Its role as an adjunct on the inner or peritoneal surface of non-absorbable meshes is speculative.

Marlex[§] knitted mesh, manufactured from polypropylene monofilament, is now the most widely used prosthesis in hernia repair. The mesh is pliant and easily cut, it is resistant to infection and excites very little biological response in the host. After implantation it remains supple indefinitely. It is invaded by fibroblasts and forms a latticework for repair. Reoperation through Marlex mesh is easy and resuture can be made using conventional techniques. The mesh should be fixed in position with monofilament polypropylene sutures; braided or biological sutures should not be used because they can become the focus of persistent sepsis and sinus formation. Marlex is the recommended prosthesis in open hernia repair, incisional hernia and uncomplicated preperitoneal inguinal hernia repair.[17, 20] Where there is

a risk that a prosthesis may be exposed to the peritoneum or bowel or to direct contact with intra-abdominal viscera in laparoscopic surgery or complicated preperitoneal hernia repair, then ePTFE may be the material of choice.

Techniques of placement of prosthetic mesh

Prosthetic mesh repair of abdominal wall defects can be accomplished by the following techniques:[526, 527, 938, 939] (a) extra-aponeurotic – subcutaneous; (b) sub-aponeurotic and extraperitoneal or preperitoneal; (c) sub-aponeurotic and intraperitoneal (Figure 6.8). Additionally, intraperitoneal placement of the mesh can be supported by an extra-aponeurotic stent (Figure 6.9).

Summary – recommendations

The patient must be fully resuscitated before any operation is undertaken.

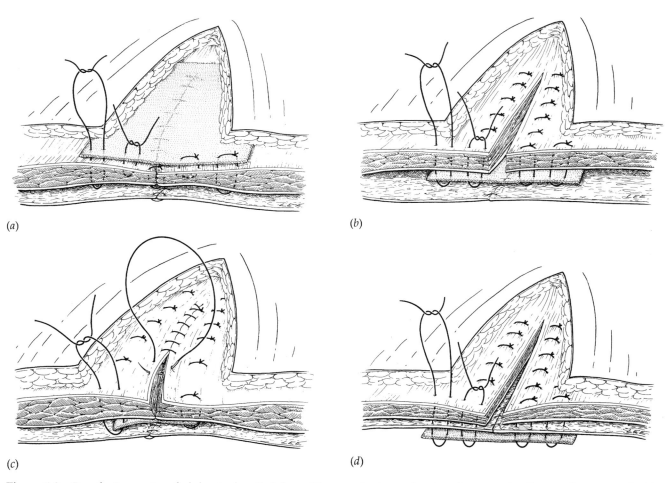

(a) (b) (c) (d)

Figure 6.8 Prosthetic repairs of abdominal wall defects. The prosthesis can be placed extraparietally or subcutaneously (**a**), subaponeurotically, extraperitoneally, or preperitoneally leaving any aponeurotic defect open superficial to the prosthesis (**b**), subaponeurotically with closure of the defect (**c**), or intraperitoneally (**d**)

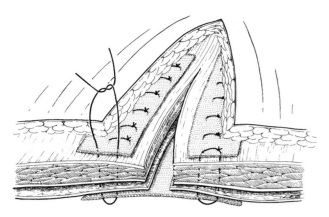

Figure 6.9 Intraperitoneal placement can be reinforced by an extra-aponeurotic stent

Aponeurosis must be closed by a method which maintains tissue strength in excess of three months – a method that causes little tissue reaction and does not cause persistent sinuses if infected. A monofilament non-absorbable synthetic should be used. Number 3 metric monofilament polypropylene is recommended. The technique of deep irregular close bites (to avoid splitting the aponeurosis) is employed. It is important to knot the suture carefully. A double throw double tie square knot is the minimal requirement if knot failure is to be avoided.

The subcutaneous fat must be closed so that there is no dead space and the suture material employed must cause little if any reaction and be absorbed fairly rapidly. Polyglactin or PGA sutures are suitable for this layer.

Closed suction drains should be inserted if there is any possibility of haematoma formation.

In the skin, desirable features of the skin closure technique include a neat scar with no skin markings from sutures on it, a minimal reaction to material used in suturing and, above all, a low instance of infection and subsequent sinus formation. If the material does not require removal it has advantages. Subcuticular clear PDS monofilament is recommended.

* Laboratoires Bruneau, 204 Avenue de Marechal Juin, BP 331 92107, Boulogne-Billancourt Cedex, France.
† Ethicon Ltd, Box 408, Bankhead Avenue, Edinburgh EH11 4HE, Scotland.
‡ W.L. Gore and Associates Inc., Medical Products Division, Flagstaff, Arizona 86002, USA.
§ USCI International Division, C.R. Bard Inc., 2 Burlington Woods Drive, PO Box 436, Burlington, Massachusetts 01803, USA.

Choice of anaesthesia: local or general

Either local or general anaesthesia is suitable for the repair of most hernias. Only rarely nowadays is the patient totally unfit to undergo a suitably judged general anaesthetic. Local anaesthesia for hernia repair does have particular advantages – organizational and economic as well as clinical. Local anaesthesia can be administered by the operator, thus no medical anaesthetist is required; the patient does require shared care during an operation performed under local anaesthetic.

A nurse should be dedicated to the patient throughout a local anaesthetic operation and a qualified anaesthetist should be available to give assistance at short notice. Peripheral oxygen saturation must be monitored with a pulse oximeter, especially if intravenous sedation is being used. In addition intravenous access should be established in order that the complications of inadvertent intravascular injection of local anaesthetic agents, which may result in cerebral and cardiovascular side effects, can be counteracted. Blood pressure should be recorded on arrival in the operating theatre and after the injection of local anaesthetic, and preferably monitored throughout the procedure. This may be done by connecting the patient to a cardiac monitor supervised by the anaesthetic nurse throughout the operation and regularly recording pulse, blood pressure, and respiratory rate. Emergency resuscitation equipment, including the requirements for endotracheal intubation, must be available in the event of severe respiratory depression needing intubation. The side effects of inadvertent intravenous injection of local anaesthesia include systemic excitation of the central nervous system with excessive anxiety, convulsions, hypotension or severe dysrhythmias.

The clinical advantages of local anaesthetic include the decreased blood ooze when local anaesthetic solution with adrenaline is employed, the prolonged analgesia provided (without any central effects), enhanced definition of tissue planes afforded by the hydrodynamic dissection by the local anaesthetic distending the tissues, and lastly the patient co-operation possible in testing and identifying anatomic defects, particularly in inguinal hernioplasty. The patient is saved the anxiety of general anaesthesia and the hangover effect of recovery.

Surgery under local anaesthesia is more demanding for the operator: he or she must be more precise and less traumatic to tissue than in the unconscious patient.

Haemostasis must be more secure and the surgeon must not be overheard demanding too many swabs to wipe away uncontrolled bleeding. Above all, when surgery is completed the subject may be asked to cough or strain so that any deficiencies in technique are immediately observed.

Local anaesthesia is not a cheap option for the careless surgeon to administer. Good local anaesthesia requires knowledge and skill; it demands careful preoperative assessment, intraoperative monitoring and adequate facilities for recovery from its effects. The complications of the local anaesthetic drugs – convulsions, dysrhythmias, hypotension and respiratory failure – are as life threatening as those of general anaesthesia. These complications are invariably caused by intravascular injection, which is the most important technical error the operator must avoid. The management of these complications is as demanding as the conduct of a general anaesthetic. Unless the surgeon understands these complications and unless the facilities are on hand to manage them, the single-handed surgeon–local anaesthetist is putting the patient to hazard. Prudence dictates that surgeons should not uncritically indulge in major local anaesthetic administration.

Hernia surgery requiring extensive dissection, major intra-abdominal manipulation, fluid shifts or blood transfusion is rarely advisable under local anaesthetic. When the diagnosis is in doubt, or subject to revision during surgery, it is best to avoid local anaesthesia. It follows that incarcerated or strangulated hernias should rarely be operated under local anaesthesia. The 'poor risk patient' requires that the risk of operation be shared by the surgeon with a skilled anaesthetist; for instance, local anaesthesia is not automatically safer than general anaesthesia after a myocardial infarct. All local anaesthetics have cardiovascular effects. Similarly, the patient with liver failure or hepatitis is not immune from the toxic effects of those local anaesthetic agents which are degraded in the liver.

Patient preference in the choice of anaesthetic cannot be discounted; the Canadian and American literature suggests that patients prefer local anaesthesia, or are at least indifferent in the choice, when they undergo surgery for a simple uncomplicated hernia.[167, 329, 354] This preference is not universally expressed by British patients. Whereas there are enthusiasts for local anaesthesia in the UK, experience and research suggests that if patients are given an entirely free choice the majority prefer to sleep throughout the procedure. Modern general anaesthesia makes it possible for safe operations to be performed on patients who are to go home 2 h or so later. The need for tracheal intubation is no longer a contraindication to day surgery. The speed of recovery from general anaesthesia is paramount to facilitate full and rapid recovery to consciousness and a degree of physical performance commensurate with returning home by private car or taxi. The introduction of new anaesthetic agents that are either exhaled without degradation or excreted or metabolized rapidly has extended to selection of patients for general anaesthesia at both ends of the age range. General anaesthesia may be provided by inhalational or intravenous drugs, or a suitable combination. Propofol is accepted by most anaesthetists as the intravenous agent of choice for use in out-patient surgery: it provides the swiftest recovery (compared with barbiturates such as methohexatone), less excitatory phenomena, and smoother induction.[411] There is little to choose between the inhalational agents (halothane, enflurane and isoflurane), particularly in terms of safety. In most patients optimal general anaesthesia for day-case inguinal hernia surgery will comprise propafol infusion supplemented with isoflurane and nitrous oxide inhalation for maintenance. Such a regimen provides a stable technique and rapid recovery and return to 'street fitness'.[230]

The time taken to infiltrate the local anaesthesia sufficiently to gain satisfactory analgesia has been thought to add significantly to the length of the operative procedure, but this is not so. Two randomized studies have investigated this.[14, 505] In one study, a small study with 45 patients in each arm of the randomization, the operating time was significantly lower in the local anaesthetic group. In the other (earlier) study it was claimed that local anaesthesia needed 3 min more operative time. Certainly, enthusiasts for local anaesthesia have never claimed that it takes significantly less time than general anaesthesia.

There are disadvantages in introducing opioids such as fentanyl or alfentanyl into the anaesthetic sequence because of the incidence of nausea and vomiting, apnoea, occasional awareness, and muscle rigidity. Benzodiazepines have proved useful for sedation; however, recovery from intravenous midazolam is not as rapid as recovery from intravenous propafol, which may be used during general anaesthesia.

Finally, the administration of a general anaesthetic should not be underestimated, irrespective of technique there is a high incidence of side effects that may persist for up to 24 h, such as drowsiness, headache, cognitive effects, muscle pain, nausea and vomiting. Whatever the type of anaesthesia, the recurrence rate is low and the long-term outcome is uninfluenced by whether local or general anaesthesia is used. The advantages of early ambulation to prevent thrombo-embolism are negated by the speed of recovery, and hence early ambulation, that can be achieved with modern general anaesthesia.

Patients for both general and local anaesthesia are transported to and from the operating room on trolleys. The walk to the operating table and the walk away after local anaesthesia is dramatic, but does not necessarily confer any benefit on the patient.

Thus, while the advantages and disadvantages of local or general anaesthesia must be considered for each and every patient, for open operations the patient's views should not be overruled by the surgeon's personal preference.

Local anaesthesia

HISTORY

The use of local anaesthesia for the repair of groin hernia has a rather exciting history. Cocaine was isolated as a pure alkaloid from the leaves of the coca plant, *Erythroxylum coca*, by Niemann in 1860. It was then exploited by the Austrian Karl Koller in 1884 when he instilled it into the eye of a rabbit. This latter discovery is attributed by some to Sigmund Freud, who had been experimenting with cocaine but who deserted his experiments, and the reporting of them, for his fiancee.[612] Freud later wrote:

In the Autumn of 1886 I began to practise medicine in Vienna and married a girl who had waited more than four years for me in a distant town. Now I realize it was my fiancee's fault I did not become famous at that time. In 1884 I was profoundly interested in the little known alkaloid of coca, which Merck obtained for me to study its physiological properties. During this work, the occasion presented itself of going to see my fiancee, whom I had not seen for two years. I hurriedly finished my work with cocaine, confining myself in my report to remarking it would soon be put to new use. At the same time I suggested to my friend Konigstein, the ophthalmologist, that he should experiment with cocaine in some eye cases. When I came back from holiday, I found it was not to him but to another friend, Karl Koller, that I had spoken about cocaine. Koller had completed the research on the eyes of animals and demonstrated the results to the ophthalmological congress in Heidelberg. Quite rightly, the discovery of local anaesthesia by cocaine, of such importance in minor surgery, was thereafter attributed to Koller. But I bear my wife no grudge for what I lost!

William Stuart Halsted, in 1885, demonstrated that cocaine could block impulses through nerves and in the process became a lifelong cocaine addict himself. He underwent sanatorium treatment for his addiction before his translation to the chair of surgery at Johns Hopkins. He apparently was never truly cured of this addiction, for he continued to require daily cocaine until his death in 1922. Halsted's resident, Harvey

Cushing,[210] pursued the development of local anaesthesia for groin hernia repair and in 1900 published the original authoritative paper on the nervous anatomy of the inguinal region and his experiences of local anaesthesia in the repair of these hernias. Local anaesthesia is mentioned in many treatises on hernia, but it has never become as popular in the UK as elsewhere. It is difficult to discover why this is so. Ogilvie's influential book *Hernia*, published in 1959, devotes only two sparse pages to the topic and describes a technique which would have given the patient little comfort throughout some of the extensive surgical repairs. Ogilvie goes on to elaborate. Perhaps the brevity of Ogilvie's description of local anaesthesia can be forgiven in the light of his qualifying sentence: 'Operations for inguinal hernia must often be undertaken urgently in patients whose age or general condition would prohibit such a step were it not for the greater danger of some threatened complication. The risks are largely eliminated by the use of local anaes-thetics.'[713] Are local anaesthetics, therefore, only recommended in dire circumstances?

More recently, Glassow has recorded the experience of local anaesthesia from the Shouldice clinic in Toronto, an experience beginning in 1954 and including over 25 000 patients.[356] Barwell has described similar results using local anaesthesia in the UK.[69] The use of local anaes-thesia in the fit patient for hernia repair is associated with few complications, and if the anaesthetic is carefully administered no complications attributable to it should occur.

Less experienced hernia surgeons should be introduced to the technique of local anaesthesia with caution. Unless the novice is well supervised and fully conversant with the subtle refinements in technique required to operate under local anaesthesia, recurrence rates may escalate.[497, 667] In a retrospective review Kingsnorth and colleagues demonstrated that the factor most strongly influencing recurrence was the experience of a particular surgeon with local anaesthetic technique.[497] They suggested that a trainee surgeon should be supervised for a minimum of six operations under local anaesthesia before being allowed to operate solo. Nevertheless, Britton and Morris have reviewed the international data and conclude that inguinal hernia repair under local anaesthesia should enable any careful surgeon to achieve low recurrence rates at low cost.[122]

Local anaesthesia is becoming more popular for two reasons. First, the prolonged analgesia which persists if bupivacaine is employed has enabled patients to walk sooner and go home sooner than after a general anaesthetic. Secondly, convalescence for patients with severe cardiorespiratory decompensation, or patients with liver disease for whom an inhalational anaesthetic would be inadvisable, is easy.

LOCAL ANAESTHETIC AGENTS

Two local anaesthetic agents are widely used. In the 1970s lignocaine was the drug of choice but since 1980 lignocaine has been superseded by bupivacaine. However, some surgeons use a combination of both agents in order to achieve the advantages of rapid onset of action and longer duration of anaesthesia. Adrenaline is used with both drugs to protract their duration of activity.

The maximum safe dose of lignocaine is 3 mg/kg body weight and with adrenaline 7 mg/kg. For bupivacaine the maximum dose is 2 mg/kg body weight and 4 mg/kg with adrenaline. Bupivacaine is more potent and longer acting than lignocaine and maintains the analgesic block for 8–10 h, which is a major advantage in day-case surgery.[33] The safety margin in the recommended maximum safe dose is wide, as illustrated by serial postoperative plasma concentrations following doses approaching the maximum recommended for lignocaine or bupivacaine. For instance, administering lignocaine with adrenaline to the maximum dose of 7 mg/kg, peak lignocaine concentration ranged from 0.23 to 0.9 mg/l, the toxicity threshold being 5 mg/l.[482] The administration of 20 ml of 0.5% plain bupivacaine resulted in peak venous plasma concentrations of 0.07–1.14 m/l, the cardiovascular toxicity occurring at plasma concentrations greater than 4 mg/l.[485]

Prolongation of the duration of local anaesthesia by the addition of agents designed to prolong absorption from the local tissues has been explored by several investigators. Loder recommends 1% lignocaine in 10% dextran 150 with l:250 000 adrenaline added to the solution.[575] He reports that the large numbers of big molecules (10% dextran of average molecular weight 150 000) retards the absorption of the local anaesthetic. Others have evaluated 0.25% bupivacaine with dextran 40 without adrenaline and have reported no enhancement or prolongation of the local anaesthetic effect. Simpson *et al.* (1982), in a small study comparing initial general anaesthesia with field infiltration to control postoperative pain, suggest that the addition of heavy dextran to bupivacaine and adrenaline solution prolongs its effect.[861] This confirms the earlier work of Loder. However, their conclusion, 'It would seem prudent, therefore, in clinical work to combine bupivacaine with high molecular weight dextran and adrenaline', is perhaps a little too enthusiastic on the basis of their small experience. In their series of 40 patients this mixture was only administered to five subjects, casting doubt on the clinical validity of the study. Kingsnorth and colleagues in a similar study could not confirm this recommendation and conclude that the addition of heavy dextran to bupivacaine confers no benefit.[499]

More recently, in a study of 30 men undergoing inguinal hernia repair under general anaesthesia, postoperative pain, patient rating score or morphine consumption did not differ between patients who had preoperative inguinal nerve block with bupivacaine 0.5% plain and those who received a similar block with bupivacaine 0.5% plain supplemented with 40 mg triamcinolone acetanide. For the present, therefore, it is recommended that local anaesthetic agents are used plain or with adrenaline, and not supplemented with additional agents which are of no proven advantage in prolonging their duration of action.[631]

Barwell, who has the largest UK series of repairs of inguinal hernias under local anaesthetic, uses 0.5% lignocaine without adrenaline. He reports 2066 patients operated on under this local anaesthetic, two of whom had to be converted to general anaesthetic in the early days of his programme. He has had no cases of anaesthetic toxicity and perhaps the worst complication is 'the occasional haematoma at the site of injection for the field block.'[69] Glassow, reporting the experience of the Shouldice clinic in Toronto, recommends 150 ml of 2% procaine without adrenaline,[354] whereas Ravitch from Pittsburgh recommends 0.5% lignocaine[772] and Wantz a mixture of lignocaine and bupivacaine with adrenaline.[357] Wantz also claims that the burning pain caused by the administration of local anaesthesia can be eliminated by neutralizing the agent.[967] The addition of 1 ml of 8.4% sodium bicarbonate solution to 9 ml of plain local anaesthesia brings the pH to a comfortable 7.5, which also enhances the anaesthesia and reduces the quantity required. The pH of local anaesthetic with adrenaline is 4, and therefore 2.5 ml of the sodium bicarbonate solution is required for neutralization. Ponka and Sapala[755] conclude that bupivacaine is superior to chloroprocaine. They report that 0.25% bupivacaine provides anaesthesia consistently lasting longer than 6 h, and as a result of this sustained release the requirement for postoperative analgesia is reduced. Chloroprocaine with 1:200 000 adrenaline was a safe agent, but its action lasted only up to 2 h.

Flanagan and Bascom, initially using 0.25% lignocaine with 1:400 000 adrenaline and currently using bupivacaine 0.125% with 1:400 000 adrenaline, have reported detailed results from Eugene, Oregon. In a prospective study 170 patients, adults with an age range of 12–82 years, with groin hernia, were given local anaesthesia as out-patients and 163 were given general anaesthesia. They found good patient satisfaction with local anaesthesia, few complications and enormous economic and social benefits.[306] Baskerville and Jarrett reported a study of local anaesthesia for day-case inguinal hernia repair undertaken in Kingston, UK in 1980.[71] One hundred and thirty-five patients were operated on using 40–60 ml 0.25% bupivacaine with 1:200 000 adrenaline. There were no complications of the local anaesthesia. Patient acceptance of the regimen was high, with 96% of patients stating that

they would have another hernia repair performed in the same way. Acceptance of this regimen by the family doctors was also tested and 100% of the family doctors expressed satisfaction with this management of their patients.

Nicholls (1977),[700] reporting his experience from the Seychelles Isles, which are geographically isolated, has commented on the economics of ambulatory surgery under local anaesthesia for groin hernia. He reports 136 adult male and female patients treated using 80 ml of 0.5% lignocaine in saline solution as a field block. He administers 70–100 mg of pethidine 1 h before surgery and 5–10 mg of diazepam intravenously at commencement of the operation. His results are impressive and confirm the acceptability and adequacy of local anaesthesia. The complications attributable in part to the local anaesthesia include a thrombosis of the dorsal vein of the penis during infiltration of the local anaesthetic. There are savings in anaesthetic gases and the salaries of anaesthetists. These, together with the high costs and difficulties of transportation to the Seychelles, are seen as distinct benefits. Patient acceptability was also recorded and found to be high.

Another Third World experience is reported by Wijesinha. In this study 100 patients in a military hospital were operated on over a three-year period under local anaesthesia.[985] The stated advantages are less work for nursing staff, less morbidity for patients and less strain on scarce health resources. Patients included soldiers, sailors, airmen, and persons from such diverse trades as cooks, clerks, nurses, drivers, bandsmen, and even the army barber!

While the advantages, and disadvantages, of general and local anaesthetic have been advanced by protagonists of one or other method, such advocacy usually being based on personal experience, only one group have put the argument to the test of a prospective randomized trial. Teasdale and his colleagues from Bristol reported, in 1982, 103 adult patients randomly allocated to general anaesthesia (50) and local anaesthesia (53).[912] Both groups were administered intramuscular papaveretum and either hyoscine or atropine as a premedicant, and general anaesthesia involved endotracheal intubation and positive pressure ventilation of the lungs. Local anaesthesia was with plain lignocaine solution. The groups were evenly matched for age, obesity and type of hernia. Significant differences in outcome were observed between the groups. Local anaesthetic patients were able to walk, eat and pass urine sooner than those having general anaesthesia. Those having general anaesthesia experienced more nausea, vomiting, sore throat and headache. Ninety per cent of patients were discharged at 24 h. Eighty-five per cent of patients having local anaesthesia would consent to its use again.

In Teasdale's trial, 13 patients had to be excluded prior

to randomization and the authors rightly make the point that neither technique is suitable for all patients. The local anaesthetic patients complained of intraoperative pain and required more postoperative analgesia than the general anaesthetic patients; perhaps the choice of the short-action agent lignocaine without enhancement by adrenaline may have been responsible for this unusual observation. The use of tracheal intubation and controlled ventilation may be unnecessary in elective hernia patients having a general anaesthetic and could account for the postoperative sore throats.

More recently, Behnia and colleagues have compared the haemodynamic changes, recovery events and economic impact in 20 patients of ASA grade I and 20 patients receiving regional field block local anaesthesia with bupivacaine 3.5 ± 0.5 mg/kg.[82] General anaesthesia was induced with thiopentone and following tracheal intubation maintained with enflurane in 50% nitrous oxide and oxygen. Patients in the group receiving regional block did not require parenteral medication for relief of postoperative pain, whereas all those receiving general anaesthetic did. However, no postoperative inguinal field block was administered to these patients. This study concluded that significant cost benefits were realized by the group receiving regional block because of elimination of general anaesthesia and reduction of recovery room fees.

This study and the earlier studies of Knapp and Alsarrage do, however, show that in a randomized sample of patients both local and general anaesthesia are satisfactory and the exclusions on clinical grounds from the study confirm that both techniques are clinically important and that the operating surgeon should be acquainted with both.[505]

Morris and Tracey have reported adverse effects of lignocaine on the healing of experimental skin wounds. A dilute solution of 0.5% lignocaine had little effect on wound healing. Increasing the concentration to 2.0% caused a considerable retardation of wound healing. Adrenaline potentiates this effect.[669] For many reasons, toxicity, dispersion of anaesthesia and wound healing, weak solutions of local anaesthetic are preferred.

Ponka lists the advantages and disadvantages of local and general anaesthesia (Table 7.1).[752] Local anaesthesia is specific in his experience for some patients with poor cardiorespiratory function, and hepatic or renal disease. General anaesthesia is equally specific for the young, the psychotic, the neurotic and the nervous. Lastly, some surgeons prefer one or other anaesthetic technique. Local anaesthesia is only successful if the surgeon is gentle and patient and has confidence in his ability to maintain the patient's morale throughout this procedure. Don't ask, for example, 'Is that hurting?' or mention 'pain'; instead, ask the patient 'Are you quite comfortable?'

Although complication rates are low and hernia recurrence rates lower in many reported series using local anaesthesia, it is difficult to suggest that the anaesthetic has a direct effect on the recurrence rate, which is governed so much by surgical and technical factors.

There is no consensus on the optimal local anaesthetic agent – procaine, lignocaine and bupivacaine each have their devotees. The addition of adrenaline is practised by the majority of operators. With bupivacaine, the anaesthesia lasts some 8–10 h; the inadvertent infiltration of the femoral nerve with prolonged paralysis delaying discharge has been reported.[904] If lignocaine is employed, it is wise to administer atropine preoperatively to reduce the chance of bradycardia.

Local anaesthesia for inguinal hernia repair is well recorded in the literature. It has been shown to be satisfactory for the patients and their carers in the community.[19]

Table 7.1   Advantages and disadvantages of local anaesthesia (After Ponka, 1980[752])

Advantages	Disadvantages
(1) Safer for poor risk patient, especially those with severe active cardiac and pulmonary disease	(1) Some patients dislike being conscious during surgery; neurotic and psychotic patients, and children, may be unsuitable for local anaesthesia
(2) Postoperative respiratory disorder and coughing are rare	(2) Surgery under local anaesthesia takes longer and demands more patient and gentle surgical technique
(3) Patient is conscious and can co-operate in testing the repair during surgery	(3) Wound complications, haematoma and skin necrosis may occur if care is not taken
(4) Urinary retention is rare because voiding reflexes are undisturbed by anaesthesia	(4) Drug toxicity and sensitivity may occur. All patients should be screened for these risks and monitored throughout the procedure
(5) Earlier mobilization decreases the risk of deep vein thrombosis and pulmonary embolization	(5) If a complicated surgical problem is found, it is more difficult to deal with under local anaesthesia

Technique

The recommended local anaesthetic agent is bupivacaine hydrochloride (Marcaine). The addition of adrenaline prolongs the action and possibly reduces local haemorrhage. In practice, up to 2 mg/kg body weight of bupivacaine plain or 4 mg/kg body weight with adrenaline, can be safely used; the 0.25% solution with adrenaline 1:400 000 is used and it is diluted with 0.9% saline. For an adult male, 3 × 10 ml ampoules of bupivacaine 0.25% = 75 mg, diluted by addition of 120 ml 0.9% saline, gives an anaesthetic solution of 150 ml which is always adequate. Bupivacaine anaesthesia is slow in onset, so a 20 min break between injection and operation commencement is recommended. The dose should be reduced in the elderly and care taken to avoid direct intravascular injection during infiltration. The patient should be weighed preoperatively and the safe maximum dose calculated. The safe maximal dose of bupivacaine must **never** be exceeded.

Although pre-anaesthetic drugs are unnecessary, patient morale may be improved by intravenously giving midazolam just before the start of the procedure. It is essential to monitor the patient carefully throughout injection of the local anaesthetic; reading the blood pressure before and after injection of bupivacaine is mandatory, and a pulse oximeter and an electrocardiograph monitor should be used throughout. The importance of monitoring the patient's oxygen saturation, blood pressure, and ECG, particularly as the bupivacaine is injected, must be stressed. An experienced anaesthetic nurse should supervise the patient throughout the surgery. The surgeon should not do this **and** operate. Equipment for tracheal intubation should be available and skilled anaesthetic support must be on hand should the patient require it.

MONITORING

Because oxygen desaturation is common in procedures carried out under sedation[169] oxygen supplementation and measurement of arterial oxygen saturation by a pulse oximeter is mandatory. Oxygen saturation and clinical monitoring should be supplemented by devices that continuously display the heart rate, pulse volume or arterial pressure and electrocardiogram.[45] The patient must be able to respond to commands throughout the procedure: if they are unable to do so the sedationist has become an anaesthetist. The same standards should be applied to sedative techniques (and regional anaesthesia), when there is depression of consciousness or cardiovascular or respiratory complications. Pulse oximetry monitoring should continue until the patient meets the criteria for discharge from the recovery area. Oxygen saturation should not be permitted to fall below 90% (arterial oxygen tension of 7.9 kPa) as below this value a minor fall in oxygen tension results in a rapid fall in oxygen content.

Applied anatomy

Free nerve endings are distributed throughout the skin; stretch and pain receptors occur in each of the aponeurotic layers and in the parietal peritoneum. The skin and subcutaneous tissue are sensitive to all noxious stimuli. Pin prick, pressure and chemical stimuli (e.g. hypertonic solutions) cause pain in these tissues. The parietal peritoneum is sensitive to pin prick, stretching and chemical stimuli. In contrast, the visceral peritoneum and hollow organs are insensitive to touch, to clamp, to knife and to cautery, but the visceral arteries to these organs are sensitive. There is no pain when viscera are handled under local anaesthesia, until a clamp is placed on the vascular pedicle.

ABDOMINAL WALL

Knowledge of the fundamental physiology and neuroanatomy of pain in the abdomen is essential if adequate local analgesia is to be obtained. Local anaesthesia should achieve the following:

1. Ensure skin anaesthesia in the line of incision. Remembering the overlap and connections between the rich plexus of epidermal nerve endings, this is best accomplished by a skin weal.
2. Block the nerve supply to the aponeurotic layers which must be dissected and manipulated.
3. Ensure anaesthesia of the parietal peritoneum of the hernia and especially of the neck of the sac which is very sensitive.

The distribution of the cutaneous nerves to the abdomen, groin and thigh is familiar to all surgeons. The anterior portions of the six lower intercostal nerves are continued forward from their respective spaces onto the anterior abdominal wall, and are accompanied by the last thoracic (subcostal) nerve. Additionally the iliohypogastric and ilio-inguinal nerve (Tl and L1) supply the lower abdomen. The genitofemoral nerve (L1 and L2) via its genital branch supplies the cord structures and anterior scrotum and via its femoral branch the skin and subcutaneous tissue in the femoral triangle. All the nerves of the anterior abdominal wall communicate with each other and thus their cutaneous distribution overlaps (Figure 7.1).

The intercostal nerves run from their intercostal space forwards between the internal oblique and transversus muscles to the lateral margin of the rectus sheath. They enter the sheath on its posterior aspect, supply the rectus muscle, pierce the anterior sheath and then ramify in the subcutaneous tissue and supply the adjacent skin. Each of these nerves gives a lateral cutaneous branch which

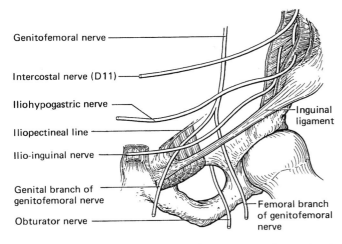

Genitofemoral nerve

Intercostal nerve (D11)

Iliohypogastric nerve

Iliopectineal line

Ilio-inguinal nerve

Genital branch of genitofemoral nerve

Obturator nerve

Inguinal ligament

Femoral branch of genitofemoral nerve

Figure 7.1 Sensory nerve supply of the inguinal, femoral and obturator regions

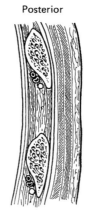
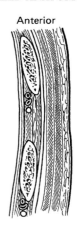

Posterior

Anterior

Figure 7.3 The relative positions of the ribs and the intercostal nerves vary. Posterior to the mid-axillary line the intercostal nerves and vessels are tucked under the rib next above, anteriorly they lie midway between the ribs in the mid-intercostal space

pierces the flat muscles and becomes subcutaneous in the midaxillary line. Once subcutaneous, this lateral cutaneous branch gives anterior and posterior branches to supply the skin and subcutaneous tissue.

For local anaesthesia nerve block to be successful, the intercostal nerve must be blocked before the lateral cutaneous branch is given off. The site of election for the local anaesthetic injection is in the posterior axillary line. If the intercostal nerve is blocked too far anteriorly, the anterior division of the lateral cutaneous branch will remain sensitive (Figure 7.2).

It should be remembered that the intercostal nerve is tucked under the lower border of the rib in its posterior third and in the centre of the intercostal space more anteriorly (Figure 7.3).

When the hernia is exposed, it is important to infiltrate the neck of the hernial sac (parietal peritoneum) to ensure adequate anaesthesia while the sac is dissected, incised, emptied and closed.

THE GROIN

Inguinal and femoral hernias lie in the borderland between the regular anatomy of the abdominal wall and

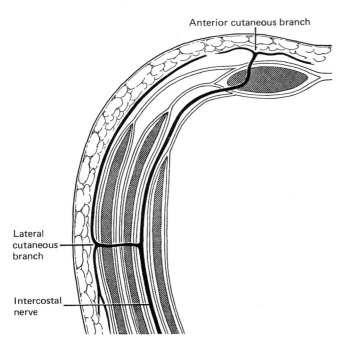

Anterior cutaneous branch

Lateral cutaneous branch

Intercostal nerve

Figure 7.2 Transverse section through the abdominal wall. the lateral cutaneous branch of an intercostal nerve gives an anterior and posterior division; the anterior division must be blocked for effective abdominal wall anaesthesia

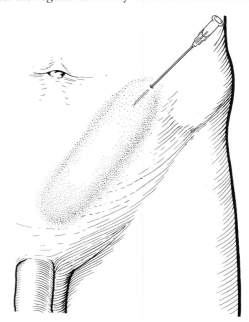

Figure 7.4 Local anaesthesia for an inguinal hernioplasty: using a long spinal needle a weal of local anaesthetic solution is made in the line of the groin incision

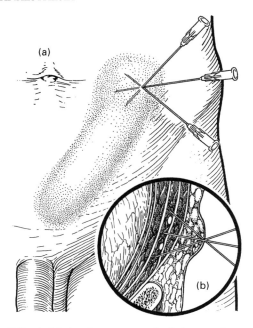

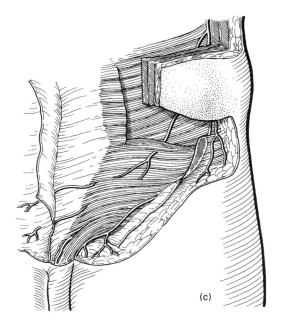

Figure 7.5 (a,b) At the upper end of the previous weal, at a point approximately 1 cm above and medial to the anterior superior iliac spine, some 3 ml of the anaesthetic solution is injected deep to the aponeurosis of the external oblique. The needle is pushed in until the external oblique aponeurosis is felt as a firm resistant structure. (c) The needle is pushed through the aponeurosis and the anaesthetic solution distributed to block the ilio-inguinal and iliohypogastric nerves which run between the external and internal oblique muscles at this point

the complex anatomy of the lower limb. However, the same technical sequence ensures adequate regional anaesthesia:

1. A local weal is raised in the line of the incision. This weal starts 2 cm above and medial to the anterior superior iliac spine. Long spinal needles are used for this infiltration (Figure 7.4).

2. An injection is made between the internal oblique and transversus muscles about 1 cm superior to the anterior superior spine in an endeavour to block the ilio-inguinal and ilio-epigastric nerves. To do this the needle is pushed in vertically; the 'give' as the needle penetrates the aponeurosis of the external oblique allows easy estimate of the depth of the injection. Five or ten millilitres of local anaesthetic are injected at this site (Figure 7.5).

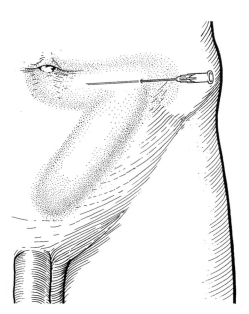

Figure 7.6 The subcutaneous tissue is lightly infiltrated to the midline in a horizontal direction to block 'overlap' from the 11th thoracic nerve

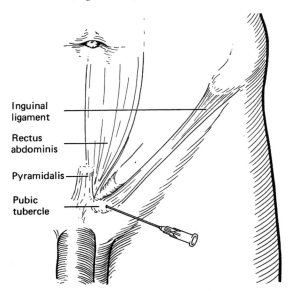

Inguinal ligament

Rectus abdominis

Pyramidalis

Pubic tubercle

Figure 7.7 The medial end of the oblique groin (incision) weal is topped up down to the pubic tubercle and origin of the rectus

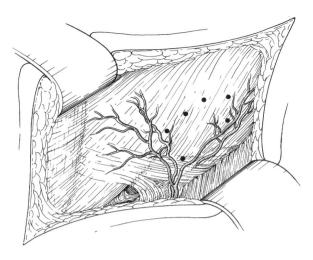

Figure 7.8 After the skin and subcutaneous tissue has been opened, and the external oblique aponeurosis (the anterior wall of the inguinal canal) exposed, further local anaesthetic is injected through it and into the cord. This should anaesthetize the peritoneum of an indirect sac and block the genital branch of the genitofemoral nerve in the cord

3. The subcutaneous tissue is infiltrated horizontally from the anterior superior spine to the midline. This is necessary to block 'overlap' from the 11th thoracic nerve (Figure 7.6).

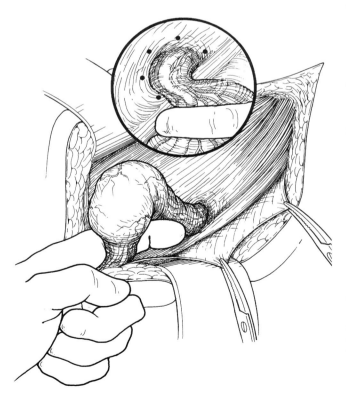

Figure 7.9 The parietal peritoneum is very sensitive. Further local anaesthetic is injected into the layers of the cord and around the neck of the sac between the fascia transversalis and the peritoneum

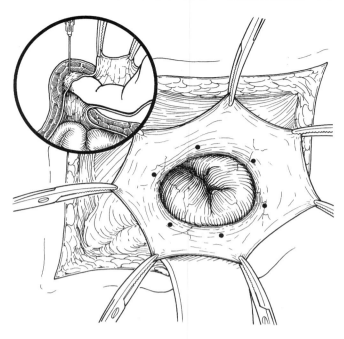

Figure 7.10 Further careful injection between the peritoneum and the fascia transversalis assists defining the tissue planes. This makes isolation and dissection of the fascia transversalis much more acceptable to the patient

4. The medial end of the oblique subcutaneous weal is now 'topped up' with 2 ml of local solution, taking care to carry the injection down to the pubic tubercle and the origin of the rectus muscle from the pubis (Figure 7.7).
5. Infiltrate the cord and adjacent peritoneum at the deep ring. Divide the external oblique and mobilize the cord and indirect sac (Figure 7.8).
6. Infiltrate the preperitoneal space around the deep ring, the direct area and around the medial end of the inguinal ligament. Do this under vision and carefully. This is an important 'trick of the trade'. Careful infiltration of this layer will accomplish peritoneal anaesthesia. More importantly, the 'hydrodissection' will separate the fascia transversalis from the peritoneum and make definition of the layers for repair much easier (Figures 7.9 and 7.10).

Complications of local anaesthetics

Complications of local anaesthetics are systemic and local:

1. Systemic: (a) excitation of the nervous system, nervousness, nausea and convulsions – these are very rare; (b) depression of the cardiovascular system with hypotension and arrhythmias; (c) hypersensitivity reactions are very rare with lignocaine and bupivacaine.

2. Local: (a) ecchymoses and bruising; (b) local ischaemia and tissue necrosis if too much adrenaline is injected at one site; (c) these local complications can compromise wound healing.

The systemic side effects are life threatening, hence patients undergoing local anaesthesia should be questioned about previous side effects from local anaesthetics. Most importantly, they should have their CNS and CVS state monitored throughout the procedure and for up to 30 min after surgery. Increased patient excitability and garrulousness, a rising pulse rate and an increasing blood pressure are the early signs of CNS intoxication. If these signs are observed, an anaesthetist should be summoned without delay.

Sedation

A small dose of intravenous midazolam (2–4 mg) reduces anxiety and makes the patient more relaxed and co-operative. In addition the useful side effect of retrograde amnesia will reduce the impact of the unfamiliar surroundings of the operating theatre following the procedure. Although recovery from intravenous midazolam is not as rapid as recovery from intravenous propofol, surgeons should not dabble with unfamiliar intravenous agents. Anecdotal evidence suggests that administration of propofol reduces local anaesthetic requirements.[169] Nevertheless, the benzodiazepine antagonist flumazenil (Anexate) should be available and used to improve recovery or combat unexpected narcosis caused by benzodiazepines. Recovery should be advanced before reversal to eliminate the likelihood of sleep reoccurring as the antagonist action wears off.

POSTOPERATIVE ANALGESIA

Effective postoperative pain relief benefits the patient by providing comfort in the period after surgery as well as modifying the autonomic and somatic reflexes to pain which delay recovery. Treatment of pain facilitates early rehabilitation and recovery.[981] Nerve blocks provide pre-emptive analgesia which may prevent central sensitization and secondary hyperalgesia after tissue damage. In a study by Harrison and colleagues[402] of 40 patients, using 10 ml of 0.5% bupivacaine for blockade of the ilio-inguinal and iliohypogastric nerves, and 20 ml of 0.5% bupivacaine for wound infiltration, the time of the first analgesic and the morphine consumption in the first 6 h postoperatively was considerably reduced. Patients given general anaesthesia do not differ in pain scores or analgesic consumption whether given inguinal field block before the surgical incision or after wound closure.[251] Spittal and colleagues have demonstrated that local anaesthetic procedures can be simplified still further in that instillation of bupivacaine into the wound provided the same degree of postoperative analgesic effect as a formal inguinal field block in patients undergoing inguinal hernia repair under general anaesthesia.[886] The benefits of supplementary bupivacaine local anaesthesia are so well documented that omission of this step should be considered suboptimal care.

Further improvements in postoperative pain relief can be achieved by the use of balanced analgesia or managed anaesthetic care (MAC). The combination of non-steroidal anti-inflammatory drugs, opioids and local anaesthesia acting at different points on pain pathways can maximize analgesic effects and minimize side effects. The non-steroidal anti-inflammatory drug diclofenac sodium (Voltarol) can reduce postoperative opioid requirements by 15–60% and reduce nausea. A suppository of 100 mg diclofenac sodium administered 1 h before surgery has now become an established part of balanced analgesia regimens. However, this drug should be used with caution in patients with previous gastrointestinal ulceration, asthma, renal failure, heart failure or bleeding diatheses.

Previously, dextropropoxyphene 32.5 mg and paracetamol 325 mg (Distalgesic) was recommended as a self-administered analgesic after day-case hernia repair. This policy has been reviewed and abandoned on account of the toxicity of this drug combination. However, perhaps the most important reason for no longer prescribing Distalgesic or its equivalent is that powerful postoperative analgesia is never required after routine repair of an inguinal hernia using current modern techniques. Regular oral paracetamol for up to one week should be recommended to supplement local anaesthetic wound blockade, intravenous midazolam and preoperative diclofenac.

In the early 1970s the use of skin clips, with the attendant removal of them, caused troublesome wound pain which patients complained of. Subcuticular sutures of fine PDS have eliminated this problem and most patients require minimal postoperative analgesics.

Local anaesthesia – incisional, Spigelian and other abdominal wall hernias

The same concept of local anaesthesia – a combination of regional block and field infiltration – can be employed for incisional, Spigelian and epigastric hernias. Important points are to adequately infiltrate the subcutaneous layer, especially cranial to the proposed incision, and then to adequately anaesthetize the intercostal nerves which run deep to the internal oblique/rectus sheath aponeurosis to within 2 cm of the midline. If a regional block is required, to repair a large incisional hernia, the intercostal nerves must be infiltrated in the posterior axillary line before they give their lateral cutaneous branch. The incidence of urinary retention following inguinal herniorrhaphy, which is the single most common cause of unplanned hospital admission, is significantly reduced by carrying out the operation under local anaesthesia.[302, 741]

Conclusions

Either local or general anaesthesia is suitable for hernia repair. Patient and surgeon preference are indications for one or the other.

Balanced analgesia should be employed.

Preoperative diclofenac sodium is recommended in selected patients.

A combination of local infiltration and field block is the recommended local anaesthetic technique.

Intravascular injection is the great hazard of infiltration anaesthesia and must be avoided at all costs.

Bupivacaine hydrochloride 0.5% is the recommended anaesthetic agent. The action of bupivacaine is enhanced and prolonged by adrenaline. The maximum dose of bupivacaine plain is 2 mg/kg body weight and bupivacaine with adrenaline 4 mg/kg body weight and must never be exceeded.

Careful intraoperative supervision and monitoring of the patient is essential for safety.

Local anaesthetic wound blockade should be performed in patients receiving general anaesthesia.

8 COMPLICATIONS OF HERNIA IN GENERAL

The complications of hernia include:

1. Rupture of the hernia – spontaneous or traumatic.
2. Involvement of the hernial sac in the disease process: (a) mesothelial hyperplasia; (b) carcinoma; (c) endometriosis and leiomyomatosis; (d) inflammation – peritonitis, acute appendicitis.
3. Incarceration, obstruction and strangulation. Reductio-en-masse.
4. Maydl's hernia and afferent loop strangulation. Strangulation of the appendix in a hernial sac. Richter's hernia. Littré's hernia.
5. Herniation of female genitalia. Pregnancy in a hernial sac.
6. Urinary tract complications, hernia of the bladder, the ureter and of a urinary ileal conduit.
7. Sliding hernia.
8. Testicular strangulation in: (a) infants; (b) adults with large giant inguinoscrotal hernias; (c) Africans.

Spontaneous and traumatic rupture

Spontaneous rupture (dehiscence) of hernia is a well-recognized though rare complication. Helwig (1958), in a comprehensive article, reported 47 cases of spontaneous exteriorization of hernial contents; of these 17 were through incisional hernia, while the remainder were through inguinal, femoral, umbilical or epigastric hernia or through recurrences of these.[417] Spontaneous rupture of an umbilical hernia with evisceration is a very rare event. Four such cases are described in the British literature and one in India. In two cases there was no precipitating cause,[637, 900] in one a bout of severe coughing precipitated rupture and evisceration,[59] in another damage to the overlying skin and trauma,[406] and in the remaining case umbilical sepsis may have been to blame.[170] All of the children were under 4 months at the time of rupture. Damage to the bowel did not occur in any of the four British cases and complete recovery followed reduction of the bowel and standard umbilical hernioplasty.

Further cases of spontaneous rupture of hernia have been described but such ruptures all follow previous surgery; they are all failures of incisional hernia scars. Such cases are described by O'Donoghue (1955) (a 56-year-old woman 13 years after a gynaecological operation);[710] Hartley (1962) (two cases – a 74-year-old man 12 years after a suprapubic prostatectomy and an 84-year-old woman 13 years after an appendicectomy through a right lower paramedian scar).[406]

Hamilton (1966) (a 76-year-old woman presenting six years after a bilateral salpingo-oophorectomy);[391] and Senapati (1982) (a 45-year-old woman who had undergone two caesarean operations 12 and 15 years previously).[843]

The majority of spontaneous hernia ruptures are in lower abdominal, inguinal and incisional hernias. Many develop insidiously and present in emergency departments some time after an apparently painless disruption. Others are associated with episodes of straining or coughing. The dehiscence would appear to be a degenerative process, with the relatively avascular and thin hernial sac undergoing progressive stretching, becoming increasingly ischaemic and finally giving way. This process is accelerated in some cases by skin ulceration due to tight corsets, or to intertrigo and skin infection in pendulous sacs.

Surprisingly, the mortality is small – no deaths are reported since 1945. The main peritoneal cavity is uncontaminated, the tight neck usually preventing reduction of the contents and contamination of the main peritoneal cavity .

Spontaneous rupture leading to fistula and then 'cure' was of course described by Cheselden (1784) (Figure 12).[175] A more remarkable example of a spontaneous cure of an incarcerated right inguinal hernia in a 7–week-old Chinese male child whose hernia remained irreducible for 10 days and who then developed a caecal fistula is reported by Stock (1951).[893]

Rupture of the intestine in an unreduced hernia in a male subjected to trauma is not excessively rare; deaths from this cause appear in nineteenth century literature (Aird, 1935).[7] Except in one case in which the colon was damaged in a sliding hernia, the perforated loop of small intestine is invariably found in the general peritoneal cavity. There is an association between small bowel rupture due to blunt trauma and inguinal hernia. Small bowel perforation is more likely to have occurred if the trauma was sustained when a hernia is 'down'.

Where the violence is applied directly to the hernia the explanation is simple – the intestine is damaged locally where it lies unprotected in the hernial sac. When blunt trauma is applied to the abdomen, loops of mobile gut slide around to absorb the violence. Fixed gut is most at risk; hence the duodenum and terminal ileum are most frequently damaged. A hernia which is 'down' is another fixed point contributing to gut immobility and predisposing to serious injury.

Involvement of hernial sac in disease process

NODULAR MESOTHELIAL HYPERPLASIA AND MESOTHELIOMA

The peritoneum has a great capacity to undergo metaplasia, to form papillary projections, pseudo-acini, squamous nests and even cartilaginous nodules in response to repeated mechanical trauma.[3] Cirrhotic ascites and collagen vascular disease are associated with marked mesothelial hyperplasia. Nodular mesothelial hyperplasia can develop in hernial sacs, particularly those subject to trauma. A truss can be an initiating factor. Nodular mesothelial hyperplasia has been described in hernial sacs in infants and children and in these cases is associated with repeated episodic incarceration or strangulation.

The pathological features are the presence in the sac of cellular nodules up to 1.0 cm in diameter. These nodules are composed of cells with a pale acidophilic cytoplasm derived from the peritoneum. The cells show a moderate to severe pleomorphism; most are round cells when lying free in the intercellular fluid, but they are polygonal when compressed together by neighbouring cells to form the characteristic nodules.[792] The nodules may coalesce to form cystic spaces grossly resembling a pseudomyxoma.[793]

If injury to the hernial sac is sustained and of sufficient intensity, the mesothelial proliferation can exceed the simple needs of regeneration and acquire pseudomalignant cytologic features. The consummate ability of mesothelial cells to simulate carcinoma should be remembered and pathologists need to be cautious in interpreting the microscopic features of hernial sacs.[793] Nodular mesothelial hyperplasia is more common in infants and children and in them it exhibits its most exuberant characteristics. The condition is entirely benign – no radical surgery is required and follow-up data confirms the harmless nature of the lesion. It is important to make the correct diagnosis to avoid pointless and potentially dangerous therapy.

On the other hand, genuine peritoneal mesothelioma has been encountered within a hernial sac.[114] The mesothelioma may be found by chance or alternatively the patient can present with a mass in the hernial sac wall. While mesothelioma generally arises in the main peritoneal cavity, it can arise from the hernial sac itself or from the cord or the tunica vaginalis. If the mesothelioma arises from the cord structures or from mesothelial remnants in them, in addition to the mass the patients usually also feature a hydrocele.

Malignant mesothelioma has been encountered in hernial sacs in patients with no history of exposure to asbestos, further evidence for a relationship with local trauma and the occurrence of mesothelial hyperplasia. Such a local origin is consistent with the relatively benign prognosis patients presenting with hernial sac mesothelioma enjoy. Survival without further symptoms to five or six years is recorded. Eventually, however, intraperitoneal deposits appear and intestinal obstruction and other complications then ensue.[114]

CARCINOMA AS A COMPLICATION OF HERNIAL SACS

Malignancy involving inguinal hernial sacs is uncommon but not rare. Suspicion should always haunt the surgeon's mind, particularly when he is confronted with an elderly patient with the recent onset of a groin hernia.[299, 795] If the sac is thickened or ascitic fluid is present in it at operation, it should be subjected to histological evaluation and the ascitic fluid to full cytology. The hernial sac offers a unique opportunity for peritoneal biopsy which should not be missed. If a suspicious sac is found at hernioplasty, immediate frozen section may elucidate the pathology, while digital laparotomy through the hernial orifice may give more information. Immediate laparotomy is not advised: repair the hernia and subject the patient to early elective operation after bowel preparation and antibiotic prophylaxis.

Lejars (1889)[549] classified malignant involvement of inguinal hernial sacs into three varieties: extrasaccular, saccular and intrasaccular. While this classification has merit it does not easily fit contemporary concepts of pathology and surgery. A better classification is:

1. Primary carcinoma: (a) extrasaccular; (b) intrasaccular.
2. Secondary carcinoma – predominantly intrasaccular: derived, by transcoelomic spread, from lung, breast, stomach, colon, ovary or any other intraperitoneal viscus.

Extrasaccular carcinoma can arise from the bladder or from a diverticulum of the bladder which is sliding into the medial side of a direct hernia. Similarly, a carcinoma may occur in the colon, which is a component of the wall of a sliding hernia. Such a carcinoma may obstruct, and a mistaken diagnosis of a strangulated hernia be made. Careful history-taking can avoid this error. In the six examples recorded in the literature, all the hernias were large and scrotal and all had been present and irreducible for some considerable time before they presented with intestinal obstruction.[546] The carcinoma is usually bulky, locally advanced and may be palpated in the sac, which is not so discreetly tender as the sac containing strangulated small bowel.[366] A liposarcoma of the cord, which invaded the adjacent hernial sac, is reported reminding surgeons that not all malignancy in groin hernias is derived from the peritoneal cavity.[795]

Intrasaccular carcinoma is a primary carcinoma arising from an organ which is a permanent denizen of a hernial sac. The most frequent examples are colon or caecal cancers. Malignant tumours arising from an appendix in a hernial sac also occur.[693]

Carcinomas in hernial sacs are often locally fixed and advanced when the diagnosis is made. This should not prevent wide local excision being successfully undertaken. Intrasaccular carcinoma can also occur in Spigelian, umbilical and incisional hernias.

Routine histological examination of hernial sacs is not recommended. Kassan and colleagues routinely examined 1020 hernial sacs after surgery; the incidence of unexpected findings, the discovery of an occult tumour, in those specimens which appeared normal to the surgeon at operation was 1 in 1020 (0.098%). The incremental cost per unexpected finding was $49 041 and the only unexpected and abnormal finding in the series was one atypical lipoma.[484] If at operation the hernial sac is seen to be abnormal or if it is thickened, then histology should always be performed. However, there is no positive benefit to be gained by the patient from routine histological examination of an apparently normal sac.

GYNAECOLOGICAL TUMOURS – ENDOMETRIOSIS AND LEIOMYOMAS

Endometriomas are not infrequently encountered in incisional hernias related to caesarean section. The characteristic cyclical pain should enable a preoperative diagnosis.

Leiomyomas arising from uterine fibroids are also encountered in inguinal, femoral, obturator[697] and umbilical hernial[185] sacs in women.

ACUTE INFLAMMATION – PERITONITIS AND APPENDICITIS AS COMPLICATIONS OF A HERNIAL SAC

Intraperitoneal sepsis producing pus and presenting as a painful distended hernial sac is an important differential diagnosis of strangulated hernia; in these circumstances the hernia is behaving as a peritoneal recess in which pus can loculate. Zuckerkandl first described this phenomenon in 1891. His patient was a 55-year-old male with a six-day history of a painful irreducible right inguinal hernia. At operation the hernial sac contained pus only and the perforated appendix lay in the peritoneal cavity just above the sac. The appendix was not removed and the patient recovered.[1009] Cronin and Ellis reported five

patients from Oxford in which a pus-filled hernia misled surgeons into a preoperative diagnosis of strangulated hernia.[205] This complication of pus in a hernial sac most frequently occurs in right inguinal,[88] then right femoral,[328] then left inguinal and, least often, in left femoral hernias.[970] The syndrome has been encountered in epigastric and umbilical hernias. Underlying pathologies include acute appendicitis (the most common), perforated peptic ulcer, pneumococcal peritonitis, acute pyosalpinx, acute pancreatitis and biliary peritonitis.[205, 280]

In acute appendicitis the appendix may itself be contained in an external hernial sac. Ryan, in 1937, collected 537 cases. An overall incidence of 0.3% of cases of acute appendicitis were found to occur in a hernial sac.[819] Although the appendix is frequently encountered within an inguinal or femoral hernial sac, it is rarely inflamed. The first reported case of appendicitis in a femoral hernial sac is that of De Garengeot in 1731.[227] Doolin (1919) described a case in which a tender femoral hernial sac was found to contain pus and the gangrenous tip of the appendix. In this patient there were no abnormal findings in the abdomen above the inguinal ligament.[258] Hernial appendicitis usually occurs in a right inguinal or right femoral hernia.[554] Claudius Amyand performed the first successful appendicectomy in 1736, which was contained in a right inguinal hernia.[716] Amyand, a Huguenot, was a pioneer of smallpox vaccination and surgeon to King George II at St George's Hospital, London – the appendix had given rise to a fistula in the right groin where it had been perforated by a pin and was discharging through an inguinal hernia. The patient was an 11-year-old boy and the operation was done without anaesthesia: it is not surprising that the hernia recurred. However, Amyand deserves the title of pioneer of surgery of the vermiform appendix, having carried out the operation of appendicectomy successfully 144 years before Lawson Tate removed an inflamed appendix through the abdomen in 1880.[849] Most reported cases of appendicitis are in femoral hernias of post-menopausal women or in inguinal hernias in males of all ages from six weeks to 88 years. Appendicitis has been reported in a left inguinal hernia,[154] in an umbilical hernia,[256] in an obturator hernia[31] and in incisional hernias.[154, 917]

The diagnosis of acute hernial appendicitis has been reported preoperatively only once, by Gray in 1910.[362] The history usually suggests a strangulated hernia with local peritonitis. The differential diagnosis is a Richter's hernia or strangulated omentum. The pain in both these conditions is classically continuous and boring, whereas in early appendicitis peri-umbilical colic is a typical feature.[197]

Treatment is operation, if possible appendicectomy via the hernial sac, with repair of the hernia. In a series of seven cases, four femoral and three inguinal, from

Bristol and Exeter, the preoperative diagnosis was a strangulated hernia in each instance; appendicitis was not suspected. Appendicectomy via the sac and hernioplasty was performed in each. All the patients recovered, although wound infection created postoperative problems in three patients. Preoperatively only three patients had right iliac fossa pain, but all had histories lasting longer than 24 h before the diagnosis was reached.[917] Acute appendicitis in a hernial sac must be distinguished from acute strangulation of the appendix in a hernia[469] (see below).

Incarceration, obstruction and strangulation

Incarceration is the state of an external hernia which cannot be reduced into the abdomen. Incarceration is important because it implies an increased risk of obstruction and strangulation. Incarceration is caused by (a) a tight hernial sac neck; (b) adhesions between the hernial contents and the sac lining – these adhesions are sometimes a manifestation of previous ischaemia and inflammation; (c) development of pathology in the incarcerated viscus, e.g. a carcinoma or diverticulitis in incarcerated colon; (d) impaction of faeces in an incarcerated colon.

Incarceration is an important finding. It should urge the surgeon to undertake operation sooner rather than later. If reduction of a hernia is performed it should be gentle; forcible reduction of an incarcerated hernia may precipitate reductio-en-masse (see below). If bowel with a compromised blood supply is reduced, stricturing and adhesions between gut loops will follow. This will lead to intestinal obstruction some weeks or months later.[597, 662] The best policy is to operate on incarcerated hernias and check the viability of the gut at operation.

Incarceration in an inguinal hernia is the commonest cause of acute intestinal obstruction in infants and children in the UK. In adults, postoperative adhesions account for 40% of cases of obstruction, external hernias for 30% and malignancy for 25% of cases. In tropical Africa, strangulated external hernia is the commonest cause of intestinal obstruction in all age groups.[218] In West Africa, strangulated inguinal hernia is the commonest cause of obstruction, with indirect inguinal hernia accounting for 85% and direct hernias 15% of these cases. In the African experience, Richter's hernias are more common with direct than with indirect sacs.[53] Incarceration of the distal stomach and pylorus in an inguinal hernia can give symptoms of gastric outflow obstruction.[219]

All patients presenting with symptoms of intestinal obstruction should have all the potential hernial sites very carefully examined. The sites of obstruction are inguinal, femoral, umbilical, incisional, Spigelian and obturator hernial orifices in that order.

A partial enterocele (Richter's hernia) is a particularly treacherous variety of hernia, especially in infancy (see below). Partial enterocele is a potentially lethal and easily overlooked complication of 'port site' hernia following laparoscopy.[518]

Strangulation is the major life-threatening complication of abdominal hernias. In strangulation the blood supply to the hernial contents is compromised. At first there is angulation and distortion of the neck of the sac; this leads to lymphatic and venous engorgement. The herniated contents become oedematous. Capillary vascular permeability develops. The arterial supply is occluded by the developing oedema and now the scene is set for ischaemic changes in the bowel wall.

The gut mucosal defences are breached and intestinal bacteria multiply and penetrate through to infect the hernial sac contents. Necrobiosis and gangrene complete a sad and lethal cycle unless surgery or preternatural fistula formation save the patient. Hypovolaemic and septic shock predicate vigorous resuscitation if surgery is to be successful.[953]

STRANGULATED EXTERNAL HERNIA

The incidence of strangulated hernia has not altered significantly in the UK over the past 15 years. The average annual incidence of strangulated external hernia is 13 per 100 000 population.[765] There are significant seasonal variations in the incidence of strangulation, the condition being most prevalent in the winter months (October to March). In the summer six months (April to September) the incidence (5 per 100 000 population) is less than half the rate for the winter.[25] Perhaps this is associated with coughing related to respiratory tract infections which are more prevalent in winter.

During the period 1991–1992, 210 deaths occurring following inguinal hernia repair and 120 deaths following femoral hernia repair, were investigated by the UK National Confidential Enquiry Into Perioperative Deaths.[148] This enquiry is concerned with the quality of delivery of surgery, anaesthesia and perioperative care. Expert advisers compare the records of patients who have died with index cases. In this group of 330 patients many were elderly (45 were aged 80–89 years) and unfit; 24 were ASA grade III and 21 ASA grade IV. Postoperative mortality was attributed to pre-existing cardiorespiratory problems in the majority of cases. Clearly this group of patients require high-quality care by an experienced surgeon and anaesthetist with skills equivalent to that of the ASA grade of the patient. Postoperative care should necessarily take place in a high dependency unit or intensive therapy unit; this may necessitate transfer of selected patients to appropriate hospitals and facilities. Sensible decisions must be made in consultation with relatives of extremely elderly, frail or moribund patients to adopt a humane approach, which may rule out interventional surgery.

The age incidence shows a peak in the very young (see Chapter 9), then a low incidence rising to a peak in the eighth decade. Males predominate until the seventy-fifth year, after which females present more frequently. Right-sided hernias strangulate more frequently than left-sided hernias; this is possibly related to mesenteric anatomy (Table 8.1). Therefore age is the main risk factor and determinant for strangulation.

Neuhauser, who studied a population in Columbia where elective herniorrhaphy was virtually unobtainable, found an annual rate of strangulation of 0.29% for inguinal hernias.[695] There is no previous history of hernia in 10% of cases of strangulation.[315] Strangulation in adults is more likely in femoral, incisional and recurrent inguinal hernias rather than primary inguinal hernias and is associated with a high morbidity and mortality. Therefore, however reluctant surgeons may be to tackle femoral, incisional and recurrent inguinal hernias electively, the greater risk of strangulation and the high complication rate when these hernias strangulate necessitate elective repair whenever this is possible[25] (Figure 8.1).

Table 8.1 Strangulated hernias: effect of hernia type on rate of bowel resection and morality in adults (From Andrews, 1981,[15] by permission)

Hernia type	Resection (%)	Morality (%)
Primary inguinal	9.5	13.6
Femoral	18.0	15.0
Umbilical	25.0	4.0
Incisional	22.0	0.0
Recurrent	40.0	18.0

Forty percent of patients with femoral hernia are admitted as emergency cases with strangulation or incarceration, whereas only 3% of patients with direct inguinal hernias present with strangulation. This clearly has implications for the prioritization on waiting lists when these types of hernia present electively to outpatient clinics. A groin hernia is at its greatest risk of strangulation within three months of its onset.[322, 663] For inguinal hernia at three months after presentation the cumulative probability of strangulation is 2.8%, rising to 4.5% after two years (Figure 8.2). For femoral hernia the risk is much higher, with a 22% probability of strangulation at three months after presentation rising to 45% at 21 months (Figure 8.3). McEntee et al. in Limerick, Ireland, questioned patients presenting to hospital with strangulated hernias about their previous history:[633] 58% had noted the hernia for one month, 23% of these had not reported the hernia to their family doctor, 24% were known by their family practitioner to have the hernia and a non-surgical approach advised, and 11% had been assessed in secondary care with a view to elective herniorrhaphy (of these half were considered fit for operation and the others were on a waiting list). A further survey indicates lack of uniformity in the approach to elective surgery in patients at high risk of strangulation.[12] A questionnaire sent to 406 senior physicians, geriatricians, surgeons and general practitioners asked if they would advocate elective surgery for a small, painless, reducible inguinal hernia in a 79-year-old man or an asymptomatic femoral hernia in a frail 80-year-old woman. The percentage of positive answers for elective surgery in the elderly man ranged from 10% (physicians) to 29% (surgeons) and for the elderly female from 38% (general practitioners)

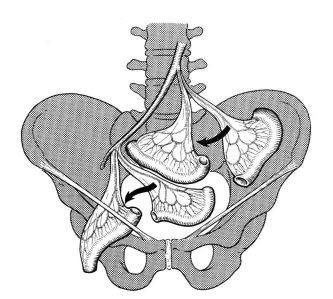

Figure 8.1 The mesenteric anatomy determines that right-sided inguinal, femoral and obturator hernias strangulate more frequently than left-sided ones

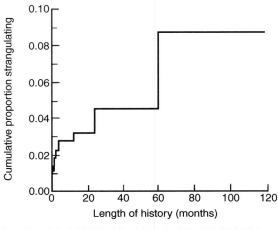

Time (months)	0.03	0.5	1.0	1.2	2.0	3.0	12.0	24.0	60.0
Patients at risk	439	433	431	411	401	369	237	151	70
Strangulations	4	1	2	1	2	2	1	2	3

Figure 8.2 Plot of the cumulative proportion of inguinal hernias strangulating versus length of history.[316] (Redrawn with permission from Gallegos et al., 1991[322])

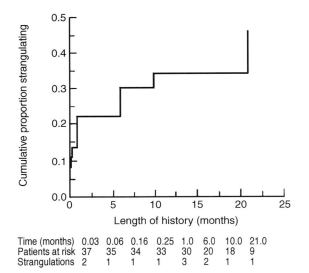

Time (months)	0.03	0.06	0.16	0.25	1.0	6.0	10.0	21.0
Patients at risk	37	35	34	33	30	20	18	9
Strangulations	2	1	1	1	3	2	1	1

Figure 8.3 Plot of the cumulative proportion of femoral hernias strangulating versus length of history.[316] (Redrawn with permission from Gallegos *et al.*, 1991[322])

to 78% (surgeons). These figures indicate that general practitioners, and to a lesser extent hospital specialists, are wrongly exercising a selective policy at the expense of the elderly. In a patient over the age of 60 years a strangulated hernia has a 20-fold increased risk of death compared with elective repair.

In both the UK and the USA the annual death rate due to inguinal and femoral hernia has decreased in the last two to three decades.[651, 989] In the UK deaths for inguinal and femoral hernia declined from 22% and 55% respectively from 1975 to 1990. The annual deaths in the USA per 100 000 population for patients with hernia and intestinal obstruction decreased from 5.1 in 1968 to 3.0 in 1988. For inguinal hernia with obstruction 88% of patients underwent surgery with a mortality rate of 0.05%. These figures could be interpreted as showing that elective groin hernia surgery has reduced overall mortality rates. In support of this contention is the fact that strangulation rates are lower in the USA than in the UK, which could be a consequence of the three times higher rate of elective hernia surgery in the USA. Even so, the available statistics show that rates of elective hernia surgery in the USA per 100 000 population fell from 358 to 220 between 1975 and 1990,[651] although this may be an artefact of the data collection systems rather than a real decline.[811]

The conclusion from these studies is that the general public, especially the elderly, should be aware of the potential dangers of a lump in the groin. Hospital physicians and general practitioners should be encouraged to refer patients with groin hernias promptly to specialists, particularly those patients with a lump that has been present for of three months or less. Indeed, patients referred with an inguinal lump or hernia (as opposed to

a femoral hernia) should receive an early out-patient appointment because of the doubt in diagnosis.[164]

Obturator hernias are very prone to strangulation; however, their elective repair is rarely feasible. To avoid confusion, primary inguinal hernias in adult males, particularly the direct spontaneously reducible 'dome' hernias, are not at significant risk of strangulation and do not always warrant an elective operation (this is discussed further in Chapter 12).

MANAGEMENT OF STRANGULATION

Diagnosis is based on symptoms and signs supplemented by abdominal radiographs when indicated. Pain over the hernia site is invariable and obstruction with strangulation of intestine will cause colicky abdominal pain, distension, vomiting and constipation. Physical examination may reveal degrees of dehydration with or without CNS depression, especially in the elderly if uraemia is present, together with abdominal signs of intestinal obstruction. Femoral hernias can be easily missed, especially in the obese female, and a thorough examination should be performed in order to make the correct diagnosis.

Preoperative laboratory investigations should include full blood count, to assess leukocytosis as an indicator of intestinal infarction and haematocrit to assess hydration. Blood biochemistry may reveal features suggestive of dehydration, such as electrolyte imbalance or raised creatinine and urea. A period of resuscitation is essential to bring these laboratory parameters in line for safe anaesthesia. In the elderly a chest radiograph and electrocardiograph will complete the preoperative workup and indicate the need for additional peroperative monitoring, such as venous pressure monitoring or atrial wedge pressure. Treatment begins with nasogastric suction, bladder catheterization and intravenous fluid replacement. Broad spectrum antibiotics to cover both Gram-negative and Gram-positive organisms should be instituted and blood cross-matched for an anticipated bowel resection. The period of resuscitation must be finely judged: the merits of optimizing the patient's state of hydration, electrolyte balance and cardiopulmonary status, must be balanced against the systemic toxic complications of unresected, infarcted bowel.

The choice of anaesthetic is dependent upon the general fitness of the patient, patient preference, and the skills of the surgeon or anaesthetist. Nevertheless, a bowel resection and anastomosis is always more safely performed through a peritoneal route; this operation should be carried out under general anaesthesia. Alternatives include regional anaesthesia (epidural or spinal) and, rarely, local anaesthetic. Inflamed skin and tissues overlying strangulated hernial sacs have a low pH and local anaesthetic solutions may be ineffective. This should be borne in mind when selecting local anaesthesia.

The choice of incision will depend on the type of groin hernia if the diagnosis is confident. When the diagnosis is in doubt a half-Pfannensteil incision 2 cm above the pubic ramus, extending laterally, will give an adequate approach to all types of femoral or inguinal hernia. The fundus of the hernia sac can then be approached and exposed and an incision made to expose the contents of the sac. This will allow determination of the viability of its contents. Non-viability will necessitate conversion of the transverse incision into a laparotomy incision followed by release of the constricting hernia ring, reduction of the contents of the sac, resection and reanastomosis. Precautions should be taken to avoid contamination of the general peritoneal cavity by gangrenous bowel or intestinal contents. In the majority of cases, once the constriction of the hernia ring has been released, circulation to the intestine is re-established and viability returns. Intestine that is initially dusky, aperistaltic or dull in hue may pink up with a short period of warming with damp packs once the constriction band is released. If viability is doubtful resection should be performed. A small Richter's hernia resulting in ischaemia of a limited area of the intestinal circumference may be adequately treated by oversewing with a serosal suture, taking care not to reduce the bowel lumen circumference.

Intestinal resection in children with strangulated hernias is rarely required. Resection rates are highest for femoral or recurrent inguinal hernias and lowest for inguinal hernias. Other organs, such as bladder or omentum, should be resected as the need requires. After peritoneal lavage and formal closure of the laparotomy incision, specific repair of the groin hernia defect should be performed. In this situation prosthetic mesh should not be used in an operative field that has been contaminated and in which there is a relatively high risk of wound infection. The hernia repair should follow the general principles for elective hernia repair. For recurrent groin hernias and femoral hernias, the preperitoneal approach is the preferred method.

REDUCTIO-EN-MASSE

Mass reduction of a hernia is nowadays a great rarity in Western nations, where elective operation is the treatment of choice and where incarcerated or strangulated hernias are subjected to early open operation. Mass reduction is, therefore, not a complication with which surgeons are well acquainted and for this reason the diagnosis may be overlooked. Pearse, in 1931, calculated that it occurred in 0.3% of strangulated hernias treated by taxis.[731]

Reductio-en-masse (mass reduction) refers to reduction of the external herniation with continued incarceration or strangulation of the internally prolapsed hernial contents. The most commonly reported instances

followed reduction of inguinal, more frequently indirect than direct, and femoral hernias. However, examples of reductio-en-masse of obturator and other rare hernias have been reported.[555]

The condition was first described by Saviard, in 1702, who reported a post-mortem examination of a patient who had died following successful taxis for a femoral hernia. Barker and Smiddy reviewed the topic in 1970 and added considerably to our understanding of the condition. More importantly, they were able to describe additional clinical signs to enable more accurate diagnosis.[62]

Reductio-en-masse is not a single anatomical entity. There are at least three varieties encountered:[731]

1. The sac still containing its strangulated contents can be forced away from the parietal muscles and come to lie in the abdominal cavity – 'arrachement de collet' (Saviard, 1702).[731] For this to occur, the neck of the sac must be small, fibrosed and unyielding, and once irreducibility has occurred, must grip the contents preventing their reduction. The neck of the sac must also be surrounded by a weak internal ring to which it is not adherent (Figure 8.4). Enthusiastic manipulation by the patient or his attendants can then force the sac and its contents from their moorings and reduce them intact inside the abdominal wall. Reduction of the hernia in these circumstances

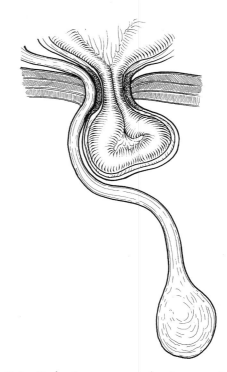

Figure 8.4 Reductio-en-masse. An incarcerated inguinal hernia with a tight unyielding neck which is not attached securely to the parieties at the deep ring can be forcefully reduced into the abdomen

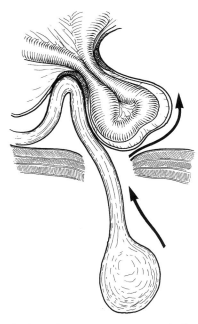

Figure 8.5 The bowel remains incarcerated; the sac and its contents are 'reduced' into the abdomen where they remain as a tender mass in the inguinal region. The spermatic cord is dragged in by its attachment to the neck of the sac at the deep ring and consequently the testicle is retracted. Attempts to reposition the testicle (traction on the cord) will elicit pain (Smiddy's sign)[62]

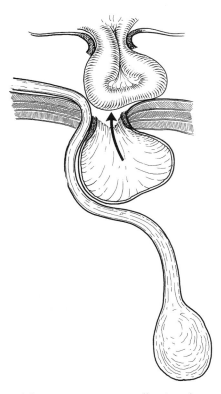

Figure 8.6 The sac may rupture allowing the contents, still strangulated by the constriction of the neck, to be reduced into the abdominal cavity. The obstruction remains, and additionally there will be extensive local bruising and tenderness

causes traction on the spermatic cord with retraction of the testis. In these circumstances the reduced mass may still be palpable in the iliac fossa, the testis will be retracted on the same side and gentle traction on the testis and spermatic cord will elicit pain – 'Smiddy's sign' (Figure 8.5).[62]

2. The sac may rupture but the constriction ring at the neck remains intact, so that although the external hernia reduces into the extraperitoneal plane, the obstruction/strangulation remains. This is the most commonly reported type, accounting for 92.8% of recorded cases[731] (Figure 8.6).

3. The contents could be reduced from an external sac into a preperitoneal communicating sac if one were present. Moynihan described apparent mass reduction of an incarcerated inguinal hernia into an associated preperitoneal sac, the obstruction at the neck of the sac where it joined the main peritoneal cavity remaining unaltered. This complication can only

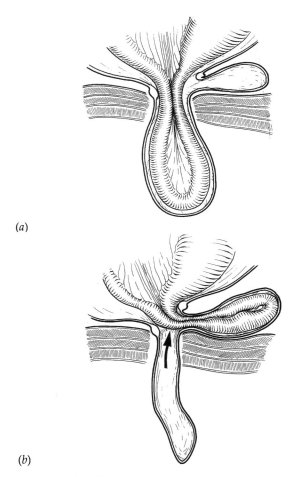

(a)

(b)

Figure 8.7 Moynihan reported reductio-en-masse as a phenomenon associated with a bilocular inguinal hernial sac. The strangulated bowel was moved from the external component of the sac to another preperitoneal component, the common neck remaining as the site of the constriction. Review of the literature suggests this is the least common form of reductio-en-masse

occur in bilocular sacs. Bilocular sacs are rare, except in patients who have worn a truss for many years and developed adhesions of the superficial inguinal ring. Hence, Moynihan's type of reductio-en-masse is also very rare nowadays[677] (Figure 8.7).

In all cases of reductio-en-masse, although the external hernial mass has gone, palpation of its egress site will demonstrate the empty ring. Usually there is adjacent tenderness around the egress ring and careful gentle palpation of the nearby abdomen will reveal the globular obstructed viscera in it. More importantly, the symptoms of obstruction will persist. Central colicky abdominal pain, increasing distension, vomiting, constipation and hypovolaemia should alert the clinician. Abdominal radiographs will point up the stigmata of intestinal obstruction, dilated loops and fluid levels.

Operation through an extraperitoneal approach to the groin will allow simultaneous hernia repair if the hernia is inguinal, femoral or obturator in type.

Maydl's hernia and afferent loop strangulation

In 1895, Maydl[624] described the *hernie-en-W* or double loop hernia, in which segments of bowel proximal and distal to an infolded loop become incarcerated within a hernial sac but without loss of viability. However, the infolded or intra-abdominal loop may become infarcted by strangulation even in the presence of viable loops incarcerated in the hernial sac. When more than one loop is gangrenous it is always the intra-abdominal loops rather than the intrahernial loops that are involved. Isolated gangrene of an intrahernial loop

without gangrene of the intra-abdominal loop has not been reported (Figure 8.8).

Maydl's hernia is commonest in men and commonest on the right side. Both small bowel and large bowel are found in these hernias of course; Maydl originally described the strangulated appendix vermiformis in a hernial sac (see below). On the left side the sigmoid colon and transverse colon have been described in the hernia.[325] One patient in whom all the loops were large bowel has been reported. This patient needed a right hemicolectomy because the loops of caecum, ascending colon and hepatic flexure were all gangrenous.[675]

Maydl's hernia is rare in Western series of strangulated hernias. Frankau (1931) reviewed 1487 strangulated hernia from centres in the British Isles; there were 654 strangulated inguinal hernias and in four of these a Maydl's hernia was found (0.6%).[315] In West Africa, where strangulated inguinal hernia is the commonest cause of intestinal obstruction, Maydl's hernia accounts for 2% of all cases.[53, 78]

In Korle Bu Teaching Hospital, Accra, Ghana, Maydl's hernia has been reported as frequently as five times in a consecutive series of 26 strangulated inguinal hernias. In this series, four sacs contained a double loop of intestine and the fifth contained three loops. All five patients were male adult Ghanaians. In three of these patients the caecum and part of the ascending colon were lying free in the hernial sac, not sliding intraperitoneally

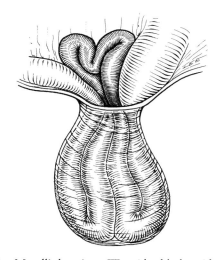

Figure 8.8 Maydl's hernia or W or 'double-loop' hernia. The infolded, intra-abdominal, loop is strangulated. It is important when operating on a strangulated hernia to inspect in continuity all the loops of gut in the sac so that an infolded loop is not overlooked

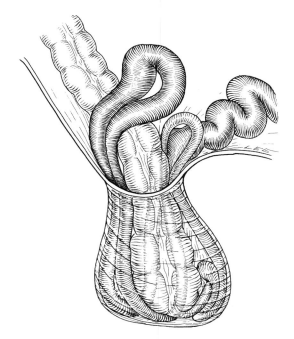

Figure 8.9 Double Maydl's hernia; described in ethnic West Africans. The caecum, appendix and terminal ileum and two loops of ileum are incarcerated in a giant inguinoscrotal sac. The two intervening loops of small intestine lying within the abdominal cavity are strangulated. Laparotomy through a paramedian incision is essential to assess the extent of bowel viability in a case of double W hernia[78]

in the lateral posterior wall as is so frequent in European patients. This arrangement allows loops of small intestine to prolapse into the sac behind and lateral to the caecum as well as anterior and medial to it[78] (Figure 8.9).

Afferent loop strangulation is a complication in which intra-abdominal strangulation of small intestine occurs proximal to an obstructed inguinal hernia. It is a common complication of right inguinal hernia obstruction in East Africa. The afferent loop is imprisoned behind the caecum which is obstructed in the inguinal hernial sac. The internal herniation of the loop of ileum passes from medial to lateral, behind the pendulous caecum which is fixed in the hernial sac. The caecum retains its circulation from the iliocaecal vessels which form the anterior component of the constriction, imprisoning the loop of ileum and infringing its mesenteric marginal blood vessels. At operation for a strangulation, if the caecum when released is pendulous and free, not sliding, the ileum for at least 1 m proximal should be checked to ensure it, has not suffered entrapment and infarction. This advice is most relevant in ethnic East African patients[742] (Figure 8.10).

Davey draws attention to these variations of strangulated hernia when the sac contains the caecum in Africans. As a precaution the surgeon should always count the loops in the sac and inspect the gut for 1 m proximal and distal. Recourse to formal laparotomy is recommended if there is any doubt. A diagnosis of stran-

gulated middle or afferent loop Maydl's hernia should be suspected in any patient who presents with a painful but not tender inguinoscrotal swelling, a tender mass in the lower abdomen and a scaphoid empty upper abdomen. Recourse to formal laparotomy is recommended if there is any doubt.[218]

In small tight-necked indirect inguinal hernia in infants, a Maydl's hernia of the appendix can occur. Appendicectomy at herniotomy is appropriate surgery[972] (Figure 8.11).

Strangulation of the appendix in a hernial sac

The appendix is seen frequently, in an inguinal or femoral hernial sac. Strangulation (as opposed to appendicitis) is rare. On clinical and histological grounds separation of the two diseases should not present difficulties. In strangulation, inflammation is accompanied by venous infarction; it involves all coats of the appendix and is clearly delimited proximally where the constriction is applied.[624] Acute appendicitis suppuration begins in the mucosa and spreads outwards. It is associated with intracavity purulent distension. A strangulated appendix behaves clinically like a Richter's partial enterocele.[205]

Richter's hernia and laparoscopy

Partial enterocele, the eponymous Richter's hernia, was not first described by Richter! And the condition has a variety of other names in the English and American literature: nipped hernia, pinched hernia, Lavator's hernia, etc.

Partial enterocele was first observed by Fabricius Hildanus in 1598 and clearly described by Lavator in 1672.[972] Littré reported cases in 1700 and 1714, Morgagni in 1723, De Garengeot in 1743 and Ruysch in

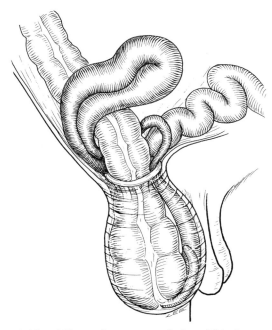

Figure 8.10 Afferent loop strangulation. This is a complication of large inguinoscrotal hernias in Africans who have a long pendulous scrotum. The caecum is incarcerated in the hernial sac; a loop of small bowel passes behind the ascending colon and is strangulated to the right of the colon. Formal laparotomy is required[742]

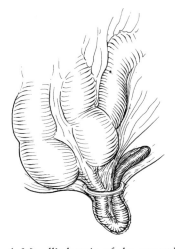

Figure 8.11 A Maydl's hernia of the appendix is a complication of an incarcerated inguinal hernia in an infant

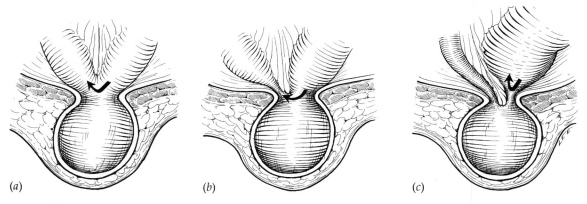

Figure 8.12 Richter's hernia (partial enterocele). The antimesenteric circumference of the bowel is first held by the rigid neck of the hernial sac, usually a femoral or obturator hernia. The situation is progressive: from (**a**) partial involvement of the bowel circumference without obstruction, to (**b**) subacute obstruction, to (**c**) complete obstruction and strangulation of the incarcerated bowel[948]

1744. The most important paper was by Richter in 1785, hence the hernia is named for him.[473, 785] Richter's hernia has recently again come into prominence, this time as a complication of CAPD, used in the treatment of renal failure,[284] and as a complication of 'port site' hernias following laparoscopy.[409]

In the partial enterocele the antimesenteric circumference of the intestine becomes constricted in the neck of a hernial sac without causing complete intestinal luminal occlusion (Figure 8.12).

Richter's hernia is most frequently found in femoral or obturator hernias, although the condition has been described at other sites.[694] Richter's hernias occur in infantile indirect inguinal hernias. Colic and distension occur, but absolute constipation for faeces and gas is a late phenomenon. Vomiting is also often absent. On physical examination there is tenderness but no palpable lump at the hernial site. Strangulation and gangrene of the bowel wall nipped in the hernial sac sets in rapidly and perforation of the gut into the sac may occur without immediate catastrophic peritonitis. It is important to recognize the condition at operation – to return the non-viable bowel to the peritoneal cavity is to precipitate disaster.

Littré's hernia – hernia of Meckel's diverticulum

Alexis Littré, in 1700, reported three cases of an incarcerated femoral hernia containing an ileal diverticulum. Littré interpreted the ileal diverticulum as a secondary phenomenon related to the hernial ring and arising from the intestine opposite it. Johann Meckel, in 1809, identified the embryological origin of the distal small intestinal diverticulum which was henceforward to bear his name. Meckel recognized that his diverticulum was a partial persistence of the omphalomesenteric duct communicating between the fetal midgut and the yolk

sac.[645] It was only after Meckel's paper that it was realized that the diverticulum in the hernia described by Littré was the diverticulum described by Meckel. The clear elucidation of these facts we owe to Sir Frederick Treves.[929]

A Meckel's diverticulum may be a chance finding in an inguinal hernia. It has been described in incarcerated inguinal hernia in infants: in infants the diverticulum frequently becomes adherent to the sac and as a consequence the hernia becomes irreducible. This can be diagnosed when after taxis of a right inguinal hernia in an infant, part of the hernia remains unreduced.[58]

Meckel's diverticulum has also been described in an umbilical hernia. This is not unsurprising when it is recalled that the omphalomesenteric duct is a component of the normal fetal umbilicus.[158] Meckel's diverticulum in femoral hernia is also described; a most unusual variant is the presentation of the diverticulum as a small bowel fistula resulting from strangulation of the diverticulum progressing to a groin abscess which discharged externally with a persistent small bowel fistula[553] (Figure 8.13).

Hernia of ovary, fallopian tube and uterus

The first case of hernia of the ovary was reported by the Greek physician Soranus of Ephesus about AD 97. Hernia of the pregnant uterus (hysterocele gravidarum) was reported by Pol (1531) and another case by Semmentus (1610). Watson (1938) reports two cases and comments that the uterus may become impregnated while in the hernial sac or the pregnant uterus may enter the sac and become irreducible as the pregnancy proceeds[972] (Figure 8.14).

The tube and ovary may also enter the hernial sac. Ectopic pregnancy in a hernial sac is reported in these circumstances.[972]

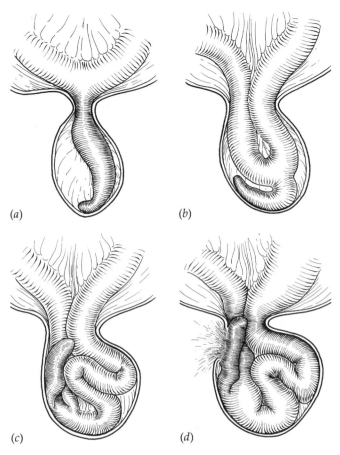

Figure 8.13   Meckel's diverticulum in a hernial sac. A Meckel's diverticulum may be the only occupant of the sac (a); alternatively, adjacent loop ileum may be in the sac too (b). A Meckel's diverticulum may become adherent to the sac (c) or form a fistula (d)[58]

In contemporary practice, internal genitalia are frequently found in inguinal hernia in baby girls. The frequency with which they occur warrants caution to open and inspect each hernial sac to exclude their presence.

In older females the tube and ovary are sometimes the contents of inguinal, femoral or obturator hernias, usually as components of sliding sacs. Pathology may complicate these hernial contents, hydrosalpinx being common in irreducible inguinal hernia.[947]

A uterus has been described in a male intersex with inguinal hernias. Routine examination of the scrotum for normal testicles should be the drill in all boys with inguinal hernias. If developmental anomalies are then found in the wall of a hernial sac, they can be excised.[98]

Urinary tract complications

The bladder is a very frequent component of the medial wall of direct inguinal and of femoral hernias (Figure 8.15). Usually the bladder is easily identified during dissection, but when difficulty is encountered the obliterated

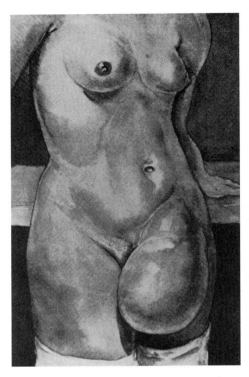

Figure 8.14   An irreducible inguinal hernia of a pregnant uterus (From Watson, 1938[972])

umbilical artery is a useful landmark. The bladder is a very common finding in the medial wall of indirect inguinal hernias in boys (see pages 116, 121).

Care will protect the bladder from trauma during surgery. If the bladder is injured, closure with two layers of absorbable polymer suture is required and then catheter drainage should be employed for several days.

The ureter sometimes presents in the lateral wall of giant sliding inguinal hernia. Knowledge, suspicion and care are all that are needed to avoid damaging the ureter. The ureter should be identified, dissected away preserving its blood supply and returned to the abdomen. If the ureter is injured or its vasculature in doubt, a pigtail ureteric catheter for several days is best advised.[737] Preoperative intravenous urogram and micturating cystogram are advisable before operation on giant inguinoscrotal hernias, to exclude ureteric complications or bladder diverticula in the hernial sac.[751]

Prolapse of an ileal conduit into an indirect inguinal hernia is described.[771] The patient presented with an ischaemic blue stoma and anuria. The ileal loop was twisted around its distal fixed point (the stoma) and prolapsed into the hernial sac.

Sliding hernia

Sliding hernia, *hernie-en-glissade*, 'landslip hernia' or 'landslide of the large intestine' are the various names for

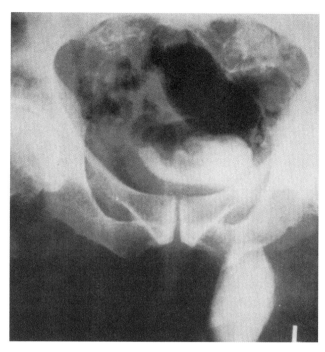

Figure 8.15 An intravenous urogram demonstrating the left wall of the bladder in a femoral hernia sac in a man with bladder neck obstruction

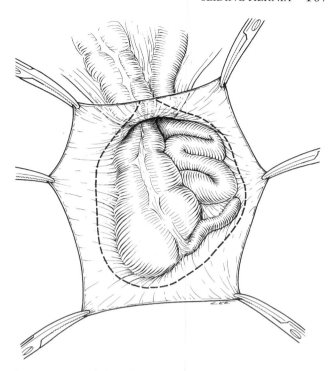

Figure 8.16 Sliding hernia. The caecum and appendix forming part of the wall of a right inguinal hernia

this hernia. With hindsight we can discover cases of sliding hernia in much ancient and Renaissance medical literature; however, it was Scarpa in 1819 who published the classic description of these conditions.[828] Carnett, in 1909, classified sliding hernias,[155] while Watson (1938) reviewed the literature comprehensively and included outstanding diagrams of the anatomic types of sliding hernias of the large intestine.[972] The most frequent sliding hernias are the caecum and appendix in indirect right inguinal hernias[794] (Figure 8.16) and the sigmoid colon in indirect left inguinal hernias[818] (Figure 8.17).

Although Cloquet in 1817[182] and Lockwood in 1893[573] had described the bladder in the medial wall of hernial sacs, it is surprising that not until 1942 did this common problem of the sliding hernia of the bladder receive detailed attention by Zimmerman and Laufman.[1007] Sliding bladder hernias in infants, so called 'bladder ears', were described by Allen and Condon in 1961.[13] The problem of congenital sliding genital hernias in females was highlighted by Gans in 1959.[326] This despite the fact that sliding hernias were mentioned by Sir Percival Pott, who also described a woman with bilateral sliding ovarian hernias in his treatise of 1757.[757] The woman ceased menstruating when Pott moved both hernial sacs including the ovarian tissues in their walls.

Moschowitz described the two most common intra-operative mistakes that bedevilled surgical intervention for sliding hernias;[674] Ponka described the third.[752]

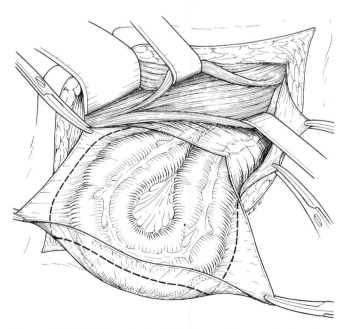

Figure 8.17 Sliding hernia. The sigmoid loop of colon in a left inguinal hernia. These hernias are sometimes very difficult to reduce and close. A muscle-splitting incision 5 cm or so above and parallel to the inguinal ligament can facilitate mobilization. The hernia is delivered through the higher incision, excess sac is trimmed away and the sac closed. Care with the colon and its blood supply is needed. The repair of the defect is described elsewhere

These are:

1. Designating a hernia to be sliding when it is merely a simple hernia in which a loop of intestine is adherent to the sac.
2. Haemorrhage caused by attempting to dissect the viscus (colon or bladder) from its blood supply. This occurs during attempts to 'create' a sac on the extraperitoneal aspect of the viscus.
3. Accidental entry into the bladder or the viscus, particularly during mobilization of the sac wall.

The solution to the management of sliding hernias owes much to the experience of the Shouldice clinic in Toronto and to the sound principles derived from this experience. Earle Shouldice, Ernest Ryan, Donald Welsh and Frank Glassow are the contributors to our knowledge. Until the Toronto group started analysing their results the series of sliding hernias published had all been small, reflecting the rarity of the problem. Nearly all the recurrence rates were high and reports had concentrated on technical innovation, usually without adequate follow-up data.

Zimmerman and Laufman described their technique in 1942, with no recurrences in a series of 24 cases.[1007] In 1956, Ryan reported the results of 313 cases repaired at the Shouldice clinic prior to 1952, with one indirect recurrence.[817] In 1961, Maingot reported his experience in 64 cases with no recurrences.[601] Welsh reported 2300 sliding hernias repaired at the Shouldice clinic with only 11 recurrences.[977]

All these authors report the same principles. The hypertrophied cremaster is removed from the sac, the cord structures are carefully dissected away from the sac up to and into the peritoneal cavity, and excess peritoneal sac is excised and closed. The hernia and its contents are then returned to the abdominal cavity. The transversalis fascia is carefully reconstructed to contain the hernia and refashion the deep ring around the cord. It is not necessary to 'reperitonealise' the viscera before they are returned to the abdominal cavity. The critical manoeuvres are to return the viscera to the abdomen and to contain them within the confines of the abdomen/fascia transversalis.

Testicular strangulation

The testicular blood supply is hazarded when a tight strangulation compresses it in its passage from the abdomen to scrotum. This may occur in three circumstances:

1. In male infants with incarcerated inguinal hernias, the venous drainage becomes obstructed at the rigid external ring. This is a not infrequent complication of infantile incarceration; it is discussed in detail on page 113.
2. In giant inguinoscrotal hernia, spontaneous infarction of the testicle has been described.[588]
3. In Africans with strangulated indirect inguinal hernia, testicular infarction due to vascular obstruction at the deep ring is reported. At operation the gangrenous testicle should be excised.[588]

The site of the vascular damage in these instances, the superficial ring in infancy and the deep ring in adulthood, emphasizes the different anatomy and structure of the inguinal canal in the pre- and post-pubertal male.

9 GROIN HERNIAS IN BABIES AND CHILDREN

Inguinal herniotomy is the operation most frequently performed in paediatric practice.[368] Neonatal practice has advanced recently with a rise in the survival of more premature babies; there is an increased incidence of inguinal hernias in premature babies and in boys with cryptorchid testicles.[733, 991]

Although inguinal herniotomy appears to be a simple operation, it is technically demanding and great harm may be done if it is incorrectly performed. It is not an operation for the occasional paediatric surgeon; there should be **no** occasional paediatric surgeons. Inguinal herniotomy will probably be the child's and the child's parents (as parents) first encounter with surgery; consequently the experience may colour their attitudes to surgeons for many years. Therefore, it behoves us not only to provide expert surgical and anaesthetic care, but to make the entire experience as pleasant as possible.

All elective inguinal herniotomies in children can be undertaken as day cases.[50, 183] Parents should accompany their child to hospital, nurse him or her themselves and thus eliminate any psychological trauma to the family unit. Inguinal hernias in children should be operated on as soon as possible after first diagnosis to avoid the hazard of incarceration.

Preterm and low birthweight babies present special risks of postoperative apnoea and bradycardia. For these reasons they need appropriate postoperative monitoring;[647] however, day-case surgery for these patients is recommended provided the gestational age is greater than 33 weeks.

Emergency herniotomy for incarcerated inguinal hernia in infants is one of the most difficult operations and should not be undertaken lightly; it is an operation for an experienced surgeon only. Sedation and taxis will reduce most incarcerated inguinal hernias.

Strangulation, or strangulation of a partial enterocele (Richter's hernia), sometimes complicates incarceration.

Aetiology and anatomy

The testicle appears at the end of the first month of intrauterine life as a ventromedial swelling at the caudal end of the genital ridge. It enlarges rapidly and by the end of the sixth week has a mesentery and bulges into the peritoneum which invests it anteriorly. The trunk of the embryo is elongating rapidly at this time, resulting in an apparent caudal shift of the gonad, so that at about 10 weeks it is found just above the groin. This is the 'internal phase' of gonad descent. The testicular blood supply directly from the aorta is stretched out by the rapid elongation of the aorta and spine which 'carries' the kidneys cephalad. From the lower pole of the testicle a finger-like column of condensed mesenchymal cells, the gubernaculum, extends behind the peritoneum down through the layers of the body wall to the scrotum.[991]

At about eight weeks a pouch of peritoneum begins to bulge down in front of and alongside the gubernaculum, pushing the surrounding muscle layers ahead of itself and stretching them all the way down into the scrotum. The stretched out layers in turn each become the 'coverings' of the cord (the internal spermatic fascia, cremasteric fascia and external spermatic fascia from the fascia transversalis, the internal oblique and the external oblique muscles serially). It is suggested that at this phase of development, when gut is forced out of the abdomen into the embryological umbilical hernia, there is raised intra-abdominal pressure due to the rapid growth of intra-abdominal organs. This raised intra-abdominal pressure forces the processus vaginalis through the abdominal wall into the scrotum, which enlarges to accommodate it.

There are two theories to explain the extra-abdominal descent of the testis. Either the gubernaculum pulls the testis down or the gubernaculum remains always the same size and the testis is pulled down by elongation of the baby. Both these theories are difficult to substantiate. The first because muscle tissue has never been demonstrated in the gubernaculum and the second because rather than a short unchanging stocky fibrous cord the gubernaculum is quite long and rambles through the inguinal canal from the testis to the base of the scrotum. Furthermore, even in normal children who have scrotal testicles at birth, they are retractile and will disappear up into the inguinal canal if appropriate stimulation is applied.

At the end of the seventh intrauterine month the gubernaculum swells markedly, owing to increase in the intracellular matrix probably brought about by hormonal influence. This enlargement dilates the internal ring and the canal then the intra-abdominal pressure probably propels the testicle along the track previously formed by the processus vaginalis through the muscle tunnel and into the peritoneal sac preformed in the scrotum.[837, 991] Boys with the 'prune belly syndrome' have undescended testicles which are not only high but look grossly normal, suggesting that intra-abdominal pressure (muscle tone) is needed to push the testis through the canal and into the scrotal space.[986] A further characteristic of cryptorchism is a small processus vaginalis or sometimes its complete absence; a further manifestation of intraperitoneal pressure failing to 'push out' the testis into the scrotum.[853]

The stimuli to the process of normal descent of the testicle and the causes of its failure or erring in its target are ill understood. It is a fault of this process that leaves the processus vaginalis, which is finely patent in 60% of normal infants at birth, as a preformed congenital hernial sac. Few, if any, of the children who present with inguinal hernia have any fascial defect. The patent processus vaginalis is a potential hernial sac but it must not be confused with a clinically evident inguinal hernia.

Normal testicular descent depends upon several factors which include: (a) a normal hypothalamic–pituitary–testicular hormone axis; (b) normal testicular production of androgen; (c) normal end organ response to androgen; (d) a normal gubernaculum; (e) a normal

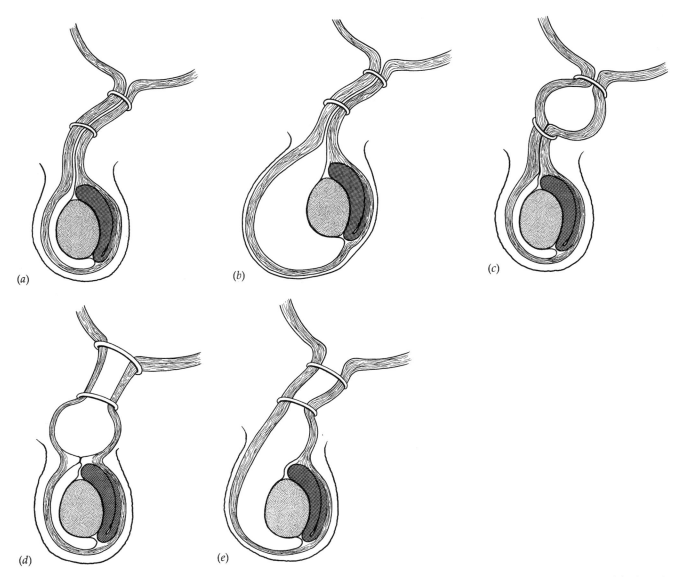

Figure 9.1 Anomalies of the processus vaginalis: (**a**) the normal appearance, (**b**) a scrotal hydrocele, (**c**) an encysted hydrocele of the cord, (**d**) an incomplete inguinal hernia, bubonocele. The sac extends part of the way along the cord. (**e**) A complete, funicular or scrotal hernia. The sac includes the tunica vaginalis covering of the testicle in the scrotum. (After Hertzfeld, 1938[973])

intra-abdominal pressure; (f) spermatic vessels of adequate length; (g) an adequate vas deferens; (h) a normal inguinal canal.[837, 853, 991]

Primary anatomic abnormalities are probably less common causes of cryptorchism than is dysfunction of the hypothalamic–pituitary–testicular hormone axis.[494, 853] Maternal oestrogen levels in early pregnancy may be a factor in determining the function of the embryonic hypothalamic–pituitary–testicular hormone axis.[177] Anecdotal clinical evidence associates vomiting in early pregnancy with cryptorchism and inguinal hernia formation.

Classification

Inguinal hernia in childhood can be divided into two types:[423]

1. Complete scrotal – total funicular hernia of Herzfeld (1938).
2. Incomplete bubonocele – partial funicular hernia of Herzfeld.

Complete hernias are present at birth, but are much rarer than incomplete hernias. About 5% of all inguinal hernias in male infants are of the complete variety.

So far we have only considered the occurrence of a hernia; remnants of the processus vaginalis, however, can remain in the inguinal canal, giving rise to an encysted hydrocele of the cord in the male or a hydrocele of the canal of Nuck in the female.

Figure 9.1 shows the following variants of the processus vaginalis: normal, hydrocele, encysted hydrocele, partial funicular hernia (bubonocele), and complete funicular hernia (scrotal hernia).[423]

Incidence – pathology

Some 3% to 5% of full-term babies are born with clinically apparent inguinal hernias, in preterm babies this incidence is substantially increased up to 30%.[60, 401, 733] Inguinal hernia is the commonest indication for surgery in early life.

The processus vaginalis was found to be open at birth in 94% of infants examined at autopsy by Camper in the 1750s. However, 94% of newborn infants do not have demonstrable inguinal hernias. Rowe et al. (1969)[790] studied the natural history of the patent processus vaginalis, reviewing 2764 patients operated on for inguinal hernia at the Children's Hospital, Columbus, Ohio: 280 (10%) had clinically apparent bilateral hernias, 83 (3%) had had a contralateral hernia repaired and 2401 (87%) had a single unilateral hernia. Of the patients with unilateral hernias, 1965 had the contralateral explored in search of a patent processus; positive explorations occurred in 946 (48%) of these patients. This number is lower than reported in most series. The usual figure of children with inguinal hernia having a patent processus on the opposite side is about 60%, but in the Ohio series some patients already had had a bilateral exploration.[495] The highest incidence of patency of the contralateral processus vaginalis occurred in the first two months of life (63%); after this there was a steady fall in incidence, until two years when the incidence was 41%, at which a levelling off developed to 16 years when a 35% incidence is recorded. Between 15% and 30% of adults without clinical evidence of an inguinal hernia have a patent processus at post-mortem.[875] Inguinal hernia presenting as a complication of CAPD confirms the incidence of persistent processus vaginalis in adulthood. Females with unilateral inguinal hernias more commonly have a contralateral patent processus vaginalis than males (57% vs. 42%); the incidence of clinical bilateral hernias is the same in both sexes (about 10%), suggesting that the presence of a patent processus is not the sole determinant of development of an inguinal hernia (Figure 9.2).

The incidence of inguinal hernia in children in England has fallen in this century. Sir Arthur Keith, in 1924, reported the incidence of inguinal hernia in the first year of life to be 44 per 1000 live births, from the second to fifth year 9 per 1000, from six to 10 years 6 per 1000 and from 11 to 15 years 9 per 1000, giving an overall incidence of approximately 60 per 1000 children up to the age of 12 years.[487] Among children of Newcastle upon Tyne, Knox found that operation for primary inguinal hernia was performed on 10.2 per 1000 children surviving at the age of 12 years. The ratio of boys to girls was 12:1, so that the incidence of inguinal hernia in boys in this community was 1.9%.[507]

In the nine years 1970–79 prior to the explosion in neonatal resources, in Stockton-on-Tees, there were

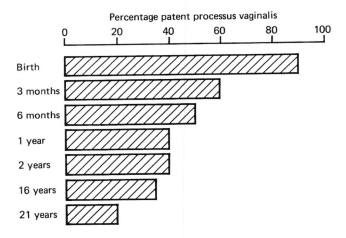

Figure 9.2   The incidence of a patent processus vaginalis falls during the first year of life; nevertheless 15–30% of adults have evidence of a patent processus vaginalis which can dilate if these persons go on to CAPD

29 094 live births; of these children, 570 (24 per 1000), 512 males and 58 females, required operation for inguinal hernia. The ratio of boys to girls was 9:1, which yields an incidence in male children of 4.2%. Of the 570 children requiring operation, some 10% required emergency admission for incarceration or strangulation. Similar statistics are recorded by Thorndike and Ferguson (1938),[920] by Lynn and Johnson (1961),[584] by Daum and Meinel (1972)[217] and by Harvey, Johnstone and Fossard (1985).[408]

The incidence of inguinal hernia is increased in preterm infants.[401, 733] Hernias occur with increased frequency in infants under 32 weeks gestational age or below 1250 g birthweight. Among infants below 32 weeks' gestational age, intrauterine growth retardation significantly increases the risk for development of inguinal hernias, especially in male infants. Thirty per cent of surviving premature infants weighing less than 1000 g develop inguinal hernias. There is an association between neonatal inguinal hernia and intrauterine growth retardation.

The incidence of inguinal hernias is higher in twins, especially in early infancy.[60] This higher incidence in twins persists throughout the childhood years and is higher in males than females: dizygotic female twins do not have the same high incidence. Inguinal hernias have a higher incidence in children with other birth defects. Inguinal hernias show a familial incidence, suggesting a polygenic defect. The incidence of inguinal hernia in African children is higher than in European children but there is no significant association of the incidence of inguinal hernias with race in a sample of American premature babies studied.[733]

Scorer and Farrington,[837] in common with most other authors,[368] report that there is a marked preponderance of right-sided hernia in boys – 70% right-sided, 26% left-sided and 4% bilateral – whereas in girls the incidence of right-sided hernia is 50%. Of the children who develop a right-sided hernia before reaching one year, 50% will develop a contralateral hernia; in contrast when the hernia develops after one year of age only 10% will develop a contralateral hernia.

Left inguinal hernias are associated with contralateral hernia twice as often as right-sided ones. Atwell, reviewing 3107 cases from Oxford and from Great Ormond Street Hospital, London, reports that the male to female ratio is 10.3:1. Of his personal series of 262 patients, 31% presented a groin lump in the first year of life, 60.6% were right-sided and 15% bilateral. After simple herniotomy, no cases of recurrence were found at follow-up.[49]

Incarceration and strangulation

Ten per cent of children with inguinal hernias present as emergencies with incarceration or strangulation.

Incarceration or strangulation has its highest frequency in the first three months of life; thereafter the incidence falls off so that incarceration is very rare after the sixth birthday. The incidence of incarceration is higher in premature and low birthweight children. Incarceration or strangulation are 10 times more frequent in male than in female children. Seventy-five per cent of the incarcerated hernias in the first three months of life present in children in whom no hernia had previously been noted.[28, 221, 321, 371, 720, 765, 883] Hernias which appear after birth are more likely to strangulate than those present at birth, the presumption being that hernias present at birth have wider necks than those that develop later by opening of the processus vaginalis.

Incarcerated and strangulated hernias are five times more frequent on the right than the left side.[25, 221, 720, 765] In boys, small gut is the most frequent viscera to be incarcerated. In girls the frequency of incarceration is the same for right and left-side hernias and the ovary and fallopian tube are most likely to be incarcerated. Adhesions between the sac and its contained viscus are very rare, except in Littré's hernia.

While incarceration is not infrequent, strangulation (an irreducible hernia containing viscera with a critically compromised blood supply) is very rare.

All series report very low resection rates: Nussbaum (1913)[705] reported two cases of strangulation in 54 000 children cared for, Maclennan (1921–22) 4 in 1038,[593] Thorndike and Ferguson (1938) 5 in 1740 (106 of which were incarcerated),[920] Smith (1954) 2 in 50,[872] and Harvey, Johnstone and Fossard (1985) none in 71 emergency presentations.[408]

Cases of strangulated hernia requiring resection of small bowel have been recorded at 12 days[423] and at 25 days.[872] Spontaneous cure by caecal fistula after 10 days' strangulation in a 7-week-old Chinese infant is reported.[893]

Strangulation, or strangulation of a partial enterocele (Richter's hernia), can complicate incarceration. Infants with incarceration require hospital observation for at least 24 h after reduction of the hernia, in case strangulation has occurred and complications of intestinal gangrene become apparent later.

Treatment by sedation and gallows traction (Solomon position) is recommended initially. Eighty per cent of incarcerated hernias reduce spontaneously if the child is adequately sedated.[683] The incidence of testicular infarction and atrophy (see below) is less with this form of treatment than with emergency surgery on the day of operation. However, if the incarceration does not reduce spontaneously, after 4 h of gallows traction with good sedation, or if the testicle is persistently tender (ischaemic orchitis) and the scrotum oedematous, surgery should be undertaken (Figure 9.3).

It is unlikely that strangulated, as opposed to incarcerated, bowel will reduce on non-operative suspension

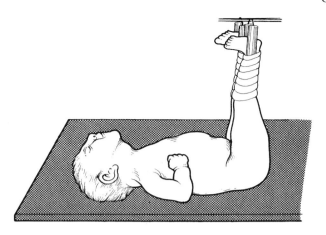

Figure 9.3 Gallows traction in the 'Solomon position' allows most incarcerated inguinal hernias in children to reduce spontaneously

treatment. At the induction of anaesthetic, incarcerated bowel will reduce spontaneously. If taxis under anaesthetic is needed, the operation should proceed and the bowel be inspected for viability. The extraperitoneal approach allows scrutiny of the intestine without the necessity of a second laparotomy/incision and is, therefore, strongly recommended for all irreducible hernias.[472, 934]

Prompt elective operation for inguinal hernia in infants is recommended, the probability of incarceration being 1:4 for hernias in male children diagnosed under 12 months of age.

There is some confusion and overlap in the literature between the terms 'irreducible', 'incarceration', 'strangulation', 'infarction' and 'gangrene'. An irreducible or incarcerated hernia in a child is one whose contents cannot be replaced back into the abdomen even with sedation . . . these are common in practice. Strangulation and infarction are terms that imply interruption of the blood supply to the organs in the irreducible or incarcerated hernial sac. This is rare in children (except to the testicle – see below). Gangrene is tissue death; tissue death of viscera contained in an irreducible or incarcerated hernial sac is very rare in children. Gross records 63 incarcerated hernias in 3874 treated in one decade, with a single mortality from strangulation.[371]

THE VASCULAR COMPROMISED GONAD

The blood supply to the testicle can be compromised in the male child with an incarcerated or strangulated inguinal hernia.[648, 763] Similarly, in female children the ovary and tube may prolapse into the hernia or be a sliding component of it and undergo a similar hazardous sequence. In males, the risk of strangulation of the testicle is due to pressure on its vessels at the superficial ring and in the canal when the testicle is incompletely

descended. The duration and completeness of the strangulation influence the viability of the testicle. If incarceration is known to have been present for a long time, greater than 12 h, emergency operation is probably indicated. Interestingly the incarcerated hernia in a female carries greater risk to the gonad, the ovary, than a similar situation in the male.

Infarction of the testicle in a 6-week-old child with an incarcerated inguinal hernia was reported by Sturdy (1960)[903] and in a 3-month-old male child with incarcerated hernia by Deshpande (1964).[237] Murdoch (1979) reported 120 boys with incarcerated inguinal hernia treated in a 3-year period.[683] In his series, there were six instances of testicular strangulation related to the hernia; strangulation of the testis occurs almost exclusively in infants aged less than three months. The strangulation is due to hernia pressure on the cord vessels as they pass through the rigid boundaries of the superficial inguinal ring.[645] When a strangulated testis is discovered at operation, it should be left undisturbed. Full recovery of most strangulated testes can usually be anticipated, although up to 5% of strangulated testicles may ultimately atrophy.

Although the outlook for both incarcerated gut and the ischaemic testicle in an irreducible inguinal hernia is good, strangulation and gangrene of the gut and testicle is recorded.[96] Operation is mandatory for the persisting irreducible hernia. If vomiting and obstruction are present, extra careful resuscitation is needed prior to operation.

Clinical diagnosis of inguinal hernia in a child

A lump in the groin of a child is a common condition that presents to surgeons. In making a diagnosis, the sex and age of the patient and the history of the onset of the lump are critical determinants. Physical diagnosis usually only confirms what can be discovered by careful history-taking.

Sixty per cent of inguinal hernias are apparent within the first three months of life; the remainder are discovered in well baby clinics or at school medical examinations. Few inguinal hernias are first noticed after five years of age.

Inguinal hernias may present at birth or at any date after that, and they are more frequent on the right side than the left side. Their early history often distinguishes them from other lumps. In the infant or child the lump is most often noticed by the mother. The lump is more prominent when the child screams or moves about vigorously, whereas it often disappears in the relaxed child; indeed when the child is brought to be examined in the clinic it may not be apparent. The mother's word alone is enough to make a diagnosis. The lump appears initially as a 'bulge' at the medial end of the groin. It increases in size and may progress down into the scrotum. Episodes of irreducibility are frequent.

The lump disappears in the sleeping child. Persistence of the lump, associated with screaming and local pain, should raise the spectre of incarceration.

The inguinal hernia in the male child should be distinguished from the hydrocele. The symptoms are similar, except that with hydrocele the mother will have noticed the swelling in the scrotum before there was a swelling in the groin. She may notice that the swelling is only in the scrotum.

On clinical examination the hernia extends from the superficial ring to the scrotum. The hydrocele extends from the scrotum towards the superficial ring; it may not extend as far as the groin crease and external ring. The hernia is reducible and if it contains gut it will reduce with a gurgle. In older children the cord will be thickened after the hernia is reduced – the 'rolled silk sign'.[123] The hydrocele is readily transilluminable. Some hernias in the newborn are said to be transilluminable (Figure 9.4).

Male and female children both present diagnostic pitfalls. In either sex the lump may come and go, it may be unilateral or unilateral on the right at one time and on the left at another time, or it may be synchronously bilateral. It may appear at any moment after birth, and there may or may not be associated pain. If there is pain the child usually has screaming fits, during which the lump becomes more prominent and tender. The lump we are describing is a congenital indirect inguinal hernia. Early operation should be recommended for all cases that are clinically apparent.

The problem of the inguinal 'bulge', usually associated with screaming which causes great alarm to the parents, must be mentioned. Sometimes it is impossible to demonstrate a hernia in the clinic, but in many of these cases if a hernia is present careful palpation will

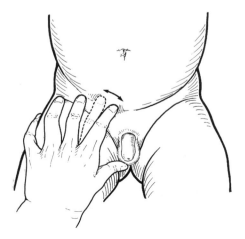

Figure 9.4 The 'rolled silk' sign. The hernia is reduced; the examining index finger rolls the cord over the pubic bone. If a hernial sac is present, its thickened walls can be felt rubbing against each other like silk in a fine garment

demonstrate a thickened cord. The index finger is placed over the cord as it emerges over the pubic bone; the cord is rolled and the thickened sac is felt rubbing against itself with a sensation like two layers of silk rubbing together. This is the 'rolled silk' sign. It is suggestive, rather than pathogenic, of an inguinal hernia and its reliability as the sole indication for groin exploration for hernia is questionable.[369] If there are no clinical findings, but the mother's description of the hernia is convincing and accurate, the groin is best explored.

It is important to examine both sides of the scrotum in male children to ensure that concomitant undescended testicles are not overlooked. An overlooked undescended testicle has bleak prospects because the scarring of the herniotomy will compromise subsequent operation.

Differential diagnosis

Always examine both groins and both sides of the scrotum with the child relaxed and supine, and then with the child upright (standing or held by the mother). An inguinal hernia in a child must be distinguished from:

1. Inguinal lymphadenitis. The irregular 'matted' nature of enlarged inguinal nodes should give the true diagnosis. Examination of the watershed area may reveal the cause, especially in acute lymphadenitis.
2. Femoral hernia. Careful delineation of the anatomy – an inguinal hernia is cephalad and a femoral hernia caudal to the inguinal ligament.
3. Undescended testicle (in the male).
4. A hydrocele of the cord (in the male).
5. Hydrocele of the canal of Nuck (in the female). A 'communicating' hydrocele that comes and goes can be confused with a hernia. Many communicating hydroceles communicate with a hernial sac. In both male and female cord hydroceles the swelling has a definite upper limit and is translucent. Hydroceles vary in size.
6. Lipoma.
7. Psoas abscess. This generally appears lateral to the femoral artery.
8. Cystic hygroma.

Additionally, if the swelling is tender and the child complains of pain:

9. Torsion of an undescended testicle can closely resemble a strangulated hernia. This condition usually appears very suddenly with no previous history of a lump. Usually the absent testicle has been noticed previously. Torsion of an undescended testicle can complicate birth in low birthweight and preterm boys. Local examination reveals a tender lump with oedema adjacent to it, and there is no testicle in the ipsilateral scrotum. The gastrointestinal

symptoms of strangulation, persistent vomiting and constipation are absent. The acuteness and severity of symptoms in a case of torsion tend to decrease with time, in contrast to the progression of symptoms from incarceration to strangulation.

10. Torsion of an appendix of the epididymis can give a swollen inguinoscrotal area which can be mistaken for a strangulated hernia. The onset is sudden. However, the acuteness of the symptoms settles fairly rapidly. No swelling is palpable in the cord above the scrotum.

11. Appendicitis can occur in an inguinal hernial sac in a child.

The bilaterality question

Because inguinal hernias in children are not uncommonly bilateral, should both groins be routinely explored? In newborn children with unilateral inguinal hernia, a patent processus vaginalis is found on the contralateral side in 60%. The processus vaginalis undergoes a progressive obliteration from birth to two years, so that after two years only 40% of children with demonstrable unilateral inguinal hernias have a contralateral patent processus vaginalis.[106, 461, 860] Whether contralateral exploration should be routinely undertaken when a left hernia is found is a moot point, remembering that a contralateral hernia is twice as likely to be found with a left hernia as with a right-sided one. It must be clearly understood that there is a hazard to the vas and vessels whenever an inguinal hernia is explored. Does this risk outweigh the advantages of exploration? In children over two years old the case against routine contralateral exploration has been powerfully made.[119, 494] On the other hand, the opposite argument has been advanced powerfully, too.

In infants less than six months old, and especially in girls, who have a left inguinal hernia when the right side is explored a sac is almost always found, and because so many infants present with complications of the sac some surgeons routinely explore the right side. In boys who are older, over two years old, the risks of damage to the vas and spermatic vessels probably outweigh the advantages of the inexperienced operator performing a prophylactic dissection.[344]

What is the authors' recommendation? If the contralateral cord is thickened – the 'rolled silk sign' – it should be explored. The chance of the hernia being bilateral is greater if the presenting lump is on the left side, and in such instances it is well to question the parents carefully when the child is initially examined: have they seen a lump in the right groin? Making the child cry and then carefully examining both groins is a useful clinic manoeuvre.

As anaesthesia is induced the child may strain slightly and if a contralateral hernia is present it will become apparent. In cases of doubt, the child should always be re-examined at this stage to ensure that bilateral hernias are not overlooked.

The author does not routinely explore both groins in children over six months old and only recommends bilateral surgery when there is evidence to suggest bilateral hernias.

Radiological herniography

The use of intraperitoneal herniography is advocated to decide on contralateral exploration. The radiological diagnosis of inguinal hernias using intraperitoneal contrast media was first described in Canada in 1967.[270] Using a midline infra-umbilical injection with an 18-gauge Surgicath under local anaesthesia, water-soluble contrast is instilled.[344, 376] Sodium diatrizoate (Hypaque M60) is an appropriate contrast medium.

The contrast is injected, the child 'shaken gently' and then prone radiographs taken. In a series of 562 inguinal hernias in children, 335 were clinically unilateral, 210 on the right and 125 on the left; with herniography, 77 (22.9%) of the patients were found to have significant contralateral hernias.[379] Kiesewetter and Oh (1980) compared transperitoneal exploration of the contralateral side by a bent Bakes' choledochal dilator with herniography. They found the technique using the Bakes' dilator unreliable and difficult to use, whereas they found herniography accurate and easy to use. They recommend routine herniography.[495] Clinical complications, including abdominal wall cellulitis, septicaemia, haematoma and intestinal obstruction, are reported. Routine use of herniography is not necessary and not recommended, but the technique should be available. It is accurate and simple to use.

Gas insulation and laparoscopy for the diagnosis of bilateral hernias

Intraoperative pneumoperitoneum, the Goldstein test, has been proposed to assess which children should undergo bilateral groin exploration. The concept, and the technique of gas insufflation of the peritoneal cavity, is attractive but in practice it has been associated with too many false positives.[759] Lightweight video-laparoscopic technology is an appealing technique for the surgeon. Good views of the groin region can be obtained in most patients. These new enhanced views have shown that a thin veil-like curtain often overlaps the internal opening of the processus vaginalis and prevents its distension by the intraperitoneal gas; this may be part of the explanation of the false-negative findings in the Goldstein test and may be a mechanism of the transitory distension of obtained sacs. Laparoscopy easily demonstrates an inguinal hernia or a patent processus vaginalis with a high degree of accuracy but is it worthwhile? Is laparoscopy in the infant the right way to proceed?[572]

Safe successful laparoscopy requires general anaesthesia, endotracheal intubation, catheterization of the bladder and gastric intubation, then peritoneal cannulation and insufflation with CO_2 and finally the insertion of the laparoscope. Introduction of the needle for gas input and the laparoscope into the peritoneal cavity is hazardous to intraperitoneal organs and blood vessels. However, conventional bilateral groin exploration involves making two 1-cm incisions with no intraperitoneal organ hazard and does not involve endotracheal intubation of a very small baby.[572]

Inguinal hernia in girls

Inguinal hernia in girls should raise the surgeon's suspicions about the child's nuclear sex, particularly if the condition is bilateral. Approximately 1.6% of these children, presenting with inguinal hernia and having apparent female genitalia, prove to be of male nuclear sex, with intra-abdominal testes but female external genital appearance and endocrine function – the 'testicular feminization syndrome'.[48, 480, 668, 702] All female children with inguinal hernia should have their nuclear sex ascertained, and skilled paediatric and genetic counselling advice should be sought where anomalies are found. Testicular feminization is a misnomer because the testes do not feminize the child. The reality is that the affected male has a metabolic disorder – complete androgen insensitivity syndrome (CAIS) – making him resistant to the action of testosterone and dihydrotestosterone. Binding of androgen to receptors is deficient at the cellular level so that a phenotypically female with breasts, external genitalia and clitoris develops.

The chromosome karyotype is 46 XY. Hyperactivity of the testes with high oestrogen and testosterone levels, and raised plasma gonadotrophins, lead to female sex characteristics and orientation at puberty.

Most cases of testicular feminization are sporadic mutations. The incidence is 1:62 400 live births, the probable method of inheritance being a sex-linked recessive gene transmitted through the female. Because affected persons are sterile, the syndrome is partially self-limiting. The real surgical problem is what to do with the gonad? Orchidectomy is not indicated in infancy or childhood because removal of gonad function will compromise development of secondary sexual characteristics. The gonads may be intra-abdominal and the condition go unnoticed. If a unilateral hernia is present, laparotomy with biopsy of the contralateral gonad should be performed to examine the internal genitalia and exclude other varieties of intersex.[738]

With bilateral hernia, the gonads should be saved and placed subcutaneously in the suprapubic fat. Orchidectomy should then be performed after development of the secondary sexual characteristics. After maturity the incidence of malignant change in the abnormally placed gonad, whether intra or extra-abdominal, outweighs the advantages of its endocrine function. An incidence of 8% malignant change has been recorded in one series.[668] Maintenance of secondary sexual appearances can be achieved with hormone therapy.

Sliding hernias in childhood

In both sexes transitory lateral extraperitoneal protrusions of the bladder occur as a sliding component of the medial wall of indirect hernias. These protrusions ('bladder ears') have been demonstrated on excretion urography in 9% of infants under one year old who have hernias.[13, 845] It is important to recognize the bladder in the medial wall, or the colon in the lateral wall, and to modify the operation technique to avoid damage to these structures. In girls, many indirect congenital sacs are sliding hernias containing genital structures, ovaries, fallopian tubes or even the uterus in the walls. In a series of 262 inguinal hernias in female children, an ovary and/or fallopian tube was found in 41% of those undergoing operation under two years old.[49] A primitive uterus has been described in a male child with intersex.

Littré's hernia in infancy

Littré's hernia, the hernial sac containing a Meckel's diverticulum, has been described in neonates. The condition can be diagnosed preoperatively; the hernia can be reduced by taxis but after reduction 'a smaller firmer mass remains below the external ring'. This residual mass resists all attempts at taxis and is sometimes tender. There are often adhesions between the Meckel's diverticulum and the sac. These prevent reduction and suggest that closed-loop obstruction may complicate this type of hernia.[58]

Relation between testicular tumours, undescended testicles and inguinal hernia

There is no doubt that testicular tumours occur more frequently in maldescended testicles, but the quantification of this increased risk is difficult. Campbell (1959) came to the conclusion that the undescended testicle is 48 times more likely to undergo malignant change than the normal testis,[146] whereas Wobbes et al. (1980), reviewing experience in Groningen, North Netherlands, estimated the risk to be increased about 17 times.[992] Are inguinal hernias in infancy similarly associated with an increased testicular cancer risk? Previous inguinal herniotomy was found in 3.4% of the patients with testicular tumour reported from Groningen: this figure is in accord with the usual incidence of infantile inguinal hernia. Consequently there seems to be no increased risk of testicular tumour in patients who have had an operation for inguinal hernia, although Morrison (1976) estimated that infantile inguinal hernia was associated with 2.9 times as high risk of subsequent malignant testicular tumour.[670] Another controversy!

If a testicular tumour develops after inguinal herniotomy, will inguinal node metastases occur? Inguinal node metastases develop in patients who develop testicular tumours after childhood orchidopexy, so that it seems unlikely that childhood herniotomy will influence or limit the spread of a testicular tumour.

Inguinal hernias are frequently associated with other anomalies of the testicle in male children. Chilvers et al. (1984) have reported an apparent increase in undescended testicle diagnoses by a factor of 2.3 for the period 1962–81, the diagnosis of undescended testicle to the age of 15 years rising from 1.4% for the 1952 birth cohort to 2.9% for the 1977 birth cohort.[177] The significance of this change is unclear. Whether there is a similar increase in the incidence of inguinal hernias is also unknown. However, the higher incidence of inguinal hernia in male infants in Stockton-on-Tees from 1970 to 1979, when compared with the earlier findings of Knox (1959),[507] may reflect a change in the epidemiology of the condition.

Increased intraperitoneal fluid and inguinal hernia in children

With chylous ascites or ascites due to liver disease, or following the insertion of a ventriculoperitoneal shunt for hydrocephalus, or in peritoneal dialysis for renal failure, there is an increased incidence of indirect hernias and hydrocele.[284, 370, 374] If an inguinal hernia develops in these circumstances in a child, early rather than delayed surgery is indicated.

Recurrence

Almost all recurrences of childhood inguinal hernias are due to technical failure at operation. The majority of recurrences are apparent within 12 months of operation. The most likely technical mistakes are a failure to isolate the sac completely at the neck or failure to ligate it high enough flush with the parietal peritoneum. Ligation of the sac with absorbable material, such as catgut, leads to recurrence. The sac should be sutured/closed off with one of the newer, slowly absorbable polymers. Reported recurrence rates vary from 0.1% for elective operation to 5.6% for emergency surgery. Recurrence rates are very closely related to the skill of the operator, being lowest in series operated by skilled paediatric surgeons and highest when junior general surgeons operate.[408] In a series of 118 operations for childhood hernias performed by non-paediatric surgeons in a Swedish community hospital over a 10-year period, the recurrence rate in boys was 3.8% and testicular atrophy complicated 7.5% of the operations in males.[453] Many hernias in neonates nowadays are in premature babies and skilled experienced surgeons are needed to manage them. Inexperience in dealing with diminutive structures, unfamiliarity with the anatomy, sliding hernias in girls and the bladder close by the internal ring in both sexes can cause difficulties. Connective tissue disorders and raised intraperitoneal pressure also predispose to recurrence.[369] The value of specialization should be emphasized, best results being obtained by surgeons who address the problem regularly.

Arrangements for surgery and anaesthesia

Most children with inguinal hernias can be treated on an out-patient basis. Only for compelling medical or social reasons does the child need to be admitted to hospital. In any case, the mother should be encouraged to accompany the child to hospital and to nurse him or her after recovery from the operation.

To operate on children with inguinal hernia effectively as day cases requires good hospital organization and excellent hospital-to-community communications. It is essential to have printed advice and instructions for the parents and a 'safety net' system which can cope with situations that go wrong.

The following American quotation encapsulates all the benefits of day surgery for children: 'It is relatively simple for the parents to drive to the Surgicenter . . . and park . . . and enjoy the highly personalized services.'[183]

The operation should be performed as soon as possible after the diagnosis has been established. Young, even newborn and preterm, children tolerate this surgery well, and the parental anxiety and risk of incarceration of the hernia are minimized by early operation.

Day-case surgery in young children is best performed between 10.00 a.m. and 3.00 p.m. Before 10.00 a.m. there may not be time for travel, unhurried preparation and sedation. A screaming child and an anxious mother are not the ideal prelude to elective surgery! Hypoglycaemia and dehydration are of rapid onset when small children are starved unnecessarily. These physiological 'complications' should be prevented by giving the child a normal morning feed and then a preoperative drink of maltose and metoclopramide, and by operating as early after the morning feed as is safe.[50, 320]

Operation, on a day-case basis, should always be completed before 3.00 p.m. in order to ensure that the effects of anaesthesia are gone before the child is sent home. Children should not be discharged in a sedated or semi-comatose state.[368]

Because of the increased risk of postoperative apnoea and bradycardia low-birthweight and preterm babies are conventionally treated as inpatients with appropriate ICU support and monitoring; however, some benefit from being treated as day cases.[647]

The operation

PRINCIPLES

In babies and young children, the inguinal canal has not yet developed its oblique adult anatomy. The superficial ring is directly anterior to the deep ring and the sac is indirect. There is no acquired deformity of the canal. In these cases the fascia transversalis is normal and a simple herniotomy is all that is necessary. Straightforward inguinal herniotomy should give a 100% cure rate.[50, 225, 973]

HAEMOSTATIS AND SUTURE MATERIALS

Haemostasis is secured by careful ligating of bleeding points with metric 3 braided polyglycolic acid (Dexon) or braided polyglactin 910 (Vicryl). Electrocoagulation with a fine paediatric coagulation probe is also used but great care is needed to prevent propagation and thrombosis of the small vessels in the delicate spermatic cord and cause subsequent testicular damage.

All deep suturing is carried out using Dexon or Vicryl. The skin is closed with metric 4 or metric 6 clear* subcuticular PDS or a skin dressing only. If the subcutaneous fat is closed carefully and accurately, no subcuticular suture will be required. Adhesive skin tape skin closure gives very good cosmetic results.

POSITION OF PATIENT

The child is placed on his back on the operating table. A light cotton blanket lies over the chest and upper abdomen and a similar blanket over the lower limbs. This precaution prevents heat loss during surgery.

Draping

Drapes are applied so that the groin area and scrotum are exposed throughout the operation (Figure 9.5)

---

*Clear PDS is recommended because skin tattooing can occur if a coloured polymer is used.

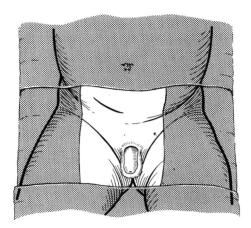

Figure 9.5   Draping should be so that the scrotum and both groins are visible to the operator

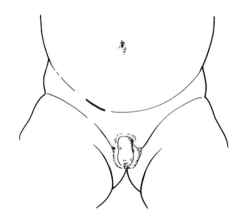

Figure 9.6   A 1.5 cm long incision is made just above and medial to the external inguinal ring

THE INCISION

A horizontal transverse incision is made in the transverse skin crease just above and medial to the superficial inguinal ring. The incision should be 1.0–1.5 cm long. The superficial ring and the emerging spermatic cord can be readily palpated under anaesthesia. The site for incision and the direction of the subsequent dissection are thus confirmed (Figure 9.6).

DISSECTION OF THE EXTERNAL RING

The superficial ring and cord, which have already been identified by palpation, are approached by gently opening the subcutaneous fat with a blunt haemostat. At this stage the superficial epigastric vessels are encountered and picked up in light haemostats, divided with scissors and ligated.

The superficial inguinal ring and cord are readily identified when the superficial subcutaneous fat has been opened (Figure 9.7).

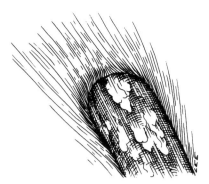

Figure 9.7 The cord is identified as it emerges from the external inguinal ring

DISSECTION OF THE CORD COVERINGS

Once the cord has been identified its coverings must be opened to give access to the hernial sac. The sac lies on the anterosuperior aspect of the cord as it emerges from the external inguinal ring.

It is covered first by the diaphanous external spermatic fascia, then by the cremasteric fascia, which is readily identified by its neat intertwining pink fascicles of muscle, and more deeply by the very delicate internal spermatic fascia. These structures – the three layers of spermatic fascia – are separated from the enclosed contents of the cord by careful blunt dissection with a fine haemostat.

A 'trick of the trade' is most useful here: a **closed** haemostat is pushed through the fascial layers into the cord and then opened slowly in the long axis so that a rent is made. If a hernial sac is present it is immediately apparent in the rent. The rent is held open with the haemostat and the sac grasped with a second haemostat placed between the open blades of the first. (Figures 9.8–9.10).

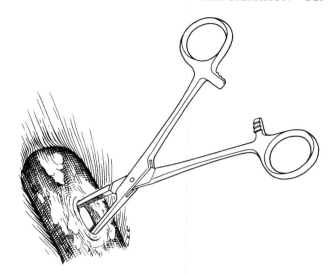

Figure 9.9 The haemostat is gently opened

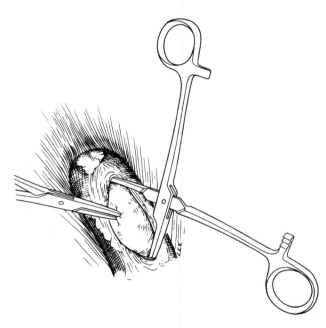

Figure 9.10 As the haemostat is opened it stretches the rent in the coverings of the cord and the bluish coloured indirect sac is immediately visible on the anterior superior aspect of the cord. The sac is grasped in a second haemostat

The sac can be identified lying on the anterosuperior aspect of the contents of the cord. It is pale blue and much thicker than the fascial coverings of the cord. The most difficult manoeuvre in the operation must now be carried out.

The sac is either 'complete' (total funicular hernia), that is it extends to the scrotum and encompasses the testicle, or 'incomplete' (partial funicular hernia), that is it extends along only part of the length of the cord.

If the sac is 'complete' its posterior wall must be separated from the other cord contents – the vas deferens,

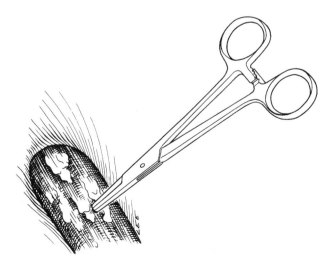

Figure 9.8 A fine closed haemostat is pushed into the cord between the easily identified interwoven bundles of the cremaster

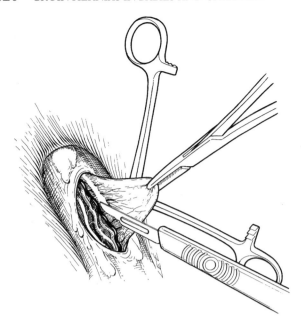

Figure 9.11   The sac being separated from the cord structures. A gentle stroke with a sharp scalpel will divide the internal spermatic fascia, opening up a plane between the sac and the cord structures

the testicular artery and the pampiniform plexus of veins. This must be done very gently. Above all, the vas or the pampiniform vessels must never be grasped in forceps. Its successful accomplishment is a benchmark by which surgical competence can be measured. First, the internal spermatic fascia fixing the pampiniform plexus to the sac is divided by a scalpel (Figure 9.11).

Then a fine haemostat is gently insinuated between each structure and the thin peritoneal sac wall in turn to push them off the sac (Figure 9.12). When each structure has been pushed off, the proximal sac is held in a

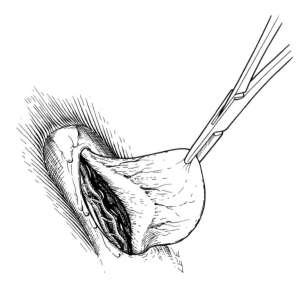

Figure 9.12   A haemostat holds up the sac and the cord structures are separated from it

haemostat and the sac divided across (Figure 9.13). The distal sac (remainder of the processus vaginalis), testicle and cord can now be manipulated back into place in the scrotum. Gentle traction on the testicle in the scrotum at this time will confirm that it has been returned to its normal site (Figure 9.14).

The proximal divided sac is now dealt with in the same manner as an incomplete sac.[106]

The fundus of an incomplete sac (or the proximal remnant of a complete sac) is held in a haemostat and the contents of the cord are gently pushed off its posterior wall using a piece of gauze, while traction is applied to keep the sac taut. The sac must be stripped of cord contents down to its junction with the parietal peritoneum.

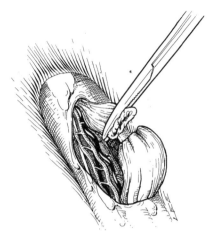

Figure 9.13   If the sac is complete it must now be clamped and divided across

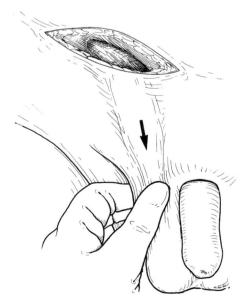

Figure 9.14   The distal end falls away towards the testicle. The scrotum is manipulated to ensure the testicle is returned to base

Difficulties dissecting the sac

If dissection of the proximal sac is difficult or obscured the lateral margin of the superficial inguinal ring should be divided for 1 cm or so to increase the exposure of the deep ring and the fascia transversalis.

Opening the sac

Once the sac has been completely separated from the cord coverings and contents it should be opened. This is most important in a female child. If any intra-abdominal contents are in the sac they are pushed back into the greater peritoneal cavity (Figure 9.15).

THE SLIDING HERNIA

Bladder, colon or internal genitalia in the female can form part of the wall of a sliding hernia. The hernial sac should be cleaned of cord structures around three-quarters of its circumference, then the sac should be divided on either side away from the sliding organ (along the dotted lines). This is made easier if the superficial ring, external oblique, is divided (as above). The sac can now be closed by a suture picking up the extraperitoneal wall of the bladder (colon, broad ligament), reducing any contents and ligating around the remainder of the sac.

THE VASCULAR COMPROMISED TESTICLE

If there is recent incarceration the venous return from the testicle will be impeded and there may even be early infarction of the testicle. Such testicles should not be removed; if left undisturbed many will recover, at least partially, and be endocrine-useful in adult life.

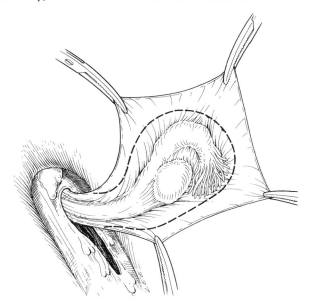

Figure 9.15 The sac should always be opened. In the female, the ovary and the tube are often sliding components of the sac wall

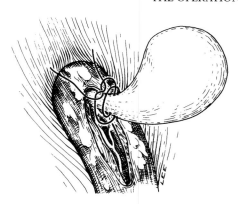

Figure 9.16 The sac is closed with a transfixion ligature

CLOSURE

The sac is now ligated circumferentially with a transfixion suture of metric 3 absorbable polymer (Figure 9.16). Catgut or catgut derivatives are not advised to suture ligate the sac; catgut loses its strength often capriciously early and precipitates recurrence. There is never any need to dislocate the testicle from the scrotum to deal with the sac, provided the proximal sac is divided across, the distal component of a complete sac can be left alone *in situ*. Protection of the distal cord and testicle will avoid trauma and vascular damage to the testicle.

The external oblique

If the superficial ring has been extended into the aponeurosis of the external oblique, the divided aponeurosis is now repaired with appropriate polymer sutures

SUBCUTANEOUS TISSUE

The subcutaneous fat is now closed with two or three metric 3 absorbable polymer sutures, carefully placed to close the dead space in the depths of the wound and its immediate subdermal layer. The knots are placed deeply (Figure 9.17).

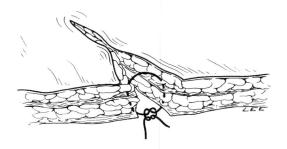

Figure 9.17 Closure of the subcutaneous fat

THE SKIN

The skin is closed with a subcuticular suture of metric 4 or 6 polydioxanone (PDS).

IATROGENIC CRYPTORCHISM

At the completion of the operation the position of the testicle in the scrotum should be confirmed. The manipulation of the sac can cause the testicle to be drawn up into the neck of the scrotum or into the inguinal region; if the testicle is not replaced into the scrotum at the conclusion of the surgery, postoperative adhesions will trap it in fibrous tissue and result in cryptorchism. Infection and postoperative cremaster spasm have also been blamed for this unfortunate complication. Vigilance will prevent it. The testicle must be easily palpable in the scrotum at the conclusion of the inguinal herniotomy; if it is not, further exploration and, if necessary, testicular fixation should be accomplished before the anaesthetic is terminated (Figure 9.18).[479]

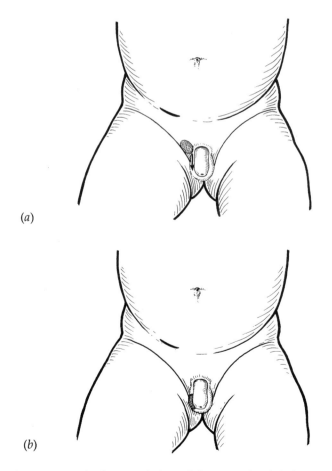

(a)

(b)

Figure 9.18 At the completion of the operation it is important to check the position of the testicle and ensure that it is in the scrotum

Postoperative care and follow-up

No postoperative care other than normal maternal nursing care is required. The child can be caressed and fed by his mother as soon as he has recovered from the anaesthetic. He can be allowed to play and be bathed as soon as necessary.

Most patients recover rapidly from these simple operations and outpatient follow up visits are probably unnecessary. Probable findings in the postoperative clinic are malposition of the testicle, atrophy of the testicle and the odd transient hydrocele. More importantly, a contralateral hernia may be discovered. Despite the vogue against routine follow up it is a valuable quality control process for the surgical team and ensures parent happiness. The authors advise it.

Complications

Some children, perhaps 10%, have bruising adjacent to the wound and in the scrotum, which resolves spontaneously. Wound infections are very rare.

Sometimes the testicle may go 'hard' after surgery. An expectant policy should be adopted with this complication. The 'hard' testicle is in reality suffering from borderline ischaemia and if left alone will recover spontaneously. Earlier techniques which involved mobilization of the testicle from the scrotum were accompanied by an incidence of up to 4% of subsequent testicular atrophy.[783] It must be emphasized again that the testicle does not require routine mobilization from the scrotum and delivery into the wound – this manoeuvre hazards the superficial pudendal anastomotic blood supply and places the testicle at increased risk of ischaemia.

Another complication is division of the vas deferens at operation. It is impossible to know how common this is. The one study of the subject in the literature reports a 1.6% incidence, or more exactly fragments of vas deferens were found in five of 313 infantile hernial sacs examined histologically after operation.[882] Care at operation – the vas should be fully visualized before the sac is ligated and excised – should prevent this complication. If the vas is damaged, immediate repair is recommended.

Personal experience

In Stockton-on-Tees experience with these operations is broadly in accord with the reported series. In the nine years 1970–79, 346 children with hernia were operated upon. Of these, 299 (86.4%) were male and 47 (13.6%) female – a ratio of 6:1. Of the 299 boys, 184 (61.5%) had right-sided hernia, 97 (32.4%) left-sided hernia, and in 18 (6%) the hernia was bilateral. The girls showed an unusual preponderance of right-sided hernia: 32 (68.1%) right-sided, 11 (23.4%) left-sided and 4 (8.5%) bilateral. No nuclear sex anomalies in the girls were identified in this series.

No major complications have been encountered and the operation has left a sound cosmetically acceptable scar. The children have been cared for by their mothers, with a minimum of psychological trauma to both. In this series of 346 cases there was only one wound infection (0.3%). This patient, a day case, required community nursing care at home after discharge.

Extraperitoneal approach to inguinal hernia

INTRODUCTION

The advantage of an extraperitoneal approach to inguinal hernia was described by Cheatle in 1921.[171] This approach to hernias in children was recommended by Boley and Kleinhams in 1966.[109]

The extraperitoneal approach can be made using a midline vertical incision, a Pfannenstiel incision or a lateral muscle-splitting incision. The midline incision gives good access but is cosmetically unacceptable and not recommended. The Pfannenstiel incision is an extensive approach but does give excellent access to each groin and is recommended if a bilateral pathology must be dealt with.

The lateral muscle-splitting approach is easy to use, gives good exposure and heals well with excellent cosmesis. This approach to strangulated inguinal hernia (and high undescended testicles) has been advocated by Jones of Aberdeen and is recommended for these circumstances.[472] Jones' contribution has significantly improved the quality of surgery available for children needing these difficult operations with potential hazard to the testicle.

This extraperitoneal approach is advised in the following circumstances:

1. For the incarcerated inguinal hernia which has failed to reduce on gallows traction. In these circumstances the oedema and early inflammation around the distended sac can obscure the delicate spermatic vessels and vas. There is no oedema proximal to the deep ring and the cord structures can thus be readily identified and preserved using the extraperitoneal approach. Furthermore, strangulated bowel needs inspection and, very rarely, resection. This is easy using this access.
2. When an inguinal hernia is associated with a high (impalpable or within the inguinal canal – so-called 'inguino-emergent') maldescended testicle. This approach facilitates dissection of the sac from the vessels and cord; the sac can be tied off flush with the peritoneum and then the vessels can be mobilized

retroperitoneally to the lower pole of the kidney and the vas fully mobilized into the pelvis. After this mobilization the testicle can be placed in the scrotum via the inguinal canal and the abdominal wound closed.
3. The extraperitoneal approach using a Pfannenstiel incision is the technique of choice for the rare instance of bilateral inguinal hernia associated with bilateral maldescent of the testicles, or for bilateral impalpable high maldescended testicles.

A note of caution

The extraperitoneal approach to inguinal hernia is unusual and the surgeon must gain experience using it in the non-emergency situation. It is not an operation for the inexperienced junior, or for the surgeon who does not have regular experience of operating on small children, to undertake on a newborn with a strangulated inguinal hernia. It must be reiterated – children should be operated on by surgeons who have experience and a special interest and training in paediatric surgery.

THE OPERATION

Principles

In babies the inguinal canal has not developed its adult obliquity; the hernial sac is a peritoneal sac passing through a congenital defect of fascia transversalis at the deep ring, thence through the canal to present at the groin.

When incarceration is present, the constriction is usually caused by the rigid aponeurotic pillars of the superficial inguinal ring. This operation exploits the potential space between the peritoneum and the fascia transversalis. It allows the peritoneal sac to be isolated before it enters the inguinal canal and before it has become oedematous and diaphanous in cases of incarceration.

The same patient position, draping, haemostasis and sutures are used as described previously.

The incision

A horizontal transverse incision is made medial to the anterior superior iliac spine across the linea semilunaris to the midpoint of the rectus muscle. This incision is 1.0–2.0 cm cephalad to the incision used for the traditional anterior inguinal herniotomy described on page 118. The external oblique muscle is split in the line of its fibres to expose the lateral margin of the rectus muscle which is retracted medially (Figure 9.19).

If bilateral hernias are to be explored: (a) a Pfannenstiel incision in the suprapubic skin crease is employed; (b) this incision should extend from the midpoint of one

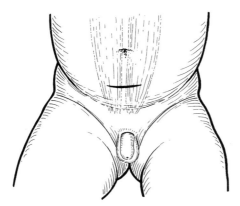

Figure 9.19 Incision for unilateral extraperitoneal exploration of a child's groin

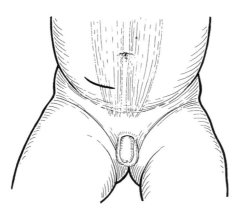

Figure 9.20 Pfannenstiel incision for bilateral groin exploration. The rectus muscles are separated in the midline

rectus muscle to the midpoint of the second – the rectus muscles are separated in the midline and the extraperitoneal space opened (Figure 9.20).

Extraperitoneal access

Access to the extraperitoneal space is gained to reveal the peritoneum. The whole of the lower edge skin, subcutaneous tissues and the musculo-aponeurotic strata are lifted up with a retractor to reveal the neck of the peritoneal sac and its contents as they plunge into the deep ring (Figure 9.21).

Defining the sac

Gentle taxis and simultaneous external pressure usually reduce the contents of the sac. If the hernia is incarcerated or strangulated the peritoneum of the neck can be opened before the attempted reduction. A soft forceps can be placed on the bowel and used to retrieve the bowel after reduction, enabling assessment of its viability. If there is difficulty reducing the bowel, a curved artery forceps can be passed alongside it through the

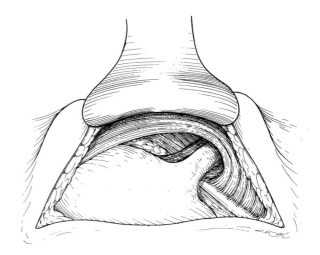

Figure 9.21 The lower aponeurotic flap is elevated with a retractor to reveal the hernial sac plunging into the inguinal canal

deep ring and gently opened to dilate rigid structures. If necessary, a superficial dissection of the lower flap will allow the superficial ring to be visualized or split laterally to enlarge it and release a strangulation.

The sac is now empty. It is now a simple matter to lift up the neck of the sac, gently pull away the cord vessels and the vas and clamp across the neck (Figure 9.22).

Dividing the sac

The neck of the sac is divided and the sac transfixed and tied off flush with the peritoneum. The distal sac (processes vaginalis) is left undisturbed. It is important not to

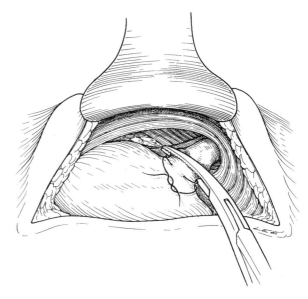

Figure 9.22 After the sac has been separated from the cord structures, the neck of the sac is clamped and the distal sac divided

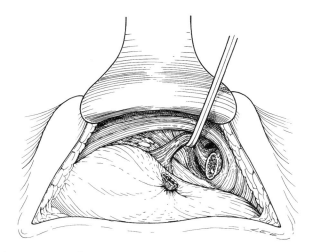

Figure 9.23 After the sac is tied flush with the peritoneum the cord structures are checked. Do not attempt to disturb the testicle or reduce it into the abdomen

attempt to manipulate the testicle into the abdomen or to attempt to remove the distal sac. If infarction and/or strangulation are present, the vascular supply to the testicle may be compromised; further manipulation and surgical viewing will not improve this! An expectant policy will be rewarded by most testicles recovering (Figure 9.23).

Closure

The aponeurotic layers, the anterior rectus sheath and the external oblique are closed with a running metric 3 absorbable polymer suture (Figure 9.24).

The subcutaneous fat is closed as before and the skin closed with a subcuticular suture of PDS.

POSTOPERATIVE CARE AND COMPLICATIONS

Postoperative management is exactly the same as for the standard herniotomy (see page 122).

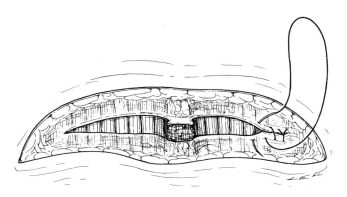

Figure 9.24 The retractors are removed, the rectus muscles spring back to position, and the anterior rectus sheath is then closed

Femoral hernia in children

Femoral hernia between birth and 14 years of age is uncommon, comprising less than 0.5% of all childhood groin hernias. In the English literature, 44 cases aged under five years are recorded. Strangulation is even rarer, 10 cases being reported in the English literature.[110, 907, 1004] The youngest victim of strangulation in a femoral hernia reported is a 5-week-old boy.[936] Of the 10 cases of strangulation reported, two contained strangulated omentum, which is surprising considering the small size of the omentum in infancy. Other contents of femoral hernia sacs in infancy include female genitalia, ovaries and fallopian tubes, and small intestine.

Femoral hernias are more frequently noticed in girls than boys.[310, 451, 565] It is suggested that the primary aetiology of infantile femoral hernia is a congenitally narrow posterior inguinal wall, fascia transversalis, attachment onto the pectineal ligament (Cooper's ligament) with a low origin of the inferior epigastric vessels; this predisposes to a wide femoral ring with weakened fascia transversalis stretched over it.[452]

Acquired femoral hernia can occur as a complication of an osteotomy for dislocation or subluxation of the hip.[823] An acquired prevascular femoral hernia can also complicate a congenital dislocation of the hip.[690]

DIAGNOSIS

Tam and Lister (1984) report 20 cases from Alder Hey Children's Hospital, Liverpool.[907] The correct diagnosis was made in only three cases by the referring physician and in only 13 cases by the consulting surgeon. This clearly illustrates the difficulty of diagnosis and, perhaps, the low index of suspicion prevailing. That the diagnostic rate improved in the second period of their study would support the argument about the suspicion index. Mistaken diagnoses included: inguinal hernia, 4 cases; lymphadenitis, 2 cases; lymphangioma, 1 case. Attention to the location of the hernia lateral to and below the pubic tubercle on clinical examination should eliminate diagnostic confusion.

In a series of 12 femoral hernias in children in Leicester, 9 were misdiagnosed: 8 as inguinal hernia and 1 as a cyst of the cord.[1004] One case was an emergency presentation of a Richter's hernia in a male 6-year-old child. Femoral hernia followed previous inguinal herniotomy in two children.

The differential diagnosis of femoral hernia in a child includes: (a) inguinal adenitis; (b) inguinal hernia; (c) ectopic testis; (d) lipoma; (e) cyst of the canal of Nuck; (f) obturator hernia; (g) cystic lymphoma.

TREATMENT

There is no uniformly agreed surgical approach to femoral hernias in childhood. The principles would seem to be to remove the sac and close the peritoneum, and then to obliterate the enlarged femoral ring either by suturing the medial inguinal ligament to the pectineal ligament or by closing the defect with pectineus fascia. If the aetiological concept of a narrow conjoint tendon attachment to the pubis is supported, it would seem logical to attach the conjoint tendon to the pectineal ligament as in the 'Cooper's ligament repair' of an inguinal hernia.[452] Whichever method of repair is favoured, it is crucially important to find and remove the sac. This can be difficult; in two of the 20 cases reported from Alder Hey Children's Hospital, failure to identify and remove the sac at the primary operation resulted in an early recurrence of the hernia.[907]

The low (crural), the inguinal or the high extraperitoneal approach can be utilized. Because of the difficulties of diagnosis and of identifying the sac, the extraperitoneal approach is probably ideal, as it allows good review of both inguinal and femoral areas at operation.

It must be stressed, however, that to avoid missing a hernial sac at operation is more important than relying on one particular method of repair.

Conclusions

Children with inguinal hernias should be operated on at the earliest opportunity after diagnosis. The operation should be performed by a surgeon experienced and interested in this surgery. There should be no children with inguinal hernias on the waiting list of general surgeons.

Emergency herniotomy for inguinal hernia in infants is one of the more difficult operations in paediatric surgical practice; this is an operation for an experienced surgeon only. Taxis and sedation will reduce many childhood incarcerated inguinal hernias. Early surgery will reduce the incidence of the condition.

The extraperitoneal approach is recommended for incarcerated or strangulated inguinal hernias in childhood. Femoral hernias are rare in children, and they will be overlooked unless diagnostic suspicion is maintained.

10 UMBILICAL HERNIA: OPERATION IN BABIES AND CHILDREN

Incidence

Minor degrees of herniation of the umbilicus are present in many neonates. These tend to regress spontaneously. However, umbilical hernias are a common source of referral to surgeons. After groin hernias and hydroceles, they are the third most frequent diagnosis paediatric surgeons deal with. Umbilical hernias occur in 4% to 5% of children, although many resolve spontaneously.[996] In Stockton-on-Tees, 2.3 per 1000 live births require surgery for umbilical hernias.

Umbilical hernias are more common in Negro people of African origin than in white, Indian or Chinese. In the West Indies 58.5% of children of African origin have umbilical hernias compared with 8% of white children, 3.3% of Indian children and 1.3% of Chinese children.[459] In East Africa 60% of African origin children have umbilical hernias, compared with 4% of Indian origin.[592] Other studies confirm that 32%[206] or 42%[286] of Negro children have umbilical hernias. Among the Xhosa tribe in South Africa 61.8% of children have umbilical hernias, some being quite large.[462] One detailed study from Johannesburg contradicts this evidence; Blumberg found the incidence of umbilical hernia to be the same regardless of race.[106] However, this is the only study that has made such a finding.

Other predisposing causes of umbilical herniation are prematurity and low birthweight, respiratory distress syndrome, rickets and malnutrition.[952, 996] Umbilical hernias occur in 84% babies weighing 1000–1500 g; 38% in those weighing 1500–2000 g; and 20.5% in those between 2000 and 2500 g.[952] Umbilical hernias often regress spontaneously by 12 months of age and do not usually require surgical correction.[40]

Indications for surgery

The usual infantile umbilical hernia is a protrusion through the umbilical cicatrix, with a small peritoneal sac and a relatively narrow neck. These hernias become very obvious when the infant cries or strains and are often a source of worry to the parents. The hernia usually is a small cone-like protrusion with the umbilical cicatrix at its apex. A more exuberant hernia with a proboscid protuberance at the centre of the belly can lead to great psychological problems and warrant urgent surgery in infancy. Tender distended umbilical hernias occur in and mirror intraperitoneal disease, peritonitis, intestinal obstruction and ascites. Umbilical hernias rarely incarcerate or strangulate. Severe abdominal wall spasm associated with an umbilical hernia incarceration during vigorous swimming has been described in two children. Breathing using the abdominal muscles is critical in competitive swimming – high intra-abdominal pressures can cause umbilical herniation and incarceration in these circumstances, such cases are often dismissed as 'cramp'.[868]

The abdominal wall around the base of an umbilical hernia should be palpated carefully. It is important to exclude linea alba hernias, interstitial hernias and cystic remnants of the omphalomesenteric duct or allantois.

Infantile umbilical hernias undergo spontaneous regression and cure as the child grows. However, if the hernia is unusually large, with a neck diameter greater than 1.5 cm, or fails to regress by school age, it should be operated upon. A small aponeurotic defect, diameter less than 1.5 cm, may be prone to incarceration and strangulation; in one large series the incidence of these complications was 5%.[529] Although infantile umbilical hernias are remarkably free from complications one very rare complication, spontaneous rupture and evisceration, requires emergency treatment. Spontaneous rupture may be precipitated by local trauma, by umbilical sepsis or by severe coughing.[59] If spontaneous rupture with evisceration occurs the eviscerated bowel should be covered with warm damp swabs and urgent repair of the hernia performed after resuscitation of the child. Complications are absolute indications for surgery. It is important for psychological reasons to preserve the umbilical cicatrix when undertaking surgery.

Arrangements for surgery and anaesthesia

Children with umbilical hernias can be treated on an outpatient day-case basis. The arrangements for this surgery are similar to those described in Chapter 9 (see page 117).

The operation

PRINCIPLES

A simple excision of the peritoneal sac and closure of the aponeurotic defect by double breasting in the vertical plane – Mayo's operation – is recommended.[626] This operation has stood the test of time, is easy to perform and is effective. The umbilical cicatrix is carefully preserved and its base sutured to the fascial linea alba to present a cosmetically attractive appearance after surgery. The alternative operation, through a vertical incision, is described by Criado but is not recommended on cosmetic grounds.[204]

HAEMOSTASIS AND SUTURE MATERIALS

These details are given on page 118.

POSITION OF PATIENT

The child is placed on his back (supine) on the operating table. A light cotton blanket is placed over the chest and upper abdomen and a similar blanket over the lower limbs. This precaution prevents undue heat loss during surgery.

Draping

Drapes are applied so that the umbilical area is exposed throughout the operation.

THE INCISION

A curved transverse incision is made below the umbilicus: a curvilinear 'smile' incision. There is usually a skin fold skirting the umbilicus and the incision can be placed in it to give the most cosmetically acceptable result (Figure 10.1).

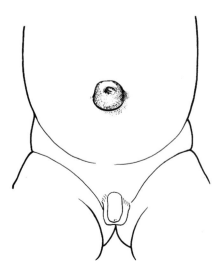

Figure 10.1 A curved subumbilical incision is recommended

SKIN FLAP AND EXPOSURE OF HERNIAL SAC

A skin flap, including the umbilical cicatrix, is dissected back to expose the hernial sac which is dissected free from the surrounding fat. When the neck of the sac is defined, the more rigid outline of the linea alba should now be easily identified (Figure 10.2).

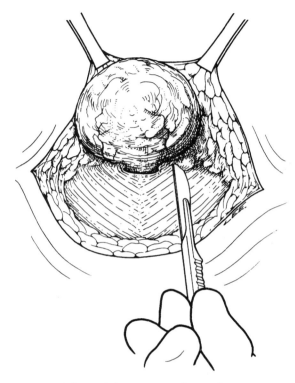

Figure 10.2 The umbilicus is raised as a flap to expose the hernia

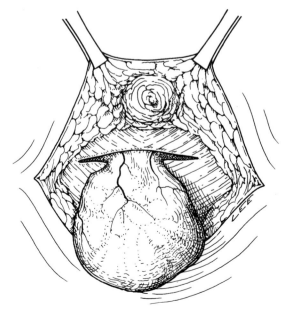

Figure 10.3 The hernial orifice is enlarged slightly on either side

Enlargement of opening

It is usually possible to reduce the contents of an infantile umbilical hernia without enlarging the opening of the linea alba. However, if the contents cannot be reduced, the opening should be enlarged by small horizontal incisions into the rectus sheath on either side (Figure 10.3)

REMOVAL OF SAC

The sac should be opened and then divided from the parietal peritoneum at its neck. As the sac is divided, its edges are picked up and held in small haemostats (Figure 10.4).

REPAIR OF LINEA ALBA

The linea alba and the peritoneum are sutured as one layer. Haemostasis must first be secured. Often in children there are some substantial vessels running between the peritoneum and the aponeurosis; these should be ligated (Figure 10.5).

A double breasting technique (Mayo) is used. The placement of the sutures is facilitated if the lateral extremities of the cut in the linea alba are held up in small haemostats. Three PDS metric 3 sutures are used; they are introduced through the upper flap, then through the lower flap and back through the upper flap. The sutures should traverse the upper flap about 0.5 cm from its margin (the condensation of the aponeurosis at the linea alba aperture). As each suture is introduced it is held, not tied (Figure 10.6).

When all three sutures have been placed, they are gently tightened and tied. Thus the lower aponeurotic flap is sutured to the undersurface of the upper flap.

The repair is now completed by suturing the edge of the upper flap to the anterior surface of the lower flap. Metric 3 PDS is used as continuous sutures (Figure 10.7).

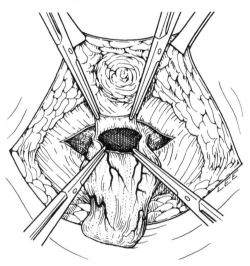

Figure 10.4 The sac is opened and checked that it is empty. The sac is then excised

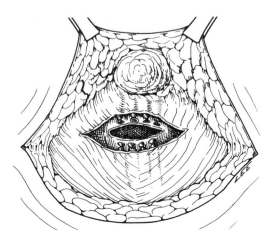

Figure 10.5 Haemostasis is ensured

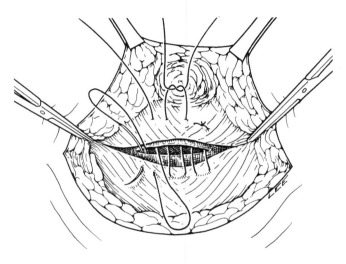

Figure 10.6 A double-breasting, 'vest over pants', Mayo operation is recommended. The first line of sutures is placed and held. Then the sutures are all tied simultaneously, pulling the lower flap up underneath the upper flap

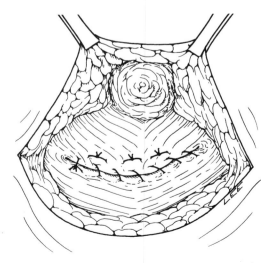

Figure 10.7 The repair is completed by sewing the edge of the upper flap to the anterior surface of the lower flap

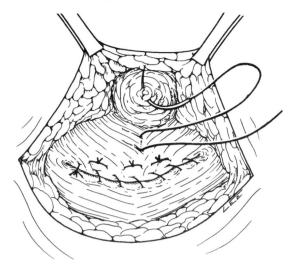

Figure 10.8 The umbilicus is reconstructed

RECONSTRUCTION OF UMBILICUS AND SKIN CLOSURE

The deepest part of the delve of the umbilical cicatrix is now sutured to the linea alba with braided polymer or fine colourless PDS, so preserving the appearance of the umbilicus (Figure 10.8).

The subcutaneous fat is closed with interrupted sutures of fine absorbable polymer, the knots being tied deeply. Skin closure is with a subcuticular suture of colourless PDS if needed (Figures 10.9 and 10.10).

Postoperative care

No postoperative care other than normal maternal nursing care is required. The child can be cuddled and fed by his mother as soon as he is recovered from the

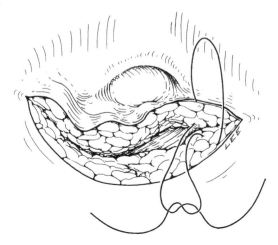

Figure 10.9 The subcutaneous fat is closed

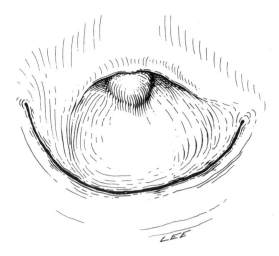

Figure 10.10 A subcuticular absorbable suture closes the skin

anaesthetic. He can be allowed to play and be bathed as soon as necessary.

The only postoperative complications are haematoma formation and minor sepsis. With careful haemostasis neither of these should be worrisome. Wound healing is usually quick and cosmesis very good.

Personal results

Because umbilical hernias generally regress spontaneously, few require operation. Consequently operations for umbilical hernias are numerically much fewer than operations for inguinal hernia in infancy and childhood. However, in Stockton-on-Tees, in the ten years 1970 up to and including 1979, 58 children (34 male and 24 female) with umbilical hernia have been operated on. There are no recurrences or major complications to report.

Conclusions

Umbilical hernias in neonates and infants should be treated expectantly. Most childhood hernias resolve spontaneously. If operation is needed, Mayo's 'vest over pants' technique is recommended.

11 DIAGNOSIS OF A LUMP IN THE GROIN IN THE ADULT

Knowledge of the anatomy of the groin and a consequently enhanced ability to differentially diagnose groin lumps is somehow projected as part of the image of surgeons. Surgical teachers are apt to regard a knowledge of groin lumps as normative for the student and aspirant surgeon. Glassow, certainly an experienced hernia surgeon, reporting his experience of femoral hernia in the female, described 8% of these femoral hernias being misdiagnosed as inguinal hernias.[347] Hardy and Costin have also drawn attention to the difficulties of distinguishing between inguinal and femoral hernias.[400] Although the distinction between femoral and inguinal hernias is difficult enough for practising surgeons, surgical teachers are obsessed with the diagnosis of groin lumps – the pursuit of the undiagnosable is, after all, an academic trail! Research shows that the differentiation between direct and indirect hernias cannot be sustained clinically.[125] In 180 patients over the age of 20 years with inguinal hernias two clinical tests were applied: the direction of the bulge and pressure on the deep ring to differentiate between direct and indirect hernia.[145] Operative findings indicated that the diagnosis of indirect hernia was correct in 92% of cases, whereas the clinical diagnosis of direct hernia was correct in only 56% of cases. These findings challenge the assumption that direct hernias are more easily diagnosable than indirect. Clinical diagnosis nevertheless remains useful as a test of a medical student's diagnostic skill.[125]

Unfortunate students had better beware; examiners will continue to ask them to distinguish inguinal and femoral, and direct and indirect inguinal hernias!

Every groin lump should be carefully evaluated and hernias must be distinguished from other lesions, but having stated this obvious truth it must be admitted that the distinction between the various types of groin hernia may often be impossible. Multiple groin hernias occur and add further to diagnostic confusion.

The Renaissance and eighteenth-century surgeons responsible for many of the clinico-anatomical descriptions we work to were coping with different clinical problems from those we deal with. We no longer have to diagnose the long-standing inguinoscrotal hernia which is carried in a wicker basket; today's patients frequently present with small lumps of recent origin. The patients are usually well nourished, not to say obese, and they expect as accurate a diagnosis as possible. But we must recognize that our clinical skills do not deliver a greater than 60% accuracy.[400, 754]

As the diagnosis is pursued from 'hernia/no hernia?' to 'hernia/femoral or inguinal?', and from 'inguinal hernia/direct or indirect?', the difficulties increase manifold. Even the experienced worker surgeon, not the academic thinker of the problem, may get the diagnosis wrong. Our differential diagnosis of these lumps demands review. The groin is an area of diagnostic uncertainty. A bizarre example of the diagnosis of a groin lump is reported by Deva *et al.* from Australia; their patient, a morbidly obese female (weight 182.0 kg, height 152.4 cm, body mass index 78.4) presented with an enlarging groin mass initially thought to be a femoral hernia. Computed tomography (CT) was not possible owing to her weight and ultrasound showed a solid lesion with no bowel demonstrated. The lesion, weighing 1650 g, was resected and found to be fat with no peritoneal sac![239]

Only one type of groin hernia can be diagnosed with any certainty; this is the broad neck direct sac in the elderly male which never strangulates, is often bilateral and rarely causes much discomfort. It is readily apparent when the patient stands and immediately disappears spontaneously when he lies. This patient is happy when told the diagnosis . . . and the need for no operation.[80] Berliner has observed patients with bilateral hernia who have needed unilateral repair only, for periods of 5–10 years. In the majority, even those doing heavy labour, the asymptomatic side did not require surgery.[93] Small, asymptomatic, direct inguinal hernias that are not enlarging can be managed with judicious neglect and remain stationary in size and continue to be asymptomatic despite heavy labour.[91]

Inguinal hernia – the adolescent and the adult

In the male adolescent or young adult the lump is most likely to be an indirect inguinal hernia. The story then is that when the lump first appeared there was acute, quite severe pain in the groin which passed off and after a day or two went away altogether. The pain may have been related to straining or lifting or playing some violent game. At first the lump comes and goes, disappearing when the sufferer goes to bed at night and not being present in the morning until he gets out of bed and stands up. The lump comes in the groin and goes obliquely down into the scrotum. The patient usually describes the sequence well. This is the classic description of an indirect (oblique) inguinal hernia in the young adult (Figure 11.1).

In the older man an indirect hernia can occur, but a direct inguinal hernia is more likely. The story here is usually of some associated strain, often at work, the lump then appearing one or two days after the initial pain in the groin has gone away. Such a hernia may not reduce spontaneously. In the older male the lump may be associated with coughing, straining to micturate or disturbances in bowel habit. In these circumstances other predisposing conditions, respiratory disease, urinary tract obstruction or carcinoma of the colon need to be excluded as potentiating factors.

Bilateral inguinal hernias in adult males are sometimes manifestations of connective tissue disorder (see page 46), ascites, carcinomatosis peritonei, heart failure or liver disease. The history may give a lead. Indirect inguinal hernias as a complication of CAPD are yet another manifestation of intra-abdominal fluid dilating the adult processus vaginalis.

A varicocele cannot easily be confused with an inguinal hernia in the male. The varicocele is invariably in the left inguinoscrotal line – it is like a mass of worms and disappears spontaneously if the subject lies down. It has no cough impulse.

Inguinal hernias are more common in adult males than adult females in a ratio of 10:1. However, inguinal hernias do occur in women; indeed, indirect inguinal hernias in women are as common as femoral hernias in women, a fact that is often forgotten in the differential diagnosis (see Table 3.3). Direct inguinal hernias are very rare in women.

The closed inguinal canal in the adult female means that small indirect inguinal hernias in women cause much stretching, and hence pain. Indirect inguinal hernias in women present with pain rather than with a lump. Even on the most careful examination a lump may be impossible to find in the suprapubic fat of an adult female.

Femoral hernia

Most femoral hernias occur in women aged over 50 years. Atrophy and weight loss are common in patients with femoral hernias. The incidence of femoral hernias, male to female, is about 1:4. The different pelvic shape and additional fat in women render them more prone to femoral hernias than are men.[347] Women with femoral hernias are usually multiparous – multiple pregnancy is said to predispose to femoral herniation. Femoral hernias are as common in men as in nulliparous women.[93] A wide variety of occupations are likely to be found in any sample of femoral hernia patients, although it is said that nurses are more prone to these hernias than other groups.[753]

Patients complain of a groin lump, groin pain or various obstructive symptoms, nausea, colic, distension or constipation. The symptoms are variable and, particularly in the obese, unless a painstaking clinical examination of the groin is undertaken a small femoral hernia is easily overlooked. Groin pain with a recent onset irreducible groin lump is the presentation in 27%, a painless reducible groin lump occurs in 10%, a painful and reducible groin lump in 7%. Groin pain with no other symptoms and no complaint of a groin lump is the presentation in 3% of patients. Six per cent of patients present with recurrent obstructive symptoms (Figure 11.2).[400, 754]

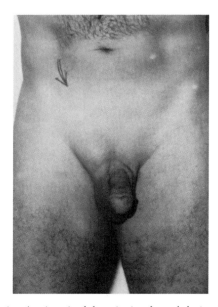

Figure 11.1 An inguinal hernia in the adult is above and medial to the inguinal ligament and pubic tubercle as the hernia emerges from the superficial inguinal ring

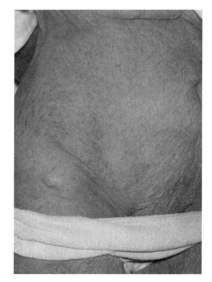

Figure 11.2 A femoral hernia is below and lateral to the inguinal ligament and pubic tubercle as the hernia emerges into the thigh

In diagnosis of a femoral hernia, distension of the saphenous veins is an important confirmatory sign.[332] The accuracy of the diagnosis of femoral hernias in the community varies. In a retrospective review, letters of referral were traceable in 88% of elective patients with an operative diagnosis of femoral hernia. The correct diagnosis had been arrived at by the referring general practitioner in only 40% of cases.[164] Patients referred with an inguinal lump or hernia (as opposed to a femoral hernia) were given a later out-patient appointment and consequently a later operation. It would seem prudent therefore that all elderly patients referred with any groin lump should receive an early out-patient appointment because femoral hernias presenting with intestinal obstruction as an emergency have a mortality approaching 10%.

Other groin swellings

Other structures in the groin each contribute to the harvest of swellings, pains and discomforts patients complain of. These include:

1. Vascular disease. (a) Arterial – aneurysms of the iliac and femoral vessels; these may be complicated by distal embolization or vascular insufficiency which will make the diagnosis easy. Femoral aneurysm as a complication of cardiac catheterization or transluminal angioplasty is a recent arrival in the diagnostic arena. (b) Venous – a saphenovarix could be confused with a femoral hernia. Its anatomical site is the same, but its characteristic blue colour, soft feel, fluid thrill, disappearance when the patient is laid flat and the giveaway associated varicose veins should prevent misdiagnosis.
2. Lymphadenopathy. Chronic painless lymphadenopathy may occur in lymphoma and a spectrum of infective diseases. Acute painful lymphadenitis can be confused with a tiny strangulated femoral hernia. A lesion in the watershed area, the lower abdomen, inguinoscrotal or perineal region, the distal anal canal or the ipsilateral lower limb quickly resolves the argument.
3. Tumours. Lipomas are very common tumours. The common 'lipoma of the cord', which in reality is an extension of preperitoneal fat,[293] is frequently associated with an indirect inguinal hernia. Lipomas also occur in the upper thigh to cause confusion with femoral hernias. A lipoma is rarely tender; it is soft with scalloped edges and can be lifted 'free' of the subjacent fat.
4. Secondary tumours. A lymph node enlarged with metastatic tumour usually lies in a more superficial layer than a femoral hernia. Such lymph nodes are more mobile in every direction than a femoral hernia and are often multiple.

5. Genital anomalies. (a) Ectopic testis in the male – there is no testicle in the scrotum on the same side. Torsion of an ectopic testicle can be confused with a strangulated hernia. (b) Cyst of the canal of Nuck – these cysts extend towards, or into, the labium majorum and are transilluminable.
6. Obturator hernia. An obturator hernia, especially in a female. This lies in the thigh lateral to the adductor longus muscle. Vaginal examination will resolve the diagnosis. Elective diagnosis is rarely entertained.
7. Rarities. (a) A cystic hygroma is a rare swelling; it is loculated and very soft. Usually the fluid can be pressed from one part of it to another. (b) A psoas abscess is a soft swelling frequently associated with backache. It loses its tension if the patient is laid flat. It is classically lateral to the femoral artery. (c) A hydrocele of the femoral canal is a rarity reported from West Africa. In reality it is the end stage of an untreated strangulated femoral epiplocele. The strangulated portion of omentum is slowly reabsorbed, the neck of the femoral sac remains occluded by viable omentum, while the distal sac becomes progressively more and more distended by protein-rich transudate.

Inguinoscrotal pain

Inguinoscrotal pain may arise in the groin and radiate to the ipsilateral hemiscrotum, thigh, flank or hypogastrium. Such pain may be neuralgic in type and accentuated by physical exertion. If the cause is a hernia or preperitoneal fat forcing its way out through the deep inguinal ring, these structures are stretched and pain fibres are stimulated. This is thought to cause a local reflex increase of tone in the internal oblique and transversus muscles coupled with neuralgic pain from stretching of the ilioinguinal nerve. The pain due to increase in tone is intermittent, whereas the neuralgic pain leading to hyperalgesia can be constant and following hernia repair will disappear, indicating that it is neuropraxic in type.[1000]

Numerous other conditions can give rise to acute or chronic pain in the inguinoscrotal and neighbouring anatomical regions (Table 11.1). These include gynaecological and urological pathology and a variety of musculoskeletal syndromes. An important entity increasingly being characterized is the syndrome of 'broad and deep fossae' or the sportsman's hernia. Thus, patients presenting with pain, as opposed to a painless, reducible swelling in the groin, should undergo very careful clinical evaluation for urological, gynaecological and musculoskeletal disorders. In addition to a careful history and examination, a variety of radiological investigations are at the disposal of the clinician.

Table 11.1 Differential diagnosis of inguinoscrotal pain

Hernia:	direct or indirect inguinal hernia, femoral hernia, lipomas of the cord
Scrotal conditions:	epididymo-orchitis, prostatitis, urinary tract infection, torsion of the testis
Urological conditions:	tumour or stone disease, urethral extravasation
Gynaecological conditions:	pelvic inflammatory disease, uterine or ovarian tumour
Musculoskeletal disorders:	adductor tendonitis, adductor avulsion, gracilis syndrome, pubic instability, osteitis pubis, rectus abdominis tendonopathy, ilio- psoas injury
Spinal abnormalities	
Hip abnormalities	
Enthesopathy[39]	

In many patients presenting with chronic groin pain, a urological disorder is the initial working diagnosis. Chronic prostatitis or seminal vesiculitis is commonly suspected and in many patients may have been treated with multiple courses of antibiotics.

Thorough examination and investigation may reveal no underlying cause; an occult hernia should then be suspected. However, a further increasingly recognized diagnosis should be entertained: 'tennis elbow' of the groin or enthesopathy (inflammation of the insertion – enthesis – of a ligament or tendon).[39] There is frequently a history of sudden onset of pain and then of aggravation by physical exertion. The exact site of tenderness must be ascertained to differentiate the ligamentous or tendinous insertion. Careful palpation using one finger of muscles, ligaments, tendons or scars in the inguinal region will point to the origin of the enthesopathy, which may be in the adductus longus insertion, inguinal ligament insertion, rectus abdominis insertion, or along the inguinal ligament at sites where the transversalis and internal oblique muscles insert. Once the condition has been recognized, symptoms may respond to local injection of lignocaine and triamcinolone.

Clinical examination of the scrotum must be included in any assessment of inguinoscrotal pain. A small hernia protruding at the deep ring may stimulate the genital branch of the genitofemoral nerve to give scrotal pain in the male or labial pain in the female as its feature. If the patient appears acutely complaining of pain in the groin associated with the lump, the differential examination should include hernias, torsion of the testicles, spasm of the cremaster and trauma to the testicle or cord.

Other causes of inguinoscrotal pain include abdominal aneurysms, degenerate disease of the lower thoracic and lumbar spines and degenerative disease of the hip joint. The genital pelvic viscera, prostate, seminal vesicles and proximal vasa have an autonomic supply from T12 to L2 and from S2, S3 and S4; therefore referred pain from these organs may radiate via the genital branch of the genitofemoral nerve Ll and posterior scrotal nerves S2 and S3 to the groin and external genitalia.

Clinical examination

The patient should be undressed and the entire abdomen and lower limbs examined.

In the male the first step is to observe where the testicles are. Knowledge of testicle position prevents all the confusions of undescended testicles, etc.

The groin should be examined with the patient standing erect and again with the patient lying flat. Hernias are sometimes only apparent when the patient stands up or only when the patient strains or coughs.

When the patient is examined a rapid decision should be made as to whether the lump is a hernia or not a hernia – this is the crucial initial decision to make. A hernia has a cough impulse, changes in size when the patient strains or lies down and may be reducible. The other lumps in the groin do not change their disposition when the patient stands or lies down.

In the male the differential diagnosis between a direct and an indirect inguinal hernia cannot be made with any certainty, except for the elderly male who has a broad neck direct inguinal hernia which is spontaneously reducible when he lies flat. Similarly, in the female it is very difficult indeed to make the differential diagnosis between an inguinal hernia and a femoral hernia which has emerged from the saphenous opening and its fundus doubled back up over the inguinal ligament. Fortunately both of these differential diagnoses between a direct and an indirect inguinal hernia in the male and between the femoral and the inguinal hernia in the female, although interesting, are not of crucial importance. The operative approach to the groin hernias allows whichever groin hernia is encountered at surgery to be corrected. It is, therefore, better to be able to make the diagnosis of a hernia and be humble enough to acknowledge that having approached the groin the operative strategy may need modifying depending upon the anatomic type of hernia found.

It is difficult to distinguish between an inguinal and a femoral hernia, particularly in an obese person. Femoral hernias may present as 'recurrences' after repair of an inguinal hernia. In these circumstances they are often indistinguishable from inguinal hernias. The diagnostic difficulty is increased by the fact that as a femoral hernia emerges through the cribriform fascia at the fossa ovalis, the fundus comes forwards and then turns upwards to lie over and anterior to the inguinal ligament. Palpation of the external ring and the cord should enable the diagnosis to be made in the male. The difficulty is in the female. If the hernia can be reduced, careful palpation of the hernial aperture should enable the examiner to orientate it relative to the inguinal ligament. If the hernia emerges above the inguinal ligament when the patient coughs, the hernia is inguinal; if below the ligament, it is femoral.

Reducing the hernia and then using one finger to hold it reduced while the patient coughs is a useful test which will enable the inguinal canal or the femoral ring to be identified, almost with certainty. Invagination of the scrotal skin into the inguinal canal, a time hallowed test, is uncomfortable for the patient and does not provide useful information, in my experience.

Hernias which extend down into the scrotum are generally indirect inguinal. Scrotal hernias must be separated from other scrotal lumps – hydrocele, varicocele, testicular tumours, epididymal cysts, etc. If the hernia is reducible, the diagnosis is obvious. A cough impulse is a characteristic of hernias, but not of other scrotal masses.

The advent of sophisticated radiological investigation (see below) has enabled small and occult hernias to be more easily diagnosed. The chief utility of ultrasound is to enable scrotal and other swellings to be clearly differentiated.

The sports hernia

In most athletes with groin pain a musculoskeletal disorder is easily diagnosed and adequately treated. The pectineus muscle, adductors (magnus, brevis and longus) and gracilis muscle should be examined by palpation, passive abduction, adduction against resistance and hip flexion. The rectus abdominis muscle must be examined by active contraction with both legs elevated and by palpation of its origins. Next the hip should be tested using Patrick's test (pressure applied to the knee with the opposite hip stabilized and with the tested hip in a flexed, abducted and externally rotated position with the heel on the opposite knee), observing the full range of movements and by flexion, adduction, internal rotation and compression. A full range of movement should be present in the lower back, including flexion, extension, lateral reflection and rotation, and the thoracolumbar spine should be examined for tenderness. Stretch tests must be performed for the femoral and sciatic nerves, and a full neurological examination carried out of the lower limb and affected groin, with particular reference to ilioinguinal or genitofemoral nerve neuralgias. Finally, the pelvis should be examined by palpation of the pubic arches, crests and tubercles, and the pubic symphysis by compression and direct pressure.[606]

Following this thorough clinical examination, which if necessary is supplemented by plain radiographs of hips and pelvis, including views of the pubic symphysis, there will remain a group of patients who have unexplained groin pain.[374] Because the diagnosis and therapy of chronic groin pain in athletes is complex, referral to a specialist sports injury clinic is advisable. Such groin injuries account for only 5% of those attending, but are responsible for a much larger proportion of time lost from competition and work. Herniography has been instrumental in identifying the cause of the sports hernia as the syndrome of 'broad and deep fossae'.[380, 871, 944]

The history is variable. Some athletes such as runners will tend to describe an insidious onset resulting in a 'groin strain' with a persistent, dull, deep ache in the groin. Athletes involved in contact sports may describe sudden tearing sensations giving rise to continuous aching pain in the inguinoscrotal region. The pain is aggravated by physical exertion and may begin to radiate to the thigh, scrotum or lower abdomen: it is often these symptoms which have led to extensive investigation. The fact that many athletes experience exacerbation of pain with physical exertion or coughing and straining points to an abnormality of the shutter or sphincter mechanism of the inguinal region. It is useful to ask patients to shade in pain areas on an anatomical diagram, to identify the areas in which pain occurs and is developing (Figure 11.3).

The signs found on physical examination are again variable and relate more to the last period of physical exertion than to any other factor. After a period of prolonged rest, physical signs may be minimal. However, following a period of training or sporting activity, the whole inguinoscrotal region may be tender. The key to diagnosis is palpation of the external ring by invagination of the scrotal skin and palpation from inside the inguinal canal. An area of exquisite tenderness is felt, which is aggravated by coughing, and a slight impulse can be detected.

The history, exclusion of all other pathologies, and characteristic physical signs as outlined above will enable the diagnosis of the sports hernia. However, many clinics will insist on objective evidence, either from a herniogram or supplemented with other radiological investigations (see below). Herniography directed hernia repair has poor specificity and the presence of an occult hernia may not necessarily identify the cause of the pain.[916]

The findings at operation are said to be characteristic: these include a dilated external ring, disruption of the conjoint tendon from the inguinal ligament, absence or attenuation of the transversalis fascia, and a plug of preperitoneal fat at the internal ring; however, it must be remembered that the detailed anatomy of the inguinal canal is very variable (see pages 20–30) and an anatomical basis for the 'sportsman's groin syndrome', 'Gilmore's groin', is elusive. Repair of the posterior inguinal wall achieves good results with 87–93% of athletes returning to full sporting activity within 3–6 months. Subsequent follow-up with pain scores in these athletes indicated a marked improvement in the level of pain.[380, 606]

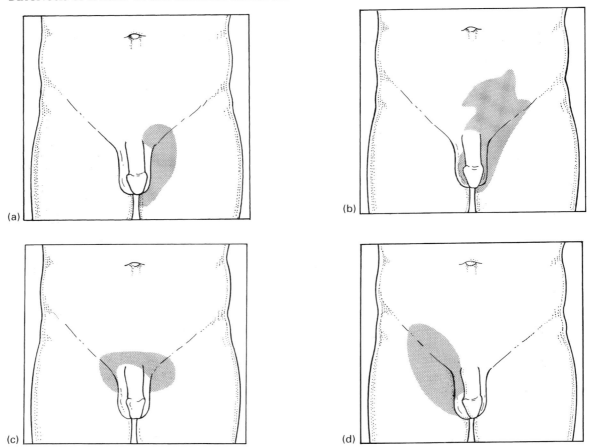

Figure 11.3 Pain diagrams, each accompanied by the instruction 'Please shade the areas where you felt pain prior to your operation'

Hidden hernias

Hidden hernias are more likely to occur in women than men. This is due to the greater prevalence of femoral hernia in women, linked to the failure to examine or the inaccessibility of the femoral opening, particularly in obese patients. In addition, certain pelvic hernias, such as obturator hernia, occur with a much higher frequency in women and internal hernias such as hernias of the broad ligament of the uterus occur exclusively in women (see Chapter 20).

In a woman, the non-palpable, hidden or occult inguinal and femoral hernia is an infrequent cause of pain.[55, 881] Symptoms are likely to be similar to those of the sports hernia: dull inguinal pain is the predominant symptom. There may be tenderness on palpation over the deep inguinal ring, tested either by inversion of the scrotal skin or the skin of the labia majora, and the Valsalva manoeuvre exacerbates this tenderness. The deep inguinal ring is often abnormally wide and there is hyperalgesia in the distribution of the ilioinguinal or genitofemoral nerves.

Herniography may establish the diagnosis, although a dilated internal ring plugged by preperitoneal fat will obscure radiographic findings. More invasive radiological techniques include a combination of herniography and femoral vein phlebography to establish the diagnosis of occult femoral hernia.

Herniography can clinch the diagnosis of obturator hernias; the hernia is seen to protrude downwards anteriorly through the obturator foramen beneath the pubic bone (Figure 11.4). The typical shape is similar to that of a femoral hernia, but the sac is situated more medially. A CT scan with contrast may help in differentiation.[911]

Hernias of the broad ligament of the uterus can occur through the ligament itself into the mesometrium, through the mesosalpinx, or under the round ligament or suspensory ligament of the ovary. Subacute or acute intestinal obstruction is the mode of presentation of this internal hernia, which can occur in women of all ages.[22] Obstetric trauma may be a causative factor and the diagnosis should be considered in any woman presenting with intestinal obstruction and no obvious cause.

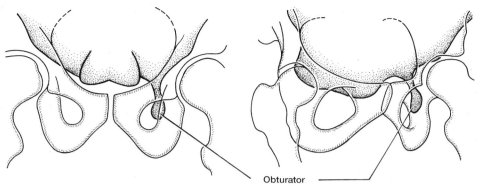

Obturator

Figure 11.4 Obturator herniogram

RADIOLOGICAL DIAGNOSIS OF OCCULT HERNIA

Herniography

Herniography is an excellent and sensitive diagnostic tool, capable of demonstrating hernias in the groin, especially when physical examination is negative.[55, 270, 273, 376, 944] Indirect herniography by injecting contrast medium into a hollow viscus and observing the position of the contrast-filled viscus has fallen into disuse because of the considerable morbidity. Nevertheless, Allen and Condon found that lateral protrusion of the urinary bladder ('bladder's ears') into the deep inguinal ring developed in 9% of 406 patients undergoing intravenous urography and cystograms.[13]

Direct herniography was first performed in experimental animals by Sternhill and Schwarz[891] and subsequently performed clinically by Ducharmé in children.[270] Herniography with fluoroscopy and peritoneography, performed by puncture of the abdominal wall and injection of non-ionic contrast medium, is now the preferred method of investigation.[376] Indications are principally symptoms indicative of a hernia but no palpable lump, obscure groin pain (other diagnoses having been excluded by appropriate investigation), and evaluation of patients who remain symptomatic following primary hernia repair.

Technique is important and will be successful only in experienced hands.[376] The patient must be placed on a tilt table with fluoroscopy, enabling tangential views of the pelvic floor and groin. The bladder should be empty at the time of the examination. Through a small skin incision a catheter is inserted through the left lower quadrant of the abdomen into the peritoneal cavity. After screening to confirm the presence of the catheter within the peritoneal cavity, it is advanced towards the pelvic floor. Contrast medium is then introduced, which should be non-ionic in nature, and adequate filling will be obtained with 60–80 ml. The X-ray table is then rotated to the upright position and contrast medium allowed to pool in the various fossae and hernial orifices. The table is then lowered to 25° foot down and the patient is moved

to the prone position. The symptomatic side is then turned downward in an oblique position and the patient asked to strain. Hernial sacs should then be screened in several positions to allow full evaluation, including several projections for optimal evaluation of all the fossae. A thorough examination of the entire surgical anatomy of the pelvic and inguinal floor should be performed for exact verification of all potential hernial orifices. A normal herniogram is shown in Figure 11.5.

Classical herniograms for direct inguinal, indirect inguinal and femoral hernia are shown in Figure 11.6. These hernias can be diagnosed from their shape, relation to the pelvic peritoneal folds and the resulting pelvic fossae. Five pelvic peritoneal folds in the pelvis and groin (lateral umbilical, medial umbilical and median umbilical) divide the pelvic cavity into three fossae: supravesical, medial umbilical and lateral umbilical (see Figure 11.7). An indirect hernia protrudes lateral to the lateral fold through the lateral (inguinal) fossa. A direct inguinal hernia protrudes lateral to the median fold through the medial (inguinal) fossa. A femoral hernia protrudes through the median umbilical fossa in a lateral direction through the femoral canal.

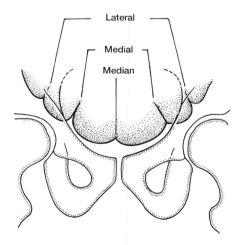

Lateral

Medial

Median

Figure 11.5 Normal herniogram, showing lateral, medial and median umbilical folds

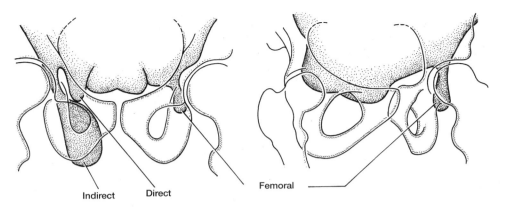

Indirect   Direct   Femoral

Figure 11.6 Herniograms; direct, indirect and femoral

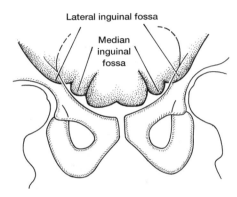

Lateral inguinal fossa
Median inguinal fossa

Figure 11.7 Herniogram showing the lateral and medial inguinal fossae

Herniography is also valuable in the postoperative evaluation of patients with persistent symptoms in whom clinically detectable hernias are not evident on physical examination.[392] Hamlin and Kahn performed herniograms in 46 subjects with 54 symptomatic sites:[392] 10 recurrent hernias were found, although only two were symptomatic. In addition, they found 14 hernias in the contralateral, asymptomatic, groin and the herniogram was negative in one patient with a clinical hernia. A herniogram can therefore corroborate clinical findings and eliminate the need for re-exploration. Herniography can also identify patients in whom recurrent hernias have developed that are not detected on physical examination.

Inguinal and femoral hernias are best demonstrated by herniography. Anterior wall defects, ventral, Spigelian and obturator hernias should be evaluated both by herniography and cross-sectional imaging techniques.[403] Herniography should be combined with other imaging techniques to avoid pitfalls caused by contrast not entering and outlining intermittent hernia defects; for this reason post-exercise and oblique and tangential radiographs are essential to enlarge the diagnostic field.

Complications of herniography occur in approximately 6% of patients and are usually minor because it is a minimally invasive procedure. The minor risks include haematoma of the anterior abdominal wall, adverse reaction to the contrast medium, bruising of the pelvic viscera and extraperitoneal extravasation of contrast medium. More serious, infrequent complications include bowel perforation, mesenteric haematoma formation, and pelvic peritonitis. These complications are unusual in experienced hands.

Essentially herniography is a sensitive and reliable investigation which can be used to diagnose hidden hernias, aid in the diagnosis of the cause of obscure groin pain, and diagnose occult hernias. The investigation can be performed under local anaesthesia on an outpatient basis with minimal complications.[589]

Ultrasonography

Ultrasound examination of the abdominal wall and inguinal region has been used to a lesser degree in the diagnosis of occult hernia and obscure groin pain.[931] The preferred method is real-time ultrasound for short-focus adjustment, using a linear scanner to clarify surface anatomy. The patient is placed supine with an empty bladder and further examination is performed in the upright position, with the patient passive, or in the Valsalva manoeuvre, and comparisons made between sides in two vertical planes.

This technique has a sensitivity of 100% and specificity of 97.9% in determining the nature of a lump in the groin. False interpretation is more likely to occur in cases of femoral hernia. The typical findings and interpretation of an inguinal and a femoral hernia are shown in Figures 11.8 and 11.9.

The antenatal diagnosis of abdominal wall defects is now a successful part of obstetric/paediatric surgical practice. Patients born with herniation can then be readily transferred to a paediatric surgical service.[252]

Ultrasound assessment of the contralateral groin accurately diagnosed a patent processus vaginalis in only 15 of 23 infants, with four false positive and four false negative cases.[536] Lawrenz and colleagues concluded

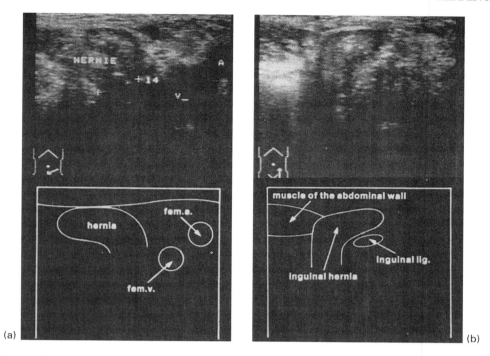

Figure 11.8   Ultrasound examination localizing an inguinal hernia sac in transverse (**a**) and longitudinal (**b**) section. (Reproduced with permission from Truong *et al.*, 1995[931])

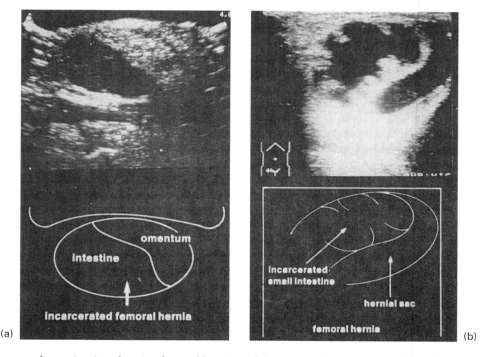

Figure 11.9   Ultrasound examination showing femoral hernia with incarcerated omentum and small bowel. (Reproduced with permission from Truong *et al.*, 1995[931])

that ultrasound can not be used alone to plan the management of the contralateral groin in infants.

Computed tomography

Cross-sectional imaging by CT scanning has the potential for evaluating disorders of the abdominal wall, including hernias. The diagnosis of hernia is based on the identification of the fascial defect rather than visualization of hernial contents. Preliminary investigations by Hahn-Pedersen and colleagues have shown that examination of the pampiniform plexus during the Valsalva manoeuvre can differentiate direct from indirect hernias.[381] The practical usefulness of this finding is unknown. The introduction of contrast medium by intubation of the small intestine followed by CT scanning is a very helpful investigation in cases of intestinal obstruction and suspected but occult external hernia.[55, 932] Contrast medium appears in the entrapped loop between the external obturator and pectineal muscles in the case of obturator hernia (Figure 11.10). Inguinal and femoral hernias may not be detected unless they are obstructed because the patient is usually scanned in the supine position.[403] Femoral hernias are distinguished from inguinal hernias because of their location inferior and lateral to the pubic tubercle.[974]

Magnetic resonance imaging

Magnetic resonance imaging (MRI) and retrograde air insufflation has been used to evaluate bowel obstruction. Using this technique Chung-Kuao Chou clearly demonstrated an internal supra-vesical hernia.[178]

Conclusions

Every effort should be made to distinguish inguinal from femoral hernias before surgery. Careful identification of the pubic tubercle, the anterior superior iliac spine and,

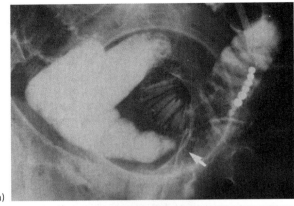

(a)

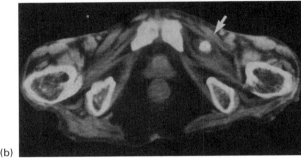

(b)

Figure 11.10 CT scan of strangulated obturator hernia after intubation and small bowel infusion of contrast. Obstructed small bowel (a) and contrast in mass between external obturator and pectineal muscles. (Reproduced with permission from Tsutsui *et al.* 1994[932])

between them, the inguinal ligament is the prerequisite. Inguinal hernias emerge from the fascia transversalis above this line, femoral hernias below it. Femoral hernias never pass from the abdomen into the scrotum or labia majora as indirect inguinal hernias do. Direct inguinal hernias are almost unknown in women.

The diagnosis of inguinoscrotal pain can be a challenging clinical problem. A diagnosis can often be achieved with appropriate radiological investigation.

12 INGUINAL HERNIA IN ADULTS (I) – THE OPERATION

Operation or truss?

Operation must always be advised for incarcerated or strangulated inguinal hernia. A truss is only an option if the hernia can be readily and completely reduced. A large hydrocele encroaching on the external ring which interferes with fitting a truss is also a contraindication to management by a truss.

A truss is sometimes advised (ill advised) in the older patient with a reducible hernia when without real justification the risks of hernia repair are considered to be excessive. Open repair of a groin hernia does not involve major exploration of a body cavity, manipulation of viscera or haemodynamic hazard. There are no metabolic complications either. Sepsis is rare after groin hernia repair. For these reasons surgery should be advised; a truss is a poor alternative to surgery. Wearing a truss does not guarantee that an indirect inguinal or femoral hernia will remain reduced. A truss increases the patient's chance of developing complications; it may obstruct the venous and lymphatic drainage of intrahernial viscera and precipitate strangulation. In addition, particularly with the large direct hernia the pressure of the truss leads to atrophy of the muscular and fascial margins of the defect enlarging the hernial orifice promoting enlargement of the hernia and making surgical repair even more difficult.

Sir Geoffrey Keynes in 1927, commented on the complications of a truss:[491]

> The tissues underlying such a truss will be found to be matted, thinned out and the muscles almost entirely converted to fibrous tissue. It is impossible to look upon the truss as anything but an antiquated piece of apparatus, the very existence of which is a sorry testimonial to progressive surgery, the use of which generally results in gradual injury to the wearer, and the results of which tax the surgeon's best efforts to undo when the time comes that the truss is no longer able to hold up the protrusion.

A more recent evaluation by Law and Trapnell assessed 250 consecutive patients referred for surgical repair of a hernia, 52 of whom were fitted with a truss before attending the out-patient clinic. The mean age of these patients was 70 years, the truss had been worn for a median of 35 months (range 2–240); 11 (21%) had been prescribed a truss before referral to a surgeon, and 23 (44%) had received no instructions, with the result that 35 (77%) fitted the truss while standing. Partial or complete control of the hernia was achieved in only 16 patients (31%) and 33 (64%) had found the truss to be uncomfortable.[533] The authors expressed concern that 40 000 trusses were being sold annually in the UK, mostly through retail outlets, yet advice to patients was incomplete which could result in an increase of complications and morbidity such as atrophy of the spermatic cord and testicle, tissue atrophy and neuritis and a considerably lower quality of life than might be expected from adequate inguinal hernia repair.

Cheek, Williams and Farndon further reviewed the use of trusses in England in 1995, they confirmed that 40 000 trusses were being issued nationally and that the evaluation of the effectiveness of trusses was inadequate. The rate of truss supply in England, 700 per million, is considerably higher than elsewhere in the developed world. Nowadays with modern anaesthesia no patient should be denied surgery, nonetheless there is an urgent need for some research on the value of trusses.[173]

Neuhauser, writing in 1977, has compared the outcome of elective herniorrhaphy in the elderly to management with a truss. His study is important if only because it highlights the difficulties of surgical decision-making and points to the value of more sophisticated option appraisal when advising patients. Neuhauser assesses what effect the choice of truss versus elective herniorrhaphy has on the life expectancy of a 65-year-old person.[695]

Reviewing data for (a) the mortality of elective surgery, (b) the mortality of emergency surgery, (c) the probability of recurrence, (d) the yearly probability of strangulation and (e) the life expectancy of the patient, he calculates and compares the effects of using a truss, and thus running the risk of obstruction followed by an emergency operation and its higher mortality, with having an immediate elective operation with its low mortality and the risk that the hernia will recur and need additional elective operations. The most recent data used for these calculations of probabilities are from 1974.

Although these data have been superseded – the mortality rate for elective hernia repair in the elderly is now approaching zero and the mortality rate for emergency hernia operation in the 60–69 decade is probably less than the 1% figure used in this study – the conclusion reached is very important. On the data available, elective inguinal herniorrhaphy does not prolong life in the elderly. It may or may not improve the quality of life.

What has changed in the past 30 years is the reduction in the mortality of emergency operation for strangulation. Although much improvement has been gained in the mortality for emergency operation, the need for elective operation to save lives in the elderly has not been eliminated.

Elective inguinal hernia repair in the elderly must be undertaken as a well-planned procedure with full medical support for any co-morbid conditions. An appropriate choice of analgesia between general, local or regional anaesthesia must also be taken. Finally the surgery must be undertaken with precision and care to avoid surgical complications, which are poorly tolerated in the elderly.[340] Gilbert reported on 175 patients over the age of 66 years, in whom elective inguinal or femoral hernia repair was performed. Of these patients 50% were ASA grade III (severe systemic disease that limits activity but is not incapacitating), and 22% had undergone coronary artery bypass grafting, indicating that vascular disease is the most common co-morbidity in these elderly patients. Most of the operations were carried out under local or epidural anaesthesia; only 17 operations being undertaken under general anaesthesia. The preoperative control of symptoms of systemic or medical disease was undertaken in conjunction with a qualified physician. However, exercise tolerance was judged by the simple ability to climb one flight of stairs if local anaesthesia was being considered, although more extensive investigations were required if general anaesthesia was to be administered. Aspirin and anticoagulants were withdrawn temporarily and heparin cover instituted. In this series there were no deaths and minimal complications. Gilbert emphasizes that there are misconceptions concerning elective inguinal hernia repair in the elderly, based on the premise that the patient has numerous medical complaints and the hernia is a minor, non-life-threatening secondary phenomenon, or that the patient is on multiple medications which would complicate anaesthesia, and lastly that the type of anaesthesia required is general anaes-thesia. These myths should be dispelled and all patients assessed and considered for hernia surgery if the hernia itself merits repair.

A not quite so optimistic overall picture was painted by Gardner and Palasti.[327] In this series of 304 patients over the age of 80 years, the overall mortality for elective hernia repair was 8.9%, with deaths resulting from complications of the primary disease rather than associated medical disorders. The mortality rate, however, was 19.9% when operation was carried out as an emergency, and the authors suggest that health resources should be directed at treating hernias before complications develop. In the USA in 1967 death from the complications of hernia in patients over the age of 60 years was one of the ten leading causes of death.[426] This represents a 20–fold increased risk of dying from attempted inguinal hernia repair when complications develop compared with patients who undergo surgery on an elective basis.

So the argument about whether to recommend an elective operation for an inguinal hernia, or to recommend a truss, must take into account the patient's assessment of his own quality of life.

The operation will not prolong his life, but it may make it more comfortable. However, will a truss prove 'dirty, tight, uncomfortable, hot and smelly'? Will it represent a horrible affront to a man's self-image? Will wearing a truss have strong negative sexual overtones? Confronted by a male with a hernia, should we allow the patient to choose between truss or operation?

The incidence of strangulation of inguinal hernia is not known with any accuracy; the usual cited rate is 4% over the entire time the patient has the hernia;[512] rates from 1.7% to 6% are quoted, but are unhelpful because they are not based on a time period.[602, 1005]

In a retrospective study Gallegos and colleagues studied the cumulative probability of strangulation in relation to the length of history calculated independently for inguinal and femoral hernias at the Middlesex Hospital over a three-year period.[322] Of 476 hernias (439 inguinal, 37 femoral) there were 34 strangulations (22 inguinal, 12 femoral). After three months the cumulative probability of strangulation for inguinal hernias was 2.8%, rising to 4.5% after two years. For femoral hernias the cumulative probability for strangulation was 22% at three months and 45% at 21 months. They concluded that the rate at which the cumulative probability of strangulation increased was in both cases greatest in the first three months. For femoral hernia there is no question that the risk of strangulation is greater; 40% being admitted as an emergency with strangulation or incarceration.[989] The age-standardized rate of incidence for strangulation is 13/10 000 population.

The delay in treatment of patients with groin hernia is multifactorial.[633] In patients presenting with strangulation more than half had noted the presence of a hernia for a month, a quarter had not reported it to their family doctor, and a further quarter were known by family practitioners or non-surgical medical personnel to have a hernia but had not been referred to a specialist. Although 10% had been previously assessed with a view to elective repair, half of these were considered unfit to undergo operation. There remains, however, a group of patients representing approximately 40% of the whole, who present primarily with strangulation within days of developing a hernia.

The only data available on untreated hernia relate to Paris in the 1890s and to contemporary Latin America. In both these series very low incidence rates are recorded for strangulation.[89, 696] The yearly probability of incarceration and strangulation for all ages was 0.0037 in the 1890s

French series and 0.002 90 for all ages and 0.100 291 for those over 65 in Colombia. Although these low probabilities and the relatively high frequency with which inguinal hernia occurs in the adult population (5–8% of the elderly male population) would seem to make hernia repair an unattractive option to the elderly male with a symptomless rupture, today lives could be saved.

In a district general hospital, doing more elective operations for primary inguinal hernias did not alter either the incidence of emergency operation for strangulated inguinal hernia[765] or the mortality of strangulated hernia.[924]

Allen, Zager and Goldman attempted to investigate the reasons why elective surgery is not being undertaken to prevent emergency admissions.[12] A questionnaire was sent to 406 senior physicians, general practitioners, geriatricians and general surgeons. Although 71–90% would not advocate elective surgery for a small, painless, reducible inguinal hernia in a 79-year old male; only 49% (physicians) to 78% (surgeons) would advocate elective surgery for an asymptomatic femoral hernia in a frail 80-year-old woman. Elective surgery in the latter case can be carried out with virtually no morbidity or mortality, yet a strangulated femoral hernia in an elderly patient carries a mortality in excess of 25%. This study concluded that general practitioners, physicians and surgeons are wrongly exercising a selective policy at the expense of the elderly.

Statistical data from the National Center For Health Statistics in the USA from the decades ending 1968, 1978 and 1988 investigated mortality from hernia.[651] In 1971 Medicare discharges for inguinal hernia without intestinal obstruction showed that 94% of patients had surgery with a probability of death of 0.005 (5/100 000). However, for inguinal hernia with obstruction, 88% underwent surgery with a mortality rate of 0.05, which represents a ten-fold increased risk of death. Encouragingly, the death rate from hernia with obstruction fell from 5/100 000 (1968) to 3/100 000 (1988), indicating that elective surgery had contributed to a reduction in the mortality rate of complicated hernia.

The mortality of strangulated inguinal hernia remains significant because of late diagnosis and referral, and increasing co-morbidity in elderly patients.[25, 128] The low probability of strangulation with the low mortality of early emergency operation has offset the need to advise elective operation for all patients with inguinal hernia to save lives in the elderly. Elective operation may or may not improve the patient's quality of life. The patient must make an informed decision, aided by the surgeon.

A truss is very rarely a useful short-term option; for instance, the patient with an inguinal hernia of recent onset when there is severe cardiovascular or respiratory disease which is not yet controlled by physic, or a recent onset groin hernia in a woman with a third trimester pregnancy.

Truss design

The adder-headed spring truss is the standard for an inguinal hernia (Figure 12.1). If the hernia is large, or if it extends to the scrotum, a rat-tailed truss with a perineal band to prevent the truss slipping is used. Sir Astley Cooper comments that if the customer has a 'very protuberant abdomen' the perineal band may not be necessary. The head of the truss should rest over the inguinal canal, not over the external ring; it should exert its pressure inwards and upwards. When the truss is worn it should control the hernia easily when the patient stands with the legs apart and coughs violently.

Different gauges of spring are needed, depending on the physique and occupation of the patient. Lightweight trusses to wear in bed – 'evening' or 'French' trusses – used to be popular. The head of the truss will need designing for individual needs, too (Figure 12.2). The hernia must be completely and easily reducible by the patient if a truss is to be worn. A truss will predispose to strangulation if the hernia is not fully reduced. Another problem with a truss is the difficulty of controlling a

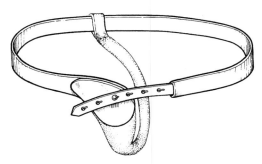

Figure 12.1   The spring truss is the standard truss for an inguinal hernia. A truss with a perineal band is used in inguinoscrotal hernia or in persons whose physique predisposes to slipping of the head of the truss

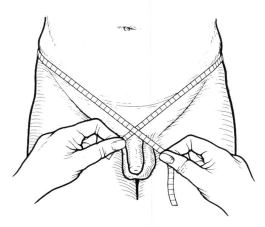

Figure 12.2   Measuring for a truss. The head of the truss should be centred over the midpoint of the inguinal canal; the circumferential spring should be worn about 3 cm below the iliac crest

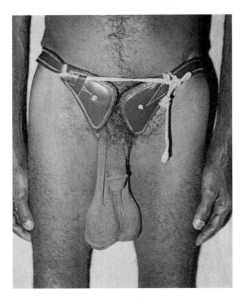

Figure 12.3 Habitual wearing of a strong truss results in matting of the abdominal wall tissues and atrophy of the cremaster muscle and other cord structures, with pendulous testicles as a consequence. (Courtesy of Professor Rajan, Manipal, India)

large direct hernial opening close to the pubis, the proximity of the bone making occlusion of the opening by the truss difficult.

The adult patient should only remove his truss after he is in bed, and he should put the truss on again before he stands. It is most important that habitual truss-wearers keep their hernias permanently reduced and controlled by the truss. There is said to be an increased risk of strangulation if the hernia normally controlled by a truss prolapses. The skin beneath the truss head needs great care. Local tissue atrophy, cremaster atrophy leading to pendulous testicles (Figure 12.3), ilio-inguinal neuritis causing pain, varicocele and testicular atrophy are complications of a truss.

Older textbooks credit 'cures' to prolonged treatment – the London Truss Society recorded that of 96 886 patients treated with a truss 4387 (4.53%) were 'cured'.[491]

The operation

The surgical literature abounds with descriptions of operations for inguinal hernia (Table 12.1). However, few of these essays describe new or original principles. The foundations underlying the modern approach to inguinal hernia were laid by Marcy, who observed the anatomy and physiology of the deep inguinal ring and correctly inferred the importance of the obliquity of the canal.[609] Bassini, who had heard Marcy's lecture in 1881, grasped the significance of the anatomic arrangement and, in particular, the role of the fascia transversalis and transversus abdominis tendon.[73]

Table 12.1 Techniques for inguinal hernia repair

Single-layered closure
  Halsted I (1890)
  Madden (1971)
Multi-layered closure
  (Bassini–Halsted principle)
  Bassini (1887)
  Ferguson (1899)
  Andrews (1895)
  Halsted II (1903)
  Fallis (1938)
  Zimmerman (1938, 1952)
  Rienhoff (1940)
  Tanner (1942)
  Glassow (1943) Shouldice repair
  Griffith (1958)
  Lichtenstein (1964, 1966)
  Palumbo (1967)
Cooper's ligament repair
  (Lotheissen–McVay principle)
  Narath (cited by Lotheissen, 1898)
  Lotheissen (1898)
  McVay (1942, 1958)
Preperitoneal approach
  Cheatle (1920)
  Henry (1936)
  Musgrove and McGready (1940)
  Mikkelson and Berne (1954)
  Stoppa (1972)
  Condon (1960)
  Nyhus (1959)
  Read (1976)
  Rignault (1986)
  Paillier (1992)
Primary repair with prosthetic materials
  Koontz (1956)
  Usher (1960)
  Lichtenstein (1972)
Plug repair
  Lichtenstein (1970)
  Bendavid (1989)
  Gilbert (1992)
  Robbins and Rutkow (1993)
Laparoscopic repair
  Ger (1990)
  Corbitt (1991)
  Ferzli (1992)

Many surgeons have contributed to the recognition of the essential role of the transversalis fascia in the pathology of groin hernia, resulting from degeneration and a change in structure and function.[778, 809]

Bassini stressed the importance of dividing the fascia transversalis and reconstructing the posterior wall of the canal by suturing the fascia transversalis and transversus muscle to the upturned, deep edge of the inguinal ligament. In his repair, Bassini included the lower arching fibres of the internal oblique muscle where they form the conjoint tendon with the transversus muscle. He called the upper leaf of his repair the 'triple layer' that is, fascia transversalis, transversus abdominis and internal oblique.

Bassini's original observations about the fascia transversalis and 'triple layer' have somehow been lost from the later literature. Many of the failures of 'Bassini's operation' occur in cases where the fleshy conjoint tendon only has been sutured to the inguinal ligament.

Division of the cremaster muscle and the posterior wall of the inguinal canal are essential components of the original Bassini hernia operation. Many surgeons, however, still perform the Bassini operation, dividing neither the cremaster muscle nor the posterior wall of the inguinal canal, possibly because Bassini did not actually describe these steps in his original papers.[778] Attilio Catterina, a colleague of Bassini's, later described and depicted the operation in a book illustrated with numerous watercolours. This atlas, although it was published in many languages in the early 1930s in Europe, was never published in North America, nor disseminated widely to European sur-geons, possibly accounting for the inaccurate dissemination of Bassini's technique.

Wantz has accurately traced the history of the relationship between Bassini and Catterina, which resulted in the enthusiastic promulgation of Bassini's technique through his atlas, illustrated by the surgeon artist O. Gaigher, and numerous lectures across the European continent.[965] Catterina, a protégé and colleague, and latterly Professor of Surgery at Genoa, recognized the importance of Bassini's quantum leap in surgical technique and the fact that Bassini had failed to get the technical points across to his surgical audience. Figure 12.4 indicates specifically that Bassini described dividing the cremaster muscle and the posterior wall of the inguinal canal.

The Bassini operation without these two essential steps gives poor results; hence in America this corrupt Bassini operation was abandoned in favour of the McVay–Cooper's ligament repair, Marcy's simple ring closure, or Nyhus preperitoneal approach. Bassini was also the first surgeon to insist on the use of non-absorbable suture material to repair his triple layer.

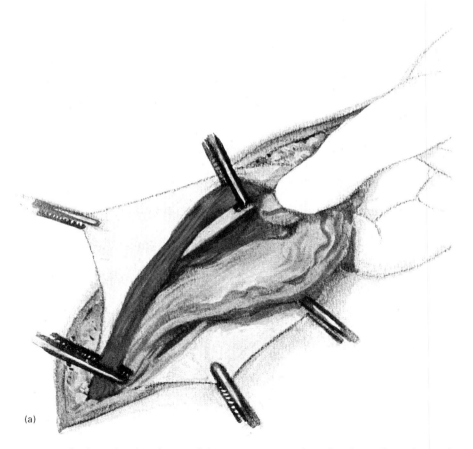

(a)

Figure 12.4   (a) Bassini completely isolated and excised the cremaster muscle and its fascia from the cord. He thus ensured complete exposure of the deep ring and all the posterior wall of the inguinal canal, an essential pre-requisite to evaluate all the potential hernial sites.

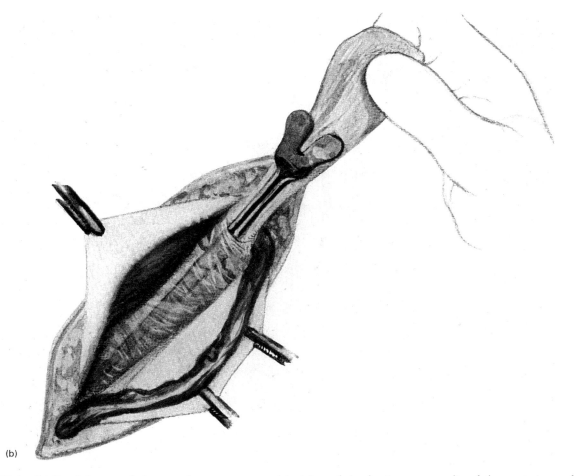

(b)

Figure 12.4 (b) Bassini stressed the complete exposure and incision of the fascia transversalis of the posterior wall of the inguinal canal. To complete the repair he sutured the divided fascia transversalis, together with the transversus muscle, and the internal oblique muscle, "the threefold layer" to the upturned inner free margin of the inguinal ligament. (From Catterina, The Bassini Procedure, published by H.K. Lewis, 1934)

The third person in seminal herniology is Halsted. Halsted's original input was to advise drawing the external oblique down behind the cord in order to strengthen the repair.[384] He later abandoned this. His major contribution is really two-fold: he insisted on scrupulous atraumatic technique and he emphasized, as Bassini had, the importance of adequate follow-up. In a more general sense, Bassini and Halsted are epoch persons because they introduced quality control and audit to surgeons. Florence Nightingale's exhortation that 'to understand God's will we must study statistics' was translated into surgical science by Bassini and Halsted![385]

Operative technique

The choice of technique will reflect the surgeon's training, the type of hernia and the age of the patient.

The Shouldice operation[357, 846]

The main principles are:

1. The normal anatomy should be reconstituted as far as possible. The deepest layer to be defective, in either indirect or direct hernias, is the fascia transversalis. This should, therefore, be repaired first.
2. All the potential hernia sites must be assessed and repaired if necessary. The 'missed' hernia is a cardinal mistake.
3. Only tendinous/aponeurotic/fascial structures should be sutured together. Suturing red fleshy muscle to tendon or fascia will not contribute to permanent fibrous union of these structures; nor will it result in anything resembling the normal anatomy.
4. The suture material must retain its strength for long enough to maintain tissue apposition and allow

sound union of tissues to occur. A non-absorbable or very slowly absorbable suture material must therefore be employed.[93, 846]

The tension in the Shouldice operation continuous suturing is low – initial suture tension is 100 g on spring balance, which falls to 50 g with the next suture – falling to 25 g. Even in large direct hernias it is only 25 g distributed.[846] The suture tension similarly is low in bilateral hernias repaired asynchronously 48 h apart.[962] This low tension maintains tissue apposition throughout healing and promotes sound repair.

SUTURE MATERIALS

The suture material of choice for the repair is metric 3 polypropylene. In the original Shouldice series from Toronto, monofilament stainless steel wire was used. Myers and Shearburn[687, 846] and Devlin et al.[244, 247, 248] originally used stainless steel wire, but have subsequently used polymers. Stainless steel wire is a most effective suture material, but it is difficult to use, whereas polypropylene is as effective and is much easier to handle.

INDICATIONS AND CONTRAINDICATIONS TO SURGERY

Elective surgical repair is the treatment of choice for inguinal hernias in adults. Operation is recommended for all hernia patients from pubescence to retirement. Surgery is advised because inguinal hernias (a) cause discomfort, (b) are at risk of obstruction and strangulation, (c) cause disfigurement, and (d) give rise to scrotal skin problems

With the elderly male aged over 75 years a less definite policy must be adopted; if the hernia is direct and spontaneously reducible the patient often has few if any symptoms attributable to it and surgery is not mandatory. Indeed, the risks of anaesthesia and surgery in this age group may be greater than the chances of developing complications necessitating urgent surgery.

ADMINISTRATIVE AND MANAGEMENT ARRANGEMENTS FOR INGUINAL HERNIA SURGERY

A careful administrative policy is necessary if the greatest benefits (for the patients and the community) are to be obtained from a policy of elective surgery for inguinal hernia. This is discussed on pages 51–60. Three regimens are mainly used:

1. Day-case – 8 h stay – applicable to all healthy males who have good home circumstances.
2. Overnight – less than 24 h stay – applicable to healthy males with less appropriate social status.

3. Five-day stay – most suitable for older patients, patients with contemporaneous medical conditions or patients who are socially disadvantaged.

About one-third of patients fall into each of these categories.

ANAESTHESIA

Local or general anaesthesia may be employed. (see pages 83–93)

POSITION OF PATIENT

The patient is placed on his back on the operating table. Access is improved if the head of the table is tilted downward by about 15 degrees; the head-down tilt is an important method of improving access (Figure 12.5).

THE INCISION

The incision is placed 1 cm above and parallel to the inguinal ligament. Laterally the incision begins over the deep inguinal ring, runs to the pubic tubercle, then curves caudally (vertically) and runs down over the pubic tubercle. It is important to keep the knife at right angles to the patient's skin on this curve in the incision in order to avoid undercutting the flap on its lower outer side. More importantly, the extension provides good access to the cord as it emerges from the superficial inguinal ring.

A skin crease incision gives a cosmetically more sound scar and is preferred by some surgeons, but to expose the pubic tubercle and Cooper's ligament the lower end of the incision needs underrunning, with the

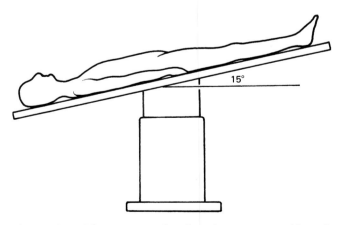

Figure 12.5 The patient is placed on the operating table with a head-down tilt of 15°. The head-down tilt improves access by emptying the lower abdomen of contents so that the upper wound edge does not continuously overhang the operating field

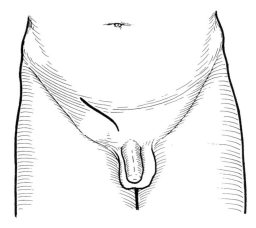

Figure 12.6   An incision is made 1 cm above and parallel to the inguinal ligament; the incision should expose the superficial inguinal ring. Incision and dissection medial to the pubic tubercle is unnecessary and harmful

attendant additional dissection, haematoma formation, etc. For these reasons the uncosmetic but surgically more acceptable incision described is preferred. It is important not to dissect in the subcutaneous fat superficial and medial to the pubic tubercle. Dissection in this area hazards the cord to pudendal anastomosis and may predispose to testicular ischaemia (see Chapter 24) (Figure 12.6).

EXPOSURE

After the skin has been divided the subcutaneous fat is opened in the length of the incision down to the external oblique aponeurosis. Careful haemostasis must be attained. The superficial pudendal and superficial epigastric vessels are tied and the smaller vessels dealt with by diathermy. A self-retaining retractor is now introduced and opened. This retractor serves two purposes: it opens the wound to facilitate access, and the slight traction it exerts on the skin ensures haemostasis in the small vessels in the immediate subdermal tissues.

After the subcutaneous fat has been opened down to the external oblique aponeurosis, the deep fascia of the thigh is opened to allow access to the femoral canal. The femoral sheath is exposed below the inguinal ligament and checked to make sure it is intact. It is important not to overlook a concomitant femoral hernia, which may present in the postoperative period (Figure 12.7).

DISSECTION OF THE CANAL

The external oblique aponeurosis is next opened in the long axis of the inguinal canal. This incision extends down to the superficial inguinal ring, the margin of which is divided. With the ring opened, the upper medial

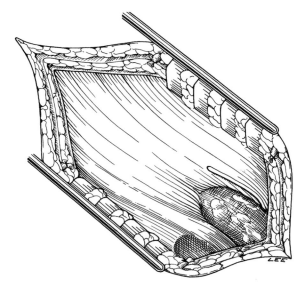

Figure 12.7   The external oblique aponeurosis exposed

flap of the external oblique is grasped in a haemostat and lifted up off the underlying cremaster fascia. The incision in the external oblique should commence at the most superior point of the superficial ring. The optimum site is to divide the external oblique about 2–3 cm cranial to the inguinal ligament; this 'high' incision allows maximal tissue for final closure and reconstitution of the inguinal canal (Figure 12.8).

The aponeurosis is gently freed from underlying structures by careful dissection up to its fusion into the lateral anterior rectus sheath.

Similarly, the lower lateral leaf of the external oblique is mobilized and freed of the underlying cord coverings down to the up-turned deep edge of the inguinal ligament, which is exposed (Figure 12.9).

Thus the whole of the cord is exposed.

DISSECTION OF THE CORD

The cremaster muscle/fascia is now divided in its long axis from its proximal origin down to the level of the pubic tubercle.

The cremaster is made into two flaps – an upper medial and a lower lateral flap. These flaps are raised off the pampiniform plexus of veins, the other contents of the cord and the vas deferens. The flaps of the cremaster are each traced proximally to their origin from the internal oblique and the adjacent fascia, and distally to the pubic tubercle. The cremaster is clamped, divided and ligated at its origin and similarly dealt with distally at the level of the pubic tubercle (Figure 12.10). The genital branch of the genitofemoral nerve should be carefully sought, routinely separated from the cremaster muscle and cleanly divided. This manoeuvre reduces the incidence of chronic genitofemoral nerve neuralgia.[968]

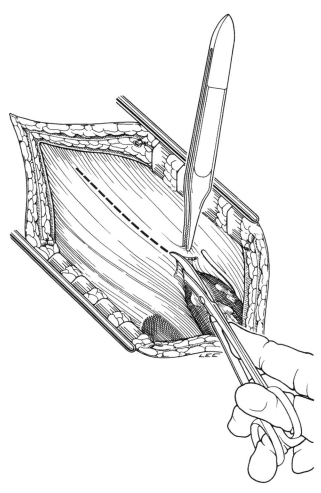

Figure 12.8   Opening the inguinal canal

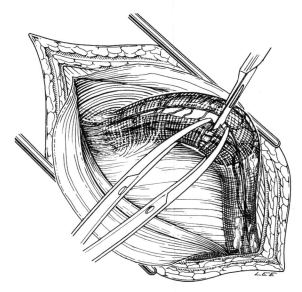

Figure 12.10   Division and removal of the cremaster

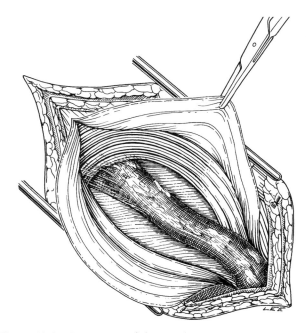

Figure 12.9   Dissection of the canal

After the cremaster has been removed, the contents of the cord and any hernia contained therein should be visualized. If there is a 'lipoma' – extraperitoneal fat around the fundus of an indirect sac[293] – in the cord, it is usually excised at this stage. Removal of a lipoma must not be used as an excuse to strip out all the fat and areolar tissue in the cord; if this is done the patient will suffer considerable postoperative testicular oedema and may develop a hydrocele. Caution and prudence are necessary when dealing with an extensive lipoma; too extensive a dissection can hazard the testicular blood supply, particularly the veins.

IDENTIFICATION OF THE FASCIA TRANSVERSALIS

After the contents of the cord have been adequately visualized, they are lifted up and the continuation of the fascia transversalis onto the cord at the deep ring is identified. The condensation of the fascia transversalis about the emerging cord is the deep ring and it must be dissected accurately. The correct identification and dissection of the deep ring is crucial to the subsequent repair operation – a technical detail emphasized by Bassini[73, 356] and more recently by Lytle.[585]

The internal spermatic fascia must be dissected off the deep ring all around the cord. Only when the cord is fully dissected like this can the deep ring be assessed.

The medial superior margin of the cord needs careful inspection now to identify any indirect sac. However small – even a tiny crescent of peritoneum entering the cord between the vas and medial margin of the deep ring – such a sac must be dissected clean and removed, otherwise it will enlarge postoperatively and appear later as a fully developed indirect hernia. A peritoneal crescent

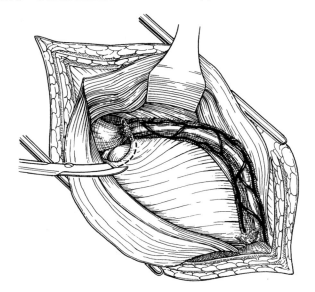

Figure 12.11 The deep ring is freed from the cord by sharp dissection

is the herald of an early recurrence if it is not treated adequately[769] (Figure 12.11).

It is important to check all the hernial sites at operation. A femoral or a direct inguinal hernia may easily be overlooked if exposure is inadequate. If a hernia is missed it will either appear postoperatively or later as 'a recurrence'. Whether the recurrent hernia is through a repaired portion of the inguinal region or not is immaterial to the patient; it is 'a recurrence' from the patient's perspective and most importantly necessitates another operation. Careful inspection of all hernial areas must be carried out at each operation.

Hernial sacs

INDIRECT

If an indirect hernial sac is present it should easily be found now. It lies on the anterosuperior aspect of the cord structures. To minimize the risk of postoperative ischaemic orchitis, scrotal sacs are transected at the midpoint of the canal, leaving the distal part undisturbed (see Chapter 24). The anterior wall of the distal sac can be incised to prevent postoperative hydrocele formation. Further management depends on the presence and nature of the contents of the indirect hernial sac (Figure 12.12).

No contents

If the sac is empty and does not extend beyond the pubic tubercle, it is lifted and freed from the adjacent

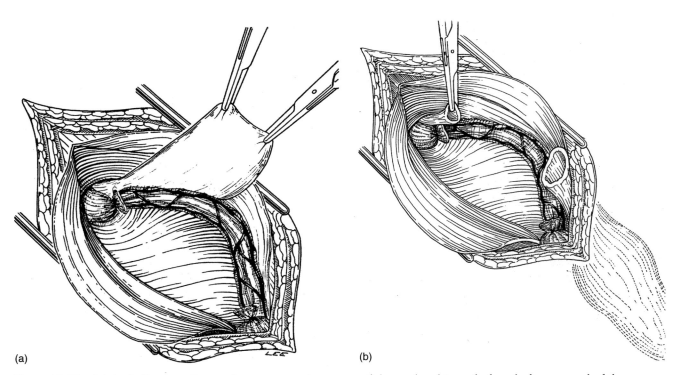

(a)   (b)

Figure 12.12 (a) An indirect sac lies on the anterosuperior aspect of the cord and is easily found after removal of the cremaster. If the sac is only in the canal and does not emerge beyond the superficial inguinal ring it is removed completely. (b) If the indirect sac extends beyond the inguinal canal it must never be dissected beyond the pubic tubercle, instead the proximal sac is identified across and ligated flush with the peritoneum at its neck. The distal sac is left *in situ* to preserve the rich anastomosis of vessels that occur in the cord and prevent ischaemia of the testicle.

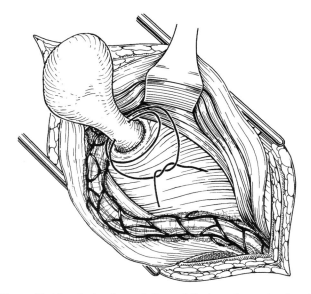

Figure 12.13 A simple sac is ligated flush to the parietal peritoneum

structures by careful dissection. It is traced back to its junction with the parietal peritoneum, transfixed with an absorbable polymer suture which is tied around it securely and the redundant sac excised (Figure 12.13). If an indirect hernia sac extends beyond the pubic tubercle the sac is transected and the distal sac left *in situ* (Figure 12.12b).

Small bowel and/or omentum, with or without adhesions

Unless the hernia is strangulated and the small bowel non-viable, any adhesions are divided and the small bowel is returned to the abdominal cavity. Strangulated omentum or small bowel can be resected at this stage. The diagnostic decision as to what should be done about very adherent and frequently partially ischaemic omentum is difficult. If there is any doubt about omentum it is best excised, because to return omentum of doubtful viability to the peritoneal cavity invites the formation of adhesions.

Sliding hernia

Such a hernia may contain the caecum and appendix (on the right side) in its wall, the sigmoid colon (on the left side) or the bladder (in the medial wall on either side). The following guidelines apply in these circumstances:

1. No attempt should be made to separate caecum or sigmoid colon from the sac wall. This may compromise their blood supply and lead to further unnecessary problems.
2. The appendix must not be removed, as this could introduce sepsis.
3. Appendices epiploicae must never be removed from

the sigmoid colon – they may harbour small colonic diverticula, excision of which will precipitate sepsis.
4. On the medial side of a sac there should be no attempt to dissect the bladder clean. If the bladder is inadvertently opened, a two-layer closure with absorbable polymer and urethral drainage are required. Recovery will obviously be delayed.

A sliding hernia is dealt with by excising as much peritoneal hernial sac as possible and then closing it using an 'inside out' pursestring suture. When it is closed it is pushed back behind the fascia transversalis (Figure 12.14).

DIRECT

The direct sac may be either a broad-based bulge behind and through the fascia transversalis or, less commonly, it may have a narrow neck. In the first type, interference with the peritoneum is not needed – the sac should be pushed behind the fascia transversalis, which will subsequently be repaired (Figure 12.15). In the second, which is usually at the medial end of the canal, extraperitoneal fat is removed, the sac carefully cleared, redundant peritoneum excised and the defect closed with a polymer transfixion suture. Care must be taken to avoid the bladder which is often in the wall of such a sac (Figure 12.16).

COMBINED DIRECT AND INDIRECT

Lastly, a combined direct and indirect 'pantaloon' sac straddling the deep epigastric vessels may be found. In such a case the sac should be delivered to the lateral side of the deep epigastric vessels and dealt with as described for an indirect hernia (Hoguet's manoeuvre).[430, 767]

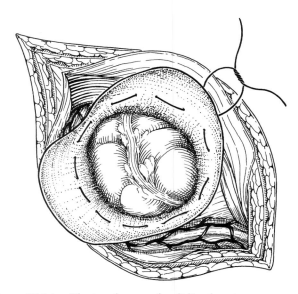

Figure 12.14 Closing the sac of a sliding hernia

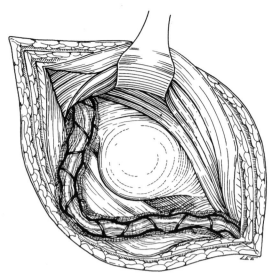

Figure 12.15 The dome-shaped direct bulge; there is no need to open this sac

The indirect sac is completely freed from the vas, spermatic vessels and the adjacent fascia transversalis at the deep ring. It is best then to mobilize the fascia transversalis medially so that the whole of the sac can be drawn laterally. Whether or not the direct sac should be opened at this stage is a question of judgement. The hazard of wounding the bladder must be acknowledged. Any opening into a direct sac must be commenced laterally; care must be taken to identify the bladder margin medially and any peritoneal incision must stop short of this. Alternatively the direct sac can be opened – a finger inserted into the peritoneal cavity through the indirect sac will identify the dimensions of the direct sac and facilitate dissection and mobilization.

Once the indirect and direct sacs are mobilized

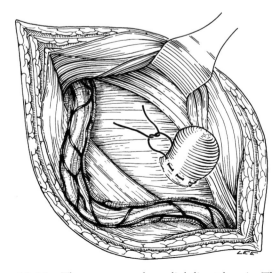

Figure 12.16 The narrow neck medial direct hernia. The sac is isolated, closed and excised

redundant peritoneum is excised and the peritoneal defect closed. Repair of the fascia transversalis is then undertaken (Figure 12.17).

DISSECTION OF FASCIA TRANSVERSALIS

The most essential part of the Shouldice operation is the repair of the fascia transversalis. This structure should already have been identified at its condensation around the cord forming the deep inguinal ring. The condensed medial margin of the deep inguinal ring is freed from the emerging cord by sharp dissection. When this is completed the medial margin of the ring is grasped in a dissecting forceps or a haemostat and lifted up off the underlying extraperitoneal fat. Dissecting scissors are now passed through the ring between the fascia and the underlying fat. By this manoeuvre the fascia is separated from the underlying structures, particularly the deep epigastric vessels. If there is no direct herniation and no gross distortion of the deep ring only the margin of the deep ring, the 'sling' of the deep ring, needs dividing, if there is a direct hernia and attenuation of the fascia transversalis, the fascia transversalis is now divided along the length of the canal, beginning at the deep inguinal ring and continuing down to the pubic tubercle. The upper medial flap is lifted up away from the underlying fat.

Attention is now turned to the lower flap. If it is penetrated by cremasteric vessels arising from the deep epigastric vessels these should now be divided and ligated close to their origin. If care is not taken with the cremasteric vessels they may be torn off the deep epigastric vessels and troublesome haemorrhage will follow. If a direct hernia is present it will bulge forward at this time and must be pushed back in order to free the lower lateral flap of the fascia transversalis. This flap must be freed down to its continuation as the anterior femoral sheath deep to the inguinal ligament. The lower, condensed fascia transversalis as it merges to the anterior femoral sheath is the iliopubic band (see page 33). Any grossly attenuated fascia transversalis about a direct sac is excised. With the fascia transversalis opened and developed the femoral canal should be checked again (Figure 12.18).

REPAIR OF FASCIA TRANSVERSALIS

If the previous dissection has been carried out carefully, and if haemostasis is now complete, the remainder of the operation should be easy. First, the fascia transversalis is repaired and the deep ring is carefully reconstituted using a 'double breasting' technique. The posterior wall of the canal must be reconstituted so that all of the peritoneum and the stump of a hernial sac are retained behind it. To do this, the lower lateral flap of the fascia transversalis is sutured to the deep surface of the upper

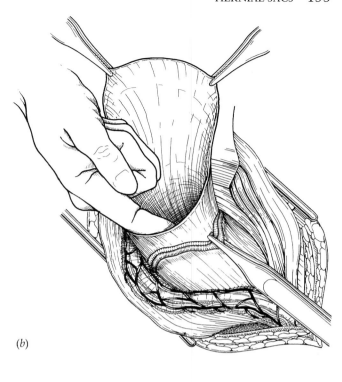

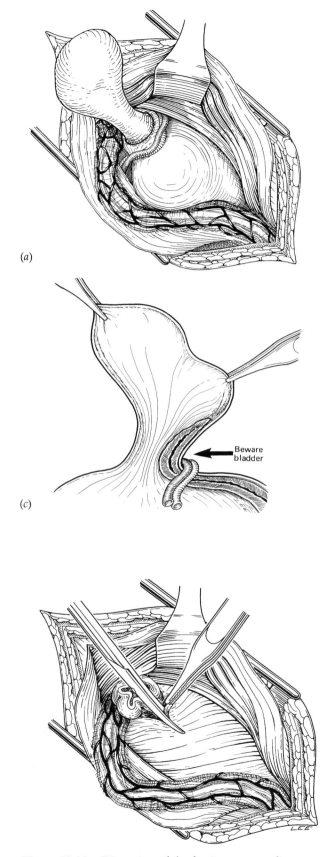

(a)

(c)

Beware
bladder

Figure 12.17 Hoguet manoeuvre. The combined direct/indirect sac (pantaloon hernia) is delivered lateral to the deep epigastric vessels. Any redundant peritoneum is excised and the sac closed

medial flap. The repair is begun towards the medial end of the canal. Where the medial margin of the deep ring only has been divided and the more medial aspect of the posterior wall of the canal shown to be sound, no direct herniation, only the divided fascia transversalis at the medial margin of the deep ring, the 'sling', will need careful two layered reconstruction with a non-absorbable suture, Lytle operation[587] (Figure 12.19). If there is a direct hernia the whole of the posterior wall of the canal will have been divided and will need repair, the first suture being placed in fascia transversalis where that structure becomes condensed into the aponeurosis and periosteum on the pubic tubercle. The lower lateral flap of the fascia transversalis is then sutured to the undersurface of the upper flap at the point where the upper flap is just deep to the tendon of the transversus abdominus (conjoint tendon). At this point there is a thickening or condensation of the fascia transversalis (the 'white line' or 'arch') which holds sutures easily.

Care must be taken with the closure of the fascia transversalis as it approaches the lateral rectus sheath, which must be adequately repaired to the fascia transversalis

Figure 12.18 Dissection of the fascia transversalis

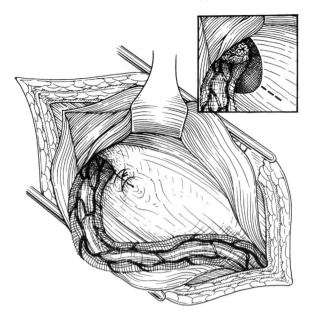

Figure 12.19 After the neck of the sac has been divided at the deep inguinal ring the fascia transversalis of the deep opening is identified and assessed. If ring is normal sized the stump of the sac is reduced and no more need be done. If the ring is marginally dilated (stretched) it should be carefully dissected and possibly divided slightly (inset) and then sutured tightly around the medial side of the cord with polypropylene to reconstitute a competent deep inguinal ring

and the pubic tubercle. The anatomy here is variable and the falx inguinalis (see page 29) should be included in the repair.

The fascia is sutured laterally until the stump of an indirect hernia lies behind it and it has been snugly fitted around the spermatic cord (Figure 12.20).

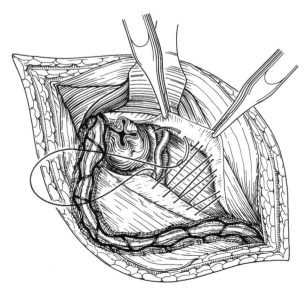

Figure 12.20 Suturing the lower lateral flap of fascia transversalis to the undersurface of the upper medial flap along the 'white line' or 'arch'

The direction of suturing is then reversed. The free margin of the upper medial flap is brought down over the lower lateral flap and sutured to the fascia transversalis at its condensation (the iliopubic tract), just above the upturned deep edge of the inguinal ligament in the floor of the canal. Suturing is continued back to the pubic tubercle, where the suture is tied. By this manoeuvre the fascia transversalis is 'double breasted' on itself, the 'direct area' of the canal is reinforced and the internal ring carefully reconstituted and tightened.

It is important not to split the fascial fibres. Sutures should be placed about 2–4 mm apart and bites of different depth taken with each so that an irregular 'broken saw tooth' effect is produced.

The repair of the fascia transversalis is the crucial part of the operation. The fascia must be dissected and handled with care if its structure is to be maintained (Figure 12.21).

A 'trick of the trade' sometimes facilitates this suturing of the fascia transversalis: after the upper medial and lower lateral leaflets of fascia transversalis have been

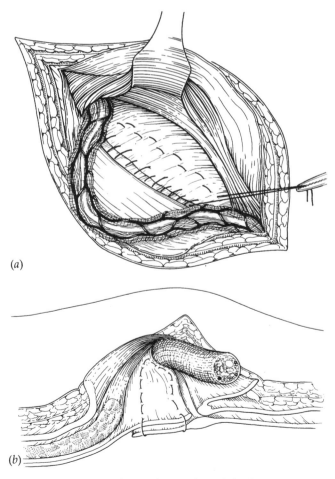

(a)

(b)

Figure 12.21 Completing the overlap of the fascia transversalis repair. The margin of the upper medial flap is sutured to the anterior surface of the lower lateral flap. A neat closure up to the cord makes a new deep ring

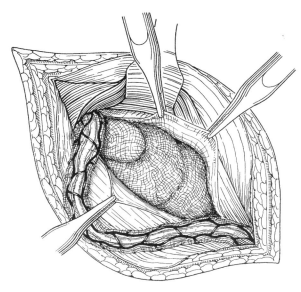

Figure 12.22 If the subjacent extraperitoneal fat and peritoneum is bulging, a 'trick of the trade' is to pack it down with a gauze swab. This must be removed before the sutures are snugged tight

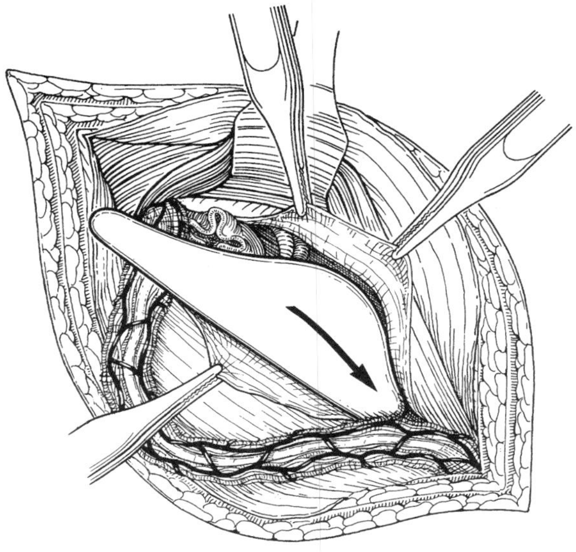

developed to clearly show the 'white line' of the transversus tendon through the fascia above and the iliopubic tract below, a loose swab is pushed into the dissection to keep the extraperitoneal fat out of the way when the first sutures are introduced (Figure 12.22) When these sutures are loosely in place the swab is removed and the suture tension adjusted to give tissue closure. A plastic extractable retractor has been invented to place deep to the fascia transversalis to achieve the same purpose*
(Figure 12.23).

Reinforcement with the conjoint tendon

The conjoint tendon is now used to reinforce the repair of the fascia transversalis medially. A suture is started laterally through the upturned deep edge of the inguinal ligament medial to the margin of the reconstituted deep inguinal ring and continued to the deep tendinous surface of the conjoint tendon, which is directly to the medial side of the deep ring. Sometimes, particularly if the cord is bulky, it is easier to proceed in reverse by passing the needle first through the undersurface of the conjoint tendon and then under the cord and through the upturned edge of the inguinal ligament.

At the point where this suture is inserted, the deep surface of the conjoint tendon is just beginning to become aponeurotic (the tendon of the transversus muscle) and it should hold sutures easily. The suture is continued in a medial direction, picking up the upturned edge of the inguinal ligament and the undersurface – the

Figure 12.23 shows the Shouldimat retractor.

Figure 12.23 The Shouldimat. This plastic retractor is placed extraperitoneally while the first layer of sutures is placed in the fascia transversalis

aponeurotic part – of the conjoint tendon down to the pubic tubercle (Figure 12.24) The direction is then reversed, suturing the aponeurotic part of the conjoint tendon, the internal oblique tendon now, loosely, to the external oblique aponeurosis about 0.5 cm above the inguinal ligament. The 'broken saw tooth' technique previously mentioned is again used, and as it is done the suture is gently pulled snug, not tight, so that the

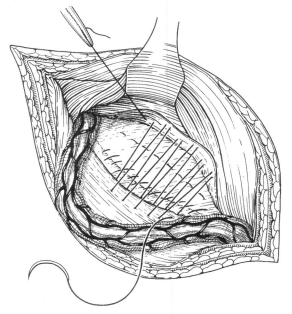

Figure 12.24 The aponeurotic, white part of the internal oblique tendon and the conjoint tendon are used to reinforce the repair

---

*Shouldimat®. J.L. Peters FRCS, CliniMed Ltd., Cavell House, Amersham Hill, High Wycombe, Bucks, HP13 6NZ.

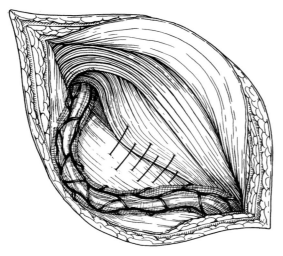

Figure 12.25   The anterior aponeurotic surface of the internal oblique aponeurosis is loosely sutured to the aponeurosis of the external oblique medially

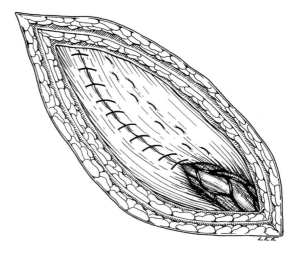

Figure 12.26   The external oblique aponeurosis is closed, double breasted, anterior to the cord. Thus the inguinal canal is reconstituted with the cord obliquely traversing it

conjoint tendon and rectus sheath are rolled down onto the deep surface of the external oblique aponeurosis. Suturing is continued laterally until the conjoint tendon ceases to be aponeurotic at the medial edge of the emergent spermatic cord. The suture is then tied.

The reconstruction of the posterior wall and the floor of the inguinal canal is now complete. The cord is now placed back in the canal (Figure 12.25).

CLOSURE

External oblique aponeurosis

Now that the cord has been replaced the external oblique aponeurosis can be closed over it. Again a 'double breasting' technique is used. Remembering that aponeurotic wounds are slow to regain strength, polypropylene sutures are used for this layer. The suturing is commenced medially, the lower lateral flap being sutured to the undersurface of the upper medial flap. Suturing is from medial to lateral and back again, so that the upper flap is brought down over the lower flap and a new superficial inguinal ring is constructed at the medial end of the canal. Care should be taken to close any secondary clefts in the external oblique (see page 22).

The repair is now complete, and if all the layers have been sutured exactly as described the loads on the suture lines should be well distributed; there should be no undue tension and no splitting of fibre bundles. Indeed, the structures should have just 'rolled together' (Figure 12.26).

Subcutaneous tissue

The subcutaneous tissue is carefully closed with interrupted sutures. No 'dead spaces' should be left and the fat should be closed so that the skin is closely approximated.

If there is much tissue trauma or dead space, a closed drain is useful in this layer[79] (Figure 12.27). The skin is closed with a subcuticular absorbable suture (Figure 12.28).

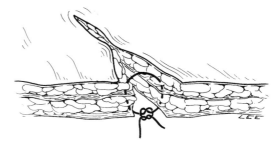

Figure 12.27   Closure of the subcutaneous tissue

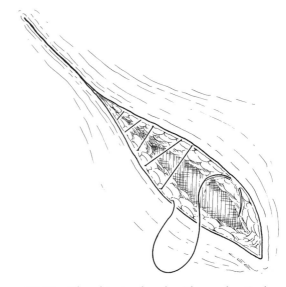

Figure 12.28   The skin is closed with a subcuticular continuous absorbable polymer suture

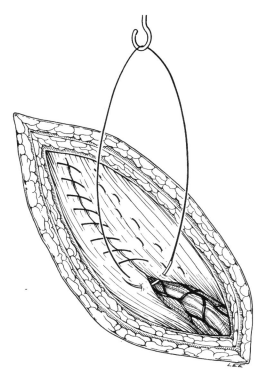

Figure 12.29   Technique of suturing with monofilament wire

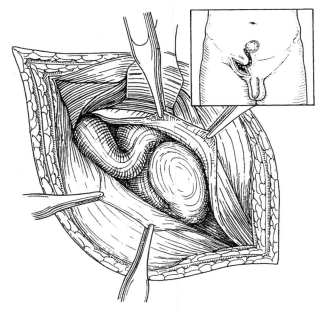

Figure 12.30   Orchidocleisis

Suture technique if monofilament stainless steel wire is used

As an alternative to polypropylene, 34-gauge stainless steel wire can be used. This is the original material used by Shouldice himself. Stainless steel is an excellent suture material as it is strong, and causes little tissue reaction. However, special attention must be given to the technique if it is not to be broken or kinked in use. It is best to carry the wire as a loop on a long hook between each suture. The assistant must wield the hook carefully while at the same time keeping out of the operating surgeon's way and simultaneously maintaining the tension in the loop constant (Figure 12.29).

Orchidocleisis

Intra-abdominal placement of the testis (orchidocleisis) allows closure of the deep ring and complete obliteration of the inguinal canal. This technique has been recommended in elderly poor risk men, the testis being placed in an extraperitoneal pouch superiorly and laterally to the internal ring. The possibility of inducing neoplastic changes in the testis can be ignored in elderly men, especially those who have severe concomitant disease.[501] In our experience the regular Shouldice operation described is always possible and it is never necessary to carry out this manoeuvre (Figure 12.30).

Inguinal hernia in women

During the 26-year period 1945–71, more than 75 000 hernia repairs were performed in the Shouldice clinic, Toronto; of these 1672 (2.2%) were primary inguinal hernias in women and 414 (0.05%) primary femoral hernias in women. Of the inguinal hernias, 1548 were indirect and only 124 were direct. Thus primary indirect inguinal hernia is 13 times more common than direct hernias. Direct inguinal hernias in women are very rare, and when they do occur they present usually in the lateral part of the posterior wall close to the deep epigastric vessels rather than in the medial canal as they do in men.[347, 353] Recurrent inguinal hernias in women are more frequently indirect than direct – medial direct recurrences are a complication of previous groin surgery, Pfannensteil incisions, or of the high repair of femoral hernia.

In women, the round ligament should be excised and the inguinal canal closed.[347] The fascia transversalis is sutured down to the iliopubic tract and medially onto the iliopectineal line as in the McVay/Cooper's ligament operation, thus reducing the risk of subsequent femoral herniation (Figure 12.31).

Bilateral hernia

Bilateral hernias should not usually be repaired simultaneously, for three reasons:

1. If sepsis occurs it may be bilateral if introduced at the same operation.
2. After simultaneous bilateral herniorrhaphy there is

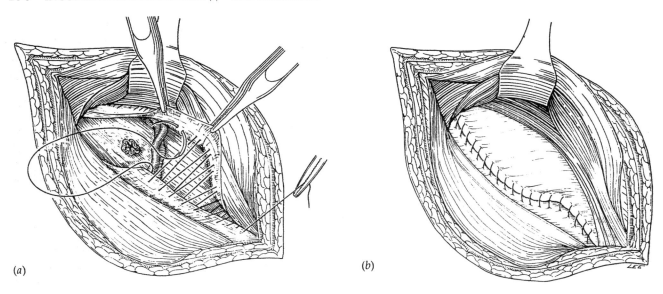

(a)   (b)

Figure 12.31   Inguinal hernia in women: the sac and the round ligament are excised and then the canal closed by suturing the fascia transversalis to the iliopectineal ligament

often much oedema and swelling of the penis and scrotum, which can make voiding tiresome and will delay convalescence.

3. There is evidence that simultaneous bilateral herniorrhaphy using the Shouldice technique may stretch the fascia transversalis unduly and predispose the patient to subsequent femoral hernia[351, 352] (see Chapter 24).

A small study by Serpell and colleagues investigated 31 patients undergoing bilateral simultaneous inguinal hernia repair, and five patients undergoing bilateral sequential repair, and compared these two groups against 75 patients having unilateral inguinal hernia repair. There were no differences in wound complications, postoperative respiratory complications or other adverse effects between the three groups.[844] However, operating time and hospital stay was reduced by two days in those patients undergoing simultaneous repair.

A larger but retrospective study from the Mayo Clinic, of patients undergoing hernia repair, compared 333 patients who underwent sequential unilateral repair against 329 who underwent simultaneous bilateral repair. Although there was greater morbidity in the bilateral group, these complications for specific events were not significantly different between the two groups, except for urinary retention, which occurred in 6.1% of the unilateral group, and 15% for the bilateral group. These results have a cautionary note: bilateral synchronous inguinal hernia repair in the elderly has a relatively high incidence of urinary retention, moreover the recurrence rate reported from the Mayo Clinic was 8.5%.[653]

It is better to allow an interval of 3–5 weeks between operations in elderly patients with bilateral hernias.

Recurrent inguinal hernia

Recurrent inguinal hernias are always difficult and operation should only be undertaken by an experienced surgeon who is interested in this problem. If there is sepsis or sinus formation, operation should not be undertaken until it has settled. It may be necessary to remove all foreign suture material from the wound at a first operation and then wait some months before attempting the repair. For a first-time recurrent hernia the technique is identical to that described above. Generally, tissue planes can be identified if a slow and gentle dissection is made. If the hernia is multiple recurrent or if there has been much sepsis or scarring, or a major tissue deficit exists, the extraperitoneal approach (pages 167–176) is advised. It should never be necessary to divide the cord in order to repair a recurrent hernia.

The Lichtenstein technique

The true tension-free hernioplasty using mesh and no suture closure of the hernial defect was introduced in 1984 by Irving Lichtenstein and colleagues.[854] Lichtenstein's experience with the use of polypropylene mesh in inguinal herniorrhaphy, however, began much earlier.[559] In a personal experience of 6321 cases reported in 1987 with a 91% follow-up over a period of 2–14 years, a recurrence rate of 0.7% was achieved. At this time apart from the innovation of polypropylene mesh, Lichtenstein had abandoned high ligation and excision of indirect sacs, but continued to use single-layer approximation of the transversus abdominis and the inguinal ligament with a relaxing incision. After a period of evolution the perfected tension-free hernioplasty was reported by Lichtenstein, Shulman, Amid, and Montelier in 1989.[564]

Repair of the posterior abdominal layer with a suture line was abandoned, except for a simple imbrication suture for large sacs that aided flattening of the posterior wall before placement of the mesh. The recurrence rate in over 1000 cases was 0% at 1–5-year follow-up, with no mesh infections and the authors stated that the technique was simple, rapid, relatively pain-free allowing prompt resumption of unrestricted physical activity. This report prompted a campaign of popularisation of the tension-free hernioplasty.[727]

Like the Shouldice Hospital the Lichtenstein Institute surgeons have written multiple publications in the surgical literature, repeating their experiences with a gradually enlarging number of patients.[18, 856, 857] The authors emphasize that the hernial defect edges are not co-apted and the sole strength of the repair is based on blocking the defect with a tension-free patch. Over 3000 patients have now undergone repair with this operation at the Lichtenstein Institute; the operation being performed under local anaesthesia and patients discharged within a few hours of operation with minimal discomfort, for which mild analgesics are prescribed. Unrestricted activity is encouraged and patients discharged from the Unit are able to resume normal activity in 2–10 days. A postal survey performed by Shulman of 70 surgeons utilizing this technique who did not have a special interest in inguinal hernia surgery indicated similar results in 22 300 repairs.[18]

The use of prophylactic antibiotic cover in the form of powder instillation or a single perioperative intravenous bolus is a vexed question. The Lichtenstein Institute have used both methods, but have not made a firm recommendation. However, Gilbert and Felton in a co-operative multicentre prospective study of 2493 inguinal hernia repairs by 65 surgeons found a wound infection rate of less than 1% whether or not biomaterials or antibiotics were used.[345] Moreover, the removal of biomaterials from infected wounds was not necessary to eliminate infection and indeed is not recommended because of technical difficulty and inevitable recurrence. The authors conclude that the expense incurred for routine prophylactic antibiotic cover in inguinal hernia operation when biomaterials are used could not be reconciled by any benefits obtained.

The ease of performance, rapid recovery and excellent results of the tension-free hernioplasty have been confirmed in a small study by Davies and colleagues from Liverpool.[222] Many of the operations in this study were performed by junior trainee surgeons whose results were equal to those of the specialist hernia surgeon. Kark and colleagues, reporting from a specialist hernia centre on 1098 tension-free hernia repairs, reported only one recurrence after primary repair and an overall sepsis rate

of 0.9%.[483] This report emphasized the cost savings associated with the operation and the rapid return to activity: with 50% of office workers returning to work in one week or less, and 60% of manual workers in two weeks or less. Nevertheless, the operation can present technical difficulties to the novice, as illustrated by a report from Brussels in which 139 primary inguinal hernias were repaired by tension-free hernioplasty and a 4.6% recurrence rate was reported during a mean follow-up of 12.7 months. The probable technical fault was failure to overlap the pubic tubercle and the entire posterior inguinal wall by a wide margin of mesh.[816] These authors reported a 50% saving of resources by utilization of the tension-free hernioplasty.

The first randomized trial reporting a comparison between the tension-free hernioplasty and the Shouldice operation was reported by Kux and colleagues, verifying the low recurrence rate (one recurrence in the Lichtenstein group over a 30-month period), and a reduced requirement for postoperative pain relief. Patients under the age of 60 years were excluded from this study.[520]

Rutkow and Robbins report a modification of the tension-free hernioplasty using a plug to block the defect in the posterior inguinal wall supplemented by a sutureless swatch or patch as an overlay on the posterior inguinal wall.[372, 812, 857] The authors have extended the technique to treat all inguinal hernias, femoral hernias, recurrent groin hernias, and small incisional hernias. Only in a large defect is the plug sutured to the fascial margins to maintain its position. In 1563 cases two recurrences were recorded with an average follow-up of 82% at 2.4 years. Until this technique has been adapted and promulgated by surgeons in general, it cannot be recommended for routine use outside specialist hernia centres.

THE LICHTENSTEIN TENSION-FREE HERNIOPLASTY

The incision, exposure, dissection of the canal and cord and the dealing with indirect hernial sacs is identical for that described for the Shouldice operation (see pages 147–152). In the case of large direct sacs, in order to flatten the posterior inguinal wall to facilitate placement of the mesh, a running, inverting, absorbable suture is applied to the transversalis fascia.

Since a considerable degree of overlap is required of Hesselbach's triangle, the pubic tubercle and laterally beyond the internal ring, the external oblique aponeurosis needs to be lifted up and dissected further from the underlying internal oblique muscle high enough to accommodate a 6–8 cm wide patch. Medially this dissection should be taken beyond the pubic tubercle to the midline (Figure 12.32).

Polypropylene mesh precut to 8 cm × 16 cm is now tailored to the individual patient's requirements. This

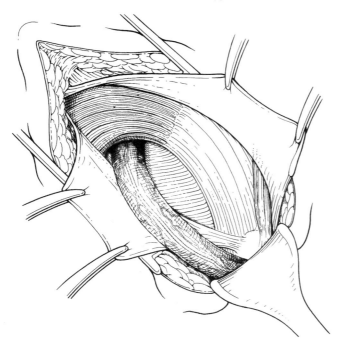

Figure 12.32 Wide dissection of the posterior wall of the canal

will involve trimming 1–2 cm of the patch's width and the upper medial corner so that it will tuck itself between the external oblique and internal oblique muscles without wrinkles (Figure 12.33).

The cord is now retracted downward and the mesh aligned into the inguinal canal such that its inferior border lies parallel with the inguinal ligament, and its medial border overlaps the pubic tubercle by 1–2 cm. Using a non-absorbable monofilament running suture beginning at the upper, medial, rounded border of the mesh, the suture is placed into the tough aponeurotic tissue of the midline and secured with a knot. This suture then continues around the edge of the mesh taking bites of firm connective tissue under direct vision, but avoiding the periosteum of the bone.

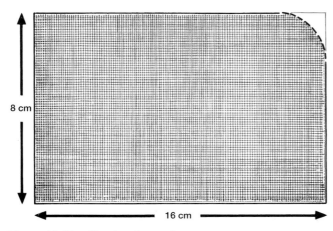

Figure 12.33 Shaping the mesh

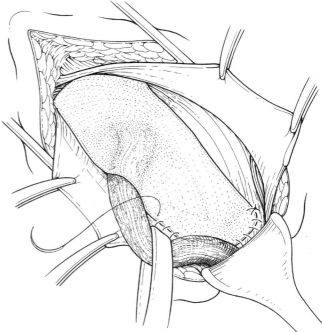

Figure 12.34 Initial half of continuous suture to allow mesh to overlap pubic tubercle and appose to inguinal ligament

As the suture continues it picks up the lower edge of the shelving margin of the inguinal ligament. Having secured the mesh medially and also secured it to 1–2 cm of inguinal ligament, this suturing is temporarily halted. (Figure 12.34). A slit is now made at the lateral end of

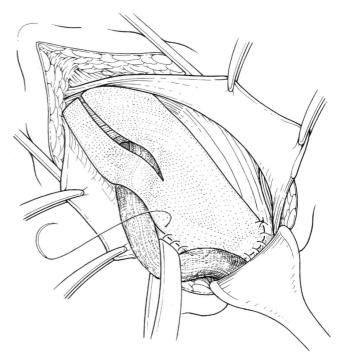

Figure 12.35 The mesh is slit (one third below; two-thirds above), up to the medial margin of the internal ring

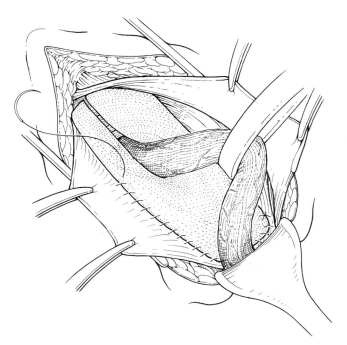

Figure 12.36 The lower 'tail' of the mesh is flipped behind the cord, followed by the continuous suture with needle, and the cord is retracted upwards

the mesh creating two tails, a wider one (two-thirds above) and a narrow one (one-third below) (Figure 12.35). The lower, narrower tail together with the needle and its running suture are now passed behind the cord which is then retracted upwards (Figure 12.36). The

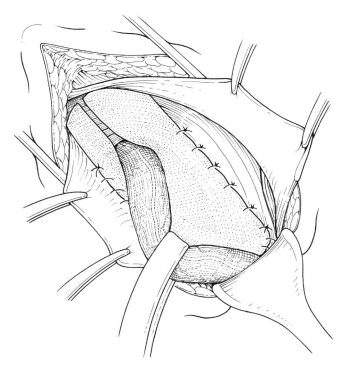

Figure 12.37 The continuous suture line along the inguinal ligament is now continued to the lateral border of the internal ring

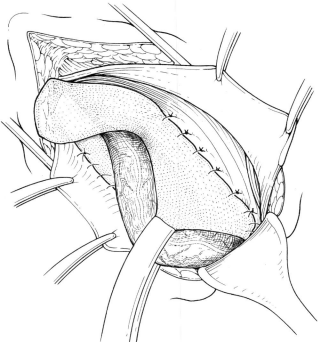

Figure 12.38 Three or four sutures tack the mesh cranially

wider upper tail and the narrow lower tail are over-lapped and grasped in a haemostat to retract the mesh and prevent unnecessary wrinkles.

The running suture between the lower edge of the mesh and the shelving margin of the inguinal ligament is now completed to a point just lateral to the internal ring (Figure 12.37). The upper leaf of the external oblique aponeurosis is now retracted strongly upward and the upper edge of the mesh is sutured to the underlying internal oblique aponeurosis or muscle with a series of interrupted sutures approximately 2–3 cm apart. Care is taken to avoid underlying blood vessels and sensory nerves, such as the ilioinguinal and iliohypogastric nerves (Figure 12.38). The mesh should not be com-pletely flattened, but should be seen to have some degree of anterior convexity in order to remain tension-free. The last fixation suture is placed laterally at approxi-mately the same level as the internal ring.

The lower edges of each of the two tails are now fixed to the inguinal ligament at a point just lateral to the completion knot of the lower running suture. A point is chosen in the lower edge of the upper tail approximately 1 cm beyond the lateral margin of the internal ring to avoid unnecessary buckling of the mesh (Figure 12.39). Having created a new internal ring with cross-over and overlap of the two tails, excess patch on the lateral side is now trimmed in order to leave approximately 3–4 cm of mesh beyond the internal ring. This lateral tail is now tucked underneath the external oblique aponeurosis and may be prevented from movement, curling up or

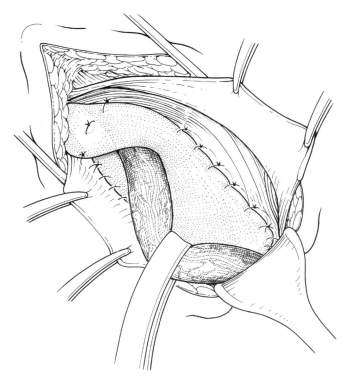

Figure 12.39 'Tails' are overlapped and crossed and a single suture placed to create a new 'internal' ring

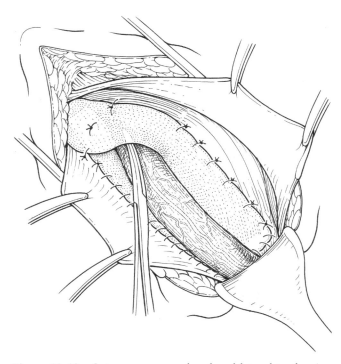

Figure 12.40 Sutures may now be placed lateral to the ring to prevent shifting and curling. An artery clip is run down between the mesh and new internal ring to ensure an adequate aperture

wrinkling by placing sutures between it and the underlying muscle (Figure 12.40). The size of the new internal ring is now tested with a haemostat, which should pass easily between the cord and the mesh. If this gap is too wide it may be closed loosely with a non-absorbable suture (Figure 12.40).

Having completed repair of the posterior inguinal wall with the polypropylene mesh, the cord is placed back into the canal, and wound closure is identical to that described for the Shouldice operation (see page 156).

Strangulated hernia

The Shouldice operative technique is recommended to treat a strangulated inguinal hernia. The additional risk of infection in this situation militates against the use of mesh, infection of which may cause morbidity. If additional access is required to deal with gangrenous gut, the deep ring can be enlarged medially by dividing the deep epigastric vessels between ligatures, taking care to avoid the bladder. It is, however, preferable to perform an additional standard paramedian incision for access to the main peritoneal cavity rather than to have to do an awkward resection of gangrenous tissue through the groin incision.

Postoperative care

Immediate active mobilization is the key to rapid convalescence. The 'client with a hernia' must not be allowed to become institutionalized into the 'postoperative patient'. If the operation has been performed under local anaesthesia, the patient should be helped to walk as soon as he is returned to the ward. If general anaesthesia has been used, the patient must be made to get up and walk as soon as he is conscious. There may be slight pain after surgery and a suitable mild analgesic should be prescribed. Analgesics with narcotic properties are never needed.

If social circumstances allow, patients should be discharged within a few hours of operation with minimal discomfort for which mild analgesics are prescribed. Unrestricted activity is encouraged, and indeed most patients should resume normal activity in 2–10 days. 'Take it easy' is the wrong advice.[858] Integrity of the hernia repair depends on good surgical technique, rather than any supposedly deleterious, premature physical activity undertaken by the patient. Return to full activity does not increase recurrences and indeed caution will engender anxiety and perhaps justify the patient's decision to remain off work for up to six weeks.[372] It is contradictory and counterproductive to warn against strenuous activity and is a recipe for long-term disability. Troublesome wound soreness is rare 7–10 days after the operation.

The wound dressing is removed by the patient on the fifth postoperative day. After the dressing is removed the patient can shower or bath normally.

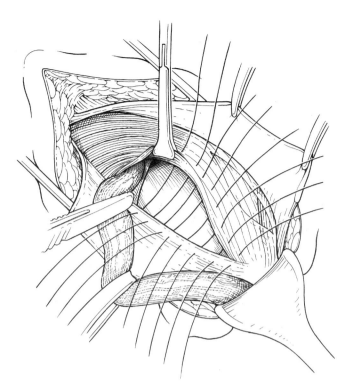

Figure 12.41 The McVay/Cooper's ligament operation: clearing the anterior femoral sheath

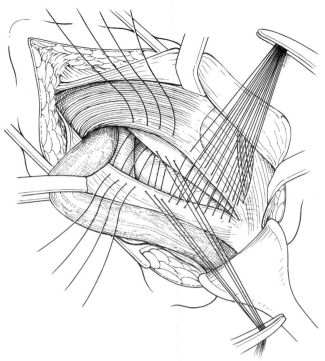

Figure 12.42 Sutures are placed between the transversalis abdominis arch and Cooper's ligament as far as the femoral vein

Light office or professional work can be resumed after about one week and most other heavier jobs after about 2–4 weeks. Patients are told that they may undertake any work which does not cause pain to their wounds.[652, 801, 804]

McVay/Cooper's ligament operation

The McVay/Cooper's ligament repair is most useful in the management of concomitant femoral and inguinal hernias.[642] In this operation the anterior femoral fascia (sheath) is carefully dissected to clear the anterior wall of the femoral artery and vein, and all fat and lymph nodes are removed from the femoral canal to eliminate any potential femoral hernia (Figure 12.41). If a femoral sac is found it is converted to an inguinal sac and then dealt with.

The incision, exposure, dissection of the canal and cord are identical to the two approaches (Shouldice and Lichtenstein) described above. The cord is dissected free, but no dissection is necessary medial to the pubic tubercle. The transversalis fascia is incised and the posterior wall of the canal is resected. The dissection is then taken deeper to expose and free the iliopectineal (Cooper's) ligament. Next, the anterior femoral fascia is exposed, beginning the dissection lateral to the femoral artery, progressing medially across the anterior surface of the artery and vein. The femoral canal is then cleared

of fat and lymphatics, taking care to identify any abnormal obturator circulation, and to carefully ligate any collaterals. After the inferior dissection is completed the tendinous portion of the transversus arch is developed. Any attenuated fascia transversalis and internal oblique is cleared from the transversus aponeurosis. A generous relaxing incision (see page 164) is made as medial as possible in the internal oblique aponeurosis – anterior rectus sheath – deep to the external oblique aponeurosis before the two aponeuroses fuse (see below). In obese females this dissection will involve the placement of deep Deaver retractors, with the patient placed in the Trendelenburg position.

The cord is opened and any indirect sac dissected free, ligated high and excised. If no indirect sac is immediately apparent the anterior medial part of the canal is dissected further to identify any small peritoneal tab that is present to ensure that an indirect sac is not overlooked.

The sacs are then opened, excised and closed, or if there is a direct bulge it is inverted and the extraperitoneal fat closed over it. Anyway, the extraperitoneal tissue is 'tidied up' by inverting it all with an absorbable polymer suture.

The repair is now initiated by bringing the transverse abdominis arch down to the inguinal ligament. This is best achieved with a layer of interrupted sutures, beginning at the pubic tubercle and continued laterally to the medial edge of the femoral vein. Each is placed carefully under direct vision and held before serial knotting (Figure 12.42) and are placed between the transversus

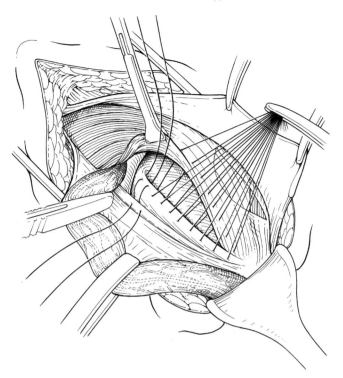

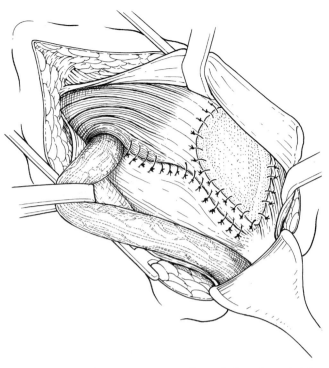

Figure 12.43 The femoral canal is closed with two or three transition sutures between Cooper's ligament and the anterior femoral fascia

Figure 12.44 The sutures are tied, medial to lateral. The defect of a relaxing incision can be filled with polypropylene mesh

completed by closure of the subcutaneous fat and skin (see pages 155–156).

arch the 'white line' and the iliopectineal (Cooper's) ligament. The femoral vein is retracted and protected by a retractor.

The femoral canal is then closed by placement of two or three transition sutures of non-absorbable sutures between Cooper's ligament and the anterior femoral fascia (sheath). The lateral suture is placed just lateral to the last suture in Cooper's ligament; the medial two or three are medial to this and go between the Cooper's ligament sutures (Figure 12.43) The repair is now continued laterally between the transversus abdominis arch and the anterior femoral fascia with the line of sutures just displacing the internal ring laterally, but not placing any sutures lateral to the cord. These sutures are of monofilament, non-absorbable material. The sutures are now tied beginning medially and a new internal ring created such that a haemostat can be inserted between the last tied suture and the cord (Figure 12.44).

Attention is now turned to the relaxing incision. This may be secured with sutures of monofilament, non-absorbable sutures or a polypropylene mesh patch can be used to repair the defect (Figure 12.45). Rutledge states that he reinforces the basic repair with an onlay graft polypropylene mesh in approximately 10% of patients (Figure 12.46).

The cord is replaced and the external oblique aponeurosis closed anterior to the cord. The operation is

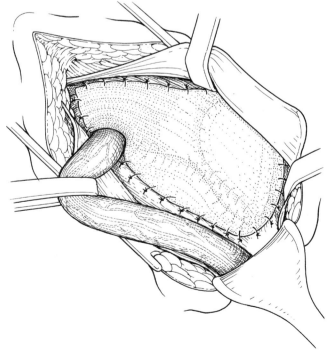

Figure 12.45 Onlay mesh can be used to reinforce the basic repair

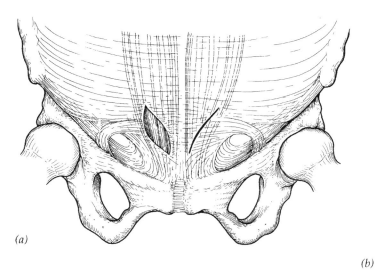

(a)

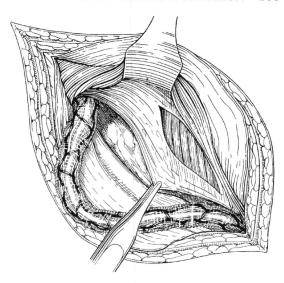

(b)

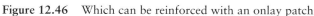

Figure 12.46 Which can be reinforced with an onlay patch

RELAXING INCISION

The employment of a relaxing incision to avoid tension at the suture line in inguinal hernioplasty is an old concept (Figure 12.47). Many surgeons do not use this technique either because they do not understand the concept or because they extensively mobilize the fascia transversalis/transversus tendon for their primary repair (as in the Shouldice operation). If this mobilization is adequate and if sutures are placed closely and at even tension, the repair can be effected without a relaxing incision. However, a relaxing incision is useful; Halsted

recommended its use for the more difficult ruptures and Halsted's former resident Bloodgood recommended it when the conjoint tendon had been obliterated. Even earlier, Wolfler and Bloodgood had separately recommended incision of the rectus sheath so that a flap of its aponeurosis could be turned down and sutured to the inguinal ligament to reinforce the direct area.[103, 994] Fallis (1938),[291] Reinhoff (1940)[784] and Tanner (1942)[908] also emphasized the usefulness of this manoeuvre. Although in the UK the operation is known as 'Tanner's slide', it does have a long international pedigree to recommend it. Mattson (1946) has stressed the importance of rectus sheath in repair of large and recurrent direct hernias[623] and more recently McVay (1971) has emphasized that a relaxing incision is mandatory if a 'Cooper's ligament' repair is to be secure.[641]

McVay prefers the 'slide' technique to the flap method of utilization of the rectus sheath; not only does the slide technique allow fixation of the strong musculo-aponeurotic rectus sheath to Cooper's ligament, but in doing so it replaces the posterior wall of the inguinal canal with a strong viable aponeurosis exactly where the fascia transversalis is weak. The slid down transversus tendon is fixed inferiorly to Cooper's ligament as the virgin fascia transversalis would be. It must be re-emphasized that the relaxing incision is used to allow an adequate repair in the transversus abdominis/transversalis layer.

In McVay's experience of the Cooper's ligament repair, a recurrence rate of under 1% in 1000 cases over 16 years is recorded. In part these excellent results are due to the securing of an adequate viable posterior wall for the inguinal canal (the intact rectus sheath with its blood supply) to the firm anchorage of Cooper's ligament. This tissue is superior to any transplanted fascia or prosthetic material.

Concern is expressed by some surgeons that an

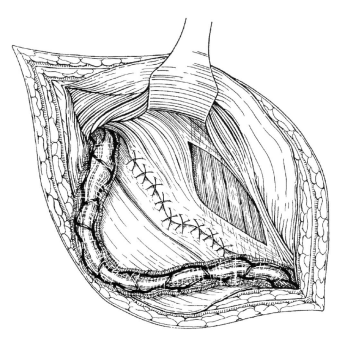

Figure 12.47 Anatomy of the relaxing incision

adequate slide, that is an incision adequate enough to allow easy apposition of the transversus aponeurosis to Cooper's ligament, leaves a triangular defect lateral to the rectus through which a hypogastric hernia could develop.[611] This is not a complication reported by exponents of the Cooper's ligament repair. Moreover further consideration of the anatomy will remind surgeons that the lateral margin of the rectus sheath is strong below the semilunar line of Douglas. This is the area where the fascia transversalis is most dense. Fears of herniation at this site can be discounted; both McVay and Ponka, who regularly employ this technique, recall no instances of pararectal herniation after using a relaxing incision.[752]

The technique for the relaxing incision is important. The upper medial flap of the external oblique is raised and then dissected medially where it overlies the anterior rectus sheath. At this site the anterior rectus sheath consists of the interdigitated aponeurotic fibres of the internal oblique and transversus muscles. They form one continuous lamina in the lower abdomen caudal to the semilunar line of Douglas and they are loosely attached to the more superficial external oblique aponeurosis. This loose attachment allows the two laminas, the superficial external oblique and the deep rectus sheath, to move independently in axis at right angles to each other – a mechanism of importance in closing the inguinal canal shutter.

In any event, a few deft scalpel strokes and blunt dissection will separate the external oblique aponeurosis from the internal oblique rectus sheath almost as far as the midline. The external oblique lamina is firmly retracted medially, the relaxing incision is then made in the deep lamina of the rectus sheath which is the continuation aponeurosis of the internal oblique and transversus muscles after they have merged to become the conjoint tendon. The relaxing incision should be about 1.5 cm from the midline: it should commence about 0.5 cm cephalad to the pubic crest and extend upward and very slightly lateralward for 7–8 cm. Care must be taken to avoid the iliohypogastric nerve. The conjoint tendon and the underlying fascia transversalis can now be slid down to make the repair. Haemostasis must be secured: failure to gain first-class haemostasis can lead to bleeding into the rectus sheath which can fill with much blood before spontaneous clotting and compartment haematoma pressure will arrest the surgeon's carelessness.[777]

The hernia repair is now made. This will draw the conjoint tendon and adjacent tissues downwards and laterally, causing the relaxing incision to gape and expose the red belly of the rectus muscle. Do not be alarmed – when the external oblique is closed, the 'gap' in the rectus sheath is adequately closed and no rectus herniation will result.

There are mistakes to be avoided; no incision must ever be made medial to the red muscle belly of the rectus. This area is the linea alba, where all the layers fuse and

no slide of one layer or another can occur. An incision in this most medial area will lead to iatrogenic herniation in the lower midline. Similarly, dissection and exploration of the lateral margin of the rectus, the Spigelian fascia, where the internal oblique and transversus muscles are banding together and, most importantly, where the fascia transversalis fuses with the aponeuroses, will lead to weakness here and be prone to a postoperative pararectus hernia. It is the continuity of the fascia transversalis posterior to the rectus muscle, the rectus muscle itself and the intact external oblique aponeurosis anteriorly which prevents herniation after the relaxing incision has created a defect in the deep lamina (internal oblique) of the anterior rectus sheath.

The employment of a 'slide' does not exonerate the surgeon from an adequate repair of the inguinal canal. All the authors who employ a slide also stress it is no alternative to a full-scale inguinal repair. McVay and Ponka use a Cooper's ligament repair, whereas Tanner repairs the fascia transversalis as a separate layer before reinforcement by conjoint tendon. The 'slide' or relaxing incision permits approximation of the fused portions of the fascia transversalis, the transversus abdominis aponeurosis and the internal oblique aponeurosis (the transversus arch, the conjoint tendon or the 'triple layer of Bassini' – principles repeating themselves under different definitions!).

Conclusions

For primary inguinal hernia in adults the method of repair will reflect the surgeon's training, the type of hernia and the age of the patient.[502]

The Shouldice operation and the Lichtenstein repair conform to the principles of good repair surgery, namely careful and accurate identification of anatomic planes and the use of appositional suture material or implanted mesh to repair the defect. When combined with good management policies, both techniques are cost-effective.

The Shouldice operation gives excellent results in Toronto, Philadelphia and Stockton-on-Tees, and the results are significantly better than those of other techniques reported in the British literature. However, the operation is technically demanding.

The Lichtenstein repair is simpler, but its track record is shorter: long-term morbidity of mesh placement in the groin is unknown.

The McVay/Cooper's ligament repair gives good results and utilizes the transversalis transversus layer, as does the Shouldice operation.

The relaxing incision (Tanner slide) is rarely needed if adequate dissection is undertaken.

The recurrence rate after inguinal hernia repair is operator dependent: the choice of operator is as important as the choice of operation.[502]

13 EXTRAPERITONEAL OR PREPERITONEAL OPEN REPAIR OF GROIN HERNIAS USING PROSTHETIC REINFORCEMENT

The technique outlined in this chapter extends the extraperitoneal approach of Annandale,[27] Cheatle[171] and Henry[418] to access all the hernial sites in both groins simultaneously and then repair the defect(s) in the fascia transversalis by inserting a sheet of prosthetic mesh between the peritoneum and the parietes to replace any deficiencies in the fascial layer. The technique was originally described by the Amiens herniology team of Stoppa and colleagues in 1972.[171, 896–898] Read has described a similar technique using Marlex mesh to repair large direct and recurrent inguinal hernias.[775] More recently the Reims Group led by Rives and colleagues have been the principal protagonists of the unilateral preperitoneal approach. They describe two or three stitches to approximate the transversus abdominis arch to Cooper's ligament in order to close the myopectineal orifice. The mesh is not sutured in place and only intra-abdominal pressure maintains its place over the hernial defect(s).[788] This approach has been further championed by Wantz for both recurrent complex and primary groin hernia.[966] A further variant has been described by Nyhus, exclusively for a recurrent inguinal hernia in which anatomical repair of the defect by approximation of the transversalis fascia to the ilio-pubic tract or Cooper's ligament is performed before reinforcement of the defect with polypropylene mesh placed in the preperitoneal space with suture fixation.[709]

As originally described, the French do not attempt any repair of any of the hernial orifices; the prosthesis is placed in position and held there by the intra-abdominal pressure of the peritoneum against the parietes, like ham in a sandwich. There are two objections to this sublime technique: first, if hernial orifices, particularly large direct inguinal defects, are left open they bulge postoperatively and although they are not true hernias patients do complain of the unsightly 'rupture'; secondly, it is technically difficult to introduce the mesh into the pelvis over the femoral vessels on each side adequately if it is not fixed down as the operator retreats upward to close the parietal wound. For these reasons, suturing, and then quilting the prosthesis into position is recommended.

Indications

The prosthetic reinforcement technique via the extraperitoneal route is indicated in:

1. Intricate (combination) groin hernias where there are multiple defects either unilateral or bilateral; for instance, combinations of prevascular, femoral, indirect and direct inguinal and low Spigelian hernias.
2. Giant inguinoscrotal hernias, either unilateral or bilateral, where replacement of abdominal contents through a groin incision only would be tiresome.
3. Recurrent or multiple recurrent groin hernias. Incision through the virgin extraperitoneal plane makes these operations simpler.
4. Incisional herniation after Pfannenstiel incisions and incisional hernias through the lateral rectus sheath (acquired Spigelian hernia). Repair is difficult because the posterior rectus sheath is absent, but placement of prosthetic mesh in the extraperitoneal layer resolves this.

The disadvantages of the extraperitoneal prosthetic operation include the need for general anaesthesia with good relaxation to enable access to the lower pelvis. It requires a more extensive dissection, and therefore causes more pain and immobility than the anterior operation. A skilled assistant who can handle a retractor deftly is all important.

A potential problem with this technique is sepsis, which will prejudice the outcome; sepsis with polypropylene (Marlex) mesh will always resolve without removal of the prosthesis. Attention to aseptic technique and absolute haemostasis are critical factors in the success of this operation. The French, and Wantz in the USA, always employ Mersilene mesh, which is more supple than Marlex. Mersilene, a multistrand material and more prone to sepsis, has a more doubtful track record with British surgeons.

A common postoperative complication is oedema of the lower flap and genitalia. This oedema is sometimes quite considerable; it does, however, always settle.

Calne (1967) has described an alternative strategy to cope with bilateral inguinal or femoral hernias without resorting to the extraperitoneal approach via a Pfannenstiel incision.[144] Both inguinal canals are opened by incising the external oblique aponeurosis. Oblique and narrow neck direct sacs are excised and their necks closed. Large direct sacs are left undisturbed. Femoral sacs can be dealt with at the same time. Bilateral orchidectomy will facilitate the operation but is not essential. The extraperitoneal space is opened behind each rectus and the internal oblique and transversus muscles displaced cephalad. Polyester mesh (Mersilene) is then threaded behind the rectus. The mesh is then fixed by four strong sutures to the periosteum of the anterosuperior iliac spines and pubic tubercles on either side. The mesh is stretched out and fixed under some tension. Excess mesh is trimmed. The edges of the mesh are sutured to the inguinal ligament inferiorly, allowing a small space to transmit the cord if it is to be left intact, and to Cooper's ligament, when there is femoral herniation, to close the femoral canal. The mesh is also sutured to the posterior layer of the anterior rectus sheath and the inferior borders of the internal oblique and conjoint tendons.

Ten operations are recorded; one patient who had a bladder diverticulum excised at operation developed a wound infection and persistent sinus. There was one unilateral recurrence at 16 months postoperatively. The longest follow-up was 4 years in a woman with bilateral recurrent femoral hernias; the other follow-up periods are short, the maximum being 11 months.[144]

The bilateral operation

PREOPERATIVELY

The patient must void urine immediately prior to operation; the urinary bladder must be empty to allow adequate exposure of the anterior pelvis. If the anatomic situation is complex and compromised by much scarring, the operation may be slow and take a long time. An in-dwelling catheter is advisable in these circumstances.

POSITION OF PATIENT

The patient is laid on his back on the operating table. The table is tilted to 15 degrees, head down; this empties the pelvis of intestine to allow the operator to work on the anterior pelvic parietes. Draping should allow a lower midline or Pfannenstiel incision.

THE INCISION

Access must be gained to the entire groin regions on both sides. A skin crease horizontal Pfannenstiel incision

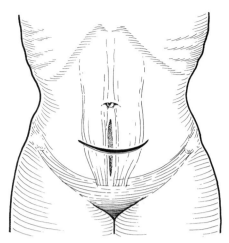

Figure 13.1 Access through a Pfannenstiel or a vertical incision separating the rectus muscles

gives the best cosmetic result and should be used for preference. Where there are scars from previous operations on groin hernias it is best to avoid these and the delayed healing that may occur in reopened skin scars. In these circumstances, a midline skin incision with midline incision of the linea alba and separation of the rectus muscles is recommended (Figure 13.1).

DEVELOPMENT OF EXTRAPERITONEAL SPACE

The red bellies of the rectus muscles are separated from the underlying peritoneum by finger dissection. A self-retaining retractor is inserted to hold the wound open. With a combination of sharp scissor dissection and blunt dissection the plane between the peritoneum and the parietes is opened behind the pubis down to the anterior

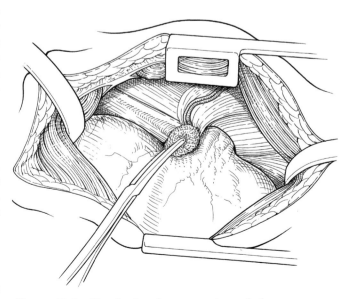

Figure. 13.2 Developing the extraperitoneal plane

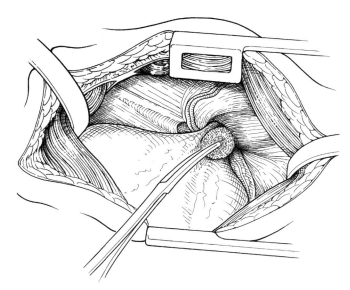

Figure 13.3 Mobilizing indirect sacs. These sacs are 'milked' out of the cord at the deep inguinal ring

prostatic capsule. This plane is extended laterally behind the pubis and obturator internus muscles. Hernial sacs may now be encountered entering the various potential defects in the parietes (Figure 13.2).

MOBILIZATION OF INDIRECT INGUINAL HERNIAL SACS

The necks of indirect sacs are identified as they spring from the main peritoneal sac. Dissection is made around them – a pledget in a curved artery forceps is a useful implement here. Once the sac is identified contents

should be reduced, if possible before the sac is opened. The sac should then be dissected back from the internal hernial orifice (deep ring). In the usual bubonocele the whole sac can easily be milked back from the canal. The sac is then opened and any remaining contents reduced. The sac is now transfixed and ligated so that the stump is closed off flush with the peritoneum (Figure 13.3).

DISCARDING DISTAL INDIRECT SACS

When a scrotal hernia is present, the proximal 2 or 3 cm of the sac should be milked back as before. The neck can now be divided across and closed flush to the parietal peritoneum with a transfixion suture. Before the distal sac springs away into the canal, its anterior wall should be slit for several centimetres, to prevent fluid accumulation within it and formation of a scrotal hydrocele. It can then be left in the scrotum with impunity. Attempts to milk all of a scrotal sac back into the abdomen and then peel it out of the scrotum will result in damage to testicular vessels, bleeding and an unpleasant and troublesome scrotal haematoma (Figure 13.4).

MOBILIZATION OF DIRECT INGUINAL AND FEMORAL SACS

Direct inguinal and femoral sacs are usually easily reduced, although if they are recurrent sacs some easement with careful scissors dissection may be required (Figure 13.5).

PARIETALIZATION OF CORD STRUCTURES

After the hernial sacs have been dissected, the stump of the indirect sac is grasped in a long haemostat. Traction

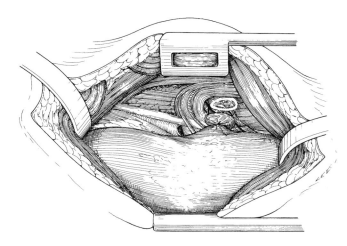

Figure 13.4 Distal sacs, which extend into the scrotum, should not be forcibly pulled up; if they are there will be excessive bruising and haematoma in the scrotum. The neck of the sac is isolated, cleaned of tissue and cord structures, and divided across. The distal end is left open to fall back into the undamaged scrotum

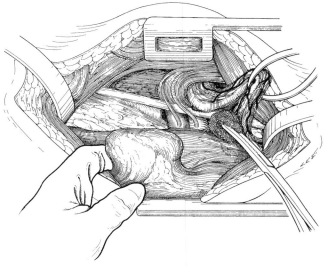

Figure 13.5 Direct inguinal and femoral hernias are dealt with; they are reduced out of their parietal defect. Direct sacs are broad necked and do not require formal amputation

upwards on the stump will display the testicular vessels and vas running on the peritoneum posteriorly. These structures should now be mobilized away from the peritoneum for 4 or 5 cm (parietalization). This will allow the cord structures to be placed against the parietes and the prosthesis to be placed between them and the peritoneum so that the deep ring is closed by the mesh. Great care must be taken during this dissection to avoid the femoral nerve which lies lateral to the deep ring. Ordinarily the femoral nerve is buried in and protected by the dense iliac fascia and is easily avoided, but if there has been previous surgery the dissection will be through much fibrous tissue and the nerve is at risk. Similarly, after vascular operations the nerve may be displaced and at risk (Figure 13.6).

CLOSURE OF DIRECT ORIFICES

If large direct defects are present these may now be closed with continuous metric 2 polypropylene sutures, picking up the iliopubic tract inferiorly and the white condensation of fascia transversalis superiorly (Figure 13.7). The Shouldice operation inside out!

MEASURING AND CUTTING OUT THE PROSTHESIS

The prosthesis should reach from the anterior superior iliac spine to the same point contralaterally. Vertically it should reach down behind the pubis and behind the pubic rami on either side. Cephalad it must extend 3.0 cm above the lower margin of the conjoint tendon (the transversus arch). It will need to extend higher if a Spigelian hernia or incisional hernia is to be repaired. If a Pfannenstiel incisional hernia is present the mesh should extend up almost to the umbilicus. In practice, the transverse size of the prosthesis usually measures the

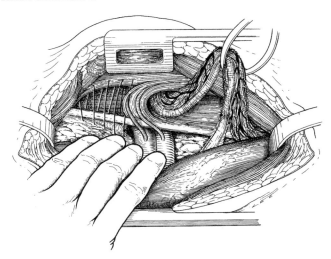

Figure 13.7 If direct defects are prominent, it is useful to suture them loosely across before inserting the mesh. A suture to approximate the conjoint tendon to the pectineal ligament medially will prevent bulging immediately postoperatively

distance between the anterosuperior iliac spines, and the height should be equal to the distance from umbilicus to the pubis. The lower lateral corners of the prosthesis are trimmed back about 2.0 cm on each side and rounded to accommodate the basin-like shape of the pelvis (Figure 13.8).

PLACEMENT OF PROSTHESIS

The prosthesis is grasped along its lower margin in four long artery forceps. Using these forceps, the prosthesis is placed on the peritoneum in the pelvis.

Suture to pectineal (Cooper's) ligament

Laterally the pectineal ligament is identified close to the femoral vein; the prosthesis is fixed to the pectineal

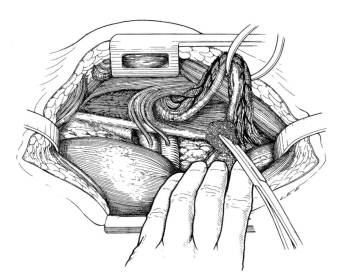

Figure 13.6 The testicular vessels and the vas are mobilized for 4 or 5 cm from the deep ring. These structures are then spread out, 'parietalized', before insertion of the mesh

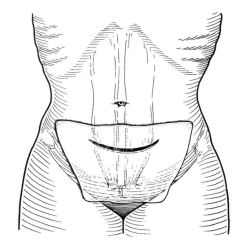

Figure 13.8 Measuring out the prosthesis

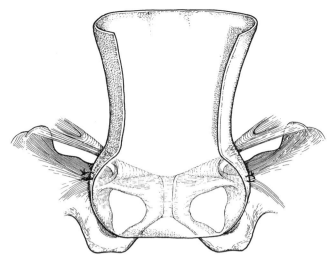

Figure 13.9 Suturing the prosthesis to the pectineal ligament

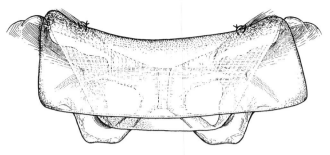

Figure 13.11 Suturing the prosthesis to the conjoint tendon

ligament at this point with a single interrupted polypropylene suture which is held untied in a haemostat. Further untied sutures are placed medially. When a series, at least three on each side, of sutures have been placed they are tied. After these sutures have been tied, the prosthesis should overlap the bony pelvis by 2 or 3 cm, extending down into the pelvis to the prostatic capsule (Figure 13.9)

Suture to lateral inguinal ligament

The lateral extremity of the prosthesis is now fixed to the deep surface of the inguinal ligament lateral to the deep ring and adjacent to its attachment to the anterior superior iliac spine. Care must be taken to avoid the cord structures and the femoral nerve which lies on the iliopsoas muscle beneath. There is a hazard to the lateral

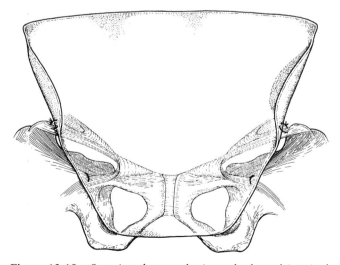

Figure 13.10 Suturing the prosthesis to the lateral inguinal ligament

cutaneous nerve of the thigh, which must be avoided. This manoeuvre completes the closure of the deep ring and the parietalization of the cord (Figure 13.10).

Suture to conjoint tendon and rectus sheath

The prosthesis is next sutured to the arch of the conjoint tendon – two interrupted sutures of polypropylene are sufficient (Figure 13.11). It is possible to achieve this fixation to the parietes cephalad to the deep ring and the direct area by a quilting suture from one lateral margin of the prosthesis to another.

With experience and careful placement technique a single polypropylene suture to the pectineal (Cooper's) ligament may suffice, thus avoiding any danger to the nerves.

CLOSURE

Suture to anterior rectus sheath

The linea alba is reconstituted, starting at the pubis and picking up the prosthesis in the midline. A continuous polypropylene metric 2 suture is used for this (Figure 13.12).

Closure of midline

The midline linea alba is closed in front of the prosthesis so that the linea alba closure is reinforced (Figures 13.13 and 13.14).

Closed suction drains should routinely be placed into the pelvic extraperitoneal space.

Subcutaneous tissue and skin closure are very important and should be carried out as described earlier (see pages 155, 156).

POSTOPERATIVE CARE

The patient is mobilized as early as possible after the operation. Oedema of the lower flap of the Pfannenstiel incision is common; it resolves slowly but spontaneously The drains are removed at between 24 and 48 h. Convalescence is smooth, but care must be taken to identify any

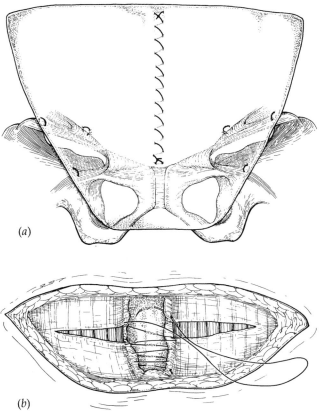

(a)

(b)

Figure 13.12 Closure: the prosthesis is sutured to the linea alba

signs of sepsis, which must be treated vigorously with appropriate antibiotics. If the patient shows a temperature above 38.5°C blood cultures should be taken and antibiotics started immediately. The antibiotic regimen will need adjusting if positive blood cultures are obtained.

The extraperitoneal, or preperitoneal, approach to groin hernias has already been described in children (see page 123) and now in this technique for extensive herniation.

The unilateral operation

Preoperative preparation and positioning of the patient is the same as for the bilateral operation.

THE INCISION

A half-Pfannenstiel incision placed two fingers-breadth above the pubic symphysis and extending from the midline laterally for 8–10 cm, is positioned well above the deep inguinal ring. Next, the rectus sheath is incised to expose the red belly of the underlying rectus abdominus muscle and the incision carried laterally into the aponeurosis of the internal oblique/transversus abdominus muscles for 1–2 cm (Figure 13.15).

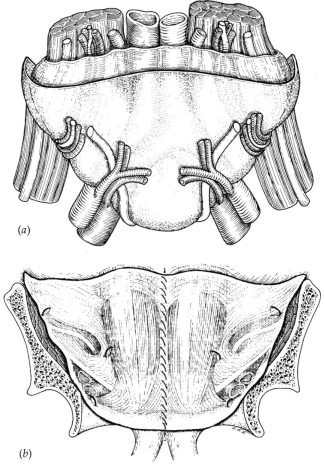

(a)

(b)

Figure 13.13 The completed operation: the mesh lies in the extraperitoneal layer and completely encloses the anterior pelvic peritoneum

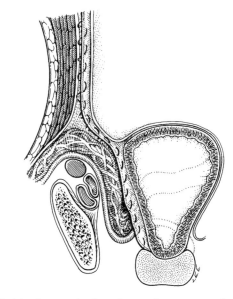

Figure 13.14 Parasagittal section to demonstrate the mesh in the extraperitoneal layer and lining the pelvis down to the prostatic capsule

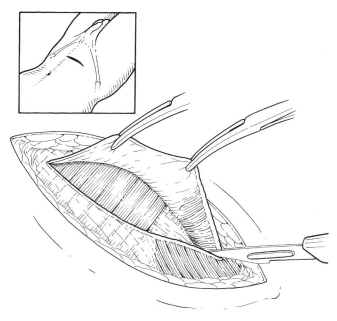

Figure 13.15 A transverse incision is made two fingers-breadth above the pubic symphysis from the midline, deepened to incise the rectus sheath and laterally into the aponeurosis of the oblique abdominal muscles.

An assistant then retracts the rectus muscle medially and it is dissected from the underlying filmy transversalis fascia. It will usually be necessary to divide and ligate the inferior epigastric vessels which cross the operative field (Figure. 13.16)

DEVELOPMENT OF EXTRAPERITONEAL SPACE

Following incision of the transversalis fascia the preperitoneal space is entered. The underlying viscera are retracted manually with the non-dominant hand and the preperitoneal space is developed by blunt dissection using a pleget mounted on a deep haemostat (Figure 13.17). The exposure should bring into view the oblique muscles of the abdominal wall, the superior pubic ramus, the posterior wall of the inguinal canal and the structures of the cord entering and leaving it, the femoral opening, and the pectineal (Cooper's) ligament.

Indirect inguinal hernia sacs, direct inguinal and femoral sacs are mobilized and managed surgically as for the bilateral operation.

PARIETALIZATION OF CORD STRUCTURES

Wantz emphasizes this manoeuvre in order that the spermatic cord is dissected away from the peritoneum to permit these structures to be placed against the pelvic wall so that the prosthesis can be laid between them and the peritoneum.[967] This step, however, is not performed by Rignault,[788] nor does he carry out any approximation of the margins of the defect with sutures. Nyhus[709] closes the defect, but does not parietalize the

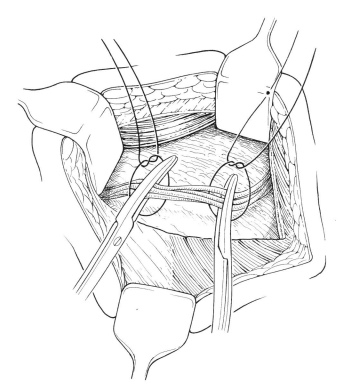

Figure 13.16 The rectus muscles retracted medially. The transversalis fascia is incised and the inferior epigastric vessels ligated and divided

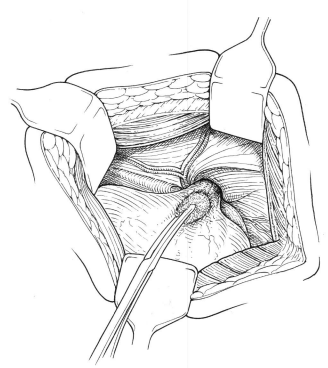

Figure 13.17 The prepositioned space is exposed in all directions, in preparation for the mesh

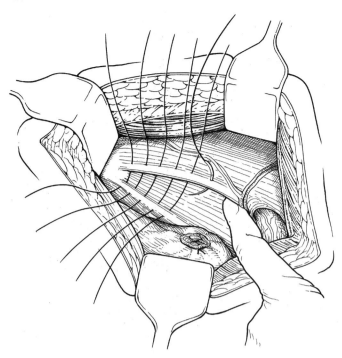

Figure 13.18   Redundant peritoneal sac has been excised. The fused transversalis fascia–transversus abdominis layer is approximated to the iliopubic tract (below)

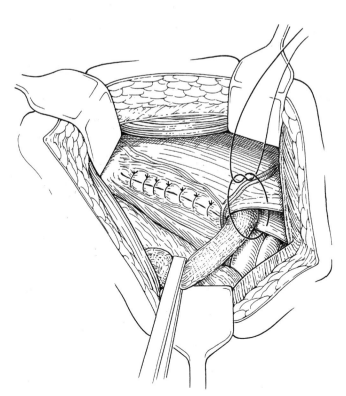

Figure 13.19   The transversalis fascia sling lateral to the cord is closed to reconstruct the internal ring

cord before placement of a supplementary polypropylene mesh prosthesis.

The Nyhus technique of closure of the defect without parietalization is illustrated in Figures 13.18 and 13.19. The upper margin of the defect is thickened transversalis fascia and the arch of the aponeurosis of the transversus abdominus muscle; the lower margin is iliopubic tract. The more medial sutures also pick up Cooper's ligament inferiorly and lateral sutures can be placed lateral to the internal ring.

MEASURING AND CUTTING OUT THE PROSTHESIS

As for the bilateral operation, wide coverage of the myopectineal orifice is necessary. The optimal shape is trapezoid (Figure 13.20). The final position of the prosthesis is shown in Figure 13.21. The essential points of fixation by sutures are:

1. Medially to the pectineal (Cooper's) ligament by two or three interrupted sutures.
2. Laterally to the fascia over iliacus.
3. Behind the abdominal wound with two or three tacking sutures (Figure. 13.22).

CLOSURE

It is essential to close the anterior rectus sheath with a continuous, non-absorbable monofilament suture which also repairs the lateral extension into the internal oblique/transversus abdominus muscle; failure to do this could result in an incisional hernia or acquired Spigelian hernia lateral to the rectus sheath.

RESULTS

The Stoppa bilateral operation, termed the 'Great Prosthesis for Reinforcement of the Visceral Sac' (GPRVS), was reported by the Amiens group in 1984.[896] Of 255 operated patients 218 (84.2%) had an uncomplicated postoperative course. The haematoma rate was 7.9% and the local sepsis rate was 5.8%. Many of these patients were elderly or poor risk and had undergone multiple previous operations. Late results, with a follow-up rate of 91.3% at 2–10 years, revealed a recurrence rate of 2.5%. All the recurrences occurred during the first postoperative year, indicating that the pattern of recurrence does not follow the same course as anterior repairs. Few of the infections were deep and related to the prosthesis, and superficial suppuration was treated by antibiotics or a combination of antibiotics and drainage, with eventual healing. The merits of Dacron mesh (Mersilene) used by the French surgeons are discussed in Chapter 6. Rignault, utilizing large sheets of mesh without closure of hernial defects, reports similar results; during a 14-year period 767 patients underwent

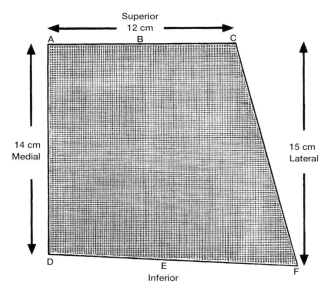

Figure 13.20   Trapezoid shapes of mesh to be inserted in preperitoneal space. The letters A–F illustrate the position of the mesh after placement (Figures 13.21 and 13.22)

preperitoneal prosthetic inguinal hernioplasty with a 2% sepsis rate and a 1.2% recurrence rate for recurrent hernias, of which there were 239 operations.[788] Once again, most recurrences were seen within the first postoperative year and were related either to sepsis or to technical mistakes made by inexperienced surgeons.

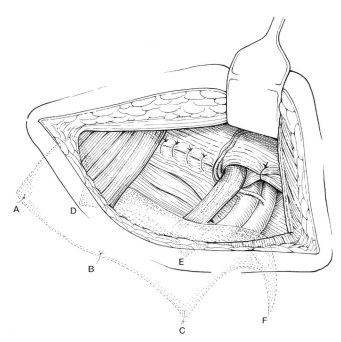

Figure 13.21   Positioning the mesh. The lower corner of the mesh (D) lies behind the symphysis pubis, the lower central part (E) is sutured to the pectineal (Cooper's) ligament and the lower lateral corner of the mesh lies on the iliacus, where it may be sutured to the pelvic fascia

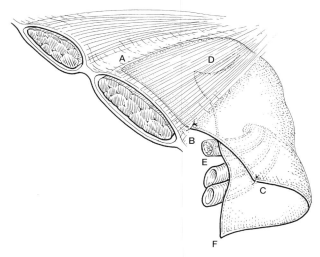

Figure 13.22   Anchoring sutures are placed into the pectineal (Cooper's) ligament and sometimes to the iliacus fascia. Superiorly the mesh is tacked to the abdominal wall above the incision (A,B and C), thus reinforcing the abdominal incision

Nyhus, reporting his preperitoneal approach and prosthetic buttress repair for recurrent hernia, assessed 203 operations in 195 patients.[709] Regional anaesthesia was used in most patients, no perioperative antibiotics were given and long-term follow-up was available for 115 hernias (56%) in 102 patients (52%) over a period of 6 months to 10 years. Eight patients had repeat recurrences at a mean of 30 months after repair but only two of these (1.7% of those followed up) have recurred after sutured repair supplemented with mesh buttress. The other six recurrences occurred in an earlier experience when no mesh buttress was being used. The authors state that the preperitoneal approach for recurrent groin hernia with reinforcing mesh buttress should be the procedure of choice for all recurrent groin hernias.

Similar results have been reported by other groups. Mozingo and colleagues treated 100 recurrent hernias in 84 men, with three re-recurrences occurring within 6 months of surgery at a follow-up of 6 months to 5 years. They reported few complications and no testicular complications.[679] Hoffman and Traverso used the technique in 175 patients with 152 primary and 52 recurrent inguinal hernias. They had one recurrence and wound complications occurred in 12 patients (5.9%).[429] Like Nyhus, these authors do not employ parietalization of the cord and close the defect with interrupted sutures before a large rectangle of polypropylene mesh is sutured to cover the entire myopectineal orifice, with fixation to Cooper's ligament, transversus abdominus medially and rectus muscle superiorly and laterally.[429] Finally, Horton and Florence[436] have described a preperitoneal approach, entering directly through the posterior inguinal wall under local anaesthesia, allowing the patient to go home within one or two hours of surgery. Because wide visualization of the preperitoneal space cannot be achieved with this approach it is likely that the mesh may shift, uncovering areas of the myopectineal orifice and causing the potential for recurrence. Additionally, suture fixation is blind resulting in a risk to vascular and neural structures in the preperitoneal space.

A further study from the Netherlands has confirmed the excellent results of the preperitoneal mesh repair in 75 patients with 150 hernias (24 primary and 126 recurrent) using Marlex mesh. The technique used placing the cord structures in a vertical slit in the mesh, is identical to that often used by one of the authors (H.B.D.) when there are difficulties mobilizing and parietalizing the cord in recurrent hernias.[81]

Advantages and disadvantages of the extraperitoneal operation

It is important to have a sense of proportion regarding the advantages and disadvantages of this approach to groin hernias.

The advantages of the extraperitoneal (preperitoneal) approach are:

1. It allows bilateral exploration through a single incision.
2. All hernial orifices are visible and easily explored.
3. Multiple sacs can be dealt with.
4. It is always easy to isolate sacs and divide and close them flush with the peritoneal cavity.
5. The anatomy of sliding hernias is more completely visualized.

6. If necessary, the peritoneal sac can be opened, e.g. if strangulation is present.
7. The layer of dissection is an unscarred virgin layer.
8. The repair is placed in the essential, fascia transversalis, plane.
9. In recurrent hernias there is no dissection of the cord vasculature and hence no risk of testicular ischaemia.

Some disadvantages of the extraperitoneal approach are:

1. It is impossible under local anaesthesia and without muscle relaxation.
2. More assistance, retraction and illumination are required than using the conventional anterior exposure of groin hernias.
3. The retraction of the rectus muscles laterally makes it difficult to identify the medial margins of direct inguinal defects.

Conclusions

The extraperitoneal mesh operation is very valuable in the surgery of complex, or recurrent, groin hernias. The approach exploits the extraperitoneal plane which is usually unscarred and easy to dissect. There need be no opening into the peritoneal cavity and no manipulation of viscera. Postoperative ileus is not encountered. With care, bleeding is minimal and a rapid convalescence the rule.

This is not a first choice routine operation for primary, uncomplicated groin hernias.

14 LAPAROSCOPIC GROIN HERNIA REPAIR

(with P.J. O'Dwyer)

Introduction

The first report of a hernia repair using laparoscopy was made by Ralph Ger in 1982.[335] In a patient with right indirect inguinal hernia the neck of the sac was closed with a series of staples using an operating laparoscope and a cannula placed in the right iliac fossa. Although this procedure was carried out in November 1979 Ger states that the first patient to be treated by laparoscopic closure of the neck of the sac was under the care of Dr Fletcher of the University of West Indies, Jamaica.

The use of prosthetic material for laparoscopic repair of an inguinal hernia was introduced by Corbitt[199] and Schultz[832] in 1991. These repairs involved the use of a polypropylene plug, patch, or both to close the inguinal canal in a tension-free manner. Because of unacceptably high early recurrence rates these approaches were abandoned in favour of laparoscopic preperitoneal prosthetic hernia repair. This repair follows the same principles as the open Stoppa repair.[897] After opening the peritoneum and reducing the hernia sac a large piece of mesh is placed in the preperitoneal space covering all potential hernia sites in the inguinal region. The peritoneum is then closed and the mesh becomes sandwiched between the preperitoneal tissues and the abdominal wall and, provided it is large enough, is held there by intra-abdominal pressure until such time as it becomes incorporated by fibrous tissue.

The intraperitoneal placement of mesh was introduced by Fitzgibbons et al.[305] as a method of laparoscopic hernia repair. This operation is performed using minimal dissection by leaving the hernia sac in situ and covering the defect with mesh, which is stapled to the surrounding peritoneum. The major concerns with this repair are the risk of injury to underlying structures from staples and of obstruction or fistula formation as a result of adhesions between bowel and exposed mesh. These concerns have resulted in this repair being performed in a few centres only under strict experimental conditions. Other materials, such as expanded polytetrafluoroethylene, are thought less likely to cause adhesions and are also being investigated with this repair.

The totally extraperitoneal approach to laparoscopic hernia repair was first reported by Ferzli[298] and later by McKernan and Laws.[636] As the peritoneal cavity is not entered with this approach it is the endoscopic equivalent of the open operation, the only difference being the size of mesh used. In open preperitoneal prosthetic approaches the mesh used is larger as it must extend up under the lower abdominal midline or transverse incision used for access to the preperitoneal space in order to prevent the subsequent development of an incisional hernia. Open preperitoneal prosthetic approaches to hernia repair are associated with low recurrence rates and considered by many to be the treatment of choice for patients with bilateral and recurrent hernias. The first investigators[298, 636] to explore totally extraperitoneal hernia repair fixed the mesh to the pectineal ligament and surrounding muscle above the iliopubic tract with staples. More recently, however, with the use of a larger mesh size many now avoid any method of fixation. This is our preference for most groin hernias and the following is a detailed description of totally extraperitoneal hernia repair with a short summary of other laparoscopic approaches.

Extraperitoneal operation

ANAESTHESIA

Although totally extraperitoneal hernia repair can be performed using either local or epidural anaesthesia, it is our preference to use general anaesthesia with complete muscle relaxation and mechanical ventilation. This ensures that the respiratory and cardiovascular changes that occur with extraperitoneal CO_2 insufflation are minimized. These changes are similar to or less than those observed with intraperitoneal CO_2 insufflation, and may be related to the size of the space created during the preperitoneal dissections.[977] All patients undergoing totally extraperitoneal hernia repair receive DVT prophylaxis. Use of antibiotic prophylaxis is controversial in this situation with little evidence for or against their use.

POSITION OF THE PATIENT ON THE TABLE

Before attempting totally extraperitoneal hernia repair it is important to ensure that the patient's bladder is empty. This can be achieved by asking the patient to micturate before entering the operating suite. The

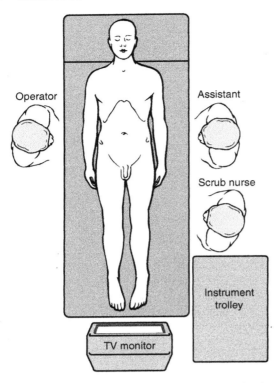

Figure 14.1 Position of operator, assistants and television monitor at the operating table for repair of a left inguinal hernia

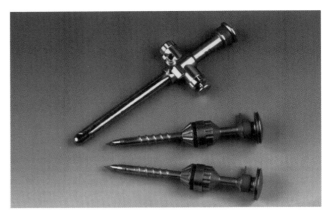

Figure 14.2 Trocars and cannulas used for totally extraperitoneal hernia repair

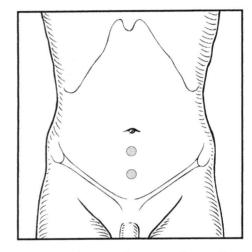

Figure 14.3 Sites of trocar placements for totally extraperitoneal hernia repair

patient should be placed on the operating table in the supine position with a 15° Trendelenburg tilt. Ideally both hands should be placed by the patient's side to allow the operator and the assistant to stand opposite each other at the patient's epigastric level. The operator stands on the side opposite to the hernia being repaired. The television monitor should be placed at the foot of the table (Figure 14.1). If two monitors are being used one should be placed at either side of the lower end of the operating table.

TROCARS AND TROCAR POSITION

One 10 mm cannula and two 5 mm cannulas are required for this operation. The 10 mm cannula should have a blunt-nosed trocar as it is inserted using an open technique. The 5 mm cannulas should have built-in fixation threads to prevent them from moving in and out of the extraperitoneal space as instruments are passed through (Figure 14.2). In addition, because of the confined operating space, the 5 mm cannulas should be short (60 mm). All the cannulas are placed in the lower midline. The 10 mm cannula is placed in a sub-umbilical position, one of the two 5 mm cannulas is placed one-third of the way between the symphysis pubis and the umbilicus and the other half way between the symphysis pubis and the umbilicus (Figure 14.3).

LAPAROSCOPE

Some surgeons substitute the 0° laparoscope for a 45° laparoscope after developing the extraperitoneal space. We find that this is not necessary and that the operation can be completed satisfactorily with a 0° laparoscope.

DEVELOPING THE EXTRAPERITONEAL SPACE

A vertical incision of 1–1.5 cm, starting in the lower half of the umbilicus and extending inferiorly in the midline, is made. The tissues are then separated with artery forceps and retracted with two Langenbuch retractors to expose the anterior rectus sheath on the side of the hernia to be repaired. The sheath is opened with a scalpel through a small transverse incision. The midline and rectus muscle are identified and the space between the rectus muscle and the posterior rectus sheath developed using artery forceps. A blunt-nosed 10 mm trocar and cannula (Figure 14.2) is then inserted into this space and

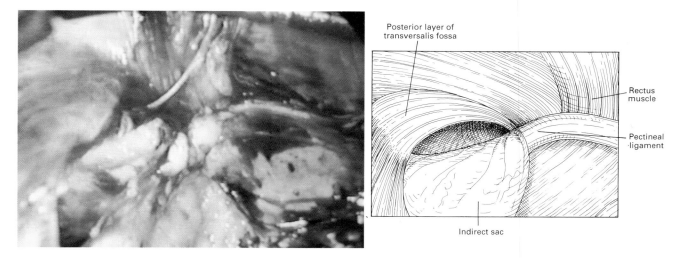

Figure 14.6 Endoscopic appearance of the deep layer of fascia transversalis

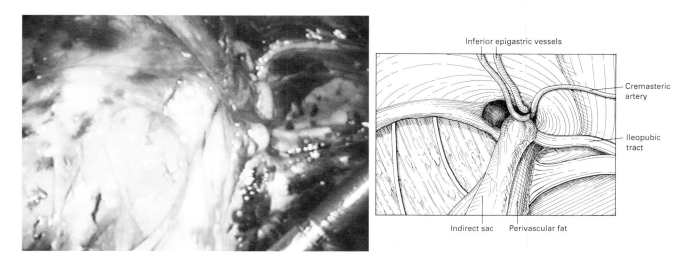

Figure 14.7 Endoscopic appearance of an indirect sac

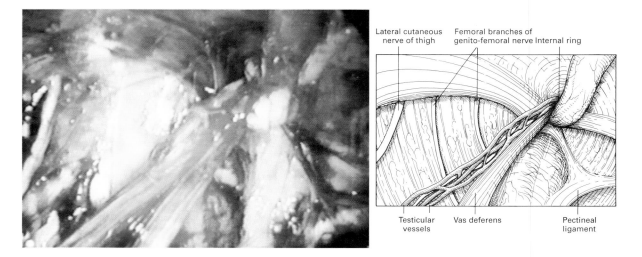

Figure 14.9 Endoscopic appearance of femoral branches of genito-femoral nerve and lateral cutaneous nerve of thigh

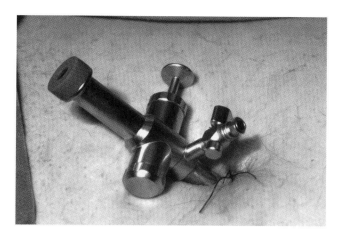

Figure 14.4 Use of skin stitch to seal the sub-umbilical cannula

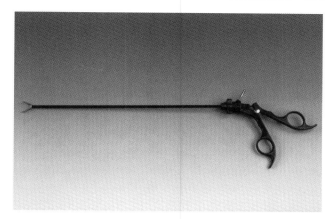

Figure 14.5 Blunt-nosed dissectors with atraumatic jaws are suitable instruments for totally extraperitoneal hernia repair

moved medially, laterally and posteriorly to develop the preperitoneal space. The skin around the cannula is sealed with a figure-of-eight stitch (Figure 14.4) and at this stage insufflation with CO_2 can commence, insufflation pressure being kept to 10–12 mmHg. A 0° laparoscope is then inserted through the 10 mm cannula and can be gently used as a blunt dissector to further enlarge the space. It is important to feel the pubic symphysis, and stay in the midline and immediately posterior to the rectus muscle with the laparoscope during this dissection. Once the pubic arch is visible, two 5 mm cannulas are inserted under direct vision in the positions previously described.

The preperitoneal space may also be developed using balloon dissection. A deflated balloon on the end of a cannula, of which many different types are available, is placed in the preperitoneal space using the access described. The balloon is then filled with air and the space developed under direct endoscopic vision. This method is helpful in the learning period when surgeons are still unfamiliar with the preperitoneal anatomy. However, balloon dissection has the disadvantage that it adds unnecessary expense to the operation. In addition, it is associated with bladder and bowel injury in patients who have had previous lower abdominal surgery.[409]

DISSECTION

Two dissectors which will grasp but not tear the peritoneum are important for this part of the procedure (Figure 14.5). A sharp pair of scissors is also helpful. It is important to identify the anatomical landmarks in an ordered fashion. The pectineal (Cooper's) ligament on the same side as the hernia should be exposed first. At this stage in thin patients you may see the external iliac vein laterally and accessory obturator vessels, if present, will be found crossing the pectineal ligament. Separation of the perivascular and extraperitoneal fat is performed

in the avascular plane between both using gentle blunt dissection, and is aided by the CO_2 insufflation. Characteristic filamentous tissue, which breaks down easily, will be observed between the two planes.

The retropubic space can now be developed in the midline and on the side of the hernia to above the level of the obturator nerve and vessels. The inferior epigastric vessels should next be identified and the space between them and the extraperitoneal fat developed. During this part of the dissection it is important to keep the epigastric vessels up against the rectus muscle using one dissector while the other is used to separate the tissues. If this is not done the epigastric vessels will come down into the operating field and small branches between them and the rectus muscles will be torn, giving rise to troublesome bleeding. Between the inferior epigastric vessels and extraperitoneal fat a fascial layer is encountered. This represents the deep layer of the fascia transversalis (Figure 14.6; see colour insert) forming its U-shaped sling around the cord and should be divided using a combination of blunt and sharp dissection to open up the space lateral to it.

INDIRECT INGUINAL HERNIAS

At this stage it should be possible to identify the sac of an indirect inguinal hernia (Figure 14.7; see colour insert). The sac will be found immediately lateral to the inferior epigastric vessels as it enters the internal ring. The sac should be grasped at the internal ring and reduced by retracting and dissecting the adhesions between it and the inguinal canal. Tension needs to be kept on the sac during this part of the dissection by using both dissectors in a stepwise fashion; otherwise as the sac is released to regrip it, it will return to the inguinal canal because of its elasticity and inguinal attachments. It is important to dissect all the tissues around the sac down to the peritoneum. These tissues represent attenuated transversalis fascia (see Chapter 2) which invests the cord and indirect sac as it enters the internal ring. Once this has been achieved the sac can be lifted up and the vas deferens will be visible at its posterior border and may be dissected off it along with the testicular vessels. The vas runs medially and crosses over the iliac vessels as it descends into the pelvis, while the testicular vessels take a course slightly lateral to the iliac vessels. In small to moderately sized indirect inguinal hernias, the apex of the sac can be identified and the sac completely reduced into the extraperitoneal space. If the sac is large and entering the scrotum, it is wise to divide and ligate it at a convenient point as one would do with open hernia repair. The testicular vessels and vas deferens should be completely skeletonized of any lipomatous material that may be in the inguinal canal. Not infrequently, a small hole may be made in the sac during its reduction. This should not impair the ability to complete the dissection and such defects can usually be ignored. Posteriorly the peritoneal dissection should be taken back until the vas can be seen descending into the pelvis. Laterally it should go to at least to the level of the anterior superior iliac spine while medially dissection should cross the midline and go well below the pectineal ligament (Figure 14.8). This is to ensure that there is adequate space for insertion of the mesh.

Lateral to the testicular vessels the femoral branch of the genitofemoral nerve and the lateral cutaneous nerve of the thigh can be identified in patients with little adipose tissue (Figure 14.9). Care should be taken not to damage these or a small branch of the deep circumflex iliac artery which lies lateral to the cutaneous nerve of thigh. Also in thin patients the external iliac vessels will be easily identified, the artery appearing between the testicular vessels and the vas and the vein lying medial to the artery. In all patients the characteristic pulsation from the external iliac vessels will be observed in this position. Small peritoneal branches arising from the iliac artery may also be noted during the dissection and as these are usually at the posterior limit of the dissection they can be preserved. As all dissection is carried out in an avascular plane there should be no need to use electrocautery during the operation. Most dissection is performed by gentle separation of tissues using atraumatic dissecting forceps.

INDIRECT INGUINAL HERNIAS IN FEMALES

These are approached as for indirect hernias in males. Once the sac is reduced the round ligament can be left *in situ* or divided and ligated at the internal ring depending on the surgeon's preference.

DIRECT INGUINAL HERNIAS

A direct inguinal hernia will be encountered during the dissection to expose the pectineal ligament. The defect lies lateral to the border of the rectus muscle and is usually medial to the inferior epigastric vessels except when a combined direct and indirect hernia is present. Sometimes a direct defect can appear to encroach on the femoral canal and in this circumstance may be confused with a femoral hernia. Patients with a direct hernia will also occasionally be found to have a femoral hernia. The direct hernia sac and preperitoneal fat are usually easy to reduce by grasping the sac with atraumatic forceps and simple pulling. While the hernia is being reduced the characteristic appearance of a pseudosac, which is attenuated transversalis fascia, will be displayed. This should be allowed to retract into the defect. As with indirect hernias, the sac is reduced into the extraperitoneal space and no attempt is made to open or ligate it. The vas and testicular vessels need to be exposed to exclude a synchronous indirect hernia and the extent of dissection should be as for indirect hernia repair. It is important to be careful during this part of the operation as the peritoneum is easily torn at the internal ring in patients with a direct hernia.

FEMORAL HERNIAS

As the pectineal ligament is exposed as far lateral as the external iliac vein in all patients a femoral hernia should not be missed during totally extraperitoneal hernia repair. This can be reduced in the same manner as for direct hernias. Once this has been done dissection should proceed as for other groin hernias.

RECURRENT HERNIAS

Considerable experience with totally extraperitoneal hernia repair is required before dealing with recurrent hernias. This is because the anatomical landmarks are

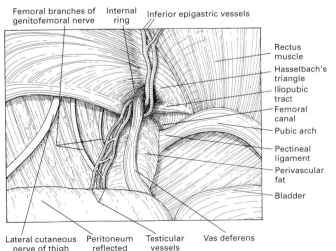

Figure 14.8 Extent of dissection required with details of anatomy observed at endoscopy

often distorted due to the previous repairs. The inferior epigastric vessels may have been divided and thus be in part absent or visible as a much smaller vessel. Dense adhesions form between the neck of the recurrent sac and the previous repair and because of this it is wise to use careful sharp dissection to free it from these adhesions. Elsewhere the peritoneum is often very thin and easily torn as stitches may have gone through it from the previous repair.

BILATERAL HERNIAS

Bilateral hernias can be repaired using the same access as for unilateral hernias and additional trocars are not required. Once dissection has been completed on one side, the operator simply switches to the other side and reduces the contralateral hernia. Although one large piece of mesh can be used for bilateral hernia repair, it is our preference to use two pieces of 15 cm × 10 cm. In this circumstance it is helpful to staple one to the pectineal ligament before the contralateral mesh is placed into position.

MESH

An open-weave monofilament polypropylene mesh should be used for this type of hernia repair. The mesh should be at least 15 cm × 10 cm with the corners rounded to facilitate placement in the preperitoneal space (Figure 14.10). The mesh is introduced blindly with a dissecting instrument through the sub-umbilical cannula and should not be rolled for this purpose. The laparoscope is then used to push the mesh into the retropubic space and in this position it can be opened, grasped at one corner and placed in the desired area. The mesh should cover all potential defects, i.e. direct, indirect and femoral canal, while its inferior fold lies on the vas and vessels for at least 2 cm. This fold must be clear of the reflected peritoneum (Figure 14.11); medially the mesh should cross the midline and go below the

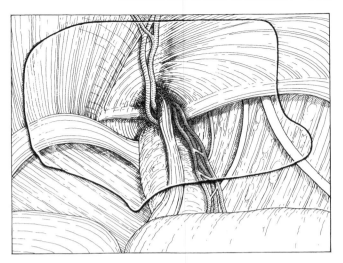

Figure 14.11   Position of mesh (darkened area) covering all potential hernia sites

pectineal ligament while laterally it should extend well beyond the internal ring to the level of the anterior superior iliac spine. If the dissection is adequate the mesh will generally, once opened, fall easily into place. When positioning the mesh, it is important that one dissector is used to grasp it, usually the one in the most proximal cannula, while the other is used to bat it into place.

For all indirect hernias and most direct hernias the mesh does not need to be stapled or sutured in place. If, however, a large direct defect encroaches upon the femoral canal or there is a femoral hernia the mesh should be stapled or sutured to the pectineal ligament to prevent the inferior border of the mesh from slipping upwards and into the defect. The mesh does not need to be divided to fit around the cord or, indeed, sutured or stapled around the cord.

On desufflating the extraperitoneal space it is important to ensure that the inferior fold of the mesh does not roll up with the peritoneum. If an adequate dissection has been carried out this will not occur. After desufflation all cannulas are removed and the rectus sheath at the sub-umbilical incision is closed with 2/0 Vicryl, while skin is closed with interrupted 4/0 nylon or absorbable subcuticular stitches and adhesive tapes.

STAPLING THE MESH

To staple the mesh one of the 5 mm cannulas is removed and replaced with a 12 mm cannula. This allows the introduction of a staple gun. Two or three staples are placed only in the pectineal ligament in the situations previously mentioned. Some surgeons staple the mesh to rectus muscle medially and the transversus abdominis laterally. These staples provide no additional support for properly positioned mesh and can be avoided in all repairs. Alternatively the mesh can be sutured to the

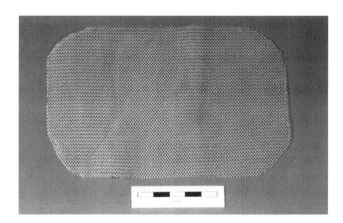

Figure 14.10   Prepared 15 cm × 10 cm polypropylene mesh

pectineal ligament with a 2/0 Prolene stitch or tacked with a 5 mm spiral tacker thus avoiding having to change cannulas.

Conversion to open repair

In 5% of cases conversion to open preperitoneal repair is required. This usually occurs as a result of a large tear in the peritoneum or, when a very large (estimated defect of 5 cm or greater) direct hernia is encountered. In the latter circumstance a 15 cm × 15 cm piece of mesh is required and is more easily placed at open surgery. If the hernia is unilateral, a small transverse incision is placed over the ipsilateral rectus muscle at the level of the lower 5 mm cannula and the preperitoneal space entered lateral to the rectus muscle. If there are bilateral hernias, a Pfannenstiel incision is made at the same level to gain access to the preperitoneal space.

Contraindications to totally extraperitoneal hernia repair

Although there are no absolute contraindications to totally extraperitoneal hernia repair in the elective setting, large inguinoscrotal or irreducible hernias are relative contraindications. Previous lower midline or ipsilateral paramedian incisions also come into this category. Extraperitoneal endoscopic repair is difficult and time-consuming in these circumstances such that it is difficult to justify attempting it in the first place.

Transabdominal hernia repair

This differs from the totally extraperitoneal approach in that the preperitoneal space is entered through a transverse peritoneal incision made above the hernia defect. The abdomen is entered using either closed or open laparoscopy and two additional cannulas are placed lateral to either rectus muscle at the level of the umbilicus. These can be two 5 mm cannulas or a 5 mm and 12 mm cannula if staples are to be used. The peritoneal incision should extend from the medial umbilical ligament medially to the level of the anterior superior iliac spine laterally. If the patient has a direct hernia it is wise to divide the medial umbilical ligament which carries the obliterated umbilical artery (see Chapter 2) to ensure adequate exposure of the pectineal ligament and retropubic space beyond the midline.

Once the preperitoneal space has been entered, dissection is as for totally extraperitoneal hernia repair. One of the important aspects of transabdominal hernia repair is adequate closure of the peritoneum after the repair. This can be accomplished by suturing or stapling

the peritoneum. A defect left between staples or sutures forms a potential source for internal herniation of small bowel. Both the umbilical and 12 mm port sites also require closure to prevent port site hernias developing.

As with the totally extraperitoneal approach there are no absolute contraindications to this repair; indeed, it can be easier to perform for patients with large inguinoscrotal hernias or with extensive lower abdominal surgery than the extraperitoneal approach.

Other methods of laparoscopic hernia repair, such as internal ring closure, plug and patch technique and intraperitoneal onlay mesh, are not based on any open technique and as such are experimental methods. The plug and patch technique has been associated with high recurrence rates and abandoned by most surgeons. Basic research continues in an effort to find a prosthesis that will not cause adhesions between it and the intestines for intraperitoneal onlay mesh techniques, while internal ring closure is limited to young patients with Nyhus Type I or II hernias.

Results

Laparoscopic inguinal hernia repair is still under evaluation and as such should not be performed except in a clinical trial or prospective audit setting. Early indications, however, are that it will become an important addition to existing methods of hernia repair, particularly for repair of recurrent and bilateral inguinal hernias. Its role in the management of unilateral primary inguinal hernias is less certain but should be answered by the various large randomized trials comparing laparoscopic with open hernia repair that are currently under way in the UK, Europe and North America.

OUTCOME DATA FROM RANDOMIZED CLINICAL TRIALS

Although there are at least ten randomized trials comparing laparoscopic with open hernia repair only six of these have randomized 100 or more patients. Short-term outcome measures from these trials show a modest benefit for laparoscopic over open approaches in terms of reducing postoperative pain (Table 14.1).[63, 165, 534, 726, 895] In a study from Glasgow[998] wound complications, particularly haematomas and seromas, were significantly reduced by the totally extraperitoneal approach. This finding differs from that of the other randomized trials and is likely to reflect the strict follow-up of all our patients at one week postoperatively by a research fellow and nurse. None of the complications in this study required any patient to be readmitted to hospital and all had disappeared by 4–6 weeks after operation. There may also be some benefit for the laparoscopic approach in terms of a more rapid return to normal activity (Table

Table 14.1   Outcome from randomized clinical trials

Authors	No. randomized	Operations compared	Pain	Complication rates	Return to normal activity/ work
Stoker et al.[895]	150 patients	TAPP vs. Darn	Less	8% vs. 21%	3 vs. 7 days
Payne et al.[726]	100 patients	TAPP vs. Lichtenstein	No difference	12% vs. 18%	9 vs. 17 days
Champault et al.[165]	181 patients	TEP vs. Shouldice	Less	No difference	12 vs. 24 days
Barkun et al.[63]	130 patients	TAPP vs. Darn/Lichtenstein	Less	22% vs. 12%	9 vs. 10 days
Lawrence et al.[534]	128 patients	TAPP vs. Darn	Less	12% vs. 2%	22 vs. 28 days
Wright et al.[998*]	120 patients	TEP vs. Lichtenstein/Stoppa	Less		2% vs. 45%
Liem et al.[567]	994 patients	TEP vs. Conventional open	Less	2% vs. 1%	14 vs. 21 days

* Compares wound haematoma and seroma rates 1 week after surgery when all patients were assessed by an independent observer; TAPP: transabdominal preperitoneal; TEP: totally extraperitoneal

14.1) although the magnitude of this is likely to be small and better assessed by larger clinical trials.

OUTCOME DATA FROM PROSPECTIVE NON-RANDOMIZED CLINICAL TRIALS

These studies[727] provide some information on what the recurrence rates are likely to be in the short term following laparoscopic hernia repair (Table 14.2). In a multicentre trial by Fitzgibbons et al.[304] overall recurrence was 4.5% after a minimum follow-up of 15 months. Recurrence rates for individual surgeons varied between 0 and 14.5% and improved with experience. The recurrence rate for 126 recurrent hernias repaired in this study was 4%.

Bladder injury occurs in 0.1% of patients while small bowel obstruction occurs in 0.3% of patients after laparoscopic hernia repair.[727] The latter complication is almost unique to transabdominal repair and occurs because of failure to close the peritoneum properly. Bladder injury has been reported following both transabdominal and totally extraperitoneal repair. In the latter circumstance this injury has been associated with balloon dissection in patients with previous lower abdominal surgery. Port site hernias have also been reported with laparoscopic hernia repair and are associated with the 10–12 mm port sites used for access for stapling instruments. The fascial defect created by such ports should be sutured to prevent this problem. Complications associated with inducing a pneumoperitoneum such as vascular and visceral injury, although rare, are potentially fatal and vascular injury can be avoided by using open rather than closed laparoscopy.

Inappropriate use of staples lead to many serious complications when laparoscopic hernia repair was first introduced. These included injury to the lateral cutaneous nerve of thigh, the femoral nerve and iliac vessels. Such injuries were avoidable and occurred because of a lack of understanding of the anatomy of the preperitoneal space combined with a poor knowledge of how preperitoneal prosthetic hernia repair works.

Complications

Most of the complications that occur in laparoscopic hernia repair can be attributed to:

1. Inadequate knowledge of the anatomy of the preperitoneal space.
2. Inappropriate use of staples to secure mesh (if required staples should only be placed into the pectineal ligament).
3. Use of the transabdominal rather than the totally extraperitoneal route for hernia repair.
4. Use of balloon dissection to expand the preperitoneal space in patients with previous lower abdominal surgery.

This suggests that with training and a better understanding of the preperitoneal approach to hernia repair, serious complications are likely to be no more frequent than with open hernia repair.

SEROMA OF THE INGUINAL CANAL

This complication deserves special mention as it can be confused with a recurrent hernia by both patient and

Table 14.2   Complications following endoscopic hernia repair[727]

Procedure	Number	Recurrence	Neuralgias	Testicular Pain	Chronic wound pain
Transabdominal preperitoneal	1944	1%	2%	0.5%	0.3%
Totally extraperitoneal	578	0%	1%	1.5%	0.3%

doctor. One to two per cent of patients will present with this problem some 1–2 weeks after totally extraperitoneal hernia repair. A well defined mass which lacks a cough impulse is palpable in the inguinal region of these patients and is treated by needle aspiration of the serous fluid.

Personal experience

Our early experience with laparoscopic hernia repair was with the transabdominal approach. Because of the increasing number of small bowel obstructions reported with this technique we changed to the totally extraperitoneal approach in 1993 and initiated a multicentre randomized clinical trial to evaluate laparoscopic hernia repair. Since January 1994 one author (P.J. O'D.) has entered 320 patients into this trial. In the open arm of the trial all primary inguinal hernias were repaired using the Lichtenstein method, while patients with bilateral or recurrent hernias underwent Stoppa repair. In the laparoscopic arm, all hernias were repaired using the totally extraperitoneal approach.

All patients were assessed by history and clinical examination at one week postoperatively and are currently being examined on an annual basis by an independent assessor for five years. The early outcome data show a significant reduction in wound morbidity in favour of the endoscopic group. Postoperative pain and analgesic consumption has also been less for the endoscopic group.[998] With 180 patients having passed their 1-year follow-up there has been one hernia recurrence in each arm of the trial. In the laparoscopic arm this occurred in a patient who had undergone totally extraperitoneal repair 12 months previously for a very large direct hernia. At reoperation a defect had occurred between the upper border of the mesh and the original hernia indicating that the size of mesh used had been too small. We now use a 15 cm × 15 cm mesh for such large hernias and will convert to open surgery to place the mesh if we are not satisfied with its position after endoscopic placement.

Disadvantages of laparoscopic hernia repair

One of the major drawbacks of laparoscopic surgery is the steep learning curve associated with its use. As with other forms of hernia repair, recurrence rates and complications are high in the learning period. Such recurrences are often not true recurrences but failure to repair the hernia in the first instance; for example, an indirect sac may be missed or inadequately reduced, mesh size may be too small or incorrectly placed. If any of these circumstances arise a persistent hernia will usually be apparent within days or weeks of the attempted repair. In a study by Liem et al.,[566] evaluating the learning curve for four laparoscopic surgeons inexperienced in totally extraperitoneal repair, the actuarial recurrence rate was 10% at six months postoperatively. Over 50% of recurrences were due to overlooking or insufficiently reducing an indirect hernia sac.

We estimate that it may take as many as 100 laparoscopic hernia repairs before a surgeon can bring the operating time for laparoscopic hernia repair into a range similar to that for open hernia repair. Since operating time is expensive this has significant cost implications. Added to this, laparoscopic hernia repair is already more costly than open repair, principally because of the use of disposable instruments. These costs, however, can be brought into a range similar to that of open repair by using reusable rather than disposable instruments and by suturing rather than stapling when indicated. A hidden cost, often not considered, is use of the laparoscopic equipment itself, which is currently less durable and more expensive than conventional instruments. These costs can be minimized by frequent use and extra care by nursing and medical staff during their use.

Some surgeons are reluctant to place mesh in patients under 40 years of age because of a potential risk of chronic sepsis or neoplastic change at the site of hernia repair. While mesh rejection due to chronic sepsis does occur, it is very rare and few cases have been reported in the world literature. There has been only one report in the literature of neoplastic change occurring at the site of a prosthesis (a sarcoma developing after a Dacron bypass graft for vascular trauma) and in this case evidence of a causal relationship was weak.[421] The relative difficulty in performing laparoscopic hernia repair using local anaesthesia is often cited as a drawback of this operation. This only applies, however, when safe general anaesthesia is not available at an institution. Despite its many proponents there is no evidence that use of local anaesthetic is safer than general anaesthesia for hernia repair.

Conclusions

Laparoscopic preperitoneal prosthetic hernia repair is technically more demanding than open anterior approaches. This, combined with a poor knowledge of preperitoneal anatomy by many, will limit its use to surgeons with a special interest in laparoscopic surgery. Nevertheless, it has modest advantages in terms of reduced postoperative pain, lower wound morbidity and a more rapid return to normal activity than open repair. These advantages need to be balanced against increased costs and a high recurrence rate in the learning curve period. Results from large randomized clinical trials evaluating laparoscopic hernia repair are likely to determine its future role in the management of the patient with a groin hernia.

15 INGUINAL HERNIA IN ADULTS (II) – THE OUTCOMES

Pre-war and wartime experience of inguinal hernioplasty

A trudge through the inguinal hernia literature from 1900 to 1986 would be, for the reader, reminiscent of the Via Dolorosa: better then to define your objective and map the Voie Sacrée only.

Thus, up to the present day there has been a continuous and inventive search for the ultimate hernia repair. Surgeons become the evangelical protagonist of one technique, whereas the more pragmatic suggest that a number of different operations must be in the armamentarium of a hernia surgeon. Nevertheless, a surgeon should adopt a single technique for primary inguinal hernia, direct or indirect, in the adult male, because there is no doubt that results improve with standardization of technique and continued practice and application.

An overview of the results of inguinal hernia repair between the two world wars is presented by Clear (1951).[180] Writing from the Veteran's Center, Dayton, Ohio, he presents 1048 inguinal hernia repairs performed from 1935 to 1938 on male ex-servicemen aged 25–78 years. All the patients were followed up for 10 years. Nine hundred and ninety-two procedures were done under spinal anaesthesia, 47 under local anaesthesia and nine under general anaesthesia. The overall recurrence rate was 11% at 10 years; 62% of recurrences occurred within five years, the remaining 38% developing between five and 10 years after surgery. In primary repairs there were 20.3% recurrences when catgut was used as the repair suture, compared with 15.5% with silk. With recurrent hernias the advantage of silk as a repair suture was further emphasized: 33.3% recurrences with silk, compared with 50% for catgut. When fascia was used on recurrent hernias, the Gallie operation, 45% recurred. The most usual operation was the Halsted I, although towards the end of the review period there was a shift to the McVay/Cooper's ligament repair.

There were only 54 complications in the entire series of 1048 operations, a remarkable achievement allowing us to quote these results as being at the 'up market' end of the USA surgical spectrum for the era. The complications were 10 wound infections and 31 transient episodes of ischaemic orchitis, with five cases of testicular atrophy. There were only three chest complications.

Wartime surgery for inguinal hernia was often unsatisfactory. Some of the controversies highlighted have been mentioned elsewhere.[718] Clear cites other reports of 10-year recurrence rates for indirect inguinal hernia from 4.2% to 8.3%, using the Halsted II/Ferguson technique; from 5.6% to 20.0%, using the 'Bassini operation'; for fascial repairs, rates from 3.0% to 9.2%, are recorded. Ten-year recurrence rates for repair of primary direct hernias range from 5.3% to 33.3%.

Moloney, writing 10 years later, after reviewing the poor results of inguinal hernia repair from Service hospitals during World War II, remarks that before the war 'the worst of hernias were capable of repair' and continues that many of 'the recurrences were the results of bad surgery by inexperienced operators'.[658]

Moloney himself was convinced of the need to repair and reinforce the posterior wall of the inguinal canal with a substantial buttress to which the tissues would take kindly. His 'darn' was accomplished with monofilament nylon which could be tailored to individual need, and was pliant and well fixed to the surrounding tissues. Moloney first repairs the fascia transversalis with a nylon suture on the medial side of the deep ring to reconstruct a secure snug sling for the cord.[649]

Then he turns his attention to reinforcing the posterior wall with his 'darn'. The darn is in two layers commencing at the pubic tubercle, darning laterally then back medially. Inferiorly the darn picks up the inguinal ligament and iliopubic tract, superiorly it is quilted up to and through the tendinous portion of the internal oblique. The darn is loose, no attempt being made to approximate the internal oblique to the inguinal ligament (Figure 15.1).

After reading and quoting from Moloney's own description three technical points need emphasizing: (a) he repairs the fascia transversalis at the deep ring; (b) only aponeurosis/tendon are used as the anchor tissues; (c) he does not distort the anatomy by approximating the internal oblique to the inguinal ligament.

Moloney originally reported 400 simple inguinal hernias repaired by the nylon darn technique. At two years' minimum follow-up he had no recurrences. In the initial 400 cases sepsis occurred as a complication seven times; all septic cases healed spontaneously without having the nylon removed. He had no cases develop wound sinuses.[658] In a subsequent letter to the Lancet in

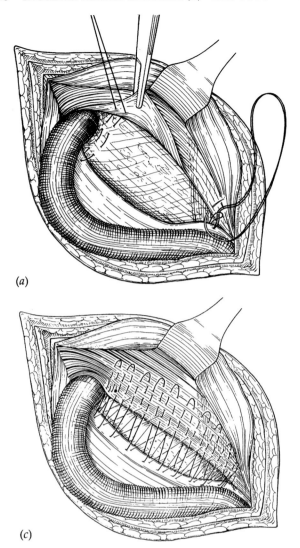

(a)

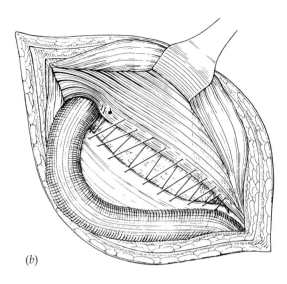

(b)

(c)

Figure 15.1 Moloney's nylon darn repair of an inguinal hernia. (a) Initial suture reinforcing and tightening the internal ring. The start of the darn medially. (b) Loose continuous suture between the lower edge of the internal oblique muscle and the inguinal ligament. (c) Second layer of continuous suture, passing through the rectus sheath medially and the tendinous portion of the internal oblique laterally (From Moloney, 1960,[659] by permission)

1960 Moloney reported that sinuses were not a problem with a properly performed nylon darn.[659]

The application of the inguinal darn by other surgeons, however, has not been so successful. In the Kinmonth modification of the Maloney darn, Lifschutz and Juler reported 115 nylon darn repairs in 100 patients followed up for an average of 62 months. The recurrence rates were unacceptably high, being 3.5% for primary hernias and 8.3% for recurrences.[568]

Simple indirect sac high ligation and excision (herniotomy) for the young soldier with an inguinal hernia was suggested as an alternative which even the most unskilled surgeon could employ. This operation gives poor results in adults.

MacLeod, in 1955, reported 161 soldiers operated on using this technique; there were 19 recurrences, equivalent to 14.3%.[594] McVay and Chapp (1958) reported a similar series, with a recurrence rate of a 5.5%.[644] Ogilvie perceptively comments that once the contents (intestine) have entered into an adult congenital sac the neck (of the fascia transversalis) is dilated and simple removal of the sac will not cure the hernia.[644]

Another corruption of fascia transversalis repair which appeared again in the stress of wartime was 'Coley's stitch', placed lateral to the cord at the deep ring. This stitch effectively abolishes the 'shutter action' of the deep ring and, because it is through red muscle, it will of necessity cut out, enlarging the defect and making the inevitable recurrence more difficult to repair.[188, 563, 686] 'Coley's stitch' must be condemned.

Invagination or imbrication without division of the fascia transversalis does not lead to sound union. Fascia or aponeurosis must be 'freshened up' or divided to initiate fibroblast activity and repair.[686]

Problems of evaluation

Our objective is to identify the best operation for inguinal hernia. To do this we need to decide rational methods of evaluating inguinal hernia operations, then define the principles involved in inguinal hernia surgery, and finally we must review the practicality of these techniques and choose our own favourite picture from the exhibition. It is no exaggeration to say there are many methods of inguinal repair, but are they all of equal merit and are they all equally valuable to the patient?

Evaluation introduces the contributions of Doran and Marsden in the UK, Palumbo and McVay in the USA and Glasgow in Canada.

Doran, in a series of major contributions over a 25-year period, used clinical evaluation and the prospective randomized trial, animal experimentation and socio-economic evaluation to elucidate aspects of the 'huge statistical slagheap' which had built up in herniology between 1900 and the end of World War II in 1945.[259, 261]

Doran and Lonsdale, in 1949, used radio-opaque markers introduced at operation and subsequent X-ray follow-up to demonstrate that if the conjoint tendon was sutured to the inguinal ligament, over the ensuing six months the conjoint tendon spread apart from the inguinal ligament in 7 out of 10 cases. Most interestingly, if the fascia transversalis was repaired deep to the suture of the conjoint tendon the hernia repair remained clinically sound, although the tendinous structures were demonstrated to have separated on the X-ray – clear evidence for the value of fascia transversalis fascia repair.[263]

Doran investigated the reliability of statistical evaluation and in a classic paper demonstrated the unreliability of many of the archival reports[261] (Tables 15.1 and 15.2). The possibility that cases 'lost to follow-up' could alter the recurrence rate by 70% was demonstrated (Table 15.3).

Doran was the first to employ the prospective randomized trial, invented by the agriculturalist Fisher, with an operation technique decided by 'lot'. This trial demonstrated again the value of simple and accurate suture of fascia transversalis around the deep ring in straightforward indirect inguinal hernia. It gave a recurrence rate of 1.96%, compared with 4.76% when an external oblique fascial sling was put around the cord and 3.5% when a fascial patch was added to the transversalis layer. Doran concluded that until a rival technique has proved its supremacy in a test conducted according to Fisher's rules, a simple suture of the fascia transversalis of the deep ring should be regarded as the operation of choice for severe primary indirect inguinal hernia with a narrow neck.[262]

The use of nylon net as a prosthetic mesh to repair the posterior wall of the inguinal canal was well researched by Doran in 1961. In this study three kinds of netting were used which differed from each other in the thickness of the strand and the closeness of the weave. The 'thin net' was fine undyed curtain netting, which was implanted in the fascia transversalis layer of 86 patients with inguinal hernias (83 males and 3 females: 50 primary indirect, 14 direct and 22 recurrent inguinal hernias). The sepsis rate was 1.2% – in one patient the net had to be removed to resolve the ongoing sepsis. At 2 years 20% of the hernias had recurred. This net and technique were abandoned.[264]

The thick net was used in 15 cases; a 53.3% sepsis rate followed – and the net had to be removed in eight patients before sepsis could be controlled. The technique is described as 'disastrous' and was abandoned.

The medium net was knitted by the author's own theatre staff and then sterilized. This net and technique gave encouraging results. Unlike the thin net this prosthesis was not perceived as a substitute or reinforcement to the fascia transversalis, rather it was sewn onto the upturned edge of the inguinal ligament below and onto the anterior surface of the conjoint tendon/internal oblique above. The cord was brought out under the

Table 15.1   To show that in 13 major series the number followed up is inadequate and the number examined unknown or grossly defective (From Doran, 1962,[261] by permission)

Author	Year	Total of series	Followed up	Examined
Bull and Coley	1907	1525	837	Not stated
Davis	1916	1756	754	614
Hoguet and Coley	1918	5525	2506	Obscure
Taylor	1920	2230	816	356
Erdman	1923	1093	978	978
Coley	1924	1155	332	332
Gibson and Felter	1930	1618	1463	Not stated
Fallis	1936	1600	800	Obscure
Grace and Johnson	1937	1115	659	659
Skinner and Duncan	1945	1126	755	'A few'
Garner	1947	2643	2220	1354
Hagan and Rhoads	1953	1082	766	766
Palumbo, Paul and Mighell	1954	1375	1176	64

Table 15.2 To show irregularity in length of the follow-up in 13 major series, and to demonstrate the rapid deterioration of efficiency of follow-up with the passage of time (From Doran, 1962,[261] by permission)

Author	Year	Span of follow-up	Gibson and Felter's series (Total, 1618: followed up, 1463)	
			Length of follow-up	Number
Bull and Coley	1907	1–14 yr	3 mth	567
Davis	1916	1 yr only	4 mth	267
Hoguet and Coley	1918	1–25 yr	5 mth	122
Taylor	1920	1–20 yr	6–12 mth	341
Erdman	1923	2 yr only	1–2 yr	99
Coley	1924	6–18 mth	2–3 yr	12
Gibson and Felter	1930	3 mth–13 yr	3–4 yr	12
Fallis	1936	2–10 yr	4–5 yr	12
Grace and Johnson	1937	1–10 yr	6–7 yr	9
Skinner and Duncan	1945	1–3 yr	7–13 yr	12
Garner	1947	1–10 yr	Died	9
Hagan and Rhoads	1953	2–5 yr		
Palumbo, Paul and Mighell	1954	1–6 yr		

Table 15.3 To demonstrate the degree of uncertainty in 13 major series due to defective follow-up, resulting in wide margin between known recurrences and possible number of recurrences (From Doran, 1962,[261] by permission)

Author	Total in series	Followed up	Known recurrences	Possible recurrences
Bull and Coley (1907)	1525	837	10(0.65%)	698(45.7%)
Davis (1916)	1756	754	67(3.8%)	1069(60.8%)
Hoguet and Coley (1918)	5525	2506	25(0.45%)	3044(55.4%)
Taylor (1920)	2230	816	46(2.1%)	1460(65.4%)
Erdman (1923)	1093	978	73(6.7%)	188(17.2%)
Coley (1924)	1155	332	28(2.4%)	851(73.6%)
Gibson and Felter (1930)	1618	1463	48(2.9%)	203(12.5%)
Fallis (1936)	1600	800	66(4.1%)	866(54.1%)
Grace and Johnson (1937)	1115	659	170(15.2%)	626(56.1%)
Skinner and Duncan (1945)	1126	755	14(1.2%)	385(34.2%)
Garner (1947)	2643	2220	177(6.7%)	600(22.7%)
Hagan and Rhoads (1953)	1082	766	42(3.8%)	358(33.0%)
Palumbo, Paul and Mighell (1954)	1375	1176	14(1.0%)	213(16.2%)

lower edge of the net at the midpoint of the inguinal ligament. This artificial reconstruction of a neo-internal ring has not been adopted by later protagonists of net or mesh repair. Neither Martin and Max, Barnes, Lichtenstein, nor Capozzi and colleagues create an artificial internal ring, rather the mesh is sutured to reconstruct the pre-existing internal ring.[64, 152, 559, 619]

Doran used the technique in 212 patients with six septic wounds (2.83%) and in each of the septic cases a second operation to remove the net was necessary before healing was achieved. Seventeen patients were lost to follow up at two years, while four recurrences were found in 189 cases whose wounds were healed soundly and who were available for follow-up at two years. This represents a recurrence rate at two years of 1.9%. Alternatively, if the early septic cases are counted as failures the rate rises in 10 out of 189 cases (5.3%) or, if the lost cases recurred, to 27 out of 212 (12.7%). They report that the more nylon inserted the greater the incidence of chronic sinus: 1.2% with thin nylon, 2.83% with medium and 53.3% with thick nylon net repairs.

Lastly, they again confirmed the essential truth of surgical asepsis and advised great care with asepsis 'in all its aspects' when nylon net is used for hernia repair.

This study is an important milestone in British surgery and must be read in the context of its time. The surgeon authors were 'workers' in a provincial district, executing a prospective trial of their day-to-day work: they were experimenting with new technology and achieving results much better than their contemporaries. They debunked prevailing surgical prejudice by demonstrating that new fibres could achieve success where failure had been demonstrated previously using meshes. The clinical research was reinforced by laboratory work with rabbits and by autopsy recovery of net from patients who died of unrelated causes after surgery.

The quest for an optimal bio-material, which should be inert, resistant to infection, achieve rapid fixation to host tissue, and be completely incorporated by fibroblastic reaction, continues. For the present knitted monofilament, polypropylene mesh (Marlex mesh) is the recommended material (see Chapter 6).

Doran and colleagues investigated the scope and safety of short-stay surgery. They demonstrated the usefulness of the technique and rightly observed that short-stay surgery would improve throughput by allowing more patients to be treated.[200]

Over 25 years, McVay has concerned himself with the anatomy and technique of inguinal hernia repair and with evaluating his methods.[642] With Halverson his review of 1211 hernioplasties performed and followed up over a 22–year period is a notable contribution.[387] This report highlights the continuing attrition of excellent early results when follow-up is purposeful and complete: in 1958 McVay reported a recurrence rate of 2.24%, but by 1969 this had increased to 3.5% – this projects to 4.2% at the end of 25 years. A humbling experience, but also a tribute to the enthusiasm of the team and to their pursuit of excellence.

From the statistical studies two important conclusions can be drawn – most (62%) of recurrences have occurred by five years, but there is a continued new recurrence rate for up to 25 years. To project the final recurrence rate to 25 years the following tabulation can be used:

All patients followed up	Multiply rate by:
1 year	5.0
2 years	2.5
5 years	1.5
10 years	1.2

It is suggested that in a group of hernioplasties with mixed durations of follow-up it is more realistic to break the series up into one year, two-year and five-year groups and then use this tabulation to derive conclusive recurrence rates. Unless a report contains the number of hernias followed up for each given time, it is misleading. Short-term studies are so misleading that most of them can be ignored. Unless the surgeon re-examines the patient, any estimate of recurrence rates is guesswork.

McVay has redefined the anatomy of the inguino-femoral region and reached the conclusion that any repair not based on a sound understanding of the anatomy of the fascia transversalis and the importance of repairing it is doomed to failure. Repairs in the plane of the inguinal ligament only are unsound and incur high recurrence rates. McVay himself has always championed the repair of the fascia transversalis to the iliopectineal (Cooper's) ligament for the larger direct hernias. For smaller indirect hernias he regards repair of the deep ring alone as adequate. His results confirm his theories. Isaac has confirmed that in direct hernias there is often a deficient attachment of the conjoint tendon and fascia transversalis to the iliopectineal line. He repairs this using a technique similar to McVay; again his results confirm the importance of the fascia transversalis/transversus lamina in inguinal hernioplasty.[455]

The McVay/Cooper's ligament operation is a standard technique with much to recommend it. It repairs the fascia transversalis and is particularly applicable to the medial end direct hernia and to the femoral hernia in the female. Rutledge records 906 consecutive primary Cooper's ligament repairs with a recurrence rate of 1.9% overall: 3.5% for direct and 1.1% for indirect inguinal hernia.[813] The patient follow-up was 97%, 80% of patients being examined, and average follow-up was nine years. The operative technique, however, is extensive, requiring deep retraction with Deaver's retractors, Trendelenburg position, and in 13% of patients a Marlex mesh overlay was used. With a 5% testicular atrophy rate in skilled hands, this operation might have medicolegal consequences.[814] Rutledge comments that the recurrence rate rises to 5.5% if the cord is brought out straight through the external oblique and transplanted subcutaneously. Testicular atrophy occurred in 7.9% of recurrent hernia repairs. In the series there were two instances of pulmonary embolism. In a further patient, femoral vein compression was demonstrated phlebographically. An alternative, less invasive, technique is to use Duplex scanning.[704]

Two clinical trials (one prospective, one retrospective) have compared the results of the Cooper's ligament operation with the Shouldice repair. Glasgow from the Shouldice Clinic achieved a 4.9% recurrence rate in 263 patients after 22 years of follow-up with Cooper's ligament repair, whereas his results with 4812 Shouldice repairs over 21 years resulted in a 0.7% recurrence rate.[355] This was a retrospective review. Panos and colleagues in a prospective randomized study, determined the recurrence rates with differing techniques performed in a surgery residency programme.[723] In 269 patients, 308 direct hernias were repaired over a six-year period, all the operations being supervised by staff surgeons. Thereafter, yearly follow-up with an 87% compliance was carried out during an average follow-up period of 36.4 months. Recurrence rate was 8.8% for the Cooper

Table 15.4 Surgical skill as a factor in recurrence of hernia (From Marsden, 1962,[615] by permission)

Status of surgeon	Type of hernia						Total	
	Primary oblique		Primary direct		Recurrent			
	Total	Recurrence	Total	Recurrence	Total	Recurrence	Total	Recurrence
House surgeon	23	3	12	3	0	0	35	6
Registrar	733	38	228	16	53	7	1014	61
Visiting staff	342	16	126	8	67	16	535	40

Table 15.5 Comparison of results of the common surgical techniques (From Marsden, 1962,[615] by permission)

Group	Type of repair*	Primary oblique hernia			Primary direct hernia		
		Total	Recurrence	Recurrence rate (%)	Total	Recurrence	Recurrence rate (%)
A	McArthur–Morrison	265	17	6.5	75	6	8
B	Bassini with artificial fibre	281	11	4	110	5	4.5
C	Wyllys–Andrews II	113	1	1	34	2	6
D	Bassini, Wyllys–Andrews III with artificial fibre	144	6	4	68	4	6
E	Bassini with catgut	104	8	7.7	19	4	20

*McArthur–Morrison. Apposition of the conjoint tendon and inguinal ligament behind the cord by a continuous suture strip of external oblique aponeurosis left attached at the symphysis pubis.
Bassini. Bassini's name has been applied quite incorrectly – but very conveniently – to simple apposition of the conjoint tendon and the inguinal ligament behind the cord in the length of the canal.
Wyllys–Andrews II. This technique consists of bringing down the upper flap of external oblique to the inguinal ligament behind the cord and bringing up the lower flap in front of the cord, so that the cord lies between the two flaps of external oblique. Behind this, the posterior wall is strengthened by the suture of fascia transversalis to the inguinal ligament – many of the registrars replace this latter step by a Bassini repair.
Wyllys–Andrews III. This has been used incorrectly, but very conveniently, for the simple suture or, more commonly, the overlapping of the external oblique behind the cord described by Halsted. In most cases the Bassini technique has preceded the Wyllys–Andrews III.

ligament repair and 6.6% for Shouldice repair. For bilateral inguinal hernias repaired six weeks apart the recurrence rate was 12.8%. Although these results would appear to be poor, the authors point out that the overall recurrence rates of 7.7% are similar to the rates reported by others for direct inguinal hernia repair by general surgeons not specializing in herniorrhaphy. However, the results must be interpreted in the light of 50% of patients being excluded, due to refusal of the patient to agree to follow-up, refusal by surgical staff to include patients because of unfamiliarity with both repairs, or failure to obtain consent. The McVay/Cooper's ligament technique is described in detail on page 163.

Controversies remain; some surgeons obtain equally good results by closing the fascia transversalis to the iliopubic tract/iliofemoral sheath (Shouldice operation). As McVay observes: they use meticulous technique and careful deep bites into the iliopubic tract to achieve this – possibly biting into Cooper's ligament medially. And the status of a rectus-relaxing incision is hard to assess. McVay recommends it and has excellent results to support his argument, whereas others never use it.

Marsden, in Liverpool, has written powerfully about the results of surgery for inguinal hernia. His database is a series of 2000 inguinal hernia repairs performed in the Liverpool teaching hospitals[614-616] (Tables 15.4 and 15.5). In retrospect, his findings are not unsurprising and are a depressing review of British surgery. Many operative techniques are employed by seniors and juniors, there is little evidence of formal review or quality assurance, and house surgeons undertake operations and achieve less good results.

Marsden in 1959 concludes that there is much to go wrong after a hernia operation: a 7% chance of recurrence in the first three years; a 6% chance of infection including a 2% chance of a continuing wound sinus; a 3% chance of continuing wound pain; and a 2% chance of testicular failure (atrophy). Duration of bed rest and the time of return to work after operation do not influence the outcome. The only technical conclusion that can be safely drawn is that catgut repairs are more prone to recurrence than repair techniques using non-absorbable material.

A recurrence is defined as 'a weakness of the operation

area necessitating a further operation or the provision of a truss'. Thus defined a recurrence is an operative failure; this is superior to descriptions of a 'bulge' or 'thrill' at the operative site. It also allows of a follow-up question: 'Do you wear a truss?' or 'Have you had a second operation?' These are questions any patient can respond to. Non-progressive asymptomatic bulges are not defined as recurrences.

Marsden's depiction of teaching hospital hernia surgery in the 1950s is confirmed by the even more depressing results of hernia repair reported in 1960 by Shuttleworth and Davies from St. Thomas's Hospital, London. In their series of 266 metropolitan policemen, fit men in the age range 21–60 years (mean age 40 years), the recurrence rate in 204 indirect inguinal hernias was 14.2%, in 94 direct repairs 18.3%, and in 37 recurrent hernias 8.1%. When house surgeons operated on indirect hernias they achieved a 20% recurrence rate.[859] Again, many techniques of repair are used and there is no clear indication which is the best. There is no doubt, however, that repairs with non-absorbable sutures, nylon or braided polyester are better than those with catgut. The duration of bed rest after operation and the time of return to work had no influence on the outcome. Postoperative sepsis and ongoing sinus infection remain important complications. A further contribution from St. Thomas' in 1974 showed some marginal improvements in results using the darn technique[143] but the results fell far short of the results published by Shearburn and Myers in the USA[846] or Glasgow from the Shouldice Hospital in Canada.[354]

Kocher's operation – invagination and lateral displacement of the sac neck – modified by opening the canal, was subjected to a careful reappraisal by Celestin (1964). Over nine years he collected 212 patients who had 223 operations. He reported a 5–9-year follow-up on 88.5% of the cases, giving a recurrence rate of 5.4%: recurrence was accentuated in septuagenarians, probably the group with the most long-standing pre-existing damage to the fascia transversalis at the deep ring.[161]

Inguinal hernia surgery is operator dependent: the wartime experience, the gloomy reports from St. Thomas' Hospital and Marsden's reports all confirm that less trained surgeons get less good results. A review of 938 hernia operations in a Swedish community hospital in 1983 observes that the recurrence rate is more dependent on operator than operation.[453] Similar less than optimal results are commonplace, even in teaching institutions world-wide, when the operations are performed by a multiplicity of surgeons without particular interest or experience in the problem.[44, 497]

Our remaining important contributions come from the Shouldice clinic in Toronto. There are many Shouldice, Welsh, Iles and most prolifically Glassow and Bendavid papers. By the end of 1952 Shouldice was able to record 8401 groin hernia repairs. With experience his recurrence rate had dropped considerably, from 6.5% in his first 461 cases followed up from 1943, 1944 and 1945–52, to 0.1% in the most recent cases followed up to 2 1/2 years from 1952.[851] Glassow, in 1984, reviewed 10 353 cases with a 10-year recurrence rate of 1.1% [356] (Figure 15.2).

The Shouldice surgeons stress meticulous anatomic repair of the fascia transversalis, the use of non-absorbable sutures and early ambulation.

The Shouldice results in different clinics yield uniformly excellent outcomes compared with other operations. The Shouldice technique, with a recurrence rate of under 1%, justifies the adoption of this operation by those surgeons adequately trained in the technique[92, 249] (Table 15.6).

A technique that competes with the Shouldice operation in the hands of experts is the McVay/Cooper's ligament repair which again depends on careful anatomic repair of the fascia transversalis and its reinforcement at the medial end by attachment to the iliopectineal line.

Standardization, even in the hands of trainees, improves results. For instance, in a general surgical service over a three-year period 1977–1979, patients were allocated to two groups of surgeons. The first were

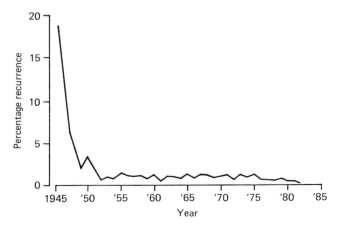

Figure 15.2 Recurrence rates of all hernias repaired at the Shouldice Clinic, Toronto, 1945–82. Each year's group of surviving patients was followed up for life and results were updated yearly (From Alexander, 1986,[10] by permission)

Table 15.6 Results of inguinal hernioplasty – Shouldice technique (After Glassow, 1984[354])

	No. repairs	No. recurrences	Recurrences (%)
Barwell (UK)	1566	28	1.8
Berliner (USA)	1084	12	1.1
Bursow (USA)	2000	70	3.5
Devlin (UK)	787	7	0.9
Dunn (USA)	2949	34	1.2
Glassow (Canada)	10353	112	1.1
Shearburn (USA)	953	7	0.7
Wantz (USA)	2470	23	0.9
Total	22162	293	1.3

general surgeons and general surgical residents with no special interest in hernia surgery utilizing the Bassini–McVay operation in 390 patients. A second group of 442 patients were assigned to a group of surgeons who had adopted a hernia service protocol. On this service a senior faculty member assisted surgical residents in the performance of all repairs using the Shouldice operation. There was no routine follow-up of the first group until the patients reappeared for care of the hernia service. The group of surgeons with a special interest in hernia repair followed up 82% of their patients for seven years. The infection and recurrence rates were higher in the general surgical service than in the hernia specialist service (5.9% versus 0.4% and 4.6% versus 0.9% respectively). This study illustrates that when junior surgeons undertake surgery, closely supervised and paying special attention to protocols, morbidity can be significantly reduced.[249, 250]

Using this argument it has been suggested that surgeons may seek to legitimize their enthusiasm for a favoured operative technique by comparing personal results in cases chosen by themselves and operated on by experienced surgeons committed to the task, with the standard results of operations performed by a typical mixture of doctors, often junior and unsupervised, who provide much of the routine healthcare[986] (Table 15.7). Specialization in herniorrhaphy is therefore best undertaken at hospital or unit level rather than at the level of the individual surgeon and practice should be based on standardized preoperative, operative and postoperative management to facilitate teaching, performance and reproducibility and to permit randomized studies.[835]

Recent results suggest that the Shouldice operation may not be the gold standard operation that it has been heralded to be for the last 20 years.[703] A retrospective

Table 15.7 Shouldice operation: a single surgeon and his trainees[986*]

	Number of primary repairs	Indirect recurrences (%)	Direct recurrences (%)
Barwell, 1974–1994	2669	0.8	2.7
Barwell trainees, 1974–1994	1293	5.2	5.0

*The recurrence rate for Barwell's trainee surgeons is similar to the cumulative recurrence rate in non-specialist units with trainees operating (Table 15.8)

review of 1936 operations performed during 1992 in eight hospitals in Sweden (catchment 761 000) revealed a 17% recurrence rate in a setting where 25% of surgeons were using the Shouldice operation.[703] The Shouldice Hospital has never performed a prospective randomized trial comparing its technique against any other. It has taken more than 40 years after the inception of this technique for the publication of the first such studies to materialize (Table 15.8).

Kingsnorth and colleagues, in a trial designed to rule out surgeon-dependent variables, prospectively randomized 322 patients with primary inguinal hernias to Shouldice repair or plication darn. Surgery was undertaken by 15 operators of whom 14 were surgeons in training who received a preliminary period of training until they were proficient with the operative techniques. After a mean follow-up of 30 months (range 24–48) there were seven recurrences in the Shouldice group (4.3%) and four in the plication darn group (2.5%). This recurrence rate is approximately five times higher than that recorded by the Shouldice Hospital, and the authors suggest that the failures were caused by collapse of the posterior wall within six months of repair, indicating that this is the area of technical

Table 15.8 Shouldice operation in non-specialist units*

	Total number (Shouldice repairs)	Median follow-up (months)	% recurrence	Selection	Predicted 5-year recurrence % (Shouldice numbers)
Kingsnorth 1992[498]	322 (151)	30	4.3	All	6.1 (9)
Panos 1992[723]	308 (154)	36.4	6.6	Direct only	8.2 (13)
Tran 1992[928]	142 (65)	24	10.8	Primary	16.4 (11)
Fingerhut 1993[301]	1593 (400)	60	3 (SSW)[a] 6 (PP)[b]	14 Centres, primary	3 (6) SSW 6 (12) PP
Paul 1994[725]	265 (119) (290)	40	1.7 / 5 (excluded patients)	Primary	2.1 (3) 6.1 (17)
Kux 1994[521]	750 (185)	40	3	All	3.7 (7)
Total (Shouldice)	(1354)				5.7 (78)

[a] Stainless steel wire
[b] Polypropylene
*In non-specialist units in which trainees often operate as the primary surgeon, the cumulative recurrence rate for the Shouldice operation is 5.7% in published series.

difficulty in reproducing the Shouldice Hospital results.[498] More trials have reproduced these results. Panos and colleagues achieved a 6.6% recurrence rate for the Shouldice operation in a residency training programme.[723] Fingerhut, reporting for the French Association for Surgical Research in a controlled trial of 1593 patients, found a recurrence rate of 6% using polypropylene for the Shouldice repair and 3% for stainless steel at five years.[301] Tran and colleagues from Cologne reported a dismal 10% recurrence rate for the Shouldice repair at two years in 142 patients with primary hernias operated on by both consultant surgeons and surgeons in training.[928] Kux and colleagues tested the standard Shouldice operation with four rows of polypropylene, and a modified Shouldice operation with two rows of polypropylene sutures against the Bassini operation using absorbable or non-absorbable sutures.[521] With an impressive personal clinical follow-up of 93.6% in surviving patients, the recurrence rate in the standard Shouldice operation group was 3.6% between 3 and 4 years, with a 2.3% recurrence rate in the modified Shouldice operation. Three board-certified surgeons and six residents performed the operations and the failure rate for recurrent hernias was 7.6%. An important observation long known to hernia surgeons was that of the 27 patients found to have a clinical recurrence, almost half were not aware of it.

The conclusion that must be drawn from these studies is the need for adequate training of surgeons undertaking the Shouldice operation, and meticulous reconstruction of the posterior inguinal wall as the cornerstone of this technique. With this caveat good long-term results can be obtained in a non-specialist setting.[463]

POPULAR MISCONCEPTIONS

Some popular myths of inguinal hernioplasty can be discarded. There are limited indications for using a relaxing incision and for dividing the cord. The preperitoneal approach (discussed on page 167) has been advocated for primary inguinal hernias. The retraction involved makes anatomic delineation of direct inguinal hernias difficult. Recurrence rates of up to 25% with direct inguinal hernia repair by this route are reported.[611] The use of insufficiently large pieces of mesh or inadequate application of the mesh on the lateral side, or both, may contribute to technical failure. Moreover, an extended learning curve for this operation seems to exist, and junior surgeons achieve considerably poorer results than senior surgeons.[829] In a study of 98 recurrent inguinal hernias repaired by the preperitoneal route, 32 re-recurrences occurred at 45 months, an exceptionally high rate of technical failure in the performance of the operation. This brings into question whether the preperitoneal route should be widely adopted, or whether it should be applied by specialist surgeons only. The preperitoneal repair is best reserved for second time or more recurrent inguinal hernias.

Techniques involving darning or suturing through fleshy red muscle give results less good than those achieved with the standard Shouldice operation. Plication of a weak fascia transversalis, posterior inguinal wall is an unsound procedure. If the posterior wall has sagged so much that it can be plicated, it should be excised and sutured, or replaced.[660] It has been argued by the protagonists of prosthetic mesh that in this situation prosthetic implant, transplant or replacement is required to overcome the primary disorder of connective tissue which cannot be achieved by approximation under tension or by continuous layers of suturing, which results in poorly vascularized healing tissues.

Return to normal activity and work

There is enormous variation in reported times for return to normal activity and work. For instance, in a socialized system of healthcare where patients' expectations and the insurance system still favour hospitalization, length of hospital stay after hernia surgery may be in excess of eight days.[372] Even in the USA, where a headlong rush for day-care surgery in ambulatory units has taken place, length of stay may be several days in institutions where reimbursement is not as strictly controlled as the private sector. Customers of the Metropolitan Life Insurance Company surveyed by a nationwide claims questionnaire revealed a length of stay that averaged 2.9 days.[811] In the US Army average hospital stay for hernia surgery is 4.6 days.[410] In reality housing conditions, distance from home to hospital, and availability of home nursing care (spouse, relative or friend) are the major factors affecting early discharge after hernia repair.[652] The French Association for Surgical Research investigated the feasibility of discharge within 48 h of inguinal hernia repair in 500 consecutive men with unilateral, uncomplicated non-recurrent inguinal hernias. Of 411 patients suitable for early discharge 107 (26%) eventually stayed longer than 48 h, early discharge was declined by 84 and contraindicated in 42 (these patients had local or general complications), which finally resulted in one-day surgery being performed in only 51 (10%) of the patients. These results emphasize the need for careful preoperative evaluation, which includes not only the hernia and the patient's general medical condition, but also any social conditions such as isolation, flights of stairs, or lack of a telephone, which may limit the ability to discharge a patient soon after surgery.

Advice concerning return to normal activity has been poorly managed by surgeons.[464] Recent studies indicate that factors limiting a patient's return to activity and work are governed principally by perceived amount of postoperative pain. Socioeconomic factors strongly influence this perception over and above the actual procedure performed or the anatomy involved.[822] In a case-controlled comparison of patients receiving workers compensation compared with patients having commercial insurance, seven surgeons from a single clinic compared 22 consecutive workers compensation patients with 22 commercial insurance patients. All patients had received open hernioplasty and the duration of postoperative pain and the days off work were compared. The differences between the two groups were striking: the median duration of postoperative pain in the workers compensation group was 27 days, with 36.5 days off work. In the commercial insurance patients the duration of postoperative pain was 7.5 days and they went back to work after only 8.5 days. Personal motivation, therefore, appears to be the most important factor affecting clinical outcome and return to activities. Return to normal activity and work is discussed further on page 58.

Stockton-on-Tees results

Since 1970 the Shouldice operation has been performed on all patients presenting with primary inguinal hernia and these patients have been followed up prospectively. The recurrence rate is 0.8% to date. The results are given in Tables 15.9–15.12.[244, 247]

These results confirm the clinical reliability of the Shouldice operation for inguinal hernia by a single surgeon with a special interest. Seven hundred and eighteen operations are recorded in this series, with six recurrences, five of these following re-interventions for complications of the suture material. The choice of suture material is important; the results with 34-gauge stainless steel wire and with metric 3 polypropylene are indistinguishable from each other and from the results of Glasgow using stainless steel wire. Stainless steel wire is difficult to handle and polypropylene is therefore recommended. The results using multi-strand braided polyester are less good; sinuses are a problem and this suture should be avoided.

Results also confirm that day cases (remaining in hospital for less than 8 h) and short-stay surgery (remaining in hospital overnight after the operation but being returned home within 24 h of surgery) using the Shouldice technique and general anaesthesia give acceptable recurrence rates. The recurrence rate and the complications rate for inguinal hernia repair are independent of the duration of postoperative stay in this series. Only 40% of patients undergoing repair of an inguinal hernia require to be hospitalized for more than 24 h (298 out of 718 in this series).

Table 15.9 Adult males (18 years): primary inguinal hernia repair, mid-1970 to mid-1982[*]

	Indirect	Direct	Pantaloon	Total
Right	256	119	20	395 (55%)
Left	210	103	10	323 (45%)
Total	466 (65%)	222 (31%)	30 (4%)	718 (100%)

[*] Anatomic type: 718 operations on 696 patients, i.e. 22 patients had metachronous bilateral repairs during the study period.

Table 15.10 Follow-up of patients in *Table 15.9* to 31 December 1983[*]

Duration of stay	Operations	Recurrences
0–8 h	198	2
Overnight	222	2
Longer than 24 h	298	2
Total	718	6

[*] 718 operations on 696 patients; 40 died during the follow-up period, 37 lost during the follow-up period.

Table 15.11 Age distribution of patients in *Table 15.9*

Age (years)	Total operations	Average duration of stay (days)
18–29	73	5.5
30–39	83	5.5
40–49	124	2.4
50–59	206	3.1
>60	232	5.7

Table 15.12 Follow-up and recurrence incidence in primary inguinal hernias in adult males[*] (see also *Tables 15.9–15.11*)

	No. operated on initially	No. died during follow-up	No. lost during follow-up	No. recurrences
At 1 year	718	5	5	1
At 5 years	521	20	14	6
At 10 years	197	40	37	4

[*] Life table analysis shows that the percentage probability of reaching 1 year without recurrence is 99.71%, 5 years 98.9% and 10 years 98.6%.

Individualized hernia surgery

Faced with many uncertainties regarding the optimal treatment of groin hernias and the requirement to develop operative strategies that are generalizable and applicable to every case, the surgical community has attempted to define the requirements in each scenario. The concept that an operation, which may give ideal results in experienced hands – the Shouldice operation for instance – may be difficult to learn and will give indifferent results in non-expert hands, while at the same time damaging normal tissue (for example dividing all the posterior inguinal canal wall in every case), has encouraged surgeons to define the different anatomic types of inguinal hernia and then match the repair to the defect found.

NYHUS CLASSIFICATION

The first attempt at classification was made by Nyhus in 1991.[706] Nyhus defined the status of the fascia transversalis in the posterior wall of the inguinal and femoral canal. He recommended minimalist repair of the medial side of the inguinal ring only when this was necessary and he warned against extensive posterior wall repair at the expense of disrupting a normal inguinal posterior wall. He railed against surgery that resulted in overtreatment of many comparatively simple hernias. Nyhus classified groin hernias into four types, which enabled individualization of surgery to be recommended.

Type I

Type I hernias are indirect inguinal hernias in which the internal abdominal ring is of normal size, configuration and structure. They usually occur in infants, children or young adults. The boundaries are well delineated and Hesselbach's triangle is normal. An indirect hernial sac extends variably from just distal to the internal abdominal ring to the middle of the inguinal canal.

Type II

Type II hernias are indirect inguinal hernias in which the internal ring is enlarged and distorted without impinging on the posterior wall (floor in American surgical anatomy) of the inguinal canal. Hesselbach's triangle (the posterior wall of the canal) is normal when palpated through the opened peritoneal sac. The hernial sac is not in the scrotum, but it may occupy the entire inguinal canal.

Type III

Type III hernias are of three subtypes: direct, indirect, and femoral.

1. **Type IIIA** hernias are direct inguinal hernias in which the protrusion does not herniate through the internal abdominal (inguinal) ring. The weakened transversalis fascia (posterior inguinal wall medial to the inferior epigastric vessels) bulges outward in front of the hernial mass. All direct hernias, small or large, are type IIIA.
2. **Type IIIB** hernias are indirect inguinal hernias with a large dilated ring that has expanded medially and encroaches on the posterior inguinal wall (floor) to a greater or lesser degree. The hernial sac frequently is in the scrotum. Occasionally the caecum on the right or the sigmoid colon on the left makes up a portion of the wall of the sac. These sliding hernias always destroy a portion of the posterior wall of the inguinal canal. (The internal abdominal ring may be dilated without displacement of the inferior epigastric vessels. Direct and indirect components of the hernial sac may straddle those vessels to form a pantaloon hernia.)
3. **Type IIIC** hernias are femoral hernias, a specialized form of posterior wall defect.

Type IV

Type IV hernias are recurrent hernias. They can be direct (type IVA), indirect (type IVB), femoral (type IVC), or a combination of these types (type IVD). They cause intricate management problems and carry a higher morbidity than do other hernias.

GILBERT CLASSIFICATION

Gilbert, another American expert, proposed another classification system based on anatomic and functional defects described at operation.[341] Gilbert classified groin hernias into five classes: types 1, 2 and 3 are indirect and types 4 and 5 direct. Type 1 has a tight internal ring through which passes a peritoneal sac of any size. When this sac is surgically reduced, it will be held within the abdominal cavity by the intact internal ring. Type 2 has a moderately enlarged internal ring which measures no greater than 4 cm. Type 3 has a patulous internal ring, greater than 4 cm, with the sac frequently having a sliding or scrotal component which usually impinges on the direct space. In type 4 hernias essentially the entire posterior wall (floor) of the inguinal canal is defective. Type 5 consists of a direct diverticular defect in a suprapubic position. Rutkow and Robbins added a sixth type to encompass those groin hernias which consist of both indirect and direct components and a seventh for femoral hernias.[811] As in any classification system, there can be numerous variations and combinations which are difficult to account for, and these variables (i.e., primary/recurrent, sliding component, reducible/incarcerated, lipoma) must be noted.

BENDAVID CLASSIFICATION[85]

Bendavid of the Shouldice Hospital has proposed an even more elaborate system, the TSD (type, staging, and dimension) classification scheme (personal communication, 1992). Five types of groin hernias are described: type 1 or anterolateral (formerly indirect): type 2 or anteromedial (formerly direct); type 3 or posteromedial (formerly femoral); type 4 or posterolateral (formerly prevascular); and type 5 or anteroposterior (formerly inguinofemoral). Each type is characterized by three stages which denote the extent of the herniation anatomically.

Type 1

Stage 1: Extends from the deep inguinal ring to the superficial inguinal ring.
Stage 2: Goes beyond the superficial inguinal ring but not into the scrotum.
Stage 3: Reaches into the scrotum.

Type 2

Stage 1: Remains within the confines of the inguinal canal.
Stage 2: Goes beyond the superficial inguinal ring but not into the scrotum.
Stage 3: Reaches into the scrotum.

Type 3

Stage 1: Occupies a portion of the distance between the femoral vein and the lacunar ligament.
Stage 2: Goes the entire distance between the femoral vein and the lacunar ligament.
Stage 3: Extends from the femoral vein to the pubic tubercle (recurrences, destruction of lacunar ligament).

Type 4

Stage 1: Located medial to the femoral vein: Cloquet and Laugier hernias.
Stage 2: Located at the level of the femoral vessels: Velpeau and Serafini hernias.
Stage 3: Located lateral to the femoral vessels: Hesselbach and Partridge hernias. (In type 4 hernias the stage does not imply the severity of the lesion.)

Type 5

Stage 1: Has lifted or destroyed a portion of the inguinal ligament between the pubic crest and the femoral vein.

Stage 2: Has lifted or destroyed the inguinal ligament from the pubic crest to the femoral vein.
Stage 3: Has destroyed the inguinal ligament from the pubic crest to a point lateral to the femoral vein.

In the TSD scheme the 'D' refers to the diameter (in centimetres) of the hernial defect at the level of the abdominal wall. Where a defect is not circular but ovoid or elliptical, the widest laterolateral measurement is recorded. There is also a series of subclassifications for type 2 hernias: the letters 'm, l, c, e' denoting whether a defect is located through the medial, lateral, central or entire portion of the posterior wall of the inguinal canal.

Examples of Bendavid's TSD scheme are as follows. An anteromedial hernia, near the pubis, 2 cm in diameter is labelled type 2, stage 1 (m), D2. An anterolateral hernia with a deep inguinal ring measuring 4 cm and extending into the scrotum is classified type 1, stage 3, D4. Where a hernia repair has failed twice, this is indicated as 2R and noted after the type; e.g. a twice-recurrent anterolateral hernia extending to the superficial inguinal ring with an internal ring measuring 5 cm would be labelled type 1 (2R), stage 1, D5. When a portion of a viscus contributes to a sliding hernia, the letter 'S' is noted after the type, as are the letters 'I' for incarceration and 'N' for necrosis. When the herniating component consists simply of adipose tissue, the letter 'L' is noted after the type and all the other characteristics of the TSD classification scheme are provided.

AACHEN CLASSIFICATION

Schumpelick from Aachen has simplified these systems on the basis of the more traditional European anatomic classification.[833] On the basis of this typing, he added a grading system of measurement of the hernial orifice. Grade I represents the normal diameter of the internal ring of up to 1.5 cm. He chose 1.5 as the measure because that is the average diameter of a surgeon's index fingertip or the length of the branches of laparoscopic scissors, simplifying the practical measurement. Indirect and direct hernias with an orifice of 1.5–3.0 cm are graded as category II. Grade III hernias are those with an orifice of greater than 3 cm. In combined hernias, the total diameter of the two defects is calculated and 'c' (for combined) is added.

The different localizations of the defect are indicated by the abbreviations L (lateral or indirect), M (medial or direct), and F (femoral) (Table 15.12).

Recommendations

On the basis of these systems of classification some principles, long since adhered to, can be appreciated:

1. If the deep ring is of normal diameter and the fascia transversalis is of normal strength it does not need to be disrupted; a simple excision of the indirect sac will suffice to cure the condition.
2. If the deep ring is stretched but the remainder of the posterior wall is normal a simple plastic operation to tighten the deep ring and resection of the indirect hernia sac will suffice; Lytle operation only is needed.
3. If the posterior wall is deficient (i.e. there is a direct hernia) a repair of the defect with reinforcement either by the Shouldice method or with mesh – the Lichtenstein operation – is needed.
4. With recurrent hernias, especially with complex recurrent hernias, an extraperitoneal mesh replacement will be necessary. Against this background of surgical requirements for individualized hernia repair the reports from personal case studies, cohort studies and randomized trials must be assessed. A key discriminant must be the generalizability of any operative recommendation. A systematic review of the literature concerning the choice of operation for groin hernia; has recently been published and confirms the recommendations in Chapters 12, 13 and 14.[174]

Conclusions

The Aachen classification is a sound basis to classify groin hernias and the individualization of the operation to repair the defects, along the lines indicated, should be applied. The operations recommended are all described in detail in Chapters 12, 13 and 14.

16 FEMORAL HERNIA

A femoral hernia is a protrusion of a peritoneal sac, covered with extraperitoneal fat, into the femoral sheath. The most common femoral hernia enters the femoral canal, which is that 'space' in the sheath medial to the femoral vessels as they proceed from the abdomen into the thigh. A femoral hernia sac may contain all or part of an abdominal viscus.

Femoral hernias occur much less frequently than inguinal hernias and are more frequent in females than males. The ratio of femoral to inguinal hernias varies: figures from 1:18 to 1:8 are recorded. A round figure of 1:10 is generally accepted. The female to male ratio of femoral hernias is 4:1.[240] Male patients with femoral hernias have frequently undergone an inguinal hernia repair.[351] Femoral hernias are more frequent on the right than left side in a ratio of 2:1 and are bilateral in 1 in 15 persons. In females femoral hernias are unknown in the young and their incidence increases with age 42% of femoral hernias are in women aged over 65 years.[811] However, it must be stressed that inguinal hernias are almost as frequent in women as are femoral hernias (see Table 3.2). Inguinal hernia is thus an important and difficult to make differential diagnosis of a groin swelling in a woman. In tropical Africa, femoral hernias are very rare; it is postulated that the frequency of inguinal lymphadenitis involving Cloquet's node in the femoral canal protects tropical Africans from femoral hernia.[186]

The aetiology of femoral hernia is ill understood. In contrast to inguinal hernia, there is no easy embryological explanation. The fact that femoral hernias are most frequently found in middle-aged and elderly females and the disparity in incidence between parous and nulliparous women suggests that intra-abdominal pressure and the stretching of aponeurotic tissue consequent on pregnancy are important factors. Chronic cough, intestinal obstruction, constipation and excessive physical labour may also contribute to raised intra-abdominal pressure. Weight loss in the elderly female is also associated with femoral hernia. Nurses are said to be more prone to femoral hernia. Ten per cent of femoral hernias follow a previous operation for an inguinal hernia; indeed, femoral hernias in men almost always occur after an operation for an inguinal hernia.[351, 753]

A very rare congenital femoral hernia in males is associated with descent of the testicle through the femoral canal into the thigh. Four well-documented cases are recorded in the literature. Absence of the ipsilateral testicle from the scrotum and an incompletely reducible femoral hernia should arouse suspicion.[892]

Anatomy

Femoral hernia has a sinister reputation because of the unyielding anatomy of the femoral canal. The whole canal (i.e. the space between the pubis and the iliopsoas muscle) is bounded anteriorly by the inguinal ligament, posteriorly by the pectineal (Cooper's) ligament at its attachment to the iliopectineal line of the pubic bone, medially by the sharp lateral margin of the lacunar ligament and laterally by the iliopsoas muscle with its overlying fascia (Figure 16.1).

The canal is divided into two compartments, the lateral being occupied by the femoral artery and femoral vein, and the smaller medial by areolar tissue, some lymphatics and a lymph node. The femoral vessels are encased in the femoral sheath of fascia transversalis. Anteriorly the sheath is continuous with the fascia transversalis deep to the inguinal ligament; posteriorly the femoral sheath fuses with the pectineal ligament. The sheath extends into

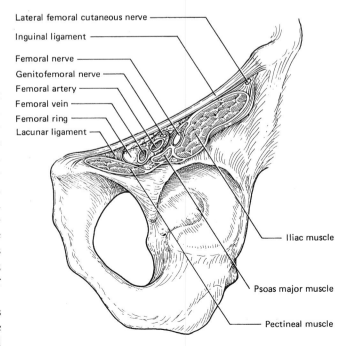

Figure 16.1 Boundaries of the femoral canal

the thigh. From the abdomen the sheath resembles a funnel extending down to the fossa ovalis where the saphenous vein penetrates the cribriform fascia (antero-inferior femoral sheath). It is through this small medial compartment or funnel that the usual femoral hernia penetrates into the thigh.[318, 586, 1005]

Once in the thigh the sac pushes anteriorly onto the relatively weak cribriform fascia – the anterior femoral sheath that surrounds the fossa ovalis opening for the saphenous vein. It carries the stretched cribriform fascia before it and bulges into the thigh. The fundus is then forced upwards to lie over the inguinal ligament. Two factors combine to make it turn superiorly: these are fusion of the femoral sheath with the deep fascia of the thigh and the repeated flexion of the hip joint (Figure 16.2).[586]

In its advancement into the thigh the hernial sac carries with it some extraperitoneal fat about its fundus and it may draw the extraperitoneal anterolateral wall of the bladder down with it on its medial aspect. Once the sac is entrenched in the thigh, the medial wall of the hernia, consisting of peritoneal sac, extraperitoneal fat and fascia transversalis, is pressed up against the sharp margin of the lacunar ligament medially, the unyielding pectineal fascia and pubic bone posteriorly, the inguinal ligament anteriorly and the femoral vein laterally. As the hernia emerges from the saphenous opening the sharp upper margin of the cribriform fascia also contributes to the structuring of the sac.[8, 1005]

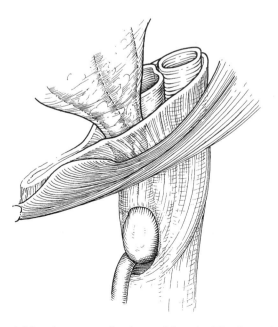

Figure 16.2 Anatomy of a femoral hernia. The hernial sac progresses down the femoral sheath 'funnel' to present in the thigh. In the thigh the fundus of the hernia carries the attenuated cribiform fascia before it

The compression of the sac leads to fibrosis in it at its neck so that it constricts any contents, omentum or intestine. This stricturing of the sac neck is an important factor in the mechanism of strangulation. Very often, the strictured sac neck is the confining structure in a strangulated hernia rather than the lacunar or pectineal ligaments.

Compression of the femoral vein and the saphenous vein by a femoral hernia may occur; indeed, visible distension of these veins is a diagnostic sign in the differential diagnosis of a femoral hernia from other groin swellings. Saphenous vein distension is particularly pronounced in cases when the femoral hernia has progressed through the cribriform fascia into the thigh and in doing so has compromised the saphenous vein at its termination into the femoral vein.[332]

Differential diagnosis

This subject is discussed in Chapter 11.

Management of femoral hernias

Operation should always be advised, for two reasons:

1. It is impossible to make and fit an adequate truss to control such a hernia.
2. The incidence of strangulation in these hernias is high. Many femoral hernias occur in elderly women, and a strangulated femoral hernia in the elderly woman carries a considerable morbidity.

Many femoral hernias present with incarceration or strangulation; in the recent North Tees series, there were 130 elective operations to 85 emergency operations. This ratio, 1.5 electives to 1 emergency, is unusual. In many series there are more emergency than elective cases and in some series the emergency cases outnumber electives by up to 10:1.[924] (In the same North Tees series there were 1720 elective inguinal hernia operations to 164 emergency operations – an elective to emergency ratio of 10.5:1.[244]) A more recent series from North Tees Hospital has confirmed the higher incidence of acute to elective admissions for femoral hernia. This study also showed the frequency of important co-morbidity in the elderly with strangulated femoral hernia and the increased mortality compared with elective cases, 8% in urgent cases compared with 0% in elective cases.[701]

When a patient presents with intestinal obstruction and a femoral hernia, if the hernia is not tender and therefore not strangulated, reduction by taxis may be employed in the short term. But if there is any local tenderness, suggesting that strangulation has occurred, taxis should not be employed. A partial enterocele (Richter's hernia) is common in femoral hernias. These patients may have confusing symptoms and signs; a high index of diagnostic suspicion should always be maintained. Urgent operation after adequate resuscitation and cardiorespiratory management in elderly shocked patients needs emphasizing.

Tingwald and Cooperman (1982) have emphasized the problems presented by the elderly with groin hernias.[924] Due to the increased risk of postoperative complications, some surgeons are becoming increasingly reluctant to perform elective procedures on these patients.[217] However, with femoral hernias delay only increases the likelihood of incarceration, and then emergency surgery in a more ill patient will be required. Elective repair of a femoral hernia is an urgency; these patients are at considerable hazard of strangulation if they have to wait for surgery. The National Confidential Enquiry in England has repeatedly warned of the high mortality of emergency surgery for strangulated femoral hernias in the female.[128, 692] All these facts are confirmed by the most recent series from North Tees; the co-existing medical morbidities in the emergency cases included respiratory disease, chronic obstructive airways disease (19%) coronary artery disease (40%) neurological disease (10%) and diabetes mellitus in 8%. The morbidity following emergency operation was also higher than elective operation, with pulmonary embolism occurring only in the emergency cases.[701]

Congenital hernia in the male

In the very rare variety of male congenital hernia mentioned previously, strangulation of omentum and small bowel in such a sac can occur as in any femoral hernia. What should be done at operation? Should the testicle be preserved? These are questions that cannot be answered from the literature. Perhaps the safest course is to excise the sac and the testicle which is always embedded in its wall (a sliding hernia) and perform a routine femoral repair.[892]

Operative approaches to femoral hernia

A femoral hernia is a variety of groin hernia – a defect in the fascia transversalis which is exploited by a peritoneal sac traversing the muscular weakness of the myopectineal orifice of Fruchaud – exactly similar to a patent processus vaginalis in an indirect inguinal hernia exploiting the deep ring in the fascia transversalis posterior wall of the inguinal canal, or a direct hernia peritoneal sac expanding into an acquired defect of the fascia transversalis. This being so, repair of a femoral hernia inexorably follows the same canons of repair as an inguinal hernia repair. Isolate and excise the peritoneal sac, repair the

fascia transversalis defect and then reinforce this repair by adjusting the local aponeurotic attachments.

In sequence, a femoral hernia occurs when the femoral sheath, a funnel of fascia transversalis enclosing the femoral vessels beneath the inguinal ligament, becomes dilated. A peritoneal sac enters the femoral funnel and then, as a plunger, causes it to dilate. As the fascia transversalis pushes onto the ligament it becomes scarred and often strictured around its neck, and in doing so pushes the attachment of the transversus abdominis aponeurosis medially along the pectineal line until the medial margin of the femoral sheath abuts on the inguinal ligament anteriorly, the lacunar ligament medially and the pectineal ligament posteriorly. After excision of the peritoneal sac, the femoral sheath must be repaired medially and the hernioplasty must prevent further herniation; to do this, the attachment of the fascia transversalis to the pectineal ligament must be broadened. This reconstruction of the medial femoral sheath can be reinforced by suturing the tendon of transversus abdominis to the pectineal line (McVay/Cooper's ligament repair) or from below by turning up a flap of pectineus fascia to close the medial femoral canal or finally by plugging it with a mesh prosthesis.[66, 642]

As an alternative, the entire operation can be conducted in the extraperitoneal (preperitoneal layer) and a mesh repair of the canal constructed in this layer.[896, 967]

Eponyms really confuse the surgeon here and are best discarded temporarily. Three approaches to femoral hernioplasty are described; because none of these is universally applicable, the surgeon must be acquainted with all three:

1. The abdominal,[906] suprapubic,[512] retropubic,[960] preperitoneal[707] or extraperitoneal[171, 418, 898] operation. This approach, developed by Henry, is often known as the McEvedy approach, although Henry used a midline incision and McEvedy a pararectus incision.[634] A Pfannenstiel incision enables bilateral hernias to be operated simultaneously by this approach. (Eponyms: Cheatle,[171] Henry,[418] McEvedy.[634])
2. The inguinal or 'high' operation. (Eponyms: Annandale,[27] Lotheissen,[579] Moschowitz.[673])
3. The crural or 'low' operation. (Eponyms: Bassini,[75] Lockwood.[573])

The extraperitoneal approach gives excellent access to the femoral canal and to the general peritoneal cavity should that be necessary to deal with a strangulated viscus. However, this approach to the pelvis is unfamiliar to most surgeons and, therefore, not to be recommended to the inexperienced surgeon operating on his first strangulated femoral hernia at the dead of night.[708]

The inguinal approach is familiar, but has the twin drawbacks of disrupting the inguinal canal mechanism and not providing adequate access to a strangulated viscus. If this approach is used, an excellent repair of the fascia transversalis (Shouldice technique) must be employed to avoid the complicating inguinal hernia. This is particularly so in women, in whom direct inguinal hernia is almost unknown . . . except as a complication of this operation.

The crural approach to the femoral sac is good and bloodless, and repair of the hernia is easy by this method. Its most significant disadvantage is that access to a strangulated viscus is often very inadequate. The crural approach is recommended for elective operation and to the occasional or novice surgeon. This is the quickest and least traumatic operation to perform.[272, 701, 915] If a visceral strangulation is present it is best to perform a standard lower paramedial incision and deal with the crisis through an incision which is familiar to most abdominal operators. With an emergency situation, or for the inexperienced surgeon, this is no place for an anatomical extravaganza.

The 'low' or crural operation

PREOPERATIVE MANAGEMENT

In the uncomplicated case no special preoperative management is required. The bladder is frequently a sliding component of the medial wall of a femoral hernia, and preoperative catheterization is a sensible precaution which will lessen the likelihood of bladder injury.

If the hernia is strangulated or obstructed, preoperative nasogastric aspiration and adequate fluid replacement is mandatory. The patient must be fully resuscitated and co-morbidities, especially in the elderly, adequately managed.

ANAESTHESIA

General anaesthesia is preferred, but local anaesthesia can be employed. Local infiltration with extra injection around the sac neck will suffice.

The operation

POSITION OF THE PATIENT

The patient is placed supine on the operating table which is tilted head down 15 degrees.

Draping

If the hernia is not strangulated, draping to allow access to the groin only is required. If strangulation or obstruction is present or suspected, towels should be placed to enable easy access to the lower abdomen if a laparotomy becomes necessary. A sterile adhesive drape is always used.

THE INCISION

A skin incision is made over the hernia. The incision is about 6 cm long and parallel to the inguinal ligament.

After the skin is divided, it is easy to separate the subcutaneous fat down to the coverings of the hernia sac. Haemostasis should be secured before the sac is mobilized.

MOBILIZATION OF SAC

The sac, having emerged from the femoral canal, carries before it fascia transversalis and extraperitoneal fat in front of which is the attenuated cribriform fascia and the femoral fascial layer of the thigh. Because of these fascial layers, the sac usually makes a forward upward turn in its path at the fossa ovalis; thus its fundus will be found lying over the inguinal ligament. It is important to appreciate this before mobilization is attempted. Once the sac is identified, the fascial layers are cleaned from it by blunt dissection, which is best achieved by breaking up the adherent scar tissue and fat with a haemostat and then wiping the fascia off with a gauze swab. These extraperitoneal coverings of the sac are frequently quite thick and fibrosed and are most often the real constricting layer when strangulation has occurred (Figure 16.3).

IDENTIFICATION OF FEMORAL OPENING

The neck of the sac is now cleared of fat and fascia so that the boundaries of the femoral canal can be identified. It is best to identify the medial and anterior margins of the canal first. The medial margin is the lacunar ligament and is easily seen as it sweeps around from the inguinal ligament to the subjacent pubic bone. Anteriorly, the rolled-over edge of the inguinal ligament

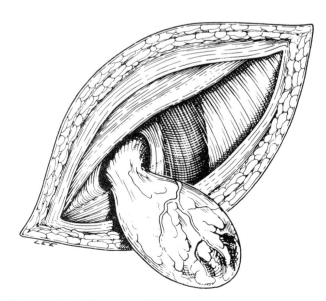

Figure 16.3   The sac mobilized

can readily be separated from the sac underneath it. The sac should next be lifted up. The fascia on the pectineus muscle is easily recognizable and if this is traced back to the ramus of the pubis, the posterior margin of the canal – the pectineal ligament – can be recognized.

Attention is now turned to the lateral boundary of the canal – the femoral vein. This is the most vulnerable structure in this area and is difficult to identify because it is covered with a quite opaque fascial sheath. One manoeuvre is to identify the femoral artery by touch; the artery lies immediately lateral to the vein so the vein must be in any space between the sac and the palpable artery. A careful dissection is made on the lateral side of the sac, preferably using 'curved on the flat' dissecting scissors and keeping close to the sac. The dissection of the sac is only complete when the entire circumference of its neck has been clearly defined (Figure 16.4).

INSPECTION OF CONTENTS OF SAC

The lateral side of the fundus of the sac should now be opened. The medial side should be avoided, as it may be partly formed by the bladder. There is always much adherent extraperitoneal fat on the fundus which generally contains many distended veins. If these bleed they can confuse the anatomy, so the fat should be gently broken through with a haemostat point and the bleeding carefully controlled.

Inside the extraperitoneal fat the true peritoneal hernia sac will be found. It is grasped in a haemostat and then opened.

Any contents of the sac can now be gently freed, adhesions divided and the contents reduced back into the general peritoneal cavity. If strangulation is present, an alternative approach to the remainder of the operation may be necessary. Often a small nubbin of strangulated dead omentum may be discovered; this should be isolated, its blood supply ligated, and then excised.

CLOSURE AND EXCISION OF SAC

When it is certain that the neck of the sac is isolated and that the sac is empty, it can be closed and excised. Traction is applied to the open sac and, using metric 3.5 braided absorbable polymer on a 40 mm round needle, a transfixion suture should be securely tied around the neck. The redundant sac is cut off, leaving a generous cuff beyond the transfixion suture. The stump of the sac will now recede through the femoral canal and out of sight (Figure 16.5).

REPAIR OF CANAL

First stage

The canal is repaired using a single figure-of-eight suture of metric 3 polypropylene on a J-shaped needle.

The femoral vein is retracted laterally and the pectineal ligament clearly identified on the superior ramus of the pubic bone. The first suture is placed through this ligament from its deep aspect at the point where the medial margin of the femoral vein would lie if it were not retracted. It is necessary to experiment with the retractor and identify this point correctly. If the suture is placed too far laterally the vein will be compromised, and if placed too far medially the repair will be unsound (Figure 16.6).

The next bite must pick up the inguinal ligament and

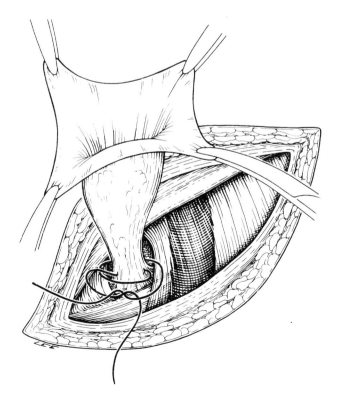

Figure 16.4　Closure of the sac

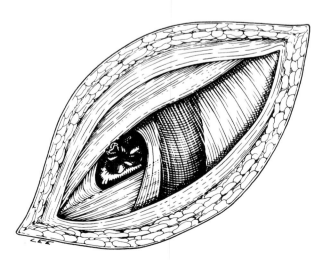

Figure 16.5　The canal after closure of the sac

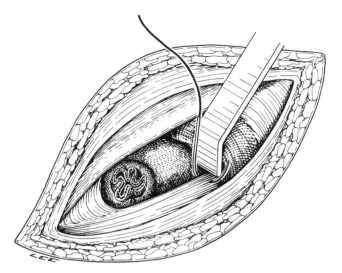

Figure 16.6 Retraction of the femoral vein laterally enables visualization of the pectineal (Cooper's) ligament. The first suture is not introduced

iliopubic tract of fascia transversalis at a corresponding distance from its pubic attachment, so that the suture forms the base of an isosceles triangle. Next, the pectineal ligament is picked up, again from deep to superficial, halfway between the first pectineal suture and the lacunar ligament and finally the inguinal ligament is picked up, again halfway between the first suture and the attachment of the ligament to the pubis.

Now the free end of the suture is passed deep to the two loops and the two ends are tied securely. When the suture is pulled tight, the medial 0.75 cm or so of the inguinal ligament will be approximated to the pectineal line and the femoral canal closed. Furthermore, if the knot is placed at the medial side, it will be away from the femoral vein which will not be damaged by it (Figure 16.7).

Second stage

So far the canal has been closed by the apposition of two tendinous structures under some degree of tension. According to the rules of biological repair, tendinous structures drawn together under tension and subject to

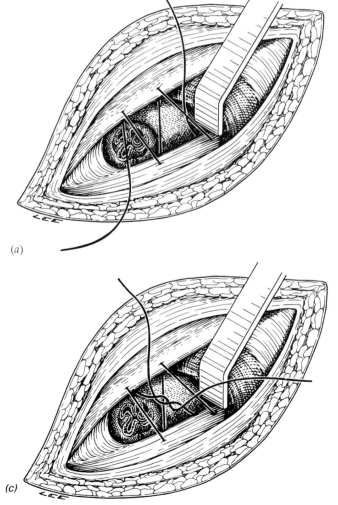

(a)

(c)

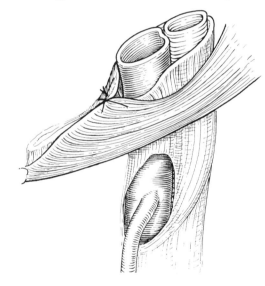

(b)

Figure 16.7 (a,b) The next suture picks up the inguinal ligament and subjacent iliopubic tract of fascia transversalis. Care must be taken to avoid the cord structures in the wall. The suture is placed to form the base of an isosceles triangle with the apex at the pubic tubercle. (c) The knot is tied deeply at the medial side away from the femoral vein

varying stresses such as respiration and movement do not heal readily. Therefore, it is advisable to reinforce the union with a further aponeurotic patch which is not under tension. This is easily achieved by raising a flap of fascia off the surface of the pectineus muscle. It is then sutured to the external oblique aponeurosis in such a way that it covers the initial repair of the femoral canal (Figure 16.8). A continuous polypropylene suture is used for this double breasting manoeuvre. As an alternative an 'umbrella' or 'dart' of mesh can be used to stop the defect.[342, 812]

COMMENT ON CRURAL OPERATION

Although the primary defect is in the fascia transversalis at the wide part of the femoral canal (the open funnel), this operation does not primarily address itself to this defect. This is the major negative feature of the operation. The fascia transversalis is, inevitably, tangled up when the sac is originally closed, the stump of sac and extraperitoneal fat blocks the medial part of the funnel, the attachment of the inguinal ligament to the pectineal ligament reduces the potential size of the femoral canal, and the patch of pectineus fascia reinforces this. However, there is still the argument that the fascial defect is not *a priori* repaired.

Prosthetic support to the medial fascia transversalis to prevent recurrence has been advocated by Lichtenstein and Shore, and Pories, who insert a Marlex mesh 'cigarette stub' obturator into the femoral canal. This is held in position by non-absorbable sutures through the inguinal and pectineal ligaments and the pectineus fascia. This prosthetic cigarette stub operation is especially useful in the recurrent femoral hernia (Figure 16.9).[562, 954]

Caldwell reports pouring 382 rubber elastomer into the medial femoral canal,[141] and Knox and Caldwell report using a rubber 'collar stud' to close the medial

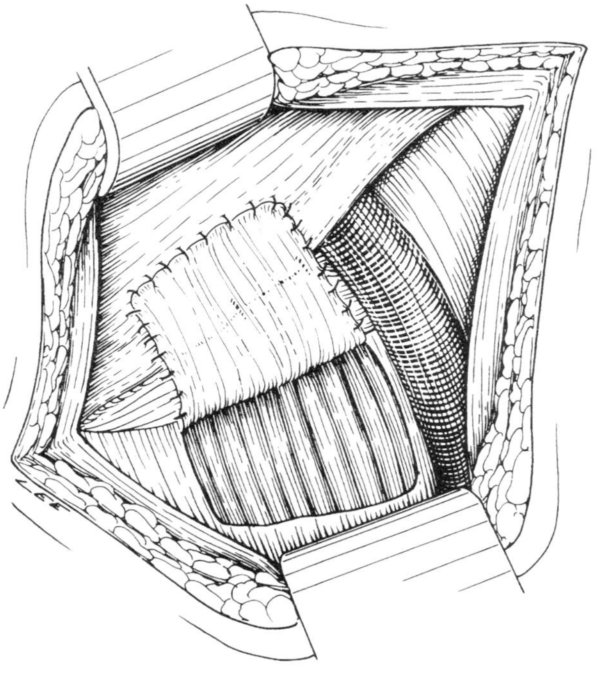

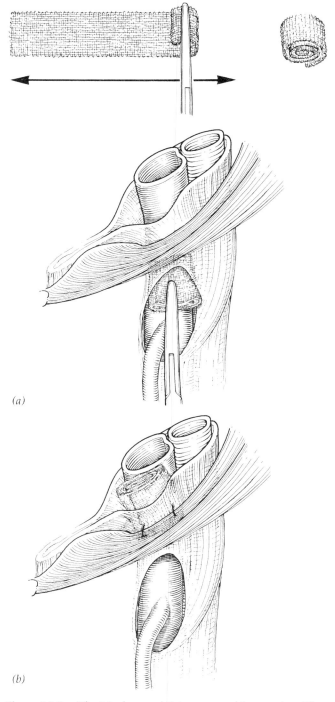

(a)

(b)

Figure 16.8 The flap of pectineus fascia sutured over the femoral canal

Figure 16.9 The Marlex mesh 'cigarette stub' operation. The insertion of a Marlex 'cigarette stub' (a) into the femoral canal (b). It is sutured into place

canal.[506] This latter technique was used 15 times, but no long-term follow-up data are reported.

The skin and subcutaneous tissues are closed as before. If the dissection has been difficult, or if there is much 'dead space', a drain should be used. Disadvantages of the 'low' approach, which are important in obstructed patients, are as follows:

1. Difficulty in delivering obstructed bowel for review. This is most relevant in Richter's hernia (partial enterocele) where the involved loop is especially liable to slip back into the abdomen and be irretrievable.
2. It is impossible to put an anastomosis, which is bulky, back into the abdomen through the femoral canal. A separate laparotomy is needed if bowel resection is necessary. This may lead to contamination of the main peritoneal cavity unless great care is taken.
3. The crural operation provides inadequate exposure if there is difficulty reducing and mobilizing the contents of a hernial sac.
4. It can be difficult to excise a thickened fibrous sac down to flush with the parietal peritoneum.
5. In long-standing hernia, access for an adequate repair is limited.

Inguinal operation

This operation achieves the same objective of closing the medial portion of the femoral canal which has been described using the crural approach. However, in the inguinal approach the femoral canal is exposed by opening the posterior wall – the fascia transversalis – of the inguinal canal and achieving initial closure, using the fascia transversalis, of the femoral cone. This repair can be reinforced by approximating the inguinal to the pectineal ligaments if the inguinal ligament is grossly stretched.

The incision and dissection for this operation are exactly the same as those employed in the Shouldice operation for inguinal hernia. After the fascia transversalis in the posterior wall of the inguinal canal has been opened, the extraperitoneal fat on the neck of the femoral hernia can be identified and removed by blunt dissection (Figure 16.10).

The sac can now either be delivered above the inguinal ligament or opened below the ligament and its contents reduced. The neck of the sac is then transfixed and ligated (Figure 16.11).

The medial extremity of the inguinal ligament is now sutured to the pectineal ligament by figure-of-eight polypropylene sutures. In this operation these are inserted from above, that is through the incision in the posterior wall of the inguinal canal.

The inguinal canal is then repaired using the Shouldice technique, care being taken to reinforce the femoral

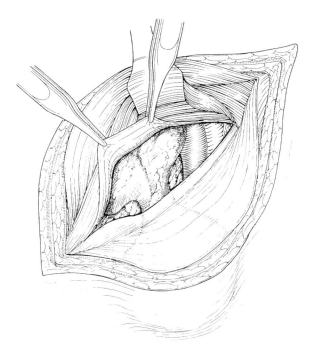

Figure 16.10 Extraperitoneal fat on the neck of the femoral hernia can be identified and removed by blunt dissection

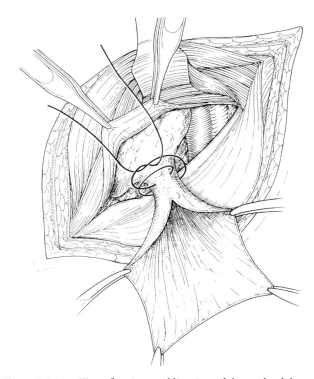

Figure 16.11 Transfixation and ligation of the neck of the sac

repair with the overlapped fascia transversalis at the medial part of the canal.

It is advisable, particularly in women with a broad pelvis, to reinforce the medial repair by suturing the insertion of the transversus muscle tendon (conjoint tendon) to the pectineal ligament (Cooper's ligament repair).

COMMENT ON INGUINAL OPERATION

The inguinal approach for the repair of femoral hernia is not recommended as the operation of choice because it is technically more difficult and more time consuming than the crural operation and because it disrupts an otherwise normal inguinal canal.

However, some experts, notably Tanner in Britain[908] and Glassow in Canada,[349] recommend this operation strongly. If this approach is used, the repair of the transversalis/transversus layer to the pectineal ligament must be adequate and must extend the tendinous attachment of the transversus muscle laterally along the pectineal ligament as far as the femoral vein. Often, to do this without tension, a generous 'medial slide' of the lateral rectus sheath/conjoint tendon must be made.

Extraperitoneal (preperitoneal) operation

This operation illustrates the genius of an expert surgical anatomist exploiting fascial plane dissection at its most elegant. Henry's extraperitoneal approach to the anterior pelvis gives an excellent exposure of both femoral canals simultaneously, but it is not an operation for the novice. In the hands of an expert it is a fine operation enabling bilateral femoral hernia to be dealt with simultaneously through one incision.[23, 418]

The patient is placed on the operating table and the bladder emptied by catheterization. A vertical midline suprapubic incision is made, the aponeurotic layer is opened vertically in the midline and the peritoneum exposed.

Alternatively, a Pfannenstiel incision, with a suprapubic side-to-side opening of the anterior rectus sheath and separation of the rectus muscles, gives good access and a much more acceptable skin scar.

The recti are retracted to either side and the space between the peritoneum and the abdominal wall muscles is opened by gentle blunt dissection in order to approach the femoral canal on either side. If only a unilateral hernia is present a pararectal vertical (McEvedy)[634] or skin crease (Ogilvie)[713] incision can be used. This latter technique is ascribed to a Cambridge surgeon, Hudson, by some authorities.[492]

Femoral sacs are dealt with by reduction of their contents, transfixion of their necks and resection of redundant sac (Figure 16.12). If strangulation is present, the subjacent peritoneum can easily be opened, the contents of the sac inspected, and so forth (Figure 16.13).

The femoral canal is repaired using a non-absorbable suture, as described in the inguinal operation. The anterior abdominal wall is closed layer by layer.

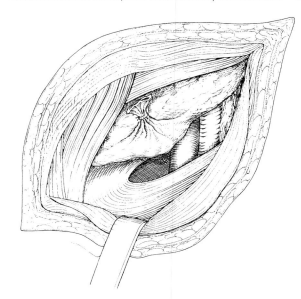

Figure 16.12   An adequate approach to a unilateral hernia can be made through an oblique or vertical pararectus incision

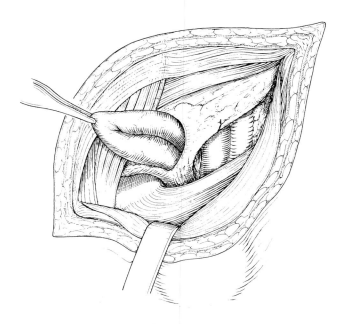

Figure 16.13   Opening a femoral hernial sac

COMMENT ON EXTRAPERITONEAL OPERATION

The extraperitoneal operation has advantages, but also disadvantages:

1. An extensive mobilization of the lower abdominal wall is required.
2. It cannot easily be performed using local anaesthesia.
3. With mobilization there is a risk of bleeding and haematoma formation between the peritoneum and the endopelvic fascia.
4. Unless an adequate repair of the abdominal wall is made, an abdominal incisional hernia can ensue.

The three approaches

The femoral hernia surgeon should ideally be familiar with all three approaches:

1. The low approach is recommended for the easily reducible uncomplicated femoral hernia especially in the thin patient, and in the frail ASA class 3 or 4 patient, when it can be undertaken electively using local anaesthesia.
2. The inguinal approach is best used when there is a concomitant primary inguinal hernia on the same side which can be repaired simultaneously.
3. The extraperitoneal approach is used when obstruction or strangulation are present, in patients who have undergone previous groin surgery, when inguinal and femoral hernias occur together, and in bilateral cases where both sides can be repaired simultaneously.[23, 960]

Strangulation

Strangulation is very uncommon in patients aged under 40 years old. Strangulation is more frequent in females than males and reaches its highest incidence and greatest morbidity in women in their seventh and eighth decades.

If strangulation is suspected, the sac is approached as described below. Once the sac is identified it will be seen to contain blood-stained fluid if strangulation has occurred.

The sac should be opened on the lateral aspect of its fundus and the contents inspected. A variety of intra-abdominal viscera may be found in the femoral hernia sac. Waddington, in 1971, reviewed 128 patients with strangulated femoral hernia; the most frequently strangulated viscera were, in rank order, small bowel, then small bowel and omentum, then omentum alone, then appendix, colon, bladder and lastly fallopian tube.[954] No viscus should be returned to the peritoneal cavity unless it is definitely viable. Viability of any viscus can only be assessed after its blood supply has been normalized by removing the constriction at the neck of the sac.

Any blood-stained fluid in the sac is sampled for microbiological culture and the remainder sucked out. The contents of the sac are gently manipulated so that the neck of the sac is revealed clearly. It is very important to be careful with a strangulated loop of gut, as operative perforation can seriously hazard the patient's recovery. Quite frequently, careful dissection of the neck of the sac and removal of oedematous extraperitoneal fat about it are all that is required to release the strangulation. The constricting agent is usually the thickened transversalis fascia and peritoneal neck of the sac and the oedematous extraperitoneal fat about it, rather than the ligamentous structures which form the anterior, posterior and medial margins of the sac. The femoral vein is

very rarely involved in the strangulation process, which confirms that the neck of the sac itself is most usually the constricting agent.

When the sac has been opened, the inguinal ligament can generally be retracted upwards and the femoral vein laterally so that the neck of the sac can be divided.

After the strangulation has been released, any contained viscera are wrapped in warm saline packs and left alone for a full 5 min before being inspected. Omentum of doubtful viability is best excised. Small intestine must only be returned to the peritoneal cavity if it has all been inspected and shown to be vital. Often there is a linear necrosis of the bowel where it has been compressed by the neck of the sac; this should be oversewn.

If a considerable segment of gangrenous small bowel needs resection, more gut is prolapsed into the wound. Alternatively, if there is technical difficulty, an ipsilateral lower paramedian incision can be made and bowel resected through the groin wound (to avoid contamination of the peritoneal cavity). Anastomosis is then carried out through the main peritoneal cavity. It is worth stressing the importance of not contaminating the main peritoneal cavity and not returning non-viable bowel into it. The use of an ipsilateral lower paramedian incision for all cases of difficulty is strongly recommended.

Waddington recommends the low, crural, approach and this was used in 119 of his 128 cases. In only one out of 14 patients needing a bowel resection and anastomosis was a paramedian incision needed for supplementing peritoneal cavity access.[954]

Wheeler (1975) reports typical results for the UK from the University Hospital, Cardiff. In an 11–year study period (1963–73), 78 patients underwent a total of 80 operations for femoral hernia. In 44 instances the operations were for acute strangulation; the remaining 36 operations were elective.[982]

In the Cardiff series, three approaches were used – the low approach gave the least recurrences, whereas the inguinal (high) and the extraperitoneal (preperitoneal) using a midline incision approaches were the least satisfactory (Table 16.1). The choice of the high approach in strangulation is interesting; this choice confirms 'traditional' British teaching that the high approach offers advantages if resection is necessary. On the other hand, the poor results with the inguinal approach demand unfavourable comparison with other series in which this approach has given excellent results.

The more recent series from Stockton-on-Tees represents English district surgical practice in the 11 years 1976–1987; during this period 145 patients (38 male, 107 female) with 146 hernias (99 right, 47 left) underwent femoral hernia repair. In the elective group all but one patient had been aware of the lump for over a month before surgery, in contrast to the emergency group in which 27 (43%) had been aware of the lump for over

Table 16.1 Femoral hernia operations undertaken at Cardiff, 1963–73[*] (After Wheeler, 1975[982])

Procedure	No. operations	No. recurrences	Percentage recurrence
Abdominal pararectal incision (McEvedy)	32 (20)	4	12.5
Midline (Cheatle)	3 (2)	1	33.3
Inguinal (Lotheissen)	7 (3)	3	43.0
Crural (Bassini)	23 (7)	1	4.4

[*] Figures in parentheses indicate emergency procedures for strangulation

one month. The most significant difference between the emergency and elective groups was age: 43 (68%) of patients in the emergency group were aged over 65 years compared with only 25 (30%) of those having an elective operation (p < 0.0001). Both groups had similar incidences of co-existing medical pathology. The preferred operation technique was the low crural (Bassini–Lockwood) operation. There were no deaths in the elective group but five in the emergency group – an overall death rate of 3.4% (8% in the emergency group). The morbidity was also significantly higher in the emergency group. The most common cause of death was pulmonary embolism. At a median follow-up of five years, five patients had a recurrence (3.4%). Three of the recurrences were direct inguinal hernias after the use of the inguinal operation.[702]

This study highlighted the problems of patients who delay in seeking medical advice and the difficulties general practitioners have in making a correct diagnosis of femoral hernia, only 35% of femoral hernias were correctly diagnosed by general practitioners in this series.[701]

Ponka and Brush report that the crural low repair gives the fewest recurrences in their experience.[754] Likewise, Duvie from West Africa reports that the low approach gives a low recurrence rate (0%), a shorter operation time and postoperative stay – although it must be commented that this report was of a very small study with no recurrences in either the 'high' or the 'low' group.[272]

Unusual variants of femoral hernia

So far we have considered the commonest variety of femoral hernia; there are, however, six rare variants, all of which pass from the abdomen into the thigh through the space bounded anteriorly by the inguinal ligament, posteriorly by the pectineal ligament and the origin of the pectineus muscle, medially by the lacunar ligament and laterally by the fusion of the femoral sheath (fascia transversalis) with the iliac investing fascia. These variants are:

1. The hernia associated with maldescent of the testis through the femoral canal (cruroscrotal hernia). This is discussed on page 199.
2. The prevascular hernia (Narath's hernia), in which the sac emerges from the abdomen within the femoral sheath but lies anteriorly to the femoral vein and artery. This hernia can be either medial or lateral to the deep epigastric vessels. Narath described this condition associated with congenital dislocation of the hip. He reported six hernias in four patients, each hernia appearing on the same side as the dislocated hip (there were two bilateral cases). Importantly, the hernias did not appear until after the dislocations were reduced by manipulation. The same condition has been described as a complication of an innominate osteotomy for congenital dislocation of the hip.[823] Similar hernias develop in adults after previous groin surgery or after vascular operations on the external iliac vessels. Repair by an extraperitoneal approach is recommended.[201, 690]
3. When the neck of the sac lies lateral to the femoral vessels – the external femoral hernia of Hesselbach and Cloquet.[182, 424]
4. The transpectineal ligament femoral hernia when the sac traverses the pectineal part of the inguinal ligament and lacunar ligament (Laugier's hernia).[530]
5. When the sac descends deep to the femoral vessels and pectineal fascia (Callisen's or Cloquet's hernia).[142]
6. When the sac, instead of progressing anteriorly and superiorly through the cribriform fascia, proceeds into the thigh deep to the investing fascia – this hernia is always multilocular and may be mistaken for an obturator hernia. A variant described by Astley Cooper in 1804 and sometimes referred to as Cooper's hernia.[193]

All these variants are best managed using the extraperitoneal mesh prosthetic operation described in Chapter 13.

Conclusions

Femoral hernia is a common clinical problem which warrants urgent elective repair to avoid the complication of strangulation.

Strangulated femoral hernia carries a high morbidity and mortality in the elderly.

The mechanism of femoral herniation, a distension and failure of the fascia transversalis in the femoral sheath, is described.

Methods of repair are outlined – the low, crural, operation is least traumatic and gives the lower recurrence rate.

The crural operation is not suitable in multiple hernias or when resection of gut is required. In these circumstances, the extraperitoneal or inguinal operations are recommended.

17 UMBILICAL HERNIA IN ADULTS

Epidemiology and pathology

Umbilical hernias in adults can be a cause of considerable morbidity and if complications supervene they can lead to death. Umbilical hernias are much less frequent in the adult population than inguinal hernias (see Table 3.2). Umbilical hernias account for 0.03% of the hernia operations performed in the UK. Of the patients with umbilical hernias, 90% are women, invariably women who are overweight and multiparous. There is no racial predisposition to adult umbilical hernias.[459] Umbilical hernias have a high risk of incarceration.[752] When these hernias incarcerate and strangulate, they contain transverse colon and/or stomach. Strangulated umbilical hernias have a considerable morbidity,[752] a morbidity dictated by the age of the patient and concomitant disease, atherosclerosis, obesity and diabetes mellitus. Umbilical herniation can complicate abdominal distension, pregnancy and cirrhosis.[166] After pregnancy these hernias can regress spontaneously. In cirrhosis the ascites must be controlled before repair is attempted. Adventitious portosystemic shunts about the umbilicus may complicate operative repair,[65] although a recent study suggests that excessive blood loss in these patients can be avoided.[740]

In a retrospective review only 11% of patients with adult umbilical hernias recalled persistence of a childhood umbilical hernia: this and other observations suggests that the adult umbilical hernia is not through the original umbilical scar but is 'para' umbilical in anatomy.[459] This view is supported by Askar, who postulates that the adult hernia is through the decussation of the fibres of the linea alba adjacent to the umbilical cicatrix.[43]

Acquired umbilical hernia following laparoscopic cholecystectomy has recently been reported from Turin.[229] Forced dilation of the aponeurotic layer is proposed as the aetiology despite primary suture of the trocar site. Such dilation should be avoided in removal of the gallbladder.

Mayo operation – historical note

William Mayo first used an overlapping technique to repair an umbilical hernia in 1895. In a paper read to the American Academy of Railway Surgeons on 4 October 1898 he publicly called attention to the impracticality of covering the defect left by excision of large umbilical hernia with muscle. He advocated overlapping the adjacent aponeurotic structures which were at hand and securing a wide area of adhesion rather than edge-to-edge union. He experimented with a side-to-side overlap and abandoned this because of technical difficulties. Mayo recommended the vertical overlap because 'on assuming the recumbent posture the stretched tissues allow of great mobility and one can often grasp the abdominal wall and overlap a number of inches without difficulty.'[626, 627]

When reporting his results and technique in 1903, he had performed the vertical overlapping operation 25 times; there were no deaths and so far he had had no recurrences. He encountered the problem of 'loss of habitation' in large hernias filled with viscera. He stressed a few operative details worthy of repetition today: he cleared the aponeurosis of fat for 'one or two inches' around the neck of the sac; he opened the sac; he extended the hernia aperture on either side to allow a better overlap, he used non-absorbable sutures (silk on this occasion, but previously kangaroo tendon) and 'rail-roaded' the upper flap down to the overlap with the lower flap. Interestingly, at this time, Mayo recommended initial closure of the peritoneum with chromic catgut prior to aponeurotic closure.

Mayo's definitive paper was given to the 54th Annual Session of the American Medical Association in 1903 – the discussants were Ochsner, Murphy and Ferguson. All three commended the operation; Ferguson went further and embarrassed Mayo by referring to it as the 'Mayo operation'.[626]

Indications for operation

Most patients with umbilical hernias complain of a painful protrusion at the umbilicus. This discomfort is indication enough for operation. Absolute indications for surgery include obstruction and strangulation. Irreducibility is not an absolute indication for surgery: many long-standing umbilical hernias have many adhesions in a loculated hernia and are thus irreducible. In larger hernias the overlying skin may become damaged and ulcerated. Skin complications may dictate the need for operation after the skin sepsis has been controlled.

Surgery is advised for all umbilical hernias unless there are strong contraindications, which include obesity, chronic cardiovascular or respiratory disease, or ascites (umbilical hernias can be manifestations of cirrhotic or malignant peritoneal effusions).

Spontaneous rupture of umbilical hernias is rare but is recorded especially in patients with ascites and cirrhosis. Cheselden's 1721 patient who developed a 'preternatural anus' is an example of the spontaneous cure of an umbilical hernia.[175] Queen Caroline succumbed to an incarcerated umbilical hernia in 1737 because of the surgical delay in lancing her hernia to allow drainage.[282]

Umbilical hernias are an important complication of cirrhosis and ascites; the ascites should be controlled either medically or with a shunt before hernia repair is undertaken. Umbilical herniation is sometimes a consequence of CAPD.[284]

Suture materials

For details see page 81

Anaesthesia

General anaesthesia with full muscle relaxation should be employed.

Patients who require an extensive intraperitoneal dissection often have considerable adynamic ileus after surgery and need postoperative nasogastric suction and fluid and nutritional support.

A further note of caution is indicated; if the patient has portal hypertension, an extensive portosystemic anastomosis will be present at the umbilicus. Careful dissection and ligation of vessels is important if massive haemorrhage is to be avoided.[740]

The operation

POSITION OF PATIENT

The patient is laid on his back on the operating table. Drapes are applied to allow good access to the umbilical area and the abdomen if extended access is required.

THE INCISION

Two semilunar incisions which are joined at their extremities are used. The ellipse of stretched skin and the enclosed umbilical cicatrix are excised.

Care must be taken not to excise too much tissue when deciding the dimensions of these incisions. Although the umbilical cicatrix is best excised, removal of too much skin will place the final wound under tension and

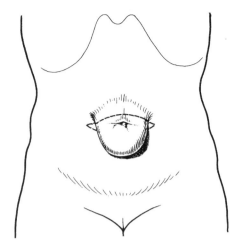

Figure 17.1 Two semilunar incisions around the hernia are made

jeopardise its healing. It is better to aim on the side of caution and take little skin away at the commencement of the operation; more skin can always be excised later (Figure 17.1).

REMOVAL OF REDUNDANT SKIN AND FAT

The area of skin and subcutaneous fat enclosed by the semilunar incisions is removed. The incisions are deepened down to the muscular aponeurosis, care being taken to ensure that the incisions are vertical and at right angles to the fascia so that the skin is not undermined and its blood supply hazarded (Figure 17.2). This part of the dissection can be very bloody, and a cautious approach and careful sequential haemostasis are recommended.

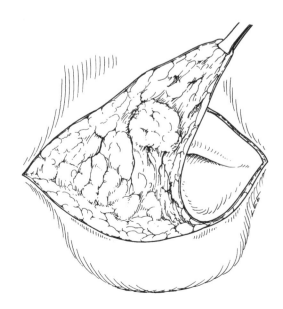

Figure 17.2 The redundant skin and scar tissue are excised

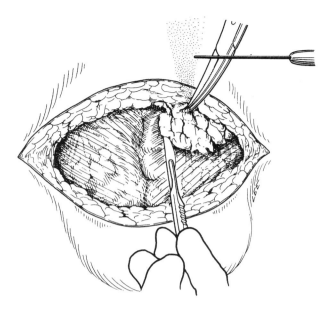

Figure 17.3 Careful haemostasis will avoid blood loss and its consequences. Absolute haemostasis is critical to optimum wound healing

The avoidance of blood loss at this stage is very important if blood transfusion and its considerable hazards in an obese and elderly patient are to be avoided (Figure 17.3).

IDENTIFICATION OF NECK OF SAC

When the incisions have been deepened to the aponeurosis, the margins of the aponeurosis about the peritoneal neck of the sac can be sought and dissected (Figure 17.4).

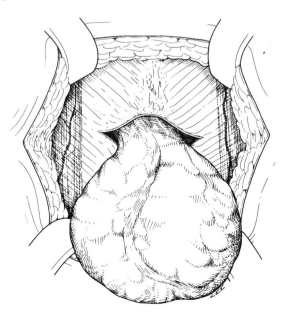

Figure 17.4 The neck of the sac is identified. The aponeuroses on either side of the neck are opened laterally for 1 or 2 cm to allow the neck of the sac to be isolated

MANAGEMENT OF SAC – I

Having isolated the neck of the sac, all the overlying fat and skin can be dissected off leaving the peritoneum of the sac protruding bare through the defect in the abdominal wall. The sac can now be opened and its contents inspected (Figure 17.5). Often the contents are densely adherent to the lining of the sac, particularly at the fundus. Adhesions must be divided and ligated where necessary to control bleeding. Again, the admonition about the avoidance of blood loss should be remembered. Densely adherent omentum, particularly if it is partly ischaemic, is best excised. All dissection should be made under direct vision. The bowel must be carefully preserved intact. Bowel puncture can lead to fistula formation postoperatively. Postoperative fistula and sepsis may precipitate death.

After the contents have been freed from the sac they are ready to be returned to the main peritoneal cavity (Figure 17.6).

MANAGEMENT OF SAC – II

If the sac is vast and multiloculated, an alternative can often usefully be employed. Once the peritoneum of the neck at any one point has been identified, it should be opened and a finger inserted. There are fewer adhesions at the neck of the sac than at the fundus, where recurrently ischaemic bowel is frequently densely adherent. A 'trick of the trade' is always to start the dissection at the

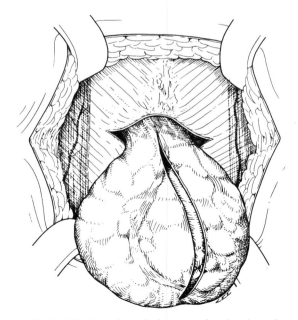

Figure 17.5 Having cleared the sac of redundant fat and fibrous tissue it is opened carefully. The incision into the sac should commence at the neck, not the fundus. Adhesions are less dense at the neck of a hernial sac; they are most dense at the fundus

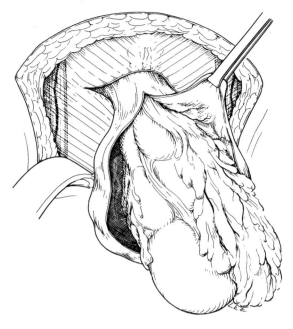

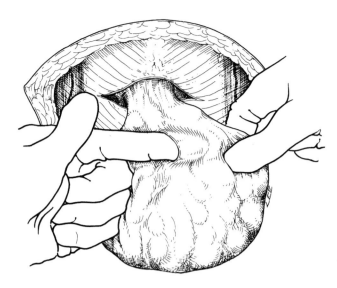

Figure 17.8 The neck of a multiloculated sac is slowly dissected and divided

Figure 17.6 The incision is extended to the fundus; adherent omentum and transverse colon are mobilized before reduction

neck; only the inexperienced operator would attempt to commence dissection at the fundus (Figure 17.7).

The whole mass of sac, contents and overlying fat and skin is then held up by assistants while the neck is dissected around, using the finger in the sac as a direction finder. This dissection can be tedious if the sac is multiloculated and the contents very adherent. It is well for the operator to change from side to side of the operating table to facilitate this manoeuvre. Once the neck

has been divided, attention can be turned to the contents of the sac. Adhesions are divided and doubtfully viable omentum excised (Figure 17.8).

ENLARGEMENT OF APONEUROTIC APERTURE

The opening in the abdominal wall is next enlarged laterally for 3 or 4 cm on either side, the rectus muscle being

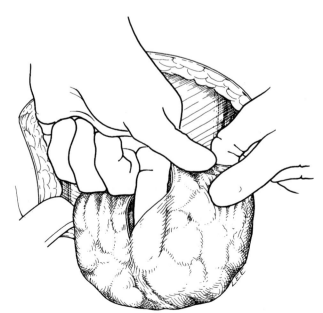

Figure 17.7 If the sac is multiloculated, a finger is inserted through the initial opening in the neck of the sac

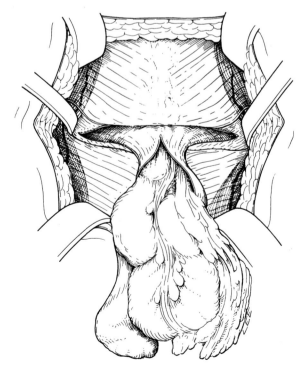

Figure 17.9 The deficit in the abdominal wall is enlarged laterally for 4 cm on either side; the rectus muscles are retracted to make this possible

retracted as the posterior rectus sheath is divided, taking care not to injure the epigastric vessels (Figure 17.9).

Once the fibrous ring of the neck has been divided, the contents of the sac can be reduced back into the abdomen. Redundant sac is excised (Figure 17.10).

REPAIR OF DEFECT – MAYO TECHNIQUE

The margins of the opening – aponeurosis, posterior rectus sheath and peritoneum – are now grasped in large haemostats and held up by assistants (Figure 17.11). The deep sutures are next placed. Strong non-absorbable material (metric 4 polypropylene or metric 3.5 nylon) are used on a round-bodied needle.

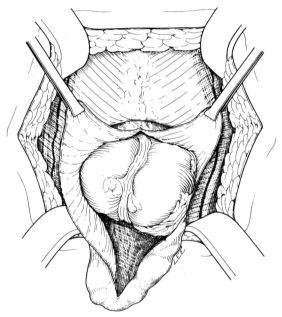

Figure 17.10 The contents are reduced after the fibrous neck of the sac has been cleared

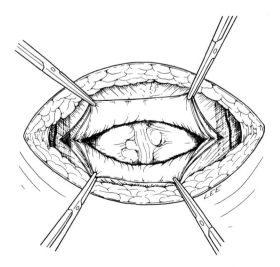

Figure 17.11 The margins of the parietal defect are now picked up in large haemostats

The suture enters the upper (cephalad) flap from without, between 2 and 3 cm from its margin. The needle is then grasped on the deep surface of the upper flap, passed across the defect and then from the outside through the lower flap. Then the needle is pulled back through the lower flap, across the defect and through the deep surface of the upper flap. The suture thus placed is held in a clip. Many more such sutures are now inserted and held untied until all are in place.

There are four useful technical points:

1. In the upper flap the sutures must all be placed further than 2 cm from the margin – up to 4 cm is permissible.
2. In the lower flap the sutures must all be at a distance greater than 1 cm from the margin.
3. It adds to the stability of the suture lines if the sutures are staggered, not all at the same interval from the margins of the defect.
4. The more sutures that are put in, the easier they are to close and tie, and the strain is more evenly distributed (Figure 17.12).

After the sutures have all been placed the flaps are brought together, the upper being 'railroaded' down the sutures until it lies overlapping the lower flap (Figure 17.13).

The sutures are now tied, fixing the tissues firmly (but not too tightly) together. A triple layer, double throw knot is used. When all the knots are complete the ends are cut short.

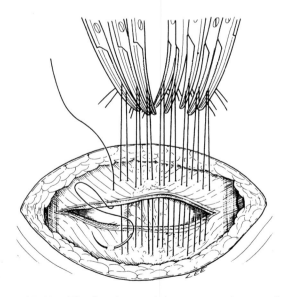

Figure 17.12 The first layer of deep sutures is now placed. The sutures enter the upper flap 3 cm from its margin. They go through both aponeurotic layers (anterior and posterior rectus sheaths) on either side and through the full thickness of the linea alba in the midline. The sutures are then carried down to and then through the lower flap 1 cm from the margin. The sutures are left lax and held in haemostats

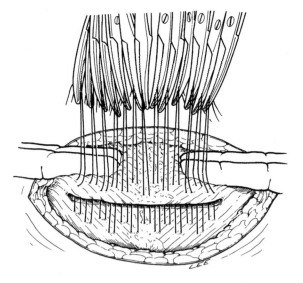

Figure 17.13 The sutures in the upper flap are all placed. The upper flap is now 'railroaded' down onto the lower flap

A fine suction drain is now placed in between the two flaps of the aponeurosis. The edge of the upper flap is sutured to the anterior surface of the lower flap using the same non-absorbable material as previously. Suture bites of over 1 cm into both upper and lower flaps are used (Figure 17.14).

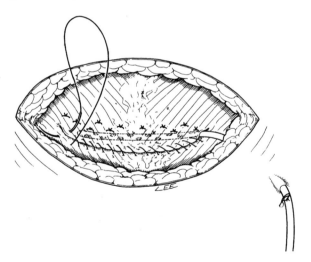

Figure 17.14 The sutures are tied and a suction drain introduced. The upper flap is sutured to the anterior surface of the lower flap. This gives the classic Mayo or 'vest over pants' overlap

CLOSURE

Meticulous haemostasis, suction drainage and obliteration of any dead space are the essential components of this part of the operation.

The subcutaneous fat is closed in terraces using fine absorbable polymer. Suction drainage is employed.

The skin is closed using a slowly absorbable subcuticular suture. Suturing of the skin is not recommended: it is often poor and infected in the vicinity of a long-standing umbilical hernia and sutures may carry skin bacteria along their tracks to the deeper parts of the wound or introduce sepsis adjacent to the non-absorbable hernia repair.

POSTOPERATIVE CARE

If there has been extensive handling and dissection of the small gut and omentum during the operation, postoperative nasogastric suction and parenteral metabolic support will be needed until normal peristalsis is re-established.

Early ambulation and breathing exercises are essential. The postoperative problem which most frequently arises is respiratory embarrassment caused by the wound pain and the newly raised intra-abdominal pressure.

Conclusions

Umbilical hernias in the adult are unsightly and painful. Incarceration, obstruction and strangulation are common. Operation should always be recommended.

The vertical overlapping operation described by Mayo is used. The operation is accomplished using non-absorbable sutures for the aponeurotic repair.

18 EPIGASTRIC HERNIA AND LAPAROSCOPIC 'PORT SITE' HERNIA

An epigastric hernia is a protrusion of extraperitoneal fat between the decussating fibres of the linea alba. These hernias usually occur in the midline of the epigastrium between the xiphisternum and the umbilicus, but small hernias can occur away from the midline and may protrude into the rectus muscle sheath. If these hernias enlarge considerably they may develop a peritoneal sac, which may be subcutaneous in midline hernia or interstitial, within the rectus sheath, in more lateral hernias.[43]

Incidence

The population incidence of epigastric hernia is undetermined. These hernias are infrequent in infants and young children, occurring in teenagers or young adults. They are more frequent in males than females in the ratio 3:1.[790] They account for 3.4% of external hernias in a series from Nigeria,[281] in the US Armed Forces they account for 5.0% of external abdominal hernias but this figure may be an underestimate because these small fatty hernias are often not classified separately in official data.[426] Other authors record a similar low incidence. They are frequently found in young men taking up physical exercise such as athletes or those in military service.

Symptomatology

Epigastric hernias cause symptoms quite out of proportion to their size. The very narrow sharp-edged opening in the linea alba predisposes to attacks of strangulation of the extraperitoneal fat which then becomes swollen, oedematous and tender. During attacks the patient will suffer severe abdominal pain.

The occurrence of such attacks is an adequate indication for operative treatment. It is, however, important to investigate the patient fully; a small innocent epigastric hernia is sometimes blamed for symptoms which are in fact due to some intra-abdominal condition, such as a peptic ulcer, cholelithiasis or hydronephrosis. At the same time it is true to say that an epigastric hernia may sometimes produce symptoms which closely resemble those due to a peptic ulcer. Pemberton and Curry, in a 1936 classic paper, reviewed 296 patients with epigastric hernia treated at the Mayo Clinic from 1910 to 1936.[735]

They concluded that no group of visceral symptoms could be said to be typical of epigastric hernia and great care must be taken to exclude intra-abdominal disease before operation is undertaken on a patient with an epigastric hernia associated with visceral symptoms. This caution needs emphasizing. The most frequently occurring intercurrent disorders causing visceral symptoms are peptic ulcer and cholelithiasis. The intermittent nature of their symptoms can be confused with other intermittent abdominal pathologies such as idiopathic hydronephroses and congenital obstructions of the small gut.

Small epigastric hernias that entrap the ligamentum teres or the adjacent extraperitoneal fat of the falciform ligament can cause symptoms similar to foregut disease. This is due to visceral afferent stimuli from the falciform ligament being transmitted via the coeliac plexus.[676] The exclusion of these diagnoses by endoscopy and ultrasound gallbladder scan should be routine before epigastric hernia repair.

Epigastric hernias are not uncommon in older children. Often, they are first noticed when the child complains of pain in them, caused by nipping of the fat in the hernia by the tight margins of the aponeurosis. In children, many epigastric hernias resolve spontaneously.

Pathological anatomy

The linea alba is an area of decussation of the three tendinous aponeurotic muscle strata of the anterior abdominal wall. At the midline these three aponeuroses, the external oblique, the internal oblique and the transverse abdominis are formed of fine tendinous fibres invested in loose areolar tissue.

The fibres of the external oblique have a downward, forward and medial inclination and additionally, especially around the umbilicus, describe a gentle upward curve (Figure 18.1). Above the umbilicus most aponeurotic fibres cross the midline and appear as the superficial fibres of the opposite side; they thus form the superficial layer of a double strata external oblique aponeurosis. When they make the cross over from one side to the other they decussate with the fibres of the opposite side; in 40% the fibres decussate only once at the midline – 'single decussation' – whereas in 60% of abdominal walls they

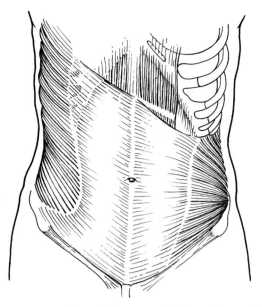

Figure 18.1 The fibres of the external oblique have a downward and medial direction. They run around the umbilicus and are almost horizontal there. (After Askar, 1984[43])

and decussating again. Below the umbilicus, except for a small area immediately adjacent to the umbilicus, this pattern of triple decussation is not seen; all the fibres of the external oblique invariably pass downwards and medially in a single stratum, then all the fibres cross the midline in a single decussation to give the external oblique a clearly defined pattern. This pattern of single or triple decussation with interlocking fibres gives the external oblique a very fine reinforced mesh structure about and above the umbilicus.

The internal oblique muscle consists of fan-shaped muscle bundles laterally. The upper fibres are directed upwards and medially, the middle horizontally and the lower arch downwards and medially. The aponeurotic bundles in both the superficial and the deep strata follow the same direction. At the midline (the linea alba) the anterior lamina fibres fuse with and are continuous with the fibres of the contralateral external oblique (Figure 18.2).

The fleshy bundles of the transverse abdominal muscle, the deepest layer of abdominal musculature, are not strictly transverse, the upper bundles go horizontal and upwards and the lowermost ones are horizontal. In 5% of specimens all the fibres go medially towards each other. The lowermost fibres of the transverse muscle are directed downwards and medially and are often parallel to the inguinal ligament (Figure 18.3).

The various muscle bundle and aponeurotic fibre directions give the anterior abdominal wall a reinforced criss-cross 'plywood' structure particularly in the upper abdomen. The anterior abdominal wall can be divided

decussate twice additionally to give three decussations, 'triple decussation'. This triple decussation is seen only above the umbilicus and never below (see Figure 18.4). In single decussation the fibres of the deep strata of one side emerge to gain the superficial status of the other side. In triple decussation the deep fibres appear superficial at the midline and then deep again after crossing the midline

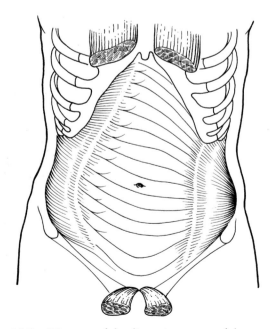

Figure 18.2 Diagram of the digastric pattern of the transversus (right) and the posterior lamina of the internal oblique (left). (After Askar, 1984[43])

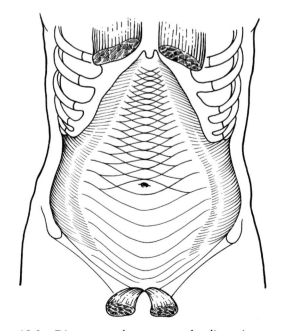

Figure 18.3 Diagram to demonstrate the digastric structure of the two contralateral transverse abdominal muscles. (After Askar, 1984[43])

into two structural–functional zones, an upper 'parachute area' aiding respiratory movement and a lower 'belly support' area. The anatomy of the midline aponeurosis is related to epigastric hernia formation. Epigastric herniation is found exclusively in patients with a single anterior and single posterior lines of decussion, this is found in only 30% of cadaver specimens examined (Figure 18.4); un-coordinated tearing strains on the aponeurotic fibres of the linea alba, for instance in vigorous sports, coughing or vomiting, will stretch the decussations and allow the development of fatty protrusions between their bundles.[41]

Repair techniques

All epigastric hernias should be repaired surgically. The only cure for the sometimes disabling and troublesome symptoms is surgical and exploration should always be advised.

Most surgeons recommend simple techniques to repair the defect. Simple suturing without tension is usually employed and is recommended. A Mayo type 'vest over pants' technique may be appropriate is some cases with larger defects, especially those that have to be extended laterally to gain control of a peritoneal sac. Askar, whose contributions to an understanding of the anatomy of this lesion are seminal, in 1978 recommended fascial darning[42, 43] of layer defects; however, the introduction of inert polypropylene mesh to repair such defects using the extraperitoneal plane has rendered fascial darning obsolete. The important operative, or nowadays preoperative, examination with ultrasound scanning principle is wide exposure of the linea alba so that multiple defects are not overlooked.

ANAESTHESIA

A general anaesthetic is usually employed, but repair can be quite satisfactorily performed under local infiltration with lignocaine or bupivacaine.

The operation

POSITION OF PATIENT

The patient is placed supine on the operating table.

SUTURE MATERIALS

For repair, metric 3 polypropylene sutures are used in adults. In children, PDS is advised.

DRAPING

Drapes are arranged so that the whole of the epigastric area from the costal margin to just below the umbilicus is exposed for surgery. Not infrequently the hernia is

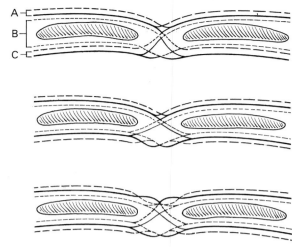

A = External oblique
B = Internal oblique
C = Transversus

Figure 18.4 Diagram of the decussation of the middle fibres of the aponeuroses. Single anterior and posterior decussation 30%. Single anterior and triple posterior decussation 10%. Triple anterior and triple posterior decussation 60%. (After Askar, 1984[43])

found to be larger than anticipated and placing the drapes widely facilitates an extended incision.

THE INCISION

A vertical incision has the advantage that the abdomen can easily be opened if this is deemed necessary. On the other hand, if the diagnosis is certain and preoperative investigations have excluded multiple defects and the hernia small a transverse skin crease incision gives better cosmesis (Figure 18.5).

The fatty hernia, which is enclosed within a fine capsule, is dissected out from the surrounding abdominal fat. The opening in the linear alba, which is usually tiny, should be enlarged by incisions from opposite sides

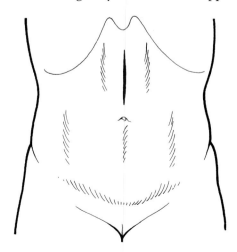

Figure 18.5 A vertical incision is made over the hernia

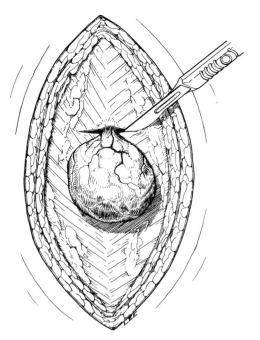

Figure 18.6 The fatty hernia is dissected out carefully

running laterally into the linea alba (Figure 18.6).

The hernia is incised at its neck to determine whether there is a peritoneal sac and to reduce contents if present into the abdomen (Figure 18.7).

The neck of the hernia is then ligated with a transfixion suture of absorbable polymer and the hernia excised (Figure 18.8).

At this stage the linea alba should be carefully examined

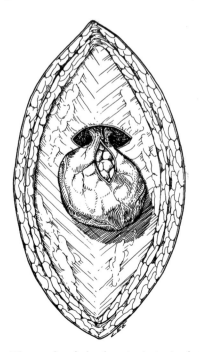

Figure 18.7 The neck of the hernia is incised. Sometimes these hernias contain small sacs with omentum in them

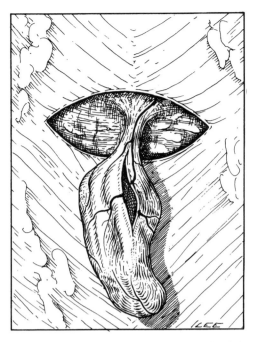

Figure 18.8 The omentum is reduced. The neck of the sac is closed with a transfixion suture. The redundant sac is then excised

for other defects. If necessary, palpation extraperitoneally may reveal other nearby aponeurotic defects that must be repaired. A small aponeurotic defect can usually be closed with a polypropylene or PDS continuous suture without tension.

Alternatively the opening in the linea alba is closed by

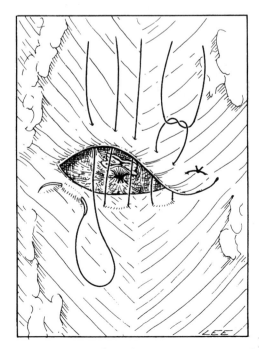

Figure 18.9 The upper flap of aponeurosis is sutured to the lower flap – the 'Mayo operation'

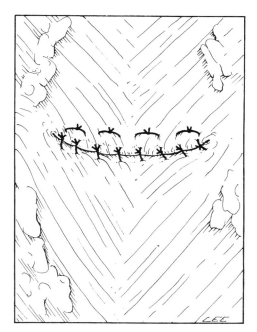

Figure 18.10   The sutures are tied with an overlap and a further line of sutures placed between the margin of the upper flap and the anterior surface of the lower flap

overlapping its edge with two rows of interrupted polypropylene or PDS – the first row inserted as mattress sutures and the second as simple sutures (Figures 18.9 and 18.10).

The subcutaneous fat and the skin are now closed (page 156)

Conclusions

Epigastric hernias usually contain extraperitoneal fat only. These hernias cause symptoms disproportionate to the hernia size. The symptoms of peptic ulcer disease or biliary disease may be confused with those of an incidental epigastric hernia.

Epigastric hernias are repaired by excising the protruding extraperitoneal fat or the rare peritoneal sac; the defect in the aponeurosis is then closed with a nonabsorbable suture.

Laparoscopic 'port site' hernias

'Port site' hernia following gynaecological laparoscopy was first recorded in 1968[294] and following the introduction of CAPD catheters in 1984.[279] The early case reports were of incarceration or Richter's type strangulation of bowel occurring within days of the laparoscopy or sometimes not for years after the initial laparoscopic intervention. The incidence of such herniation is estimated at 1 in 550 cases of laparoscopy, so it is no longer a rarity.[510] The herniation occurs most frequently after the use of the larger diameter laparoscopes (10 mm and 12 mm) although two cases following the use of 5 mm laparoscopes in gynaecological practice are recorded.[731] Most cases are recorded when the port site is through the midline, but the umbilicus, transrectal port sites and flank port sites can all give rise to herniation. Most patients present with localized pain and a lump but vomiting may occur if intestinal obstruction occurs. The importance of not dilating port sites and thus stretching the aponeurotic boundaries must be emphasized.[225] Direct suture of trocar sites avoids the hazard.[402] A comprehensive review of the subject by Krug identifies all these points.[510]

19 LUMBAR HERNIA

Anatomy

The lumbar area is bounded above by the twelfth rib, below by the iliac crest, behind by the erector spinae (sacrospinalis) and in front by the posterior border of the external oblique (a line passing from the tip of the twelfth rib to the iliac crest). Within this area two triangles are described: the superior lumbar triangle (of Grynfelt) and the inferior lumbar triangle (of Petit). The superior lumbar triangle is an inverted triangle, its base is the twelfth rib, its posterior border is the erector spinae and its anterior border the posterior margin of the external oblique, its apex is at the iliac crest inferiorly. The base of the inferior lumbar triangle is the iliac crest, its anterior border is the posterior margin of the external oblique muscle, its posterior border is the anterior edge of the latissimus dorsi muscle and its apex is superior.

Both the superior and the inferior lumbar triangles vary in size depending on the attachments of muscles to the iliac crest (Figure 19.1). The floor of both triangles is the thoracolumbar fascia incorporating the internal oblique and the transversus abdominis to a variable degree. The T12 and L1 nerves both cross the superior lumbar triangle.

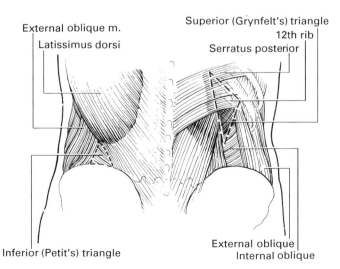

External oblique m.
Latissimus dorsi

Superior (Grynfelt's) triangle
12th rib
Serratus posterior

Inferior (Petit's) triangle

External oblique
Internal oblique

Figure 19.1 Dissection of the lumbar region to illustrate the anatomy of the inferior lumbar triangle (left) and the superior lumbar triangle (right)

Clinical features

Congenital lumbar hernia does occur and can be bilateral.[5] Such congenital hernias present as a bulge in the loin and may be associated with intestinal symptoms. Lumbar hernias may be acquired, following sepsis in the retroperitoneal tissues,[687] as a result of osteomyelitis or tuberculosis of the vertebral bodies or iliac crest which disrupts the lumbodorsal fascia,[972] or following surgical operations on the kidneys.[333] Traumatic lumbar hernias occur following direct blunt trauma[515] and seat-belt injuries in vehicle accidents.[285, 629]

Lumbar hernias may contain a variety of intra-abdominal organs; hernias of the colon are most frequent but small intestine, stomach and spleen are also likely candidates for herniation. A particular curiosity is the sliding hernia of the colon which causes intermittent obstructive symptoms.

Differential diagnosis must include tumours of the muscles, lipoma, haematoma associated with blunt trauma, abscess and renal tumours. Small fatty protrusions of retroperitoneal fat through the lumbodorsal fascia have been implicated as a cause of low back pain.[198, 289]

Backache radiating to the groin, presumably due to irritation of lateral cutaneous branches of the tenth, eleventh and twelfth intercostal nerves, has been recorded. Tiny fatty hernias along the tracks of cutaneous nerves through the lumbar fascia give rise to severe low back pain with radiation to the buttocks and thigh. These hernias are palpable and tender. They are similar to the fatty hernias that occur through the linea alba and anterior aponeurosis. Local anaesthetic infiltration abolishes the pain and confirms the diagnosis. Local excision and closure of the defect cures the condition. Nowadays the diagnosis is made/confirmed by CT scan which will delineate the defect.[285, 629]

The operation

In the acute traumatic situation, where full laparotomy to exclude intraperitoneal bleeding is mandatory, the abdomen should be explored through a midline abdominal incision.

Extensively damaged, ischaemic gut in the hernia will need resection with the formation of a stoma appropriately. The defect in the lumbodorsal fascia should be sutured with non-absorbable sutures. The defect in the fascia is best repaired with polypropylene mesh reinforcement.

When the hernia is being dealt with electively an oblique loin incision (in the line of the intercostal nerves) is made over it. Any sac is identified and the contents reduced. The peritoneum is closed and an extraperitoneal repair with polypropylene mesh effected.

20 PELVIC WALL HERNIAS, OBTURATOR HERNIA, SCIATIC HERNIA, PERINEAL HERNIA, SUPRAVESICAL HERNIA

Pelvic wall hernias

CLINICAL FEATURES AND DIAGNOSIS

Hernias through the walls of the pelvis are rare. The confines of the pelvis are compact and complex. The pelvis consists of bones and ligaments and muscles, penetrated by different nerves which supply the lower limb. Those which are sometimes accompanied by peritoneal protrusions are the obturator nerve, the sciatic nerve, the posterior cutaneous nerve of the thigh and the pudendal nerves. All the foramina which transmit these nerves can form hernial sites. Urogenital and rectal prolapse, which are examples of herniation through the floor of the pelvis, are not included in this section; neither are the iatrogenic incisional hernias which sometimes complicate operations for pelvic malignancy.

All pelvic wall hernias have similar clinical features. A peritoneal sac, closely allied to an important nerve, may contain pelvic or other abdominal organs. The hernia sac will protrude into the adductor muscles if it is an obturator hernia and into the buttock if it is a sciatic hernia. Perineal hernias present in the perineum of both sexes and in the labia in the female. Supravesical hernias present in the lower abdominal wall or into the anterior pelvis retropubically. Sciatic and perineal hernias are more prominent when the patient stands and often disappear altogether when the patient is recumbent.

These hernias may incarcerate or strangulate and are readily demonstrated on herniography[869] or CT scanning. Nowadays CT is the diagnostic modality of choice.[90] Finally all these hernias can be treated by excision of the peritoneal sac and extraperitoneal reinforcement of the defect using an inert plastic mesh prosthesis.[176]

Obturator hernia

Obturator hernia was first described by Arnaud de Ronsil in 1724. Hilton performed a laparotomy for the condition in 1848.[428] Sir Cecil Wakeley described the

anatomy of this hernia in 1939; he comprehensively reviewed the literature and described two cases of his own.[957] A further excellent review of the topic was by Craig in 1962.[202]

Obturator hernias are rare and few surgeons have seen many cases. However, the condition is curable by operation and although the clinical features are elusive, contrast herniography and modern CT scanning have transformed the diagnosis.[90, 207, 448]

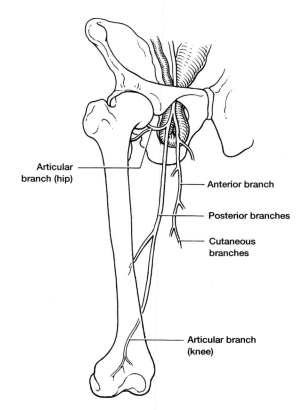

Figure 20.1 An obturator hernia develops in the obturator foramen where it is alongside the obturator nerve. A strangulated or obstructed hernia may cause groin discomfort and pain in the knee and an absent adductor reflex in the thigh

ANATOMY

Obturator hernia occurs through the obturator canal which is situated at the upper lateral part of the obturator membrane covering the obturator foramen and which transmits the obturator vessels and nerve. The obturator (adductor) region is the medial upper third of the thigh between the extensor and flexor muscle groups. The nerve is a mixed motor and sensory nerve supply to the adductor muscles of the thigh and the skin overlying them. The obturator nerve arises from the ventral rami of L2, L3 and L4. At the obturator foramen the nerve divides into anterior and posterior branches separated by a few fibres of the obturator externus muscle. The posterior branch gives a slender articular branch which penetrates the posterior capsule of the knee joint and is distributed to the anterior knee joint[363] (Figure 20.1).

The hernial sac may follow the path of the anterior or that of the posterior division of the nerve. Rarely the hernia has been found to descend beneath the superficial part of the obturator membrane. The path of the hernia is of little clinical importance; it is important to remember that the obturator nerve is posterolateral and it should be visualized and avoided if the obturator membrane requires division to release the hernial sac (Figure 20.2).

Most authorities cite anatomic variation as an aetiological factor. Obturator hernia is six times more common in females than males; the more marked inclination of the broader female pelvis, together with multiple pregnancy, are factors in the sex incidence. Obturator hernia usually occurs after the fiftieth birthday and is sometimes preceded by weight loss. The largest series recorded is 20 cases from the University of Chang Mai, Thailand – all the patients were female.[618] In another series from the Orient all five patients were women aged over 55 years.[522] Watson, in his series collected from the literature, found one case, a female aged

12 years old.[972] Obturator hernia is more common in Oriental (Chinese and Japanese) than Caucasian women.

Obturator hernia is a rare condition and can present with no obvious external signs. It should be particularly suspected in elderly women with a history of recurrent small bowel obstruction. Obturator hernia has a considerable incidence of potentially lethal complications.

CLINICAL FEATURES

Obturator hernia nearly always becomes manifest only when acute symptoms of strangulation supervene.[30, 395, 468] The rigid margins of the obturator foramen cannot stretch, so strangulation is inevitable if a hernia develops and gut or genitalia (the broad ligament and ovary) then enter the sac.[574, 862, 932, 1001]

Fifty percent of obturator hernias present with groin discomfort and with pain or parasthesiae radiating to the knee, caused by pressure on the adjacent nerve – Howship–Romberg sign.[202, 862, 876] This sign can be made more specific by noting whether coughing and thigh movements, especially extension, abduction and external rotation, make the pain or parasthesiae worse. The sign may be difficult to elucidate in the elderly dehydrated patient. Another test is an absent adductor reflex in the thigh – Hannington–Kiff sign.[396] The adductor reflex is a stretch reflex and is elicited by placing the index finger at right angles across the adductor muscles, 5.0 cm above the knee, and percussing onto the extended finger with a patella hammer. The contraction of the adductor muscle will be seen and felt. The reflex is absent in cases of strangulated obturator hernia. Comparison with the opposite side, which is often hyperactive in cases of obturator hernia strangulation, will confirm the diagnosis. The absence of the adductor reflex in a patient with a normal patellar reflex is a strong indicator of compression of the obturator nerve from whatever cause.

If infarction of bowel occurs in thin, emaciated, elderly females who present with strangulated obturator hernia, blood-stained fluid is exuded into the upper thigh and presents as a faint bruise in the femoral triangle just below the medial part of the inguinal ligament (Figure 20.3). If the infarction progresses to perforation subcutaneous emphysema develops in the upper thigh.[481] A fistula into the rectosigmoid has been described following the development and drainage of such emphysema.

Vaginal examination confirms the diagnosis, a tender mass being felt in the obturator region. Rectal examination is unhelpful because the obturator foramen is not palpable per rectum (Figure 20.4).

A partial enterocele (Richter's hernia) is often found in obturator hernial sacs. The rigid margins of the obturator membrane make early strangulation inevitable. A partial enterocele will make the clinical features more

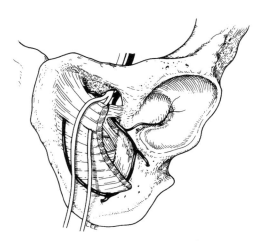

Figure 20.2 The obturator canal transmits the obturator vessels and nerve

ambiguous, and the diagnosis will be missed if a careful physical examination is not done.

Rheumaticky type pains in the groin and in the lower back can be caused by the bladder in an obturator hernia;[630] similar groin pains following a hip prosthesis have been described as causing confusing differential diagnoses with concomitant obturator hernia.[331] We can only re-emphasize the diagnostic difficulties of obturator hernia. Appendicitis in a strangulated obturator hernia sac in a Ghanaian male has been described from Accra.[31]

Modern radiographic techniques can readily demonstrate and diagnose obturator hernia. Plain abdominal radiographs will demonstrate the characteristic intestinal

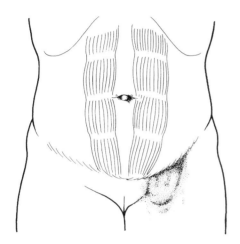

Figure 20.3   The hernia may be palpable in the upper thigh lying in the femoral triangle between the adductor longus and pectineus muscles. If the hernia is strangulated there may be a telltale area of bruising over the hernial sac in the thigh[21]

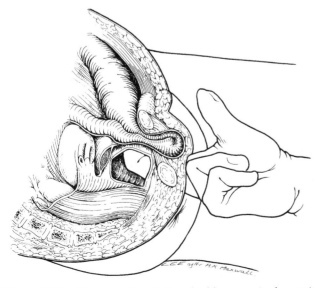

Figure 20.4   Obturator hernia is palpable on vaginal examination

gas patterns if there is obstruction. Herniography using an intraperitoneal water-soluble contrast will sometimes delineate an obturator hernia sac as a small localized diverticulum in the upper lateral corner of the obturator foramen. These hernias protrude beneath the superior ramus of the pubis.[376] In cases of obscure groin pain herniography can be particularly helpful.[156, 273, 870]

The radiological diagnosis of obturator hernia has been revolutionized by CT scanning which does not require the potentially hazardous puncture of the peritoneal cavity to instil the contrast medium in herniography.[207] This is nowadays the diagnostic modality of choice.[90, 448]

The use of modern imaging techniques has suggested that obturator hernia may be more common than previously suspected. In a series of 396 patients with suspected occult hernias, Nagahama found seven patients with symptomatic obturator hernia and another seven with asymptomatic obturator hernia, giving a frequency of 3.5% in this series.[689]

OPERATIVE MANAGEMENT

Anderson (1900) described a groin approach to the sac in the space between the adductor longus and pectineus.[21] Milligan recommended an approach through an oblique incision, splitting the fibres of the external oblique with an extraperitoneal dissection to the hernia.[654] Both these routes produce little shock but neither is adequate for bowel visualization and resection if needed. Either a paramedian incision with a supplementary thigh exploration or a Henry type extraperitoneal approach is recommended.[418] Because the diagnosis is so rarely made with certainty before laparotomy, an abdominal incision has been employed in most reported series.

Repair by suturing or darning across the peritoneal opening has been employed in most cases.[4, 971] Prosthetic repair with tantalum gauze[921] and the use of a tantalum gauze plug in a recurrent obturator hernia[737] have been described. In contemporary surgery an extraperitoneal patch with polypropylene mesh is recommended. Using adjacent peritoneum to suture across the defect or plug it is not recommended; such peritoneal repairs get reabsorbed and the hernia then recurs.[290]

PREOPERATIVELY

Haemodynamic consideration

If intestinal obstruction is present, appropriate intravenous fluid and electrolyte replacement is commenced and the patient resuscitated before anaesthesia. If extensive bowel infarction is found, whole blood replacement may be needed and this should be planned for preoperatively. A nasogastric tube should be passed and the stomach contents aspirated prior to anaesthesia if intestinal obstruction is present.

Suture materials, prostheses and haemostasis

For details see Chapter 6.

Preoperative catheterization

An in-dwelling balloon catheter is inserted prior to operation and the bladder kept empty throughout the procedure.

THE OPERATION

Position of patient

The patient is laid on her back on the operating table and drapes are placed to allow a lower paramedian incision. The drapes should be arranged so that access to the appropriate upper thigh can be gained if necessary.

Incision and exploration of abdomen

A lower abdominal paramedian incision is performed (Figure 20.5).

Nearly always it is small intestine which is caught within the strangulated obturator hernia. Dilated bowel will be seen to pass into the pelvic cavity and thence into the obturator canal, from which the collapsed distal gut is found to emerge. At this point it is necessary to tilt the operating table into the head-down position.

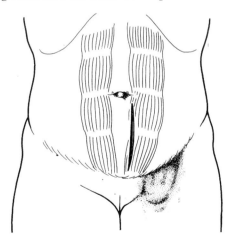

Figure 20.5   Access is through a lower abdominal paramedian incision on the same side as the hernia

Exposure

The intestinal contents within the pelvic cavity are packed off into the upper abdomen with warm wet packs. If the bowel above the obstruction is grossly

dilated, it should be decompressed by retrograde milking of the contents to the stomach and aspiration through the nasogastric tube. The bowel above and below the loop caught within the hernia should be clamped with non-crushing clamps in case the obstructed loop has either perforated or is torn during delivery; in this way peritoneal contamination will be minimized (Figure 20.6).

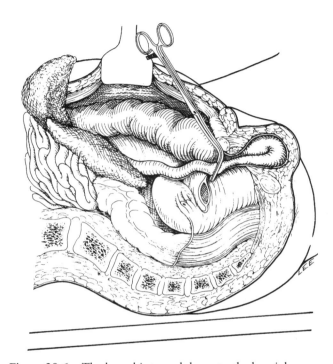

Figure 20.6   The bowel is traced down to the hernial sac

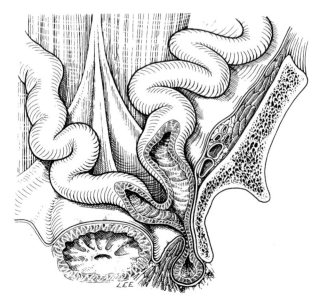

Figure 20.7   The neck of the sac lies in the obturator canal, which is quite narrow

The sac

This is formed by a narrow and usually small pouch of peritoneum lying within the tight confines of the obturator canal. Indeed, in some cases only part of the circumference of the bowel is caught within the hernia, forming a Richter type of strangulation (Figure 20.7).

Reduction of hernia

If the hernia cannot be reduced by gentle manipulation, the constricting ring should be stretched with the index finger; if this is not sufficient, then it must be divided taking particular care not to injure the obturator vessels and nerve which lie posterolaterally to the obturator foramen. These are avoided if any incision extending from the obturator foramen is made in an upward and medial direction.

Exposure in thigh

These manoeuvres will enable the occluded bowel to be released. If this is impossible, however, then the hernia must be exposed in the obturator region and its content carefully coaxed back by gentle pressure. A vertical incision is made medial to the femoral vein. The adductor longus is retracted medially and the pectineus pulled laterally or its fibres divided to enable the sac to be visualized (Figure 20.8).

When the strangulated gut has been delivered it must be carefully inspected. If gangrene of a small portion of the bowel has supervened, this area may be invaginated by a few seromuscular sutures. If the area is more extensive, resection must be performed.

Inversion of sac

The sac is inverted by inserting a pair of artery forceps into it, grasping its fundus and applying steady traction (Figure 20.9). The fundus is opened and the peritoneum gently raised from the surrounding tissues by blunt dissection in the extraperitoneal plane. A coiled up plug of polypropylene mesh is then put into the hernia defect and the peritoneum closed over it; or preferably a full polypropylene mesh patch is applied.

Mesh repair

The defect in the obturator membrane, which may be considerable, should be repaired using a patch of polypropylene mesh placed deep to the peritoneum. The hernial sac is inverted and lifted. Then the adjacent peritoneum is freed from the pelvic parietes. The sac is opened and through this opening a mesh patch, sufficiently large to overlap the defect by 2.0 cm in each direction, is placed. The patch needs layering over the defect; no suturing is necessary. The peritoneal sac is excised and closed so that the patch is left in the extraperitoneal plane (Figure 20.10).

Extraperitoneal approach

The extraperitoneal approach (see Chapter 13) through a midline lower abdominal incision will give good access to the obturator area. Repair with mesh placed in the extraperitoneal plane can be used to make a repair if the defect is large.[971]

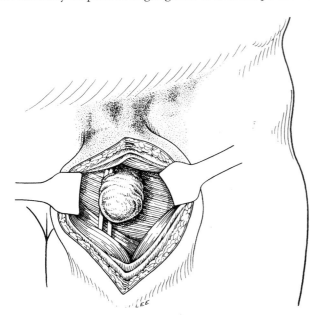

Figure 20.8 If the hernia cannot be reduced readily into the abdomen, a thigh incision and dissection is needed. An incision is made below the inguinal ligament and the sac is exposed. The adductor longus is retracted medially and the pectineus laterally. The pectineus can be divided to make adequate exposure of the neck possible

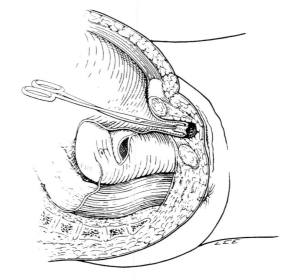

Figure 20.9 The sac is invaginated, transfixed and excised

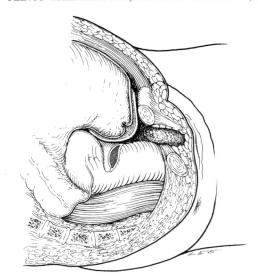

Figure 20.10 Usually the defect is small and no formal repair is used. If the defect is large an extraperitoneal patch of mesh can be placed and the peritoneum closed over it. Another example of the 'ham sandwich' technique of hernia repair

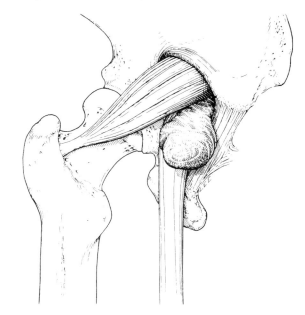

Figure 20.11 The sciatic hernia passes through the greater sciatic foramen either above or below the pyriformis muscle

POSTOPERATIVE CARE

Early mobilization should be encouraged. If intestinal obstruction has been present, nasogastric aspiration and intravenous fluid replacement will be needed until the bowel regains its function.

Sciatic hernia

A sciatic hernia is a protrusion of a pelvic peritoneum sac through either the greater sciatic foramen (above or below the piriformis) or the lesser sciatic foramen (Figure 20.11). The more common variety is through the greater sciatic foramen above the piriformis. The sac extends backwards and inferiorly deep to the gluteus maximus muscle. Sciatic hernias are very rare. In a series of 50 000 hernias from one hospital in Zaria, Nigeria, one sciatic hernia was reported.[47]

Watson in 1948 found 35 case reports[972] and concurs that sciatic hernia is very rare. Sidney Black comprehensively reviewed the subject in 1995; he noted that although the Mayo Clinic from 1944 to 1974 repaired 30 000 hernias there was no sciatic hernia in the series.[100]

Sciatic hernias may be either congenital or acquired. Congenital hernias present in children as reducible lumps in the buttock. Adult-acquired hernias are found equally in the sexes, herniation frequently being related to straining or heavy lifting. Without adequate repair these hernias may recur; indeed, a case in a 60-year-old woman which recurred three times was reported by Ivanov and colleagues in 1994.[458] Sciatic hernia related to wasting and weight loss in a young female was reported from the same unit in 1995[458] – surely a record!

CLINICAL FEATURES

The symptoms of a sciatic hernia are very variable depending upon the structures involved in the hernia sac. If there are elements of intestinal obstruction, then abdominal distension, cramps and nausea are common. Many cases present first as undiagnosed intestinal obstruction and the true diagnosis is made only when the abdomen is opened.[972] Some hernias present as bulges in the lower buttocks; bulges that characteristically are more pronounced when the patient stands, 'gurgle' and have bowel sounds in them, cause discomfort when the patient sits down and are reducible. Sciatic nerve compression can occur with pain and muscle weakness down the posterior of the lower limb. The hernia sac, and any contents, can be delineated by herniography but the investigation of choice is CT scanning.[337]

OPERATION

Operation is best through the main abdominal cavity. The patient is placed in the Trendelenburg position with the head tilted down. The abdomen is opened through a midline incision; the mouth of the hernia is situated just posterior to the broad ligament in the female and in a similar position anterolaterally to the rectum in the male. Often the hernial sac is readily identified by a loop of small intestine in the sac.

Firstly the contents are gently drawn out of the sac. If the neck is narrow it can be dilated under direct vision. If there is still difficulty with incarcerated intestine the neck can be carefully incised, taking care to avoid any underlying nerves which must be visualized. Exterior pressure on the buttock mass will expedite this process. Once the sac has been emptied of its contents forceps are inserted, the fundus grasped and the whole sac invaginated. The fundus is then amputated, thus opening up the extraperitoneal space.

A large area of extraperitoneum is opened up by blunt dissection and a prosthetic mesh placed in to cover the defect widely. It is probably best to use a polypropylene sheet for this repair but alternatives are polyvinyl sponge or a rolled up polypropylene plug. Repairs using fascia raised from the piriformis or rolled up plugs of peritoneum are no longer advocated. The peritoneum is closed over the repair. This extraperitoneal repair is a further elaboration of the Stoppa operation for abdominal wall hernias.[176]

Perineal hernia

AETIOLOGY

Perineal hernias are very rare. Acquired (incisional) perineal hernias occur in both males and females after abdominoperineal resection of the rectum and after pelvic operations for genital malignancy (radical prostatectomy and gynaecological exenteration). These acquired forms of herniation can be extremely distressing and sometimes warrant repair using gracilis or rectus abdominis flaps.

Naturally occurring herniation through the pelvic floor is five times more common in older women (40–60 years) than in men. This sex difference is due to the broader female pelvis and antecedent obstetric damage to the pelvic floor. The hernia sac may protrude anterior or posterior to the superficial transverse perineal muscles. Anterior hernias proceed into the labium majus where they present as a 'gurgling' lump. In the male only posterior hernias have been described. Posterior hernias occur between the levator ani and coccygeus muscles. If the internal fascia of the obturator internus muscle and the levator ani inferior fascia fail to fuse there is a potential space, the hiatus of Schwalbe, through which a hernia may protrude. Patients complain of a lower gluteal lump and discomfort. The hernia emerges below the inferior margin of the gluteus maximus, then extends anteriorly as a perineal lump. In the female the hernia extends into the labium majus – a pudendal hernia – where it causes discomfort. The mass is readily palpable and usually easily reducible. Intestinal sounds in the lump may be noticed by the patient.

Diagnosis is simple. Herniography will delineate the defect and the sac and contents and CT scanning confirms the picture. Operative treatment is straightforward: with the patient in the Trendelenburg position the contents are coaxed from the hernia sac. The peritoneum of the sac and surrounding areas is raised and a mesh patch inserted to cover the full extent of the levator

floor. Ivalon sponge is a particularly good prosthetic in these circumstances but polypropylene mesh could also be used. This operation is straightforward and similar to the Wells operation for rectal prolapse (Figure 20.12).

Supravesical hernia

Supravesical hernia was first described by Astley Cooper in 1804.[193] External supravesical hernias bulge through the transversus muscle aponeurosis and fascia transversalis in the most medial part of the myopectineal orifice of Fruchaud. They then present as very medial direct inguinal hernias or as interparietal hernias within the lower abdominal wall.[867] The defects in the fascia transversalis are sometimes multiple, as in the original case with six hernial openings described by Astley Cooper in 1804; two of these hernias were in the supravesical fossae (Figure 20.13). Skandalakis and his colleagues have also described two separate patients with multiple hernias.[864, 866]

Anterior (exsupravesical hernia presents with a groin lump and are usually routinely repaired as groin hernias without special difficulty.

Internal (anterior) supravesical hernias most commonly occur in the supravesical fossa whence a hernia

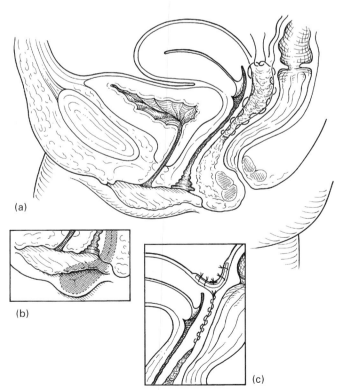

Figure 20.12 A perineal hernia extends into the labium majus through the potential space between the vagina and the rectum. (a) The hernia is reduced and the space obliterated. (b) Further obliteration of this space is ensured by a prosthetic patch

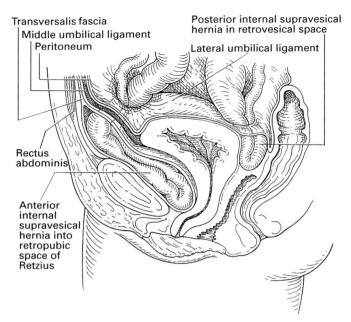

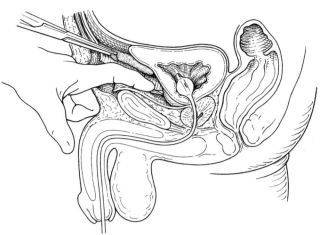

Figure 20.13 Supravesical hernias occur through the parietal peritoneum either anterior to the bladder and extending into the retropubic space, or posterior to the bladder and uterus in the female and extending into the pararectal tissues

Figure 20.14 A supravesical hernia in the male may present as a groin lump or plunge into the retropubic space. Repair using an extraperitoneal mesh technique can be employed

sac extends anterior to the bladder and posterior to the pubis into the retropubic space of Retzius. A loop of small intestine can become incarcerated and obstructed in such a hernia (Figure 20.14). Most reported cases have been in males and they usually present as urgent cases with obstruction which sometimes is associated with bladder symptoms if the bladder capacity is reduced by the hernia. Treatment is surgical because it is important to obliterate the sac to prevent recurrence. Internal (posterior) supravesical hernias traverse defects in the parietal peritoneum posterior to the bladder and into the pararectal tissue.

21 SPIGELIAN HERNIA

Definition

Spigelian hernias occur through slit-like defects in the anterior abdominal wall adjacent to the semilunar line which extends from the tip of the ninth costal cartilage to the pubic spine at the lateral edge of the rectus muscle inferiorly. The semilunar line is formed by the division of the lamellae of the internal oblique to form the rectus sheath. Anteriorly throughout its length, the semilunar line is reinforced by the aponeurosis of the external oblique. Posteriorly in the cephalad two-thirds it is reinforced by the transversus abdominis muscle which is muscular almost to the midline in the upper abdomen. This musculo-aponeurotic support prevents herniation which is, therefore, very rare above the umbilicus. In the lower third or so the posterior rectus sheath is deficient where the internal oblique and transversus form the thin margin of the arcuate fold of Douglas, halfway between the umbilicus and the pubis. Most Spigelian hernias occur in the lower abdomen where the posterior rectus sheath is deficient, but hernias have been recorded all along the semilunar line (Figure 21.1).

Morphologically, some direct inguinal hernias (parainguinal hernias) are hernias through the semilunar line below and medial to the inferior epigastric vessels. There is no useful purpose in including this more frequent variety of hernia under the heading 'Spigelian hernia'.[232, 935]

The hernial ring is a well-defined defect in the transversus aponeurosis. The hernial sac, surrounded by extraperitoneal fatty tissue, is often interparietal (interstitial) passing through the transversus and the internal oblique aponeuroses and then spreading out beneath the intact aponeurosis of the external oblique, or lying in the rectus sheath alongside the rectus muscle[15, 127, 880] (Figures 21.2 and 21.3).

The diagnosis of a Spigelian hernia is difficult; few doctors suspect it, it has no characteristic symptoms, and the hernia may be interparietal with no obvious mass on inspection or palpation.

Historical note

The semilunar line was described by Adriaan van Spieghel (Spigelius, 1578–1625),[885] who held the Chair of Anatomy and Surgery in Padua in the early seventeenth century; however, the hernia that is named for him was first described by Klinkosch in 1764.[504] Sir Astley Cooper recognized the hernia and described three cases in 1807. By 1827, Sir Astley Cooper had collected 23 cases of Spigelian hernia of which 19 occurred below

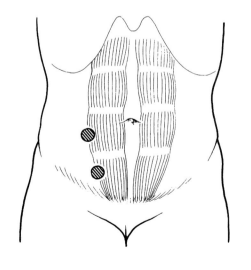

(a)

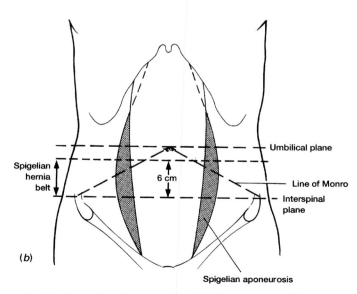

Spigelian hernia belt

6 cm

Umbilical plane

Line of Monro

Interspinal plane

Spigelian aponeurosis

(b)

Figure 21.1 (a) Spigelian hernias occur through the semilunar line just lateral to the rectus muscle. They are more frequent in the lower abdomen at or below the fold of Douglas (b) The sites of Spigelian hernias. (After Spangen, 1984[879])

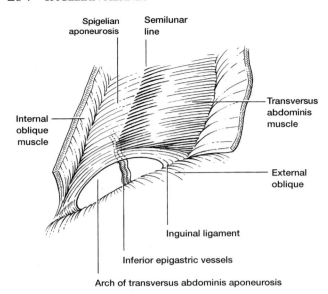

Internal oblique muscle

Spigelian aponeurosis

Semilunar line

Transversus abdominis muscle

External oblique

Inguinal ligament

Inferior epigastric vessels

Arch of transversus abdominis aponeurosis

Figure 21.2 The Spigelian aponeurosis

the umbilicus. He wrote a precise description of his findings and launched the theory that the neurovascular openings in the Spigelian fascia may become enlarged permitting herniation: 'Vascular openings are situated in the semilunar line, viscera can find an easy exit through these openings.'[193, 195]

Anatomic basis

The detailed anatomic basis for Spigelian hernia was unravelled by Anson and his associates.[1005] They have shed new light upon the predisposition to hernia of the semilunar line and drawn attention to the 'banding' of the abdominal wall muscles at this site. In a series of dissections of adult cadavers they demonstrated that in 22% the lateral abdominal wall muscles form bands or fascicles at the semilunar line and that there are slit-like deficiencies in the aponeurosis between these fascicles. Extraperitoneal fat and peritoneum can become extruded through these musculo-aponeurotic defects. Most of the hernias of the semilunar line are described as occurring at or below the level of the arcuate fold of Douglas, and this corresponds with the distribution of the defects in the muscles as described by Anson.

The Spigelian aponeurosis is widest between 0 and 6 cm cranial to the interspinous plane and 85–90% of the hernias occur within this 'Spigelian hernia' band.[879]

Incidence

Two cases of Spigelian hernia have been reported in girls under 1 year old; in one case the hernia reduced spontaneously after repair of a congenital diaphragmatic

hernia and then spontaneously closed.[961] Two cases of childhood Spigelian hernia related to the neuropathy caused by a mediastinal neuroblastoma are reported in Japan.[510] Other causes of Spigelian hernia in childhood are trauma and abdominal wall surgery. The ratio of males to females in children is 1.5:1 – quite different to the ratio in adults.

Spigelian herniation is most frequently found in adults in the age range 40–70 (mean 50.5) years. In adults the male to female ratio is 1:1.18.[880] Spigelian hernias may be related to stretching in the abdominal wall caused by previous surgery or scarring.

Richter's type strangulation is reported, the sharp fascial margins of the aperture predisposing to this complication.[847, 880] Spigelian hernia has been described as a complication of CAPD.[284]

Spigelian hernias are uncommon; in the ten years 1970–79 only four cases, two males and two females, presented in Stockton-on-Tees. The incidence reported in the literature is less than 1% of all abdominal hernias treated surgically. Stuckej *et al.* (1973) reported 43 cases, the biggest series from one department, and estimated the incidence to be about 0.1% of all abdominal hernias.[902] Spangen (1976), in a classic thesis, has reviewed the literature exhaustively.[878] He reviews 744 patients operated on for Spigelian hernia; the mean age was 50 years (49.5 for women and 50.5 for men) and the ratio of women to men was 1.4:1. The hernia was bilateral in 24 patients and the ratio of right to left was 1.6:1. In 10 cases there was more than one hernia on one side. Most of the hernias were located below the umbilicus, only 28 being situated in the upper abdomen.[878]

Diagnosis

Spigelian hernias are of interest because of the diagnostic confusion they cause. The emerging hernial sac can be deflected by the overlying, intact, external oblique aponeurosis, so that it lies interstitially and tends to be pushed laterally where it may present as a swelling adjacent to the iliac crest and may easily be palpated at the anterosuperior iliac spine. Rarely the hernia can enter the rectus sheath to lie alongside the rectus muscle: in an acute presentation it can be confused with a spontaneous rupture of the rectus muscle or with a haematoma in the rectus sheath (Figure 21.3).

Patients may complain of a lump which often disappears when they lie recumbent; they may have symptoms of acute or subacute intestinal obstruction; or they may have a variety of vague abdominal discomforts. Spigelian hernias may lie interparietally between the flank muscle layers or within the rectus sheath and not be easily palpable.[880] Often the last is worse at the end of a day's work and settles when they lie down to rest. The local discomfort can be quite severe, but is

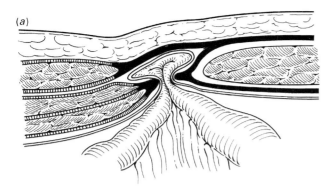

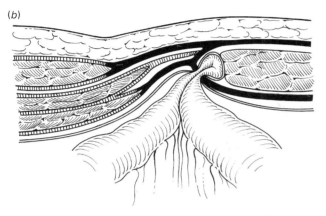

Figure 21.3 (a) A Spigelian hernia may be interstitial with a palpable mass at the linea semiluna (b) A Spigelian hernia may be occult, herniation occurring into the rectus sheath

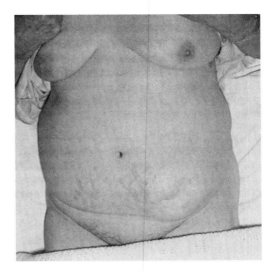

Figure 21.4 The patient may have a classical lump when she stands up. The lump is painful if the patient stretches and disappears if she lies down

sometimes only a feeling of 'something there that shouldn't be'.[959] On occasion, the pain is vague or dyspeptic and can be confused with peptic ulceration. It has been suggested that neuralgic pain is a consequence of local pressure on peripheral nerves as they pass through aponeurosis (Figure 21.4). Incarceration of the bladder in a Spigelian hernia has been reported.[839]

Classic features are localized pain made worse by stretching the arm on the affected side above the head to put the external oblique aponeurosis under tension, by abdominal straining, by defecation or by athletic exertion. Localized pain is associated with point tenderness and a reducible abdominal wall mass.

It is essential to examine the patient with the abdominal muscles relaxed; tense muscles compress an interparietal hernia and render it inconspicuous. The patient should also be examined standing because, although the external oblique muscle is tense, the general extent of the hernia may be felt on profile in this position.

Ultrasonic scanning has been advocated by Spangen.[880] With this aid he was able to obtain the correct diagnosis in 19 of 24 cases studied. Ultrasonic scanning of the semilunar line should be undertaken in all cases of obscure abdominal pain associated with

bulging of the belly wall in the standing patient. Deitch and Engel have confirmed the usefulness of ultrasound in the diagnosis of abdominal wall defects.[232] Ultrasound provides the diagnosis easily and cheaply in our experience and is recommended as the first-line imaging investigation. It is a sensible precaution to always ultrasonically scan the semilunar lines on both sides because herniation is frequently multiple.

Scanning by CT, performed with close thin sections, can visualize a Spigelian hernia. This is now the most reliable imaging technique to make the diagnosis.[432]

Many Spigelian hernias go unrecognized on clinical examination, and even after both ultrasound investigation and CT scanning patients having exploratory laparotomies in these circumstances should have careful bimanual (one hand intra-abdominally) examination of the linea semilunaris to diagnose small deficiencies.

The differential diagnosis includes appendicitis and appendix abscess, a tumour of the abdominal wall or a spontaneous haematoma of the rectus muscle.

Spigelian hernias are treacherous and have a real risk of strangulation. For this reason, operation is advised for all cases (Figure 21.5).

Preoperatively

SUTURE MATERIALS

For details see Chapter 3.

ANAESTHESIA

General anaesthesia is preferred, but local infiltration anaesthesia can be employed. If the latter is used, the operating surgeon must remember that the parietal

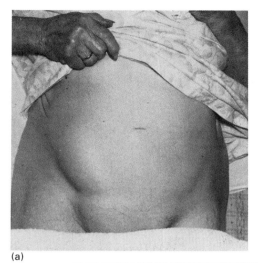

(a)

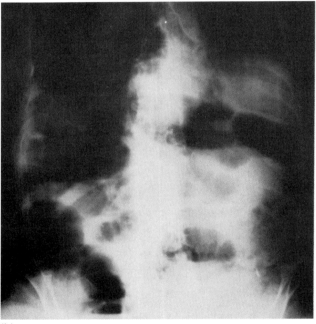

(b)

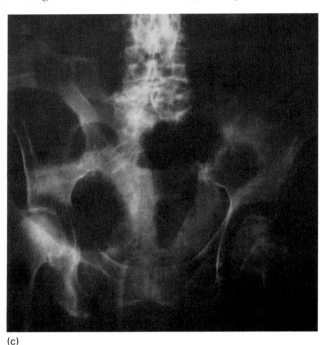

(c)

Figure 21.5 (a) An elderly woman with a strangulated Spigelian hernia and bilateral femoral hernias; (b) an abdominal film shows the features of intestinal obstruction and a gas-filled loop in the Spigelian hernia; (c) gas is also seen in a loop of small gut in the left femoral hernia (Courtesy of A.L.G. Peel)

peritoneum is very sensitive and manipulation of it can cause the patient much discomfort unless the anaesthesia is adequate (see Chapter 7).

The operation

POSITION OF PATIENT

The patient is laid on his back on the operating table.

Draping

Drapes are placed so as to allow easy access to the hernia and to the abdominal cavity if bowel resection becomes necessary in patients with strangulated or obstructed intestine.

THE INCISION

A transverse incision over the protrusion gives an excellent exposure. Only in the occasional very large hernia is it necessary to construct an elliptical incision and to remove the intervening redundant skin and subcutaneous tissue with the sac (Figure 21.6). If there is no obvious hernia protrusion, or if the diagnosis is in doubt, a midline or paramedian incision is advisable.

The dissection is deepened to the external oblique aponeurosis. The hernial sac may lie deep to the aponeurosis, between it and the internal oblique, or it may be within the sheath of the rectus muscle. In either of these situations it is necessary to incise the aponeurosis and split it in the direction of its fibres to expose the peritoneal sac (Figure 21.7).

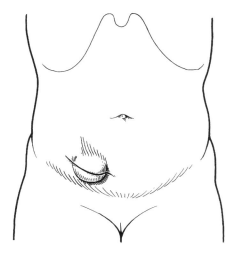

Figure 21.6   An oblique incision over the hernia gives access

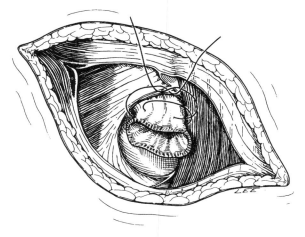

Figure 21.8   The sac is opened and the contents reduced, then the neck of the sac is closed with a transfixion suture of absorbable polymer. Redundant sac is excised

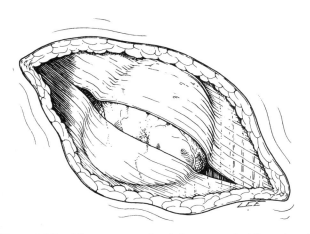

Figure 21.7   The aponeurosis of the external oblique is split to deliver the hernial sac

neck closed with either pursestring suture or by a continuous suture according to size (Figure 21.8).

CLOSURE

The opening in the internal oblique and transversus muscles is closed with a continuous suture of polypropylene. The external oblique aponeurosis is sutured with polypropylene and a suction drain is placed to the suture line (Figure 21.9). The subcutaneous fat is carefully closed. No 'dead spaces' should be left and the fat should be closed so that the skin is closely approximated.

Occasionally the aponeurotic margins of the sac are very lax and mobile; in these circumstances a 'Mayo-type' 'vest over pants' repair is preferable.

The skin is closed with a subcuticular suture.

Spigelian hernia defects may be multiple, therefore it is essential in every case to palpate the adjacent semilunar line fascia from the peritoneal surface to exclude other hernial orifices. To overlook a second Spigelian hernia could be catastrophic for the patient.

THE SAC

This is always present, even if the hernia is small. It may be globular or mushroom shaped. The most common content of the sac is omentum, which may be adherent, but small or large intestine may be found. The appendix, stomach, gall bladder, endometrium, ovary and ectopic testicle have all been described in Spigelian hernia sacs.[880]

EXCISION OF SAC

Once the sac has been adequately exposed, it is opened, its contents reduced, its redundant part excised and its

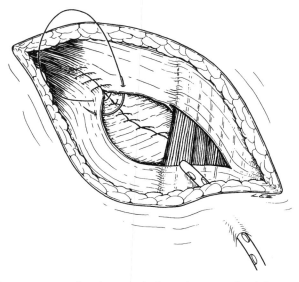

Figure 21.9   The deep and then the superficial layers of aponeurosis are separately closed with continuous sutures of polypropylene. A suction drain is always used

Postoperative care

If there has been extensive handling and dissection of the small gut and omentum during the operation, postoperative management with nasogastric suction and parenteral metabolic support will be needed until normal peristalsis is established.

Early ambulation and breathing exercises are essential. The postoperative problem which most frequently arises is respiratory embarrassment due to the wound pain and the newly raised intra-abdominal pressure.

Conclusions

Spigelian hernias are clinically elusive often until strangulation occurs. Ultrasound examination of the semilunar line is a simple and accurate method of diagnosis.

Operation should always be advised. Apart from the discomfort these hernias cause, they strangulate frequently and for this reason particularly they should be repaired.

22 INCISIONAL HERNIA (EXCLUDING PARASTOMAL HERNIA)

Historical note

Incisional hernia is iatrogenic and its incidence has increased with each increment of abdominal surgical intervention. An incisional hernia is the most perfect example of a 'surgeon-dependent variable'. The recent introduction of continuous ambulatory peritoneal dialysis has been followed by its own unique harvest of incisional hernias.[166, 284] Laparoscopic surgery has also added a new entity: 'Port Site' hernia[294] (Chapter 18, page 221).

The development of abdominal surgery in the nineteenth century – the excision of an ovarian cyst by McDowell in 1809,[632] partial gastrectomy by Billroth in 1881,[97] cholecystectomy by Langenbuch in 1882[924] – has been followed by operations to manage the incisional hernias which followed as complications. Gerdy repaired an incisional hernia in 1836 and Maydl another in 1886.[447] Judd in 1912[474] and Gibson in 1920[339] both described repair techniques based on extensive anatomic dissection of the scar and adjacent tissues. Prosthetic materials were introduced early on: autografts of fascia lata by Kirschner in 1910,[503] and fascial strips by Gallie and Le Mesurier in 1923.[324] Tendons, cutis and whole skin grafts, both homografts and heterografts, have been advocated and found to have problems. Non-biological prosthetics include stainless steel and tantalum gauze, polypropylene (Marlex, Proline), polyester (Mersilene) and nylon fabrics (these are reviewed in Chapter 6).

The ideal prosthetic material has yet to be discovered. The visionary Theodore Billroth stated more than a century ago, 'If we could artificially produce tissues of the density and toughness of fascia or tendon, the secret of radical cure of hernia would be discovered'.[815]

Symptoms and signs

An incisional hernia is defined by Pollock and his colleagues as 'A bulge visible and palpable when the patient is standing and often requiring support or repair'.[543]

Sixty per cent of patients with incisional hernias do not experience any symptoms; however, symptoms that predicate medical advice include difficulty in bending, embarrassment with the lump, discomfort from the size of the hernia, persistent abdominal pain and episodic subacute intestinal obstruction. Incarceration persisting to acute intestinal obstruction and strangulation necessitate emergency surgery.

Spontaneous rupture of incisional hernia is an unusual but life-threatening complication. This complication is more likely in infra-umbilical hernia. It may be exacerbated by friction of clothes or corsetry.[406] Hernias after gynaecological and obstetric interventions are most at risk.[843]

The demonstration of small incisional hernias may be very difficult. Patients with tiny protrusions of extraperitoneal fat and a small peritoneal sac may complain of a tender lump which is not always there but which causes quite severe localized pain when it is present. Physical examination of the patient supine and relaxed usually reveals the cause. Ultrasound examination is the most useful diagnostic test and will often reveal an impalpable defect, particularly in the obese patient. In massive complex incisional hernias CT scanning may help in defining the defect and planning the need for preoperative pneumoperitoneum or the need for replacement of a large tissue defect with prosthetic mesh.

Incidence

The overall incidence of incisional hernias is difficult to estimate. Homans, in 1887, reported that 10% of abdominal operations were followed by incisional hernias;[433] more recent studies give lower incidences – probably only 2% of all abdominal operations are followed by incisional hernia, although series which include only 'major laparotomy' wounds yield higher incidences. Certainly the reported incidence of this complication has fallen in the past 10 years, during which major sepsis has diminished, non-irritant, non-absorbable sutures have been introduced and the technique of wound closure has been emphasized. Incisional hernias are slightly more frequent in males than females (55:45) (see Table 3.2).

Until recently there were very few studies with adequate follow-up of laparotomy wounds to determine the real incidence of incisional hernia. Stanton, in 1916, reported 500 consecutive laparotomies followed up for 5–7 years. Over this period a total of 24 postoperative hernias were found (4.8%). In 260 clean cases only three incisional hernias developed, whereas in 186 contaminated cases 18 hernias developed.[887]

Although the incidence of burst abdomen has been reduced by mass closure techniques, incisional hernia remains an important problem. The strength of the abdominal wall resides in the aponeurotic layers, the linea alba and the rectus sheath. These layers are slow to heal and only regain adequate strength after 120 days from wounding.[267] On a theoretical basis, most incisional hernias would be expected to be apparent before this healing is complete. The reports of onset of incisional hernia which occur in the standard textbooks are usually based on the information gleaned from patients having repair operations for symptomatic incisional hernias, hence they probably over-emphasize these large and early onset hernias. For instance, Akman (1962) estimated that 97% of incisional hernias were apparent at five years.[9]

Long-term prospective studies of laparotomy wounds were unknown until Hughes and Ellis separately raised the question of late wound failure in the early 1980s. Ellis and colleagues from the Westminster Hospital followed up 363 patients who had undergone laparotomy but who had sound wounds without herniation when examined at one year. When reviewed between 2½ and 5½ years later, 21 patients (5.8%) had developed incisional hernias.[130, 283, 398, 681, 682]

Mudge and Hughes from Cardiff have published an important continuation of their study of incisional hernia.[682] During the years 1972–73, 831 patients aged over 40 years undergoing major abdominal surgery were entered into a long-term study. Of 564 patients surviving and being willing to enter the study at the end of one year, 337 patients were followed up for a further nine years. Of the remainder, 128 patients had died and 99 patients had an incomplete follow-up for various reasons. All the

patients were questioned regarding symptoms and incapacity.

Of the 564 patients 62 (11%) had developed incisional hernias by the definition of Pollock. Of these 62 patients developing incisional hernias, details of the original operative closure technique were known for 52 and for 408 patients who did not develop hernias. The incidence of hernia in patients having nylon closure to both peritoneum and linea alba was 11 of 143 (7.7%); for catgut to peritoneum and nylon to linea alba, 24 out of 196 developed incisional hernia (12%); for catgut to both layers, 14 out of 100 developed incisional hernias (14%); of four patients having nylon through-and-through tension sutures, two developed incisional hernias. When the 337 completing the 10-year follow-up are scrutinized 37 (11%) developed an incisional hernia and 13 of these (35%) first appeared at five years or later. One in three of these hernias caused symptoms.

More than half the incisional hernias first appeared more than one year after the initial operation. These 10-year results confirm that there is a continued attrition of the healed laparotomy wound, with incisional hernias developing up to and after 10 years. When the distress and disability of the hernias is considered, those that develop in the first three years after laparotomy cause the most symptoms; they are also the larger hernias and are more likely to require repairs.[398]

These findings from two independent groups in London and Cardiff confirm each other, the failure rate of abdominal wounds being about 6% at five years rising to 11% at 10 years.

Akman's earlier statement that 97% of incisional hernias are apparent at one year after the original surgery is not confirmed by these long-term studies. Moreover, without full-scale prospective follow-up the incidence of incisional hernia will be underestimated.

The number of incisional hernias coming to surgical operation is lower than their overall incidence. Over the

Table 22.1 Incisional hernia: initial operative procedures

Procedure	Akman (1962)[9] Total no. 500 patients (%)	Ponka (1980)[752] Total no. 794 patients (%)	Devlin (1982)[244] Total no. 214 patients (%)
Hysterectomy and other gynaecological interventions	18.6	34	19
Cholecystectomy and biliary tract operations	9.6	21	11
Appendicectomy	43.8	16	16
Colorectal operations*	7.6	9	9
Gastric operations	4.2	11	30
Caesarean section	4.2	2	12

* Colorectal operations are not defined separately by Akman: the figure quoted is the sum of 'laparotomy other than specified' and 'non-specified (i.e. non-urologic and non-gynaecologic) pelvic operations'.

15 years mid-1970 to mid-1985, 277 incisional hernia repairs were undertaken in Stockton-on-Tees. During the same period approximately 19 000 abdominal operations were performed which, if recent British reports are broadly correct, should have been followed by a much greater (10%) harvest of incisional hernias. Fortunately not all incisional hernias warrant an operation. The incidence of incisional hernias resulting from various operative procedures is given in Table 22.1.

Aetiologic factors

The important causative factors include sepsis (60% of patients developing an incisional hernia within the first year after surgery have had significant wound infection); the placement of drainage tubes through the original incision; a previous operation through the same incision within six months; initial closure with catgut alone ('inept methods of suture');[600, 905] steroid and other immunosuppressant therapy; and inflammatory bowel disease. Obesity is an important risk factor both for the occurrence of the original incisional hernia and for the likelihood of recurrence of the hernia after repair.[130, 752] Early wound dehiscence is frequently followed by incisional herniation. Needle puncture incisional hernias are described as 'satellites' of a main wound failure. These hernias may be related to the sawing effect of non-absorbable sutures on the aponeurosis.[519] Less significant factors include age and sex, anaemia, malnutrition, hypoproteinaemia, diabetes, type of incision, postoperative intestinal obstruction[607] and postoperative chest infection. Two recent retrospective reviews which included multifactorial regression analysis of putative risk factors, such as sex, age, smoking, chronic lung disease, obesity, sight, surgeon's experience, closure method and suture material have found that size of the hernia[425] and obesity[607] were the prime factors

involved in recurrence after incisional hernia repair. Many of these hernias recurred early with re-medial time between the primary operation and the first symptoms of hernia being within a year. Fifty-five per cent of incisional hernias occur in men. Incisional hernias are infrequent under the age of 40 years and their incidence increases with age. There is an association between the development of incisional hernias and the occurrence of the post-thrombotic syndrome.[680]

Of particular importance as an aetiologic factor is the wound drain. Ponka records that of 126 patients with herniation through a subcostal incision for biliary surgery, all had drains delivered through the wound at the time of the initial operation.[752]

Midline incisions are at greater risk than paramedian incisions.[51] The revival of interest in the 'lateral paramedian' incision with its considerably lower risk of wound failure should decrease the incidence of incisional herniation further.[257, 375] However, no matter which anatomic type of incision is made, the choice of suture material is crucial. Kirk compared paramedian incisions closed with two layers of catgut with midline incisions closed with nylon; the crucial difference was not the anatomy of the incision but the choice of suture – the nylon closed incisions were significantly better than those closed with catgut.[500]

Lower midline incisions seem to be at greater risk than upper midline incisions (but this may be a faulty finding; inadequate suture techniques as well as physiological factors need assessing). Many of the lower midline incisions are done for gynaecological interventions and the subsequent hernias are often not included in purely 'surgical' follow-up data; hence, there may be under-recording of the true overall incidence of this problem. Table 22.2 shows the site of some incisional hernias.

The one clear conclusion is that catgut alone is an unreliable method of closing a laparotomy wound. Of

Table 22.2 Site of incisional hernias

Site	Akman (1962)[9] n = 500 (%)	Ponka (1980)[752] n = 794 (%)
Midline:		
lower abdomen	33	26
upper abdomen	5.4	16
Subcostal: right and left	—	16
Paramedian: right and left	9.6	11
Transverse and muscle-splitting right lower quadrant: McBurney, etc.	21	9
Peristomal	—	4
Vertical:		
right upper quadrant	—	4
right lower quadrant	—	3
Vertical: midline xiphoid to pubis	—	11

107 paramedian wounds closed with two layers of catgut in the Leeds trial, there was an early wound failure rate of 14%; of 107 wounds closed with two layers of catgut reinforced by all-layers nylon tension sutures, the wound failure rate was 4.8% (P<0.05). Interrupted mass Smead–Jones closure with monofilament 28 s.w.g. wire gave a wound failure rate of 0.92% (method 1 vs. method 3, P<0.001).[359]

Mass suture with wire is the most secure method, but wire is difficult to handle and is uncomfortable for the patient. Closure with catgut either alone or with tension sutures removed at 14 days was associated with a considerable incidence of late incisional herniation. No late incisional hernias developed in the cases closed with interrupted wire.[359] Additionally, there was a higher incidence of haematoma, wound infection and sinuses when catgut was used.

The newer absorbable polymer sutures polyglactin (Vicryl) and polyglycolic acid PGA (Dexon) have been subjected to trial and are reported as less good than non-absorbables. The longer life polymer polydioxanone (PDS) is under evaluation. A controlled trial of PDS versus polyamide (nylon) in the closure of 233 major laparotomy wounds failed to show any statistically significant difference. The patients were randomized to either suture, a mass-closure technique was used and patients were followed up to six months. There were two wound failures in the PDS group and more sepsis in the PDS group. There were no wound sinuses in either group.[343]

Late hernias occur just as frequently in patients whose wounds are sutured with catgut, absorbable polymer and non-absorbable filament. At present there is no explanation of why mature collagen should yield to form a hernia so long after healing has occurred. There is no aetiological factor to account for these late hernias[398, 682] although the concept of collagen failure, metastatic emphysema, may offer an explanation (see page 46).

Epigastric incisional hernias are recently reported as a complication of median sternotomy wounds for cardiac surgery. The risk factors identified include male sex, obesity, wound infection, aortic valve replacement and left ventricular failure.[220]

In children, either a layered or a mass closure with polyglycolic acid sutures gives acceptable results and a low failure rate. Non-absorbable sutures are unnecessary in children.[493] For some unknown reason the risk of failure in children is greatest in those undergoing pyloromyotomy (Ramstedt's) operation for hypertrophic pyloric stenosis.[121] Early incisional hernias in children are likely to resolve spontaneously. The late development of incisional hernias occurs rarely in children.[493]

Principles of repair

The following principles should be followed:

1. Whenever possible the normal anatomy should be reconstituted. In midline hernias this means the linea alba must be firmly reconstructed; in more lateral hernias there should be layer-by-layer closure as far as possible.
2. Only tendinous/aponeurotic/fascial structures should be brought together. *In situ* darning over the defect without adequate mobilization and apposition of the aponeurotic defect gives a 100% recurrence rate.[398]
3. The suture material must retain its strength for long enough to maintain tissue apposition and allow sound union of tissues to occur. A non-absorbable material must, therefore, be used.
4. The length of suture material is related to the geometry of the wound and to its healing. Using deep bites at not more than 0.5 cm intervals, the ratio of suture length to wound length must be 4:1 or more.[456, 467]
5. Repair of an incisional hernia inevitably involves returning viscera to the confines of the abdominal cavity with a resultant rise in intra-abdominal pressure. It is important to minimize this. Preoperative weight reduction is the first precaution.
6. Every care must be taken to prevent abdominal distension due to adynamic ileus which will lead to additional stress on repair suture lines. For this reason, handling of the viscera should be minimized.
7. Postoperative coughing can put an additional unwarranted strain on the suture lines. Hence, pulmonary collapse, pulmonary infection and pulmonary oedema must be avoided. Restriction of preoperative smoking, chest exercises, weight reduction and avoidance of excessive blood or fluid replacement (and their haemodynamic effects on the heart) are important components in the successful repair of an incisional hernia.
8. The repair must be performed aseptically; inoculated bacteria, traumatized tissue and haematoma should not be features of these wounds.

Drawing these eight points together, appropriate preparation for operation includes measures to reduce the risk of subsequent infection: all skin lesions and erosions should be resolved before surgery: pulmonary function should be optimized. A carefully planned procedure using a tension-free repair with prosthetic reinforcement is recommended in appropriate patients.[826]

In epigastric incisional hernia repair it should be remembered that the linea alba is broad in the epigastrium – at least as broad as the xiphoid cartilage is wide – therefore efforts to draw the rectus muscles close together are unanatomic and doomed to disruption. Most of the side-to-side tension in the linea alba in the epigastrium is generated in the anterior rectus sheath which consists of two laminae, the anterior lamina being the external oblique arising from the lower ribs. The short span of this muscle makes this layer relatively inelastic and unstretchable to the midline for repair.[41] Division of one anterior rectus sheath longitudinally over the rectus muscle will allow a medial flap to be turned into suture to the contra-lateral fellow flap.[126] Alternatively, longitudinal incision of the medial scarred margins of both the rectus sheaths, the longitudinal 'releasing operation' of Gibson (1916),[339] allows the rectus muscles to spring into a straight line to cover the defect.[598, 1003] The defect in the anterior sheath can be repaired with an onlay fascia lata graft or nowadays preferably with an onlay polypropylene (Marlex) mesh.[126, 389, 938] A nylon darn is an alternative technique to reinforce the anterior rectus sheath. The darn should only be used if one layer of aponeurotic repair can be accomplished, by turning in the rectus sheath for instance.[445] Jenkins has described a similar technique of darning the anterior aponeurotic defect.[467] A similar technique using stain-less steel mesh (Toilinox) is reported from France[943] (Figure 22.1).

Incisional hernia following appendicectomy

Incisional hernias related to appendicectomy are reported in all series. Aetiological factors include severe postoperative wound sepsis and the placement of a drain through a grid-iron appendicectomy wound. These hernias occurring through the red muscle in the flank are difficult to repair adequately. If there is a well-developed fibrous margin to the defect this can be used as the basis of a Mayo-type overlap repair. Direct suture of these hernias, suturing red muscle, often fails and if an adequate overlap cannot be constructed, extraperitoneal mesh (page 243) or mesh reinforcement of the external oblique aponeurosis is advised.

Pneumoperitoneum as an aid in surgical treatment of giant hernias

Management of giant incisional hernia is often compro-mised by obesity, intrahernial adhesions and contraction in the volume of the abdominal cavity – the hernial con-tents have lost their 'right of domain'. Long operations

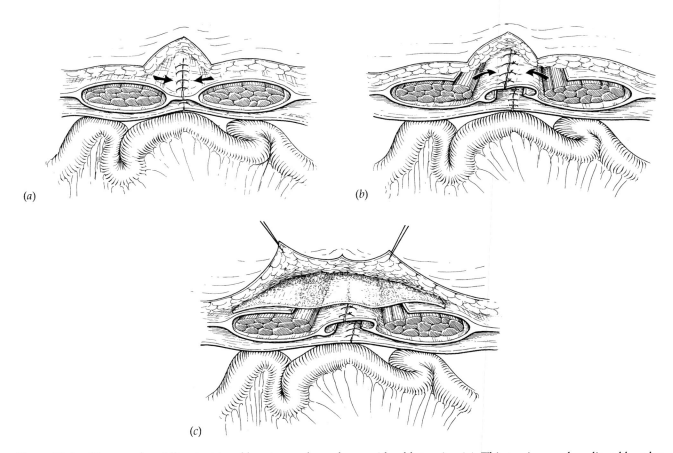

Figure 22.1 Closure of a midline incisional hernia may be under considerable tension (a). This tension can be relieved by a lon-gitudinal rectus relieving incision. The medial rectus margin can then be turned in as aponeurotic flaps to repair the defect (b). The anterior rectus sheath is replaced by mesh in the extraparietal (extra-aponeurotic) plane (c)

to free the adhesions and brutal reduction of the contents can lead to ileus, pulmonary restriction and cardiac embarrassment. After these operations, if the patient does not succumb to the cardiorespiratory complications the persistent ileus will lead to disruption of the repair.

The use of pneumoperitoneum before attempting definitive repair of giant hernias was originally suggested by Moreno in 1940 (Moreno, 1947).[664] The advantages of the technique are:

1. Stretching of the abdominal wall, creating a larger cavity into which the hernial contents can be replaced.
2. Reduction of oedema in the mesentery, omentum and viscera in the hernial sac, creating less mass to be reduced.
3. Stretching of the hernial sac leading to elongation of adhesions, making dissection and reduction easier.[388]
4. Increased tone of the diaphragm, allowing preoperative respiratory and circulatory adaptation to the elevation of the diaphragm.[313]

The technique of pneumoperitoneum is simple: under local anaesthetic an epidural catheter, an intracath or a ureteric pigtail catheter, is introduced into the peritoneal cavity. The site of puncture should be kept well away from the hernia or its margins to avoid damaging viscera fixed by adhesions. The optimum site is probably through the linea alba. Successful abdominal puncture is marked by a lessening of the pressure required to advance the needle. The catheter can then be easily threaded into the peritoneal cavity and its position checked radiologically after injection of a small quantity of contrast medium.[772] The catheter is fixed into position and about 500 ml of gas or air is injected via a micropore filter.[46] Graduated amounts of gas or air are injected on successive days, 500 ml at a time once, twice or thrice a day, until a daily volume of about 2.5 litres is obtained. Caldironi and colleagues used nitrous oxide in 41 patients with giant incisional hernias. A laparoscopic insufflator was used to top up the pneumoperitoneum every other day for a mean of 5.5 days, a total volume of 23.2 litres of nitrous oxide being injected. The volume introduced at each session was 1000/1500 ml greater than the previous session and the procedure was well tolerated in all but one patient. The good results of the subsequent repairs (only two recurrences in 40 repairs at a mean 25 months follow-up) attests to the success of this technique.[140] The abdomen will inevitably be blown up like a balloon and much patient reassurance may be needed. If the patient develops discomfort, shoulder tip pain, tachycardia or dyspnoea, the rate of insufflation can be reduced; indeed, if severe symptoms occur gas or air can be withdrawn. No attempt is made to prevent the hernial sac distending; distension of the hernial sac is helpful, stretching adhesions and allowing contents to reduce spontaneously prior to operation. Unfettered

distension of the peritoneal sac may reveal subsidiary hernial protrusions, enabling a more adequate surgical repair to be planned and undertaken.

In practice, the patient is ready for operation at about a fortnight after induction of the pneumoperitoneum, the end point being judged by the tension of the abdominal wall which should feel as tight as a drum, especially in the flanks.[67] The patient should be operated on at this stage – if possible most of the dissection should be performed with the hernial sac unpunctured and distended. Puncture of the sac at operation will allow easy reduction of contents and the slack parietes will facilitate repair. Air is only slowly absorbed from the peritoneal cavity and often after the first two or three days absorption is so reduced as to become inconsequential.

Contraindications to pneumoperitoneum include abdominal wall sepsis, prior cardiorespiratory decompensation and strangulation of hernial contents. Complications, which are very rare, include visceral puncture, haematoma and the risk of an embolism into a solid organ if the liver or spleen is needled prior to insufflation. Mediastinal and retroperitoneal surgical emphysema are rare complications.

Indications for operation

Incisional hernias produce symptoms of discomfort and pain, and often recurrent colic if subacute obstructive episodes occur. Such symptoms are reason enough for operative intervention. Irreducibility and a narrow neck are further indications for surgery. Obstruction and strangulation are absolute indications.

Contraindications to elective operation

Extreme obesity is a contraindication to surgery. Obese patients frequently have cardiorespiratory decompensation and diabetes, making weight reduction essential prior to surgery.[850] Subcutaneous and intra-abdominal obesity make the repair more difficult and postoperative complications more likely.

Continuing deep sepsis in the wound is also a contraindication to repair surgery. Such cases frequently have a history of more than one repair attempt, and the wound may be indurated with many sinuses in it. If the sepsis is long standing, calcification may be present. Usually wounds with continuing infection contain buried and heavily infected non-absorbable material; it is best to open these wounds, remove all the foreign material, drain all the pockets of pus and saucerize all the sinuses. The wound is then left to granulate over. Only when the wound has been without deep sepsis for some months should repair surgery be undertaken.

Skin infections and intertrigo beneath a vast incisional

hernia are common, and require vigorous preoperative treatment. Operation should be delayed until the skin is sound.

Choice of operative technique

It is important to make an accurate assessment of the anatomy of the hernia prior to surgery. How big is the defect? Does the size of the defect increase or decrease on movement? Are the contents easily reducible?

The sac and fibrous margins of the sac are examined with the patient supine and at ease, and then standing erect.

Finally the patient is laid flat again, and as much of the sac as possible is reduced and held reduced by the examining surgeon. The patient is then asked to sit up while the surgeon continues to hold the hernia reduced. In some hernias, particularly upper midline ones, the margins of the defect close together on movement and the contraction of the abdominal wall will then hold the sac reduced (Figure 22.2).

LAYER-BY-LAYER CLOSURE

If the sac is small, does not protrude and become pendulous in the erect patient, and if the margins can be approximated easily when the patient is relaxed and draw themselves together when the patient tenses the muscles, there is relatively normal anatomy and a layer-by-layer anatomic repair should be done. Akman and Obney, from the Shouldice clinic, recommended a layer-by-layer closure with an overlap. If the operation is performed under local anaesthetic the patient can be encouraged to breathe in synchronously with the

suturing, enabling a tight first layer of repair. Subsequent layers overlap the aponeurosis and reinforce this.

PROSTHETIC MESH OPERATION

If the aponeurotic margins of the defect cannot be approximated in the conscious patient and do not spontaneously draw together when the patient moves, it is probable that there is a tissue defect (or loss) and that a prosthetic operation will be required. The choice of prosthesis is discussed on pages 76–80. Polypropylene (Marlex) mesh is the preferred material and is used in the operative sequence described below.[557]

An important note of caution: unless the margins of the defect can be approximated in the conscious patient do not attempt a layer-by-layer repair. The sutures will cut out and the result will be failure. Some form of prosthetic repair is mandatory if there is a persisting tissue deficit in the relaxed conscious patient.[334]

ANAESTHESIA

Small incisional hernias without a tissue defect can be repaired using local anaesthetic; however, for larger hernias full general anaesthesia is necessary. Muscle relaxants will assist in reducing the contents of the sac and drawing together the margins of the defect during the repair.

The operation

POSITION OF PATIENT

The patient is placed on his back on the operating table.

THE INCISION

An elliptical incision is made to enclose the cutaneous scar. The incision must generally be extended at either end to give adequate access to all the margins of the defect. The direction of this initial incision will depend on the shape of the original scar through which the hernia has come.

Care should be taken not to excise too much skin: at this stage the minimum excision of cutaneous scar tissue is done (Figure 22.3).

REMOVAL OF OVERLYING REDUNDANT TISSUE

The redundant skin and scar are separated from the underlying hernial sac, which is often just subcutaneous especially near the fundus of the hernia. Redundant skin and scar tissue are removed (Figure 22.4).

If the hernia is very large the skin and underlying peritoneal sac may be virtually fused into one layer near the

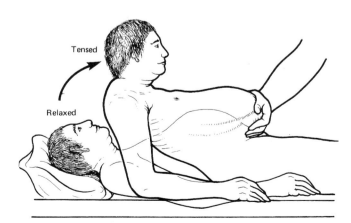

Figure 22.2 Examination of an incisional hernia. The anatomy of the sac must be known. The patient is examined laid and relaxed, and with the muscles tensed. Do the margins of the sac close or open during activity? Is there a tissue defect?

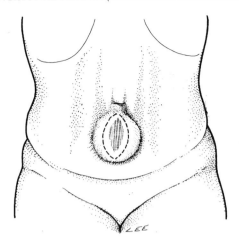

Figure 22.3 Elliptical incisions are made on either side of the hernial cicatrix

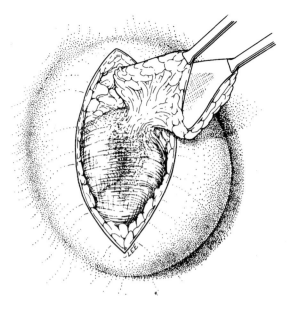

Figure 22.5 Care must be taken not to remove too much skin and not to damage the hernial sac. The cutaneous cicatrix is often closely adherent to the sac

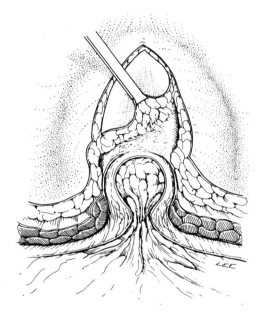

Figure 22.4 Removal of the redundant scar

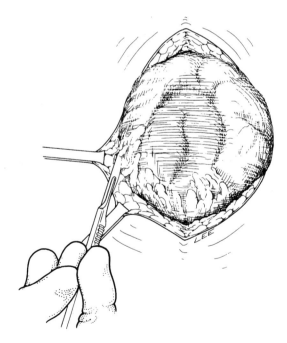

Figure 22.6 The sides of the hernial sac are dissected to the aponeurotic margins of the defect

fundus of the hernial protrusion. When removing the redundant skin, care is necessary to avoid damage to the hernia contents which may be adherent over wide areas of the inside of the sac (Figure 22.5).

EXPOSURE

The hernia is dissected from the surrounding subcutaneous fat. Its coverings are stretched scar tissue merging into the stretched abdominal wall aponeurosis at the circumference of the protrusion and a variable amount of extraperitoneal fatty tissue (Figure 22.6).

The scar tissue is incised in an elliptical fashion around the hernial neck, where it merges with the stretched aponeurosis. The peritoneal hernial sac is thus defined all around at its attachment to the muscle/aponeurotic layer (Figure 22.7).

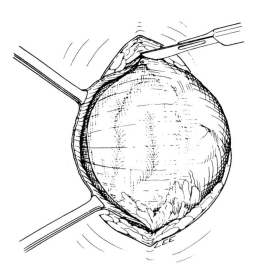

Figure 22.7 The peritoneal sac is defined at its neck; this clearly identifies the aponeurotic defect

MANAGING THE PERITONEAL SAC

If intestinal obstruction or strangulation is present the sac must be opened and its contents explored, as is the case also if a layer-by-layer or mesh repair is contemplated.

OPENING THE PERITONEAL SAC

The sac should be opened near its neck as shown. The presence of a great deal of extraperitoneal fat may make this difficult because the peritoneal sac is deeply buried in layers of fat which are often surprisingly vascular.

The peritoneum is often very thin over the fundus of the sac and the cavity is frequently loculated here by adhesions between the sac and its contents. Such adhesions are less marked at the neck of the sac. The peritoneum is usually less adherent and is thin at this point (Figure 22.8).

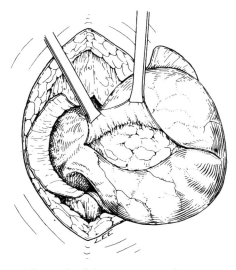

Figure 22.8 The neck of the sac is opened

CONTENTS OF THE SAC

The sac may contain almost any intraperitoneal viscus, but usually omentum, small bowel and transverse colon are found.

Unless the hernia is strangulated and the small bowel non-viable, any adhesions are divided and the small bowel is returned to the abdominal cavity. Strangulated small bowel or omentum can be resected at this stage. The diagnostic decision is now made as to what should be done about very adherent and frequently partially ischaemic omentum. If there is any doubt about omentum it is best excised; to return omentum of doubtful viability to the peritoneal cavity invites the formation of adhesions (Figure 22.9).

Particular care must be taken in manipulating and dissecting any colon in the sac. If the colon is strangulated it should be exteriorized with the formation of a colostomy and distal mucus fistula. If it is not strangulated it should be mobilized and returned to the peritoneal cavity. Any densely adherent hernial sac should be trimmed and left adherent to the bowel and returned to the peritoneal sac rather than risk perforating the bowel in a tedious dissection. The greatest care must be taken to avoid puncturing the colon. If the colon is punctured, the safest action is to exteriorize it and conclude the operation. Re-anastomosis of the colon and repair of the hernia can be performed at a later operation after full patient evaluation and colon antibacterial preparation (Figure 22.10).

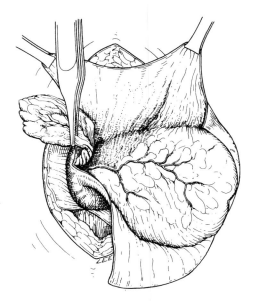

Figure 22.9 Viable bowel is freed and returned to the peritoneal cavity. If the peritoneal sac is closely attached to the bowel, most particularly the large bowel, no attempt should be made to dissect it free. Damaging the bowel is a hazard to be avoided; such fragments of adherent sac should be left alone and replaced in the peritoneal cavity. On the other hand, adherent omentum of doubtful viability is best excised

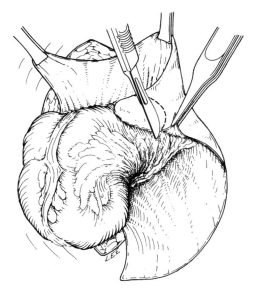

Figure 22.10   Completion of clearing the contents from the sac

EXCISION OF SAC AND SUTURE OF PERITONEUM

The redundant peritoneum of the sac is now excised and the peritoneal edges are united with a continuous suture. In the upper part of the wound it will be seen that the peritoneal layer is strengthened by the incorporation of the posterior layer of the rectus sheath, which is, of course, deficient below the semilunar fold of Douglas, halfway between the umbilicus and the pubes. A suction

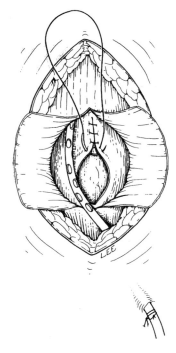

Figure 22.11   Now that the peritoneum is identified, it can be closed. Redundant peritoneum is first excised. A suction drain is placed down to this suture line

drain is now placed down to this suture line (Figure 22.11). Wide drainage should be used to eliminate dead space and fluid accumulation.[826]

CLOSURE OF APONEUROTIC LAYER

The aponeurosis must be dissected until normal aponeurosis and not scar tissue is identified. Then the full thickness of the margins of all the aponeurotic layer (i.e. the abdominal wall in midline and paramedian areas) are approximated and held together by sutures until healing is complete (Figure 22.12).

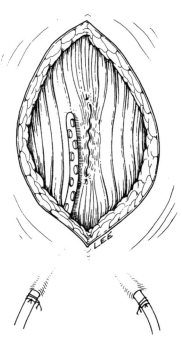

Figure 22.12   Closure of the anterior aponeurosis, rectus sheath. Only normal aponeurosis can be used in this type of repair

A polypropylene (or steel) suture is started at each end of the defect. Suturing is continued towards the centre of the defect, one suture alternating with the other and slowly being used to draw together the margins of the defect. Stitch intervals of no more than 0.5 cm are used and bites must be taken more than 2.5 cm from the edges to be sutured (Figure 22.13).

After one layer has been inserted and the margins closed together, at least one further layer of polypropylene (or steel) is inserted, taking bites in between and slightly wider than the first layer. Very large quantities of suture material, up to 44 times the length of the wound, are inserted (Figure 22.14).

When completed, the defect in the aponeurosis should resemble a very closely meshed darn. A suction drain should now be inserted down to this suture line. Haemostasis in the subcutaneous tissue is rigorously

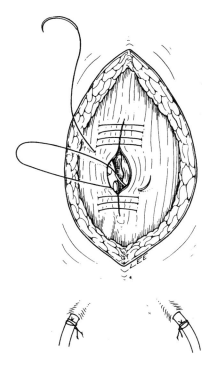

Figure 22.13 Closure of the aponeurosis, suturing from each end simultaneously to distribute the load. Notice the drains

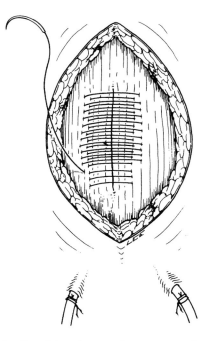

Figure 22.14 Repairing the anterior aponeurosis with many layers of 'big bite' polypropylene sutures

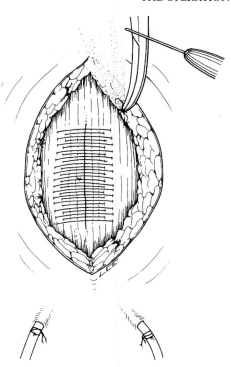

Figure 22.15 When completed this type of darn repair needs checking for meticulous haemostasis

excised at this stage. A carefully placed subcuticular suture of PDS is used. The wound is finally sealed with spray or sealant. A dressing is not applied. The suction drains are fixed with adherent tape or sutures placed well away from the main wound (Figure 22.16).

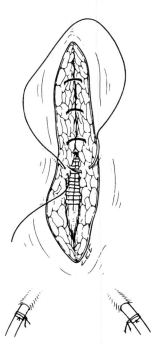

Figure 22.16 Standard closure is employed; subcutaneous fat closed with absorbable polymer and deep knots, skin with subcuticular clear PDS

checked before further closure of the wound (Figure 22.15).

The subcutaneous fat is now closed in layers with interrupted absorbable sutures. The skin margins are now approximated. Skin closure must be effected without any tension, but undue redundant skin can be

Postoperative care

Immediate active mobilization is the key to rapid convalescence.

In the absence of extensive handling of the intestines there is no postoperative adynamic ileus and no need for encumbrances such as nasogastric suction or intravenous drips. The patient is made to take deep breaths; breathing exercises and, where necessary, chest percussion are given. As soon as possible the patient gets up and walks. Fluids are given for the first day, then a light diet started. Any wound discharge and the contents of the suction drains are cultured and any incipient infection treated vigorously with antibiotics.

Alternative operative technique – polypropylene (Marlex) mesh repair

This technique is applicable to the large diffuse incisional hernia when there is a tissue defect demonstrated preoperatively. Alternatively, on-table pneumoperitoneum can be used, which assists in defining the real margins of the defect and may also reveal the presence of occult hernias.[990]

INCISION AND DISSECTION

The elliptical incision, removing the skin cicatrix, is used as previously described. The dissection is carried down to the neck of the sac. If the sac needs to be opened – because it is irreducible or its contents are compromised – this is done and the peritoneal opening is then closed. If the sac does not need to be opened, and opening the sac should be avoided if possible, it is imbricated with 'snaking' sutures of polymer.

If the hernia is in or near the midline, the anterior rectus sheath on either side should be mobilized by a lateral releasing incision.[576] The anterior rectus sheath is then reflected inward, sutured together and reinforced with a nylon darn to form the posterior layer. The lateral edges are then brought to within 3 cm of each other and sutured together to form the anterior layer (Figure 22.17).

If the peritoneum is deficient, for instance in a flank hernia, and cannot be closed over the viscera, the greater omentum should be mobilized to lie over the intestines. Alternatively, a prosthetic mesh–peritoneal sandwich technique can be used so that the mesh lies between two layers of peritoneum at the overstretched hernia sac and there is no direct contact with intestine.[621] This technique, rather than leaving the mesh in contact with greater omentum but potentially free to adhere to intestine, is preferred. With this technique the sac is exposed and freed for 3–5 cm beyond the hernia ring. The sac is then incised along its midline, the left leaf is tucked under the right leaf and the free border sutured lateral to the opposite hernia ring (Figure 22.18). The mesh is then placed superficial to this layer and sutured to the margins of the hernia ring, laid over the defect and sutured to the margin of the opposite hernia ring to complete the circumferential suture line. The right (other) leaf of the hernia sac is now stretched over the mesh and sutured to the left hernia ring (Figure 22.19). The aponeurotic sheath can then be closed and the mesh lies within a sandwich of peritoneum.

Mesh should never be in direct contact with the intestine, because of the risk of adhesion formation and fistulation.

The mesh should be fixed to aponeurosis around the margins of the defect. The greatest difficulty is usually to make the tension of the mesh equal all around the defect it is to repair. There are four approaches:

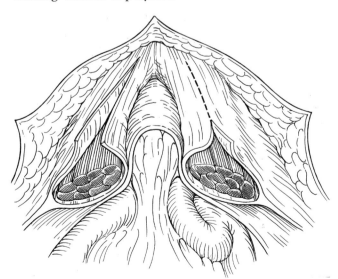

Figure 22.17 Bilateral longitudinal releasing incisions on the anterior layer of the rectus sheath

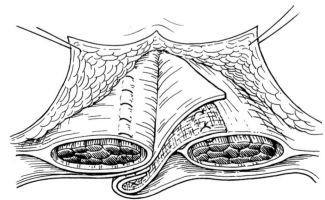

Figure 22.18 The sac has been incised along its midline and the edge of the left leaf sutured lateral to the margin of the hernia ring on the right side

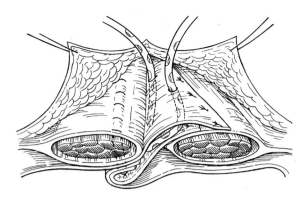

Figure 22.19 The free edge of the right leaf is stretched over the fixed mesh and sutured to the left hernia ring to complete the 'mesh peritoneal sandwich'

1. The mesh is placed over the defect and sutured in position (Figure 22.20).

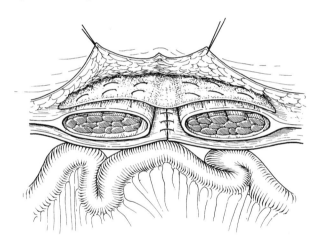

Figure 22.20 Repair using a mesh onlay

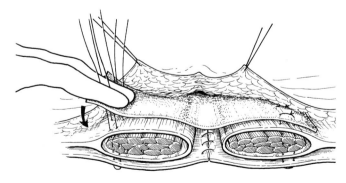

Figure 22.21 Repair by onlay mesh with all-layers fixation. The mesh is 'railroaded' down previously inserted sutures and fixed extraparietally

2. The mesh is carefully cut to size and finally 'rail-roaded' into position at the correct tension. Wagman (1985) recommends a 'through all layers' suturing of the mesh. In this technique, first sutures are placed

through all layers and the peritoneum and aponeurosis are closed. Then the sutures placed through all layers of the parietal muscle wall are pushed through the mesh which is 'railroaded' into position and fixed in the extraparietal plane[956] (Figure 22.21).

3. The mesh is divided into two halves, sutured into position and the tension adjusted by suturing the two halves together (Figure 22.22).

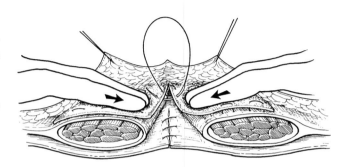

Figure 22.22 The technique of using two leaves of mesh; this allows the tension between them to be adjusted

4. Each rectus sheath is incised along its medial border and opened in the mid-line to expose the anterior and posterior aspects of the rectus muscle (Figure 22.23), which by blunt dissection is mobilized to its entire width along the length of the defect. The mesh is then placed posterior to the rectus muscles, after first closing the posterior leaf of the sheath/peritoneum with monofilament nylon (Figure 22.24). The layered closure is completed by approximation of the anterior rectus sheath.

Whichever technique is employed, the mesh must overlap each margin of the aponeurotic defect by some 4 cm and must be well fixed to the aponeurosis. This can be achieved by using continuous 'quilting' sutures, at least three lines, all around the defect.

PREPARATION OF MESH

The mesh is cut so that it is 4 cm longer and some 8 cm wider than the defect (Figure 22.25). The rectangle of mesh may then be divided into two equal halves down its central long axis if the two-leaf technique is to be used.

INSERTION OF MESH

The mesh is applied as an onlay to the external surface of the aponeurosis, or the external surface of the posterior rectus sheath if method (4) is being used, and fixed with polypropylene sutures. Generally three lines of continuous suture are placed.

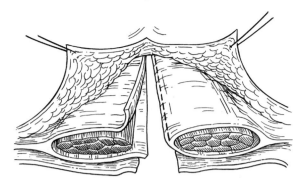

Figure 22.23 Each rectus sheath is opened in the midline

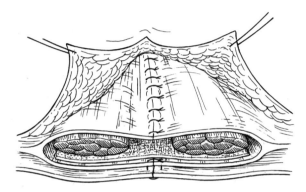

Figure 22.24 The mesh is placed anterior to the posterior sheath–peritoneum closure and posterior to the rectus muscles

The farthest one is placed first, at the margin of the mesh, which should be some 3.5–4.0 cm from the edge of the aponeurotic defect. The sutures should take good bites of the aponeurosis and mesh at intervals of not more than 0.5 cm (Figure 22.26).

With the mesh spread taut by traction by an assistant, a second line of sutures 1 cm closer to the margins of the

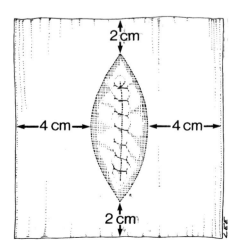

Figure 22.25 The dimensions of the mesh for repair of a midline defect

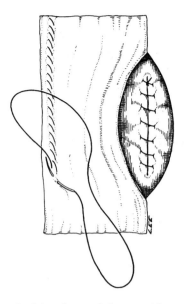

Figure 22.26 Quilting the mesh into position

defect is placed, and finally a third line of sutures at the margin of the defect (Figure 22.27).

The mesh is now put into the contralateral side using the same technique. A fine suction drain catheter is now placed to lie along the suture line in the peritoneum, deep to the mesh (Figure 22.28).

A technique of stapling the mesh in position has been described.[956] After placing the mesh in the preperitoneal space the linea alba is closed; this can be facilitated by multiple buttonholes in the anterior rectus sheath. The mesh is then placed deep to the abdominal wall muscles and fixed in place with an articulating stapler at multiple points.

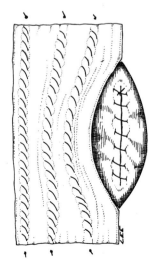

Figure 22.27 Three parallel lines of quilting are used on either side of the defect

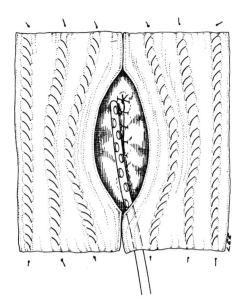

Figure 22.28   Fine suction drainage is always used

CLOSING THE DEFECT

The two leaves of mesh are apposed and sutured together with continuous polypropylene, the tension being adjusted according to the size of the defect (Figure 22.29). A suction drain is then placed down to the surface of the mesh.

The subcutaneous fat is tacked down to the underlying aponeurosis to obliterate the 'dead space'. Closure is then completed as described previously (Figure 22.30).

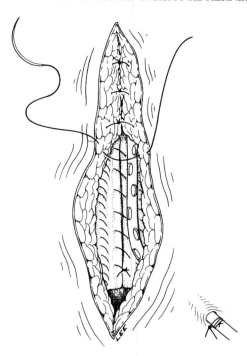

Figure 22.30   The subcutaneous fat is tacked down and 'dead' space obliterated

Another technique of extraperitoneal mesh placement

With very large incisional hernias prosthetic mesh repair can be accomplished in the extraperitoneal plane while avoiding the hazards of simultaneously dissecting the subcutaneous layer to place the mesh. A series of tiny stab wounds through the skin is used to place the sutures and railroad the mesh into position. This technique is shown in Figures 22.31–22.33.[246]

Continuously infected incisional hernia

In 1967, Ton reported the use of a novel extractable prosthesis to manage the multiple recurrent and the fistulizing incisional hernia.[926] Doeven has reported the use of this device in the non-infected incisional hernia.[254]

The device is a U-shaped loop of metal, one leg of the loop is perforated throughout its length, the other solid. The device is manufactured in a variety of sizes (Figure 22.34).

The concept is threefold: (a) to use strong non-absorbable sutures for the repair; (b) to distribute the load to the aponeurosis through the rods and thus prevent the sutures cutting out; (c) to allow all the non-absorbable material to be removed and thereby eliminate sepsis and ongoing sinuses.

Sutures are placed around the solid limb and tied through the perforated limb. When healing is complete

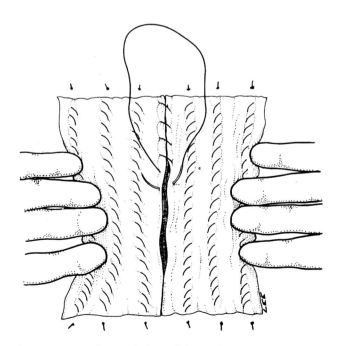

Figure 22.29   The two halves of the mesh are sutured together at the correct tension

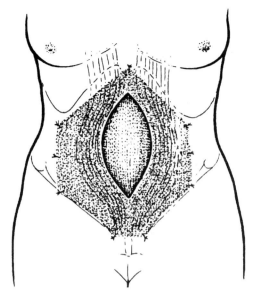

Figure 22.31 A large piece of mesh is cut so that it overlaps the margins of the defect by at least 2 cm, or over 3 cm if possible – the larger the overlap the better. The mesh should be cut with a chevron shape to go down into the pelvis behind the pubis and inguinal ligaments, and above with an inverted chevron so that it fits up to the costal margin. (Reproduced by permission from Devlin and Nicholson, 1994[246])

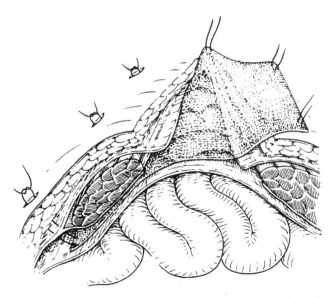

Figure 22.32 A series of tiny stab wounds is made 2 cm or more from the margins of the defect. Sutures are passed through each stab wound, through the full thickness of the abdominal wall and through the mesh. The lowermost sutures should pick up the pectineal ligament and the mesh. The sutures are held in clips and not tied until all the sutures are in position. (Reproduced by permission from Devlin and Nicholson, 1994[246])

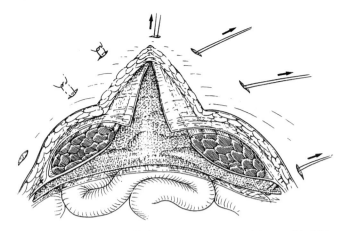

Figure 22.33 When all the sutures are in position and held in clips the mesh is slid into position in the extraperitoneal plane deep to the musculoaponeurotic layer of the abdominal wall. The sutures are then tied securely using robust non-slip knots. The stab wounds are then closed with subcuticular strands. (Reproduced by permission from Devlin and Nicholson, 1994[246])

the U-loop is removed through a small incision; removal of the loop means removal of the sutures too – they slip off the solid limb and are pulled from the wound in the perforated limb (Figure 22.35).

Doeven has advocated prophylactic use of the device in patients at high risk of abdominal dehiscence or incisional hernia. The device can be safely used in the contaminated wound.

Doeven reported the use of the device in 80 patients, 19 of whom had abdominal wall sepsis and 11 had fistulation. In 62 patients the repair healed without recurrence, but in 18 patients the hernia recurred after removal of the prosthesis. Fifty patients had an uncomplicated recovery with no ongoing sepsis and of these 11 developed a recurrent hernia. This latter result is disappointing. The device was left *in situ* for six weeks to three months, but this is clearly not long enough for mature collagen repair to take place.

The operation is performed under general anaesthesia, with intubation and full relaxation. The entire skin cicatrix is excised and all previous sutures, prosthetic fragments and other non-absorbable material is removed. The skin and subcutaneous tissues are mobilized to allow at least 3 cm access to the aponeurosis beyond the defect margin. The peritoneal sac is dissected and its contents reduced. The sac is closed with an absorbable polymer.

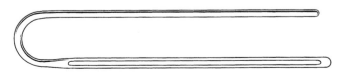

Figure 22.34 The Ton device

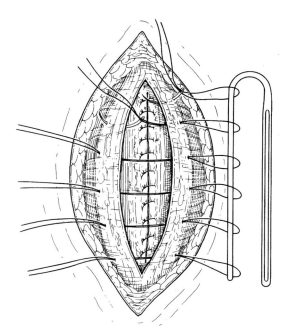

Figure 22.35 The Ton technique; placing the sutures

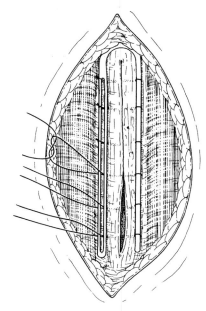

Figure 22.36 The Ton technique; fixing the device in place

Strong nylon or polypropylene sutures are threaded double on a curved needle and placed through the entire abdominal wall from one side of the defect to the other. The sutures are laid extraperitoneally across the defect and thence through the abdominal wall of the opposite side. The sutures are 2.5 cm from the edge of the hernia defect in the aponeurosis and 0.5–1.0 cm apart.

A suitably sized device is chosen. The device is positioned so that the loops of the sutures overrun its solid limb and one free end of each suture is threaded through

Table 22.3 Results of incisional hernia repair

Reference	Clinic	Technique	No. patients	Recurrence rate (%)
Suture or layer techniques				
Obney (1957)[712]	Shouldice, Canada	Layered steel wire	192	12.5
Young (1961)[1003]	Warrington, UK	Rectus-relieving incision	15	6.6
Akman (1962)[9]	Shouldice, Canada	Layered steel wire	500	1.6
Maguire and Young (1976)[598]	Warrington, UK	Rectus-relieving incision	32	18.8
Jenkins (1980)[467]	Guildford, UK	Nylon darn	50	8.0
George and Ellis (1986)[334]	Westminster, UK	Keel or mass nylon	81	46.0
Graft techniques				
Usher (1962)[937]	Houston, USA	Marlex	156	10.2
Hamilton (1968)[390]	Louisville, USA	Fascia lata	43	7.0
Usher (1970)[939]	Houston, USA	Marlex	48	0.0
Larson and Harrower (1978)[526]	Providence, USA	Marlex	53	11.3
Lewis (1984)[557]	McGill, Canada	Marlex	50	6.0
Pless (1993)[749]	Odense, Denmark	Free fascia lata transplant	32	28
van der Lei (1989)[945]	Groningen, Netherlands	ePTFE	11	18
Molloy (1991)[657]	Cork, Ireland	Marlex	50	8
Matapurkar (1991)[621]	New Dehli, India	Marlex peritoneal sandwich	60	0
Liakakos (1994)[558]	Athens, Greece	Marlex	102	8

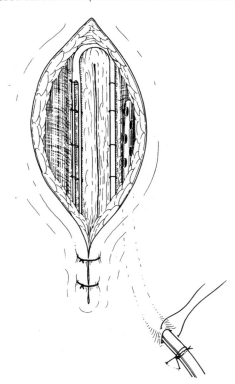

Figure 22.37 The Ton technique; closing the defect

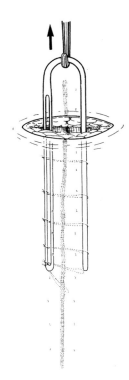

Figure 22.38 The Ton technique; removing the device under local anaesthetic

the perforated limb (Figure 22.36). The sutures are tightened and the defect closed. Then the sutures are tied. The aponeurotic defect is not approximated by the non-absorbable sutures threaded over the device. In the interval between the limbs of the device the aponeurosis is closed from side to side using an absorbable polymer. Subcutaneous suction drains are inserted (Figure 22.37).

The skin is closed over the repair. Then the device is removed by infiltrating the wound with local anaesthetic over the 'U' end of the device, incising the skin, inserting a hook and pulling the device out (Figure 22.38).

The reported results of incisional hernia repair vary; recurrence rates from 1.6% (layered steel wire) in the Shouldice clinic and 0% (Marlex mesh) from Usher in Houston compete with 19% from Warrington (releasing incision and suture) and 46% from the Westminster Hospital (keel and mass nylon technique)[5, 9, 27, 334, 938] (Table 22.3).

Conclusions

Again, the striking conclusion is that specialists who have developed an interest and experience in these operations have significantly better results than non-specialists.

Important predictors of recurrence are haematoma and wound infection, and obesity. The choice of operative technique is critical. If there is no tissue loss, layer-by-layer closure, or the overlap operation used at the Shouldice clinic, gives good results. If there is any tissue loss, prosthetic mesh reinforcement is always needed.

23 PARASTOMAL HERNIA

Parastomal hernias may present as problems of stoma care, difficulty with appliances or irrigation; or as straightforward complications of a hernia, intestinal obstruction or strangulation. The presence of a large protrusion itself may make repair a necessity irrespective of its other side effects. Herniation is less frequent with ileostomy than colostomy but the overall incidence of parastomal herniation is difficult to quantify.

Paracolostomy hernia – incidence and aetiology

Burns, in 1970, found 16 paracolic hernias among 307 colostomates, an incidence of 5%.[137] Other authors quote figures of 5–50% (Table 23.1). Burgess and colleagues in the north of England reviewed their experience of permanent colostomy with abdominoperineal resection for rectal cancer in the decade 1970–80. One hundred and twenty-four operations were performed and six patients (5%) developed paracolostomy hernias, but only one of these hernias required surgical correction.[135]

Wara et al. (1981) review their experience of herniation about temporary transverse colostomy and reported 3.9% incidence of parastomal herniation.[969]

Contrary to previous surgical dogma,[358, 925] the risk of stomal herniation is not reduced if the stoma is brought through the rectus muscle.[577, 717] The extraperitoneal technique of stoma formation described by Goligher does not slightly lessen the risk of parastomal hernia either.[577]

The worst parastomal hernias occur if the stoma is brought out through a laparotomy wound. Indeed, it should be a principle of colon surgery never to place a stoma in a laparotomy wound because of the risks of

Table 23.1 Percentage of patients developing paracolostomy hernia

Study	Date	Number of end colostomies performed	Percentage of patients developing paracolostomy hernias*	
Birnbaum[99]	1952	569	4.71	
Green[364]	1966	318	2.5	
Burns[137]	1970	307	5.2	
Saha et al.[821]	1973	200	1.0	
Kronberg et al.[517]	1974	362	11.6	
Harshaw et al.[404]	1974	99	9.1	
Marks and Ritchie[613]	1975	227	10.1	
Kodner[509]	1978	–	50	
Abrams[1]	1979	248	1.6	
Burgess et al.[135]	1984	124	4.8	
Cevese et al.[163]	1984	183	16	
Pearl et al.[729]	1985	88	2.5	(Only early complications reviewed. This report is difficult to decipher because it does not include the actual figures involved)
Phillips et al.[744]	1985	243	5	
		52	12	
Sjodahl et al.[863]	1988	79	10	
Londono-Schimmer et al.[577]	1994	203†	36.7	
Ortiz et al.[717]	1994	54	48.0	

* The duration of follow-up varies in different series.
† 289 operations performed but only 203 patients available for review at ten years.

infection, dehiscence, herniation and difficulties with appliance fitting.[358, 442, 730, 925, 926]

Para-ileostomy hernia – incidence and aetiology

The incidence of para-ileostomy hernia is between 5% and 10% and of para-ileal conduit stomas in urological practice 5–10%.[617]

Lubbers and Devlin reviewed their experience of permanent ileostomy in the years 1970–80; the incidence of para-ileostomy hernia was five out of 102 (5%).[580]

Williams *et al.*, in a study of 28 ileostomies using clinical and radiological CT evaluation, found the rate of herniation to be 35% and the same whether the ileum exited through or lateral to the rectus muscle.[988] Parastomal hernias occur most usually alongside the mesentery of the emergent gut. Thus in the conventional right lower quadrant ileostomy the hernia initially presents along the mesenteric attachment at the superomedial aspect of the stoma. Nevertheless, the most optimum site for ileostomy management is to site the stoma on the top of the infra-umbilical mound of the rectus muscle with the stoma constructed so that the bowel exits through the rectus muscle.[243, 717, 729]

Types of hernia

The anatomy of the herniation is variable. For convenience, four principal types may be identified:

1. **Interstitial.** In this instance there is a hernial sac lying within the muscle/aponeurotic layers of the abdominal wall. This may contain omentum, small or large intestine. In these cases the stoma is asymmetrical, and is oedematous and cyanosed if its vascular supply is compromised (Figure 23.1).
2. **Subcutaneous.** In this instance there is herniation alongside the stoma with a subcutaneous sac

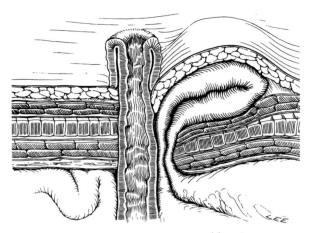

Figure 23.2 A subcutaneous parastomal hernia

containing omentum, small or large intestine. This is the commonest form of paracolostomy hernia and not infrequently colon situated just proximal to the stoma is found in the sac. Such a tangled-up stoma is very difficult to irrigate (Figure 23.2).

3. **Intrastomal.** This is a problem of spout ileostomies only. A loop of intestine may herniate alongside the stoma and lie between the emergent and the everted layer of the stoma. Intestinal obstruction has been described in such hernias by Cuthbertson and Collins[211] (Figure 23.3).
4. **Perstomal or prolapse.** All stomas can prolapse, but transverse colostomies prolapse three times more frequently than any other stoma. A prolapsed stoma contains a hernial sac within itself; other viscera, especially small gut, can enter this sac and even become strangulated. Large perstomal hernial sacs are often seen in neonates who have a transverse colostomy for anorectal agenesis (Figures 23.4 and 23.5).

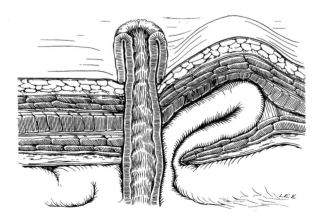

Figure 23.1 An interstitial parastomal hernia

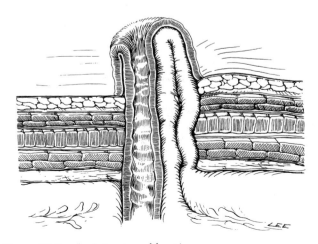

Figure 23.3 An intrastomal hernia

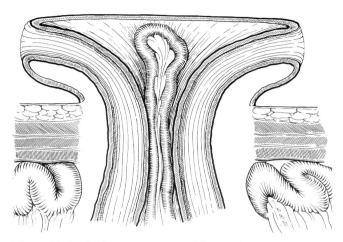

Figure 23.4 Prolapse or perstomal herniation

Strangulated small bowel requiring resection has been found in the hernial sac of a prolapsed terminal colostomy.[215] A similar strangulated small bowel hernia can be found in large prolapsed transverse colostomy. The treatment should be to expedite the closure of a transverse colostomy or to excise and refashion the bowel into an end stoma.

Causative factors

A variety of factors are responsible for the development of parastomal herniation. These may be:

1. 'Operator-dependent' – a disproportionately large aperture in the abdominal wall, placement of the stoma in the laparotomy incision or postoperative parastomal infections.
2. 'Patient-dependent' – cachexia due to advanced malnutrition or malignancy, senility or excessive obesity. Obesity and the presence of other abdominal wall hernias are important risk factors for the development of paracolostomy herniation. The latter observation suggests that paracolostomy hernia in the older patient could be a further example of failure of the fascia transversalis.[577]

Principles of management

An accurate diagnosis and assessment of the anatomy of the hernia is essential. Therefore, the patient must be examined (a) recumbent and relaxed, (b) with the muscles tense, and (c) in the erect position. Investigation of the detailed anatomy with CT scanning is useful to delineate large parastomal defects in the abdominal wall. CT scanning can also detect small impalpable defects around ileostomies that present with dysfunction.

An accurate assessment of the anatomy of the hernia should be made. Alternative stoma sites should be considered if relocation of the stoma is needed. Care must be taken if a decision to resite a stoma is made; the help of stoma care nurse (enterostomal therapist) is invaluable.[243]

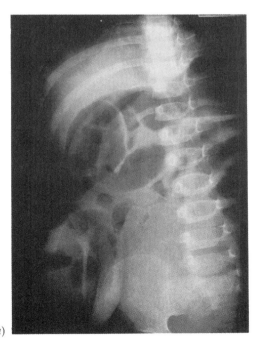

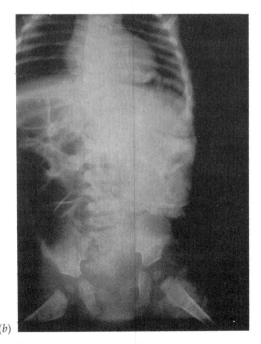

(a)   (b)

Figure 23.5 Prolapsed transverse colostomies often contain loops of small bowel; this is especially so in neonates who have transverse colostomies for anorectal agenesis. These radiographs show loops of small gut in a prolapsed transverse colostomy (Courtesy of Caroline Doig, FRCS)

Finally, the patient who has had cancer surgery must be screened for recurrence before surgery is advised. Similarly, it is prudent to exclude recrudescent inflammatory bowel disease before undertaking operation in patients with ileostomies although it should be noted that the risk of para-ileostomy herniation is similar in patients with ulcerative colitis and Crohn's disease.

There are three operative options to treat a parastomal hernia:

1. A local repair operation. The stoma is mobilized locally, the peritoneal sac identified and its contents reduced, and the peritoneum is closed. The musculo-aponeurotic defect is stretched laterally with a retractor and closed with far and near non-absorbable sutures[434] (Figure 23.6). If the skin aperture is too large it can be reduced using the 'Mercedes' technique described by Todd[925] (Figure 23.7).

   Local repair operations for parastomal hernias cannot be recommended. Horgan and Hughes report two patients and in both of these the operation failed.[434] This experience is shared by one author (H.B.D.) who employed the technique twice; on both occasions the hernia recurred within 18 months. One of these patients had a further local repair – again followed by failure. This patient then had his stoma relocated with long-term success. In this patient the aponeurotic defect extended laterally into the banding of the internal oblique, a sort of Spigelian hernia, so that the lateral margin of the stoma incision extended into the fleshy internal oblique. Sutures into these red muscle bands are unlikely to

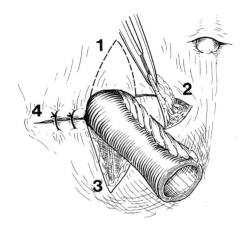

Figure 23.7 The Mercedes operation to reduce the skin aperture around a stoma[925]

hold and lead to lasting healing, particularly if the medial defect is splinted open by the emergent stoma.

   Horgan and Hughes, 1986, conclude: 'We cannot recommend [*in situ* herniorrhaphy] as both patients treated in this manner had recurrence of their hernia within two years.[434] Prian *et al.*,[762] Cuthbertson and Collins[211] and the authors agree with this observation. We do not recommend local repair of subcutaneous parastomal hernias.

2. Prosthetic repair by either an extraperitoneal or extraparietal route. Extraperitoneal placement of polypropylene mesh at open operation is a similar technique to the GPRVS operation for groin hernias. The mesh is laid around the stoma in the plane between the peritoneum and the parietal muscles. This is the recommended technique if mesh repair of a defect is needed.

   Intraperitoneal placement of polypropylene mesh around an emergent colostomy has been reported. This is a successful operative technique in the short term but long-term reservations about the intraperitoneal usage of polypropylene mesh must be noted.[138]

   Placement of the mesh in the subcutaneous plane involves mobilization of the stoma and fixation of the prosthesis to the external oblique, after threading the stoma through a window in the prosthesis. The advantage of subcutaneous placement is that no laparotomy is required. Phillips has pioneered the use of this technique using a local circumstomal incision and he reports excellent results.[890] A similar technique using a specially devised polypropylene ring set in a polypropylene mesh is used by de Ruiter and Bijen.[231]

   The disadvantage of local techniques is the risk of contamination from the stoma. No matter how the stoma is sealed, there is a risk of contamination and of subsequent sepsis. If sepsis occurs troublesome

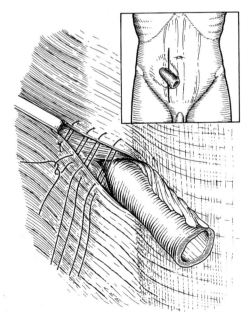

Figure 23.6 A local repair for a parastomal hernia. The defect frequently extends into the red muscle, which does not hold sutures or repair adequately

sinuses follow; such sinuses may warrant removal of the mesh. However, modern polypropylene mesh is tolerant of sepsis and simple local infection will usually settle with the prosthesis remaining in place.[890]

The extraperitoneal operation offers significant advantages avoiding sepsis.

3. Stoma relocation either with formal laparotomy or with limited transperitoneal transfer of the stoma. This is the most consistently satisfactory operation.[803] Pneumoperitoneum is a useful preoperative technique to secure increased intra-abdominal space and to stretch adhesions prior to operation on large peristomal hernia.

Indications and contraindications to surgery

Surgery is imperative in all cases of intestinal obstruction or strangulation related to parastomal hernia. Urgent emergency surgery is also absolutely indicated in all cases of paracolostomy hernia where perforation has occurred during irrigation.

Surgery is the treatment of choice when a parastomal hernia causes abdominal wall distortion and difficulties with fitting an appliance or irrigating a stoma. Surgery should also be considered if the stoma has become out of the patient's range of vision or if its site on a hernia bulge makes it unmanageable to elderly patients, especially those with arthritis. The disfigurement caused by a bulging parastomal hernia may warrant surgery for cosmetic reasons.

Contraindications to surgery include such general problems as cardiorespiratory failure, recurrent Crohn's disease, extreme obesity and disseminated malignancy.

Pneumoperitoneum

Preoperative pneumoperitoneum is a useful adjunct in the management of large parastomal hernias; this is described in detail on pages 243–244.

Technique of extraperitoneal prosthetic repair of parastomal hernia

The patient is prepared with the stoma sealed with an adherent plastic film. The original laparotomy scar is excised and reopened (Figure 23.8).

A plane of dissection is opened between the peritoneum and the parietal muscles lateral to the stoma. During this dissection the hernial contents are reduced if possible without opening the hernial (peritoneal) sac. This may not be possible. If the peritoneum is opened it

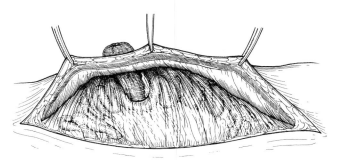

Figure 23.8   Reopening the laparotomy incision

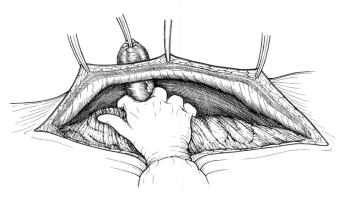

Figure 23.9   Developing the extraperitoneal plane to the stoma

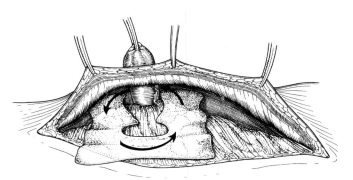

Figure 23.10   Preparing the mesh to make the repair

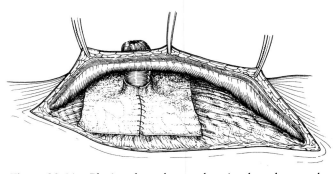

Figure 23.11   Placing the polypropylene in place deep to the muscle layer and superficial to the peritoneum – in the extraperitoneal plane again like 'ham in a sandwich'

is closed carefully around the stoma so that the mesh can be introduced into the extraperitoneal plane (Figure 23.9).

A sheet of polypropylene mesh is prepared, to repair the defect, with a hole in it to allow the egress of the stoma. A cut is made in the mesh so that it can be positioned. The polypropylene should fit snugly around the efferent bowel and should overlap the margins of the defect by 2–3 cm (Figure 23.10). The polypropylene is quilted into place (Figure 23.11). Suction drains are positioned. If there is any defect in the main wound, the margin of the mesh is extended medially to overlap and repair this defect, as described earlier.

The wound is closed carefully as before.

Subcutaneous parastomal hernia repair

An adherent wound drape is used to occlude the stoma and restrict contamination.

INCISION

An incision is made through the old incision and then laterally above and around the stoma, permitting the stoma to be raised on an 'L'-shaped flap (Figure 23.12). The incision is deepened to the aponeurosis[268] (Figure 23.13). Alternatively a circumstomal incision may be used just around the stoma. The stoma is oversewn and temporarily closed[890] (Figure 23.14).

HERNIAL SAC

The sac is found, opened and its contents reduced. The peritoneum is closed. A defect in the aponeurosis is closed.

MESH REPAIR

The mesh is introduced around the stoma and quilted down to the aponeurosis (Figure 23.14). The mesh should extend 3 cm outside the margins of the aponeurotic defect. If possible, a cuff of mesh should surround the emergent stoma (Figure 23.15); this prevents later stoma prolapse. A prosthetic mesh with a polypropylene ring used around the stoma is useful here.[231] Suction drains are inserted. Closure is as described previously.

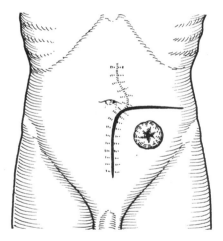

Figure 23.12 An 'L' shaped incision is made; this allows the stoma to be raised on a flap

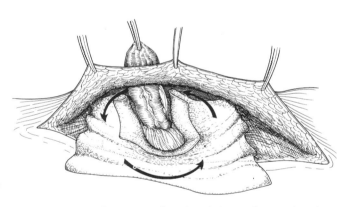

Figure 23.14 The sac is reduced and the mesh introduced

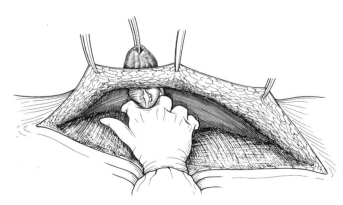

Figure 23.13 Extraparietal repair; the incision is made and the stoma then approached in the subcutaneous layer

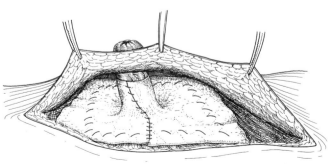

Figure 23.15 The mesh surrounds the stoma and is fixed by quilting sutures to the underlying external oblique aponeurosis

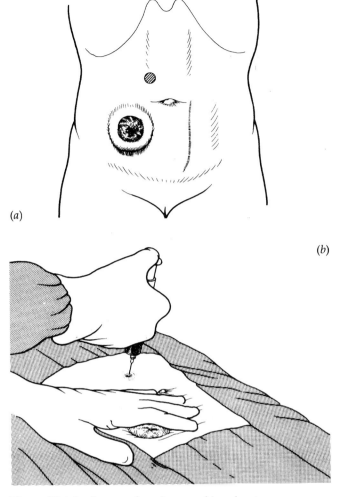

(a)

(b)

Figure 23.16   Stoma relocation: marking the site

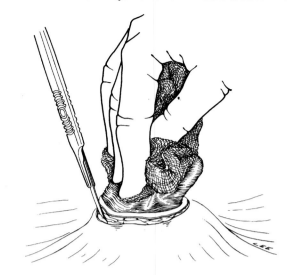

Figure 23.17   Mobilizing the original stoma (1)

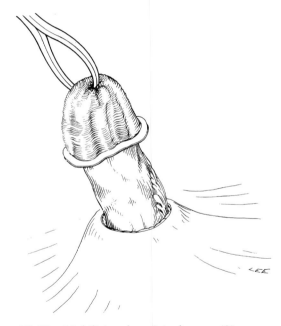

Figure 23.18   Mobilizing the original stoma (2)

Technique of stoma relocation

NEW STOMA SITE

The new stoma site must be precise and careful. One in the upper abdomen overlying the contralateral rectus muscle and away from any old incisions and delves in the skin is preferred.

The site should be selected, tested by an appliance pre-operatively and then marked.

A problem which should be foreseen is distortion of the abdominal wall by surgery after the operation has begun. Therefore, the stoma incision site is marked into each layer of the abdominal wall with the patient conscious.

The technique described by Turnbull and Weakley is recommended: the centre of the disc of skin to be removed is injected with a speck of dye – methylene blue or patent blue violet – which similarly marks each layer of the abdominal wall at right angles to the skin[933] (Figure 23.16).

MOBILIZATION OF EXISTING STOMA

A circumstomal skin incision is made. A 'trick of the trade' is to carry this incision through normal skin about 1 mm from the point of mucocutaneous fusion. Preservation of the scar tissue at the point of mucocutaneous fusion facilitates subsequent closure of the stoma (Figure 23.17). The incision is deepened until the stoma is completely freed from the skin and subcutaneous tissue (Figure 23.18).

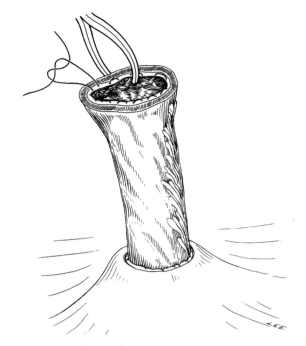

Figure 23.19 Closing the stoma

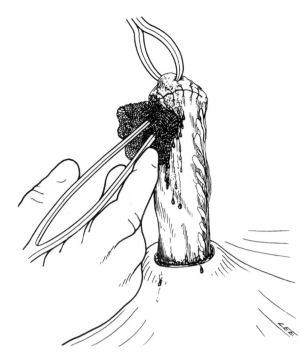

Figure 23.21 Cleansing the stoma with an antimicrobial solution

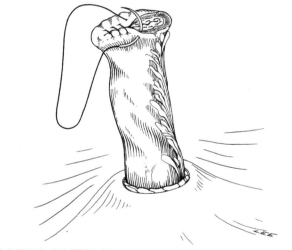

CLOSURE OF STOMA
Figure 23.20 Completing the stoma closure

The stoma is straightened out, an everted ileostomy being uneverted, and then closed.

A continuous circular suture of polypropylene is used, with small bites taken of the previously preserved scar tissue at the stoma margins. This suture is tied, closing the stoma off (Figure 23.19).

If there is doubt as to the competence of this closure a second, inverting suture can be put in. It must be stressed that the stoma closure must be adequate if contamination is to be avoided (Figure 23.20).

LOCAL ANTIMICROBIAL CHEMOPROPHYLAXIS

At this stage, before any deep dissection is undertaken, the wound and the abdominal wall should be reviewed for inadvertent faecal contamination. Cleansing of the closed stoma, the wound and the abdominal wall with povidone–iodine solution and a change of gloves, drapes and instruments, at this stage converts the operation into a clean abdominal case (Figure 23.21).

DISSECTION OF CONTENTS OF HERNIA

The incision around the stoma is deepened and the subcutaneous herniated bowel mobilized and freed from the adjacent tissue.

After the bowel has been traced down to the external oblique/anterior rectus aponeurosis, the opening in the fascia is identified and the bowel is mobilized. If necessary, this opening can be enlarged by splitting the muscle laterally in the line of its fibres (Figure 23.22).

INTERSTITIAL/INTERMUSCULAR COMPONENT

The deeper parts of the hernia are mobilized and freed, which involves the complete mobilization of the hernial contents and sac down to its junction with the parietal peritoneum. Once the contents have been mobilized, they are returned to the main peritoneal cavity (Figure 23.23).

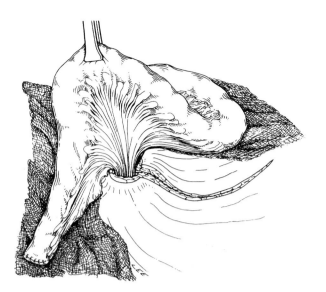

Figure 23.22 Dissecting and freeing the hernial sac contents

THE DEFECT AND THE NEW STOMA

At this stage a decision must be reached about the construction of the new stoma. If the hernial defect is large – it is in effect a major laparotomy wound – the abdomen can now be explored and the construction of the new stoma accomplished through it. If it is small or it does not afford access to the new stoma site, a paramedial laparotomy wound will need to be made. To construct the new stoma it is necessary to be sure of the following:

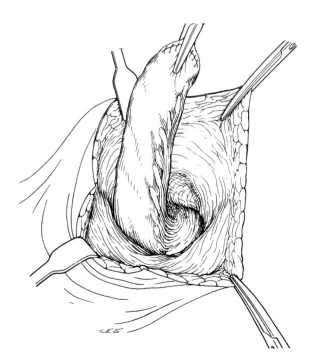

Figure 23.23 Completing the dissection to the aponeurotic defect

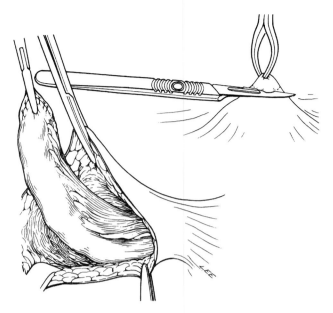

Figure 23.24 Transferring the stoma to the new site

1. A very adequate length of intestine – ileum for ileostomy, colon for colostomy – must be mobilized so that the new stoma can easily be constructed with no degree of tension.
2. There is no need to close 'lateral spaces' around a stoma in the upper abdomen. The stoma should be placed close to the middle of the rectus sheath; the 'spaces' on either side of it are then vast and are left entirely open. Postoperative strangulation of intestine in such a large defect is unlikely (Figure 23.24).

CLOSURE OF DEFECT

The peritoneum is closed with continuous polymer. Each layer of fascia/aponeurosis is closed with 3 metric polypropylene (Figure 23.25). Closure of the abdominal wall is crucial; you do not want to create a further parastomal hernia or leave a new hernia at the old stoma hernia site. It is sensible to reinforce the aponeurosis at both sites with polypropylene mesh.

CLOSURE OF WOUND

The subcutaneous tissue is carefully closed with interrupted polymer, suction drainage being placed down to the external oblique aponeurosis (Figure 23.26). The skin is closed with a subcuticular suture of PDS.

Postoperative care

Appropriate stoma care should be instituted. Some degree of postoperative adynamic ileus, probably followed by hyperactivity of the stoma, necessitates intravenous fluid replacement for 24–72 h after operation.

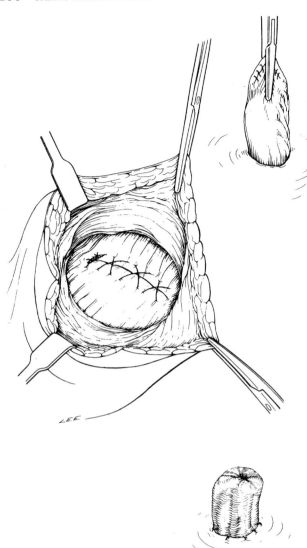

Figure 23.25 Closing the defect

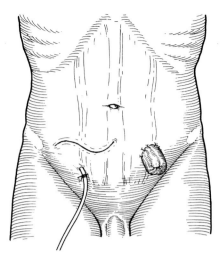

Figure 23.26 The new stoma and the wound closure. Notice a suction drain is always used

Conclusions and recommendations

The most successful operation is relocation of the stoma, but this is also the most traumatic and extensive. For the young ileostomate, stoma relocation is always advised if a parastomal hernia develops. A more conservative attitude is advised with the elderly colostomate. Many paracolostomy hernias can be managed conservatively with a corset-type colostomy appliance.

24 COMPLICATIONS OF HERNIA REPAIR

Incidence of complications

The incidence of complications of elective groin hernioplasty has been falling over the past 50 years. Important factors in this fall in the past 20 years include better nutrition and social standards, improvements in sterilization techniques for surgical instruments and, in the past 25 years, a very considerable reduction in the use of natural, biological suture materials and their replacement by inert polymers.

Dodd (1964) reviews his experience of 624 patients undergoing inguinal hernia repair over the age of 50 years. There were 568 men and 56 women. His operative technique was very similar to the Shouldice operation, with careful repair of the fascia transversalis and deep ring, but the cord was brought out through a 'neo-canal' formed by overlapping the external oblique about it. Fine black silk interrupted sutures were used. The author stresses careful technique. The complications included wound infection: six in the first 415 patients in the series from 1929 to 1950; none in 100 patients from 1950 to 1964. Dodd believes that haematoma is the most common cause of infection. There were three persistent wound sinuses, one case of osteitis pubis and two postoperative hydroceles. There were four deaths from pulmonary embolization.[253]

Gaston, reviewing 621 patients in 1970, reports very similar results: two wound infections and one scrotal infection; 11 instances of testicular oedema with consequent testicular atrophy (1.7%), three cases of pulmonary embolism and one myocardial infarction postoperatively.[330]

Alexander, from the Shouldice clinic in Toronto, reviews their experience of complications in all types of hernia repair performed in 1984. Between January and December of that year they performed 7367 hernioplasties; these operations were complicated by 16 wound infections, 12 wound haematomas and 3 episodes of urinary infection. There were no chest infections, no pulmonary emboli and no deaths during the year. Alexander stresses the value of the postoperative regimen – early mobilization and in-house exercise classes – which the Shouldice clinic employs to prevent postoperative complications.[10]

The complications of elective hernia repair are now so remote that, when performed by a skilled surgical team, it carries a negligible risk and operation can be safely offered to all patients. In the USA the results of operations performed by surgeons with a broad-based practice compared with those with an exclusive interest in hernias is significantly different.[250] National US audit figures reveal a recurrence rate of 10% for primary and 25% for recurrent inguinal hernia. Hernia specialists report recurrence rates of 1% and 5% for primary and recurrent inguinal hernias, respectively. Improvements in treatment appear to depend on standardization of technique and the adherence to protocols; nevertheless hernia surgery is generally taught and performed by surgeons with minimal attempts at standardization. In contrast, in the hernia clinics which standardize preoperative, operative, and postoperative management results are consistently good. Such an environment facilitates teaching, performance, and

Table 24.1 Classification of the complications of hernia repair

1 Operation failure
  (a) Recurrence
  (b) Missed hernia during surgery
  (c) Suture failure
  (d) Late repair failure
2 Wound complications
  (a) Bruising
  (b) Haematoma
  (c) Sepsis
  (d) Sinus formation
3 Scrotal complications
  (a) Ischaemic orchitis and testicular atrophy
  (b) Injury to the vas deferens
  (c) Hydrocele
  (d) Genital oedema
  (e) Impotence
4 Special complications
  (a) Nerve injury
  (b) Persistent postoperative pain
  (c) Femoral vein compression
  (d) Urinary retention
5 General complications
  (a) Visceral injury
  (b) Incidental appendicectomy
  (c) Pneumoperitoneum, air embolism and the Le Veen shunt
  (d) Chest infection
  (e) Deep vein thrombosis and pulmonary embolism
6 Mortality from elective hernia repair

reproducibility and can permit the performance of randomized studies. In the 3 year period 1977–79 at the Stony Brook Hospital, New York, patients were handled by two groups of surgeons.[249] In the first group of 390 patients, general surgeons and general surgical residents adopted the Cooper's ligament – McVay operation to repair primary inguinal hernias. In the second group of 442 patients a hernia service was set up with a defined protocol and consisted of a senior faculty member and junior surgical residents who performed the Shouldice operation. The senior faculty member assisted in the performance of all repairs and supervised the standardized protocol. The general surgeons and general surgical residents did not follow-up their patients until they reappeared for care at the hernia service. Annual follow-up was undertaken for 7 years in 82% of patients on the hernia service. The results showed a significant advantage for teamwork and adoption of protocols, with the hernia service team having half the incidence of wound infection (0.9% vs. 0.45%) and a lower recurrence rate (4.6% vs. 5.9%). Table 24.1 gives a classification of possible complications.

Operation failure

RECURRENCE

No operation for repair of any abdominal wall hernia is free of recurrence. Reviewing the many series of inguinal hernioplasties published,[354, 387, 766, 914] there is a striking similarity between the rate at which recurrences appear in the different series; at two years 25% of recurrences will be apparent, at 5 years 60%, at 10 years 75%. Most importantly, even a follow-up to 10 years does not give

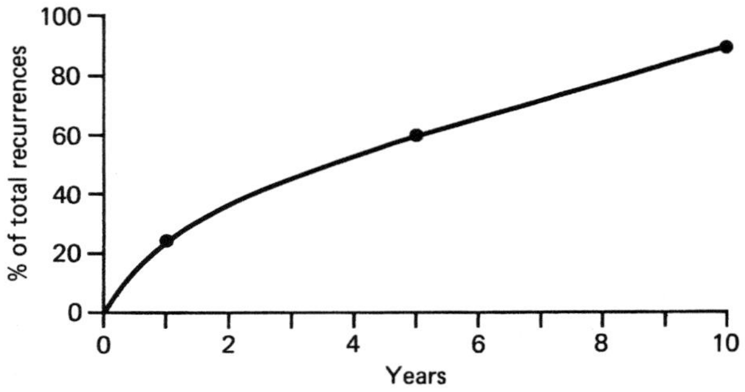

Figure 24.1 Rate at which recurrence becomes apparent. Sixty per cent of recurrences become apparent by 5 years, but there is a continued attrition rate and even after 10 years new recurrences develop

a complete picture, for recurrences occur after this time. This phenomenon of late recurrence is of most importance in the assessment of incisional hernia repair[334] (Figure 24.1).

The chance of recurrence is related to the experience of the operator. This phenomenon is most clearly demonstrated by the results of the Shouldice clinic. In their early years the recurrence rate was similar to that in general hospitals, but with increasing experience and refinement of the technique they have had, for some 30 years, consistently low recurrence rates for all types of hernia (see Figure 15.2). To have general applicability a hernia operation must have a short learning curve and be capable of reproduction in the hands of general surgeons working in district hospitals. A highly technical operation, which can achieve good results only in the hands of experts, cannot be popularized for the large volume of hernia surgery that requires to be undertaken on a day-to-day basis.

Table 24.2 Aetiology of hernia recurrence

Technical failure (early)	Tissue failure (late)
Missed concomitant hernia, e.g. a femoral in an inguinal hernioplasty	Inadequate collagen replacement as the repair heals
Inadequate dissection and reduction of the peritoneal sac, e.g. leaving the stump of an indirect sac within the cord	Inadequate tissue stretches to allow another adjacent defect to develop, e.g. a femoral hernia years after an inguinal hernia repair
Inadequate restoration of the disordered anatomy, e.g. failure to reconstruct the deep ring snugly around the cord	
Inadequate suture technique, e.g. sutures too close to the tissue margin or too far apart or pulled too tight	
Inadequate size of mesh to cover and overlap fascial margins of the posterior inguinal wall	
Wrong suture material. Aponeurosis must be closed with a non-absorbable suture	
Sepsis	

The causes of recurrence can be broadly divided into two groups – technical failure at the time of operation or tissue failure over the years after successful surgery (Table 24.2).

MISSED HERNIA

This is a most serious and most unforgivable technical failure. It casts serious doubts on the surgeon's competence. Furthermore, to the patient, a missed hernia which appears after the operation is an operative failure no matter what casuistry is advanced to disguise the truth. Even in the literature, casuistry is used to camouflage fact! The reporting technique for the Shouldice clinic is the 'gold standard' again; they report any anatomic type of hernia appearing in the related part, e.g. the groin, after operation as a recurrence. Contrast this with another report which does not classify all operation failures as recurrences.[568]

The message is to thoroughly examine all the points of potential weakness at operation and repair all deficient areas. This is most important in incisional and groin hernias. In incisional hernias, small peritoneal protrusions alongside the main hernia defect, adjacent to the sites where sutures penetrated the aponeurosis at the time of laparotomy closure, are easily overlooked. These protrusions can extend and lead to recurrence subsequently. In the groin the small crescent of an indirect sac, if overlooked, can push its way down the cord and years later present as a 'recurrent indirect hernia'. This type of recurrence is easily recognized at reoperation – the sac is within the cord, it is virgin and unscarred by previous surgery – above all, no suture material is found in its wall. The femoral hernia occurring soon after an 'inguinal repair' is most often a 'missed hernia'. It is an excellent policy to open the peritoneal cavity and through the opening to palpate all the potential hernial sites bimanually from within the abdomen.

Glasgow, in his review of 1500 femoral hernia repairs, notes that 359 of these cases had undergone a previous inguinal hernioplasty on the same side. While he acknowledges that some of these may be hernias missed at the earlier operation, he postulates that some could be due to an opening up of the femoral cone by the pull of the inguinal repair on the anterior margin of the femoral canal fascia transversalis. This possibility should be considered at primary surgery.[353] The inclusion of Cooper's ligament in the medial fascia transversalis repair will prevent this type of postoperative femoral hernia.

Inadequate dissection of peritoneal sac

If any peritoneal sac is left to protrude through the aponeurotic repair a recurrence cannot merely be predicted but guaranteed. This is important in groin and incisional hernias. In groin hernias a peritoneal stump, usually an inadequately excised indirect sac or a tongue of extraperitoneal fat penetrating the fascia transversalis close to the pubic tubercle, can force its way out and lead to recurrence. Low ligation of the indirect sac will probably only occur because dissection is incomplete, i.e. not within the abdominal cavity deep to the fascia transversalis. If this is so, the stump of the sac will not retract so that the fascia transversalis repair is not made anterior to it. The same phenomenon occurs in incisional hernia repair.

Inadequate anatomic reconstruction

This is a self-evident truth; if any orifice is left unrepaired a recurrence through it can be anticipated. In addition, if the closure of the sac is inadequate a wedge of omentum or a loop of gut can get between the sutures and act as a piston to enlarge the sac stump that remains. A careful pursestring and/or transfixion closure of the sac is mandatory.

In groin hernias an adequate repair of the deep ring cannot be accomplished unless the dissection of the deep ring is carefully made.[93, 350, 365] The superior, medial and inferior margin of the deep ring must be clearly identified. Clear definition of the ring does **not** demand the removal of the cremaster from around the ring and the cord at this site. So-called stripping of the cord by radical excision of the cremaster, cord lipomata and extraneous fat in an attempt to effect snug closure of the deep ring can cause damage to blood vessels in the spermatic cord and thus increase the risk of ischaemic orchitis.

This same golden rule of dissection and definition applies to all other aponeurotic defects. Unless the defect is skilfully defined it cannot be closed.

SUTURE FAILURE

This is discussed elsewhere (see pages 71–81). Close deep bites distribute tissue tension more adequately than infrequent bites and should always be employed. In groin hernia repair the tension is greatest in the medial part of the direct area and, if the sutures show a tendency to cut out, a relaxing incision should be employed.[139] Alternatively, such cases are ideally suitable for tension-free hernioplasty by the Lichtenstein technique.

Localized defects (recurrences), particularly in the medial area of Hesselbach's triangle are most likely caused by too tight suturing under tension.

The role of absorbable sutures in leading to recurrence and the problem of sepsis are discussed elsewhere (see page 73). After inguinal hernioplasty, 50% of recurrences are indirect, 45% direct and 5% femoral in anatomic type. These proportions vary slightly in different series, but the overall distribution of these recurrent hernias confirms the importance of checking all the anatomic areas at operation in every case. After femoral hernioplasty, recurrences are femoral in type.

In the first year after inguinal hernia repair, indirect recurrences outnumber direct ones by 2:1; however, at five years the proportion of indirect to direct becomes 1:1 and later recurrences are more likely to be direct or femoral. The maximum incidence of recurrence is in the first six months after surgery; thereafter the incidence falls off to plateau at five years. There is, however, a continuous incidence of recurrences, principally direct and femoral recurrences up to 10 years. These recurrences after five years probably indicate tissue failure.

No clear-cut anatomic factors can be deduced for direct recurrence; 55% of recurrences occur at the medial end of the canal just adjacent and lateral to the pubic tubercle. Thirty-three per cent come through the posterior wall and often through the conjoint tendon, 9% through the middle of the posterior wall and 3% just medial to the deep epigastric vessels. The fact that so many occur at the medial part of the posterior wall should alert us to check all the posterior wall, especially the area near the pubic tubercle. Berliner has demonstrated the highest suture tensions in this area and stressed the importance of careful suturing to distribute the load and avoid cutting out. Leaving extraperitoneal fat tabs protruding through the suture line can predispose to recurrences.[92, 139, 962]

Indirect recurrences are avoided by always checking the deep ring and ensuring there is no crescent of peritoneum, or proximal processus vaginalis remains in the cord at the deep ring. In repairs of 30 000 indirect inguinal hernias from 1945 to 1967 at the Shouldice clinic, there were only eight recurrent indirect inguinal hernias,[365] confirming the value of the most careful freeing of the peritoneum from the fascia transversalis at the deep ring. This facet of technique is as important as high flush ligation of the indirect hernia peritoneal sac.

With sliding indirect hernias the same principle of deep ring dissection is employed most scrupulously. The hernia should be completely freed at the deep ring and then the sac and any contents returned to the abdomen so that an adequate fascia transversalis repair can be made anterior to it. No complex manoeuvres are necessary to deal with the sac which generally need not be opened. Again the Shouldice clinic report excellence; in a series of 2000 sliding hernia repairs, their recurrence rate using this technique is less than 1%.

Recurrent direct hernias should not occur if the fascia transversalis repair and overlap are adequate, particularly at the medial pubic tubercle end. To ensure adequacy, all the posterior wall of the canal must be exposed and reviewed. With the Shouldice repair this cannot be accomplished unless the cremaster is removed to give an adequate anatomic dissection. With the tension-free hernioplasty using the Lichtenstein technique, fenestration of the cremaster to search the spermatic cord for the indirect sac is adequate and excision of the cremaster is not required. Additionally, the posterior wall must be fully assessed both visually and by digital testing, using a finger deep to the fascia transversalis or intraperitoneally to discover any small defects.

Femoral hernia may occur after inguinal repair; these hernias must be regarded (at least from the patient's perspective) as recurrences, although some perhaps are hernias overlooked at the initial intervention. The overall incidence of femoral hernia after Shouldice inguinal hernia repair is less than 0.5% in the series from the Shouldice clinic. Indifferent surgery leading to too great a tension on the anterior femoral sheath and inguinal ligament could also be responsible. Over the years the Shouldice clinic have significantly reported a decrease in this complication, pointing to the value of experience and specialization in hernia surgery.

LATE REPAIR FAILURE

The reason why late musculo-aponeurotic failure occurs after hernioplasty (and after primary laparotomy closure) is unknown. However, all series demonstrate this phenomenon, which must be related to a continuing disease process rather than incompetent surgery. Reference has been made elsewhere to the work of Peacock and Madden and of Read and his associates demonstrating collagen malsynthesis in some patients.[728, 774] Berliner has studied the structure of fascia transversalis. He has demonstrated a paucity of and fragmentation of elastic tissue fibres at the deep ring in cases of indirect inguinal herniation and around the fascial defect in direct hernia cases.[95] These changes are similar to those reported in patients with Marfan's and Ehlers–Danlos syndromes. The attrition rate and long-term failure rate in hernia repairs suggest that collagen metabolic dysfunction may be responsible. The absence of a late failure rate (up to 10 years of follow-up) in the mesh types of repair for primary inguinal hernia leads to the inescapable conclusion that replacement of the transversalis fascia by a prosthetic material overcomes any potential metabolic synthetic dysfunction.[855]

First-time recurrent hernia can usually be readily repaired using the Shouldice or Lichtenstein technique described. The skin scar should be carefully excised. Neat dissection and accurate haemostasis are needed, but with patience the layers can be identified and repaired.

When there is much scarring and multiple hernias, particularly if femoral and inguinal hernias are simultaneously present, the extraperitoneal prosthetic technique is advised.

Bilateral simultaneous hernia repair is prone to more complications than unilateral repair. These early complications include wound and genital oedema which is most pronounced if the cord has been extensively dissected superficial to the external inguinal opening on both sides. Superficial cord dissection disrupts the superficial pudendal vascular and lymphatic anastomoses to the cord. Considerable genital oedema can interfere with micturition and early mobilization.

There is also an increased risk of recurrence when bilateral hernias are simultaneously repaired by a sutured technique. No published data is available and it is too early yet to say whether mesh repair by an open or laparoscopic technique results in increased recurrence rates after simultaneous bilateral repair. In the series reported by Palumbo and Sharpe, bilateral hernias were present in 417 patients. In 78 operations simultaneous bilateral hernioplasties were performed; there were two recurrences (2.5%) in this group. The remaining 756 hernioplasties performed on 378 patients were staged to intervals of 6–10 days, with only four (0.5%) recurrences. The recurrence rate was five times higher when bilateral repairs were undertaken simultaneously.[721] Berliner and his group, whose figures for unilateral hernioplasty are outstandingly accurate and whose results are exceptionally good, report an 8% recurrence rate in a series of 114 simultaneous bilateral hernioplasties.[95] These findings have been confirmed notably by the Shouldice clinic group.[350] Glassow has specifically advised that bilateral direct hernias in men aged over 55 years old are better repaired some months apart.

There is, of course, a contrary view towards simultaneous bilateral hernia repair. Are we comparing the very low, less than 1%, recurrence rate of the modern fascia transversalis unilateral repair, with an 'acceptable' recurrence rate for bilateral repairs of less than 10%? The risks of two operations and the additional costs of two hospitalizations must be weighed in the calculation. In some circumstances a tenfold increase in recurrence rates is perhaps 'acceptable'. But should the surgeon or the patient make the decision?

The hazard of ischaemic orchitis should also be weighed as a risk associated with bilateral simultaneous groin hernioplasty, especially in a man under 50 years old (see page 274).

Wound complications

The complications of hernioplasty wounds are (a) bruising, (b) haematoma, (c) sepsis, and (d) sinus formation. Prompt and uncomplicated wound healing is most important in elective hernia repair. If wound healing is compromised, sepsis may involve the fascial repair with persistent sinuses or more extremely with failure of the repair.

BRUISING

Bruising is very common after abdominal wall and groin hernia repair. Haemostasis must be meticulous, particularly after repair using local anaesthetic infiltration if adrenaline is included in the anaesthetic infiltration. Skin discoloration following inguinal hernia repair is common.[764] Pye and colleagues studied 351 patients over a 3-year period. They observed a flair consisting of a reddened area around the wound, which blanched on digital pressure and subsequently turned yellow before fading, in one-third of patients. However, only 7.4% of these patients developed wound sepsis.

Generally bruising is of no consequence. In the groin it may track down into the scrotum, becoming most pronounced some three or four days after operation. Oedema of the scrotum may compound the patient's anxiety and discomfort. An expectant policy is correct: reassurance, a scrotal support and time always lead to a successful resolution and in the longer term bruising leaves no sequelae.

HAEMATOMA

Haematoma formation in a hernioplasty wound can spell disaster for the enterprise. Haematoma is the precursor of infection and this must be avoided at all costs. Meticulous haemostasis using fine neat exact ligatures of 3–0 polyglycolic acid (Dexon) or 3–0 polyglactin (Vicryl) are employed. For minor vessels diathermy is used.

Bassini, in 1887, advised that after closing the aponeurosis of the external oblique a tube drain should be placed in the wound and brought out through the outer end of the wound. He later particularly advised a drain in cases where dissection had been difficult or when the isolation of a large sac caused much trauma and predisposed to bleeding. Modern suction drains are very efficient and in complex inguinal hernia, inguinoscrotal, recurrent repairs, or when heparin prophylaxis is mandated by intercurrent medical conditions, fine-bore suction drains confer a significant benefit. The suction drain is only required for 24 h postoperatively. In a controlled trial of fine suction drains in groin hernia repairs, the complication rate was reduced from 48.7% to 17.6% when a fine-bore drain was used.[79]

In incisional or umbilical hernias in adults, especially in the obese, multiple fine-bore suction drains are an obligatory precaution against haematoma formation, with the ever present risk of consequent infection. Haemostasis and subcutaneous fat closure are essential to successful hernioplasty. Haematoma and its bedfellow seroma can be eliminated by careful haemostasis, the elimination of 'dead space' and the judicious use of closed suction drains.

SEPSIS

Skin closure should respect the integrity of the skin as an antibacterial barrier. Sutures should never penetrate the skin. Skin is closed with microporous ad-hesive tape or a subcuticular absorbable suture. Our preference for all hernioplasty wounds is a clear polymer subcuticular suture. This is easy to insert, does not require removal and does not cause sinuses. Coloured PDS should not be used as a subcuticular suture; there have been reports of the colour leaching out of the suture with tattooing of the wound.

Sepsis after simple clean hernia repair is a most important short-term complication and cause of prolonged hospital stay. More importantly, it is a determinant of recurrence. In the Shouldice experience, where the wound infection rate is 1.8%, recurrence is four times as likely in an infected as in an uninfected case.[348] Berliner (1984), recording 2900 elective and emergency groin hernia repairs under local anaesthesia, reveals that 'Deep wound infection has not been a problem since 1975'. Prior to then, pus discharged from the wound 10 times in 643 operations, four of the infected 10 patients subsequently developing a recurrence. Berliner uses a prophylactic irrigation of 1 g kanamycin and 50 000 units bacitracin in 400 ml of saline throughout the operation. He records 11 recurrences in 1017 primary repairs.[92, 95] Fear of infection in prosthetic and mesh materials used for the Lichtenstein technique and other mesh repairs is not justified.[345] Gilbert and Felton, in a co-operative multicentre prospective study of 2493 inguinal hernia repairs carried out by 65 surgeons using mesh repair, observed a wound infection rate of less than 1%. More than 70% of the wound infections occurred in patients over the age of 60 and prophylactic antibiotics had no effect on the infection rate. Removal of biomaterials from infected wounds was not necessary in any case and generally is not recommended, nor did recurrence occur in any infected wound.

In the Stockton-on-Tees series, one inguinal hernia recurrence in six could be directly attributed to infection.[244] George and Ellis similarly comment that haematoma and infection are the most important predictors of recurrence in incisional hernioplasty.[334] Sepsis, if it occurs, should be managed with appropriate antibiotics and drainage. Any discharge or crusting on a wound should be cultured – fine needle aspiration of the inflamed wound will give a culture in most cases. Culture material should be always obtained before antibiotic therapy is commenced. If pus does collect, the wound is opened and washed clean. Then it is allowed to granulate. Once granulation is established a Silastic foam dressing is an appropriate and convenient wound care technique. We advise these patients to bath or shower twice a day, to soak and wash the Silastic foam in an antiseptic solution, povidone-iodine or cetrimide; but there is no evidence that this enhances healing. All skin disinfectants induce some tissue injury, with impairment of blood flow in the granulation and surrounding tissue. They inhibit healing. Povidone-iodine 5% solution and hypochlorite antiseptics have both been shown to marginally inhibit healing.[115] If the wound is grossly contaminated and smelly, we recommend the use of the proprietary toiletry Badedas (an anionic cleansing and wetting agent, pH 6.5, manufactured by Beecham) or Steribath (manufactured by Stuart), an iodine-monoxylol complex which is added to bath water.

SINUS FORMATION

Using polypropylene sutures or polypropylene mesh to repair hernias simplifies the therapeutic response to sepsis. These prosthetics are biologically inert and, being monofilament, bacteria are not trapped in the interstices, if pore size is adequate (see page 76). They need never be removed on account of acute sepsis. Despite their presence in the wound, the wound will granulate and heal if it is kept cleansed. Sinus formation is rare. Braided polyester sutures or meshes, on the other hand, are prone to sinus formation. In 351 hernioplasties repaired with monofilament stainless steel no sinus formations occurred in 10 years, 274 with monofilament polypropylene with no sinuses, but of 86 patients with braided polyester three developed sinuses requiring further surgery.[216] The hostile potential of braided synthetic non-absorbable sutures has been confirmed by others.[471]

Table 24.3   29 823 hernia operations – sutures, infections and sinuses (After Shouldice *et al.*, 1961[852])

	No. operations	No. and % of infected incisions	No. and % of sinuses excised	Percentage of infections developing sinuses
Group 1: silk only	250	9 (3.6%)	8 (3.2%)	88.8
Group 2: silk and wire	974	22 (2.2%)	9 (0.92%)	40.09
Group 3: wire only	28 599	509 (1.79%)	42 (0.15%)	8.2

Earle Shouldice himself reviewed 29 823 consecutive hernia operations performed between 1942 and 1960.[852] He demonstrated that as he used less and less silk for his repairs, replacing it with monofilament stainless steel wire, the incidence of wound infection and sinus formation decreased considerably (Table 24.3).

PARAVESICAL SUTURE GRANULOMA FOLLOWING INGUINAL AND FEMORAL HERNIOPLASTY

Granulomas are a very infrequent complication of surgery, except following surgery for regional ileitis (Crohn's disease), and granulomas following groin hernia surgery are extremely rare. Kahnan described a bladder granuloma, which was relieved only when the patient passed chromic catgut suture *per urethram*.[476] Brandt reported three cases of granuloma formation in 7500 hernioplasties, but only one of these involved the bladder.[114] Patients may present months or years after hernioplasty – up to 11 years has been recorded. The aetiology of these granulomas is probably a small nidus of infection in the bladder wall associated with non-absorbable braided or multistrand suture material; most cases are related to silk sutures. An unrecognized urinary leak provides the culture medium for the bacteria that have contaminated the suture. The bladder is commonly a component of the medial wall of a direct or femoral hernia sac and sliding hernias of the bladder wall are common in the medial side of indirect inguinal hernias in male infants and young men.

Patients present with symptoms of inflammatory involvement of the bladder, dysuria, frequency and sterile pyuria or with symptoms suggestive of tumour of the bladder or urachus. Invariably there is a palpable mass above the inguinal scar. There may be a history of local wound infection that has been treated with antibiotics following the hernia repair.

Excretory urography demonstrates a normal upper urinary tract with a thickening of the bladder wall. Biopsy reveals chronic inflammation of the bladder wall with no evidence of malignancy. The urine remains sterile. CT shows a mass in the bladder wall with a central cavity.

The bladder tumour can be deeply resected transurethrally to reveal pus and the offending suture material, which should be removed. The bladder is drained, allowing the urothelium to heal. Histology of the excised tumour tissue reveals no malignancy.[214, 583]

Although paravesical granuloma is very rare, care must be taken to avoid it; the bladder component of hernias should be identified and injury to it or suture into it avoided. If the bladder is inadvertently damaged it should be repaired with polymer absorbable sutures and the bladder catheterized for 48 h. Silk sutures should not be used to tie off a hernia sac because of the risk of granuloma formation many years later.

Scrotal complications

ISCHAEMIC ORCHITIS AND TESTICULAR ATROPHY

The major blood supply of the testis is the testicular artery, a branch of the abdominal aorta. The testicular artery joins the spermatic cord at the deep ring. Additional blood supply to the cord is via the cremasteric artery, a branch of the inferior epigastric. This artery is variable in its course, sometimes entering the cord structures through the deep ring but more frequently emerging through the fascia transversalis in the posterior wall of the inguinal canal to enter the inferior portion of the cremaster muscle and then ramify through the cord coverings. A third arterial supply, the artery to the vas deferens, enters the cord at the deep ring; the artery to the vas is a branch of the superior vesical artery which is, in turn, a branch of the anterior division of the internal iliac. These three arteries form an anastomosis in the cord proximal to the testicle. At the superficial inguinal ring the cord receives additional arterial blood supply from the internal and external pudendal arteries (Figure 24.2).

During operations, all these arteries are exposed to risk. The testicular artery can be damaged in the abdomen if an extraperitoneal approach to the groin is employed, at the deep ring or in the cord during anterior mobilization. The cremasteric artery, when it pierces the posterior wall of the canal away from the deep ring, must be dissected and divided to effect an adequate repair of the fascia transversalis in the posterior wall of the

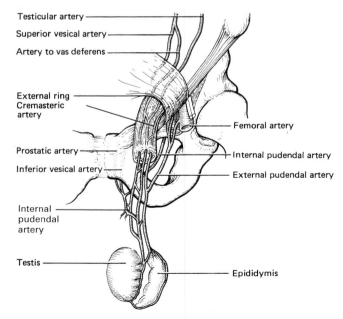

Figure 24.2 Blood supply of the testicle. The main supply is from the inguinal canal vessels, testicular and cremasteric, but the pudendal and vesical systems contribute importantly. Every effort should be made to preserve these superficial anastomoses

inguinal canal. If the cord has to be dissected to remove a lipoma or if the vas is closely adherent to a thickened hernial sac, the artery to the vas and the testicular artery are put at risk. All these arteries communicate freely with one another. This extensive anastomosis is a boon to the inguinal surgeon, for if only one of the supplies to cord and testicle are divided the testicle will survive and function on the remaining vessels. As a general rule, if the cord is being extensively mobilized, for instance in the Shouldice operation, provided the testicle is left undisturbed in the scrotum the pudendal and scrotal anastomosis will ensure its viability. However, the combination of mobilization from the scrotum and ligation of the vessels in the canal will jeopardize testicular life. If transection of the cord is contemplated, for instance to close a multiple recurrent inguinal defect, care must be taken to preserve the distal anastomotic supply to the scrotal contents. As a general rule, the testicular blood supply will be adequate if the cord medial to the pubic tubercle is left undisturbed. **Never** deliver the testicle from the scrotum during hernioplasty in either child or adult.[134] Other identifiable risk factors include previous groin or scrotal surgery, in particular a clumsy vasectomy operation which may result in disruption of the distal collateral blood supply to the testes, dissection of distal sacs with similar effects on scrotal blood supply, and concomitant scrotal surgery.[782]

The testicular veins emerge from the back of the testis and receive tributaries from the epididymis. They then unite with one another and form a convoluted plexus, the pampiniform plexus, which forms the bulk of the cord and ascends anterior to the vas. About the superficial ring these veins coalesce to form three or four veins in the cord as it traverses the inguinal canal. These veins enter the abdomen at the deep ring, where they further coalesce to generally form two veins which ascend retroperitoneally. On the right the testicular veins drain to the inferior vena cava and on the left to the renal vein. The testicular veins are valved.

The testicular veins are vulnerable during groin surgery. In the inguinal canal they are thin walled and easily torn as structures are dissected out of the cord. The same caveats apply to the testicular venous drainage as do to the arterial supply. If the testicle is undisturbed in the scrotum, adequate venous drainage is maintained even if the testicular veins themselves are ligated proximally, as may be done in a varicocele operation.

Thrombosis of the testicular veins may complicate hernioplasty. This leads to transient scrotal and testicular oedema, but provided the scrotal venous anastomoses are intact this oedema generally settles spontaneously.

Lymphatics from the scrotal contents pass within the cord generally as four to eight trunks accompanying the veins into the abdomen to the lateral and pre-aortic nodes. Lymphatic interference at surgery can precipitate postoperative hydrocele.

A syndrome of avascular inflammation may complicate inguinal hernioplasty in infants, children and adults. In infants and children, the condition most frequently follows episodes of incarceration or strangulation of the hernia. In these patients, raised pressure in the sac leads to obstruction of the testicular vessels with venous engorgement and inflammation of the testicle. In infants and children, sac strangulation is usually at the external ring which is aponeurotic and relatively rigid. After reduction of the hernia, or herniotomy, the testicle remains firm and tender, there may be scrotal oedema and slight fever. The situation resolves spontaneously, but often with some inevitable testicular atrophy, although the epididymis is spared the mass loss that occurs is in the testis. This syndrome complicates up to 10% of strangulated infantile inguinal hernias. The risk of this and the subsequent testicular atrophy is an additional reason for advising prompt operation for inguinal hernias in infants and children.[763]

Testicular atrophy as a complication of elective herniotomy in male children should occur in less than 1% of cases, although this incidence may rise if the surgeon is inexperienced or a low-volume operator.

In adults, the complication of ischaemic orchitis and testicular atrophy occurring after operation can raise more sinister problems than the spontaneous, non-iatrogenic complication in the child. Men of all ages who suffer this complication are very unhappy, even though their life-threatening hernia has been cured and even though the atrophy of one testicle does not diminish testosterone levels, or reduce sexuality or fertility.[963]

In adults, the ischaemic orchitis syndrome classically commences some three or four days after surgery but may become manifest soon after hernioplasty. Then the cord becomes swollen and tender as it emerges subcutaneously from the external ring. A tender painful testicle develops, often with minimal if any scrotal oedema. A low fever and occasional leucocytosis occurs. The severity of the signs vary greatly; sometimes there is gross swelling and discoloration of the scrotum. The signs are not related to the ultimate outcome.

The condition sometimes completely resolves, but in up to half the cases a progressive testicular atrophy develops. The atrophy can take up to 12 months to become fully established. This is important to remember, for when a patient with bilateral hernias develops this complication during his reproductive years the second side should not be operated until the final outcome of the ischaemia is settled. The atrophic testicle is ultimately painless and non-tender. The cord becomes foreshortened as the swelling resolves and the testicle is then drawn up into a high subinguinal position. Such malposition inevitably becomes permanent.

The sequence is the development of a swollen, painful and tender cord as it emerges from the superficial inguinal ring and is palpable and very tender over the pubis. The testicle then swells in the scrotum. Fruchaud operated on such cases and described the venous infarction of the cord and testicle.[317] The cord is infarcted and then becomes foreshortened and the swollen testicle is drawn up in the scrotum. The thickening and shortening of the cord distinguishes the testicular infarction syndrome from a simple haematoma in the scrotum, i.e. that following trauma or a reactionary haemorrhage after a vasectomy. The process of testicular infarction is sterile and suppuration does not occur. Very rarely the testicle may become necrotic and necessitate orchidectomy. It is important not to introduce infection by an ill-judged operation.

Histologically, in the established case there is atrophy of the seminiferous tubules. The supporting Sertoli cells and Leydig cells which produce testosterone remain normal. Atrophy of the testicle after ischaemic orchitis is not associated with an increased incidence of malignancy.

Similar atrophy, demonstrated on serial biopsy, follows elective division of the cord in the closure/repair of inguinal hernias provided the cord and testicle distal to the pubic tubercle are left undisturbed (preserving the pudendal anastomosis).[108]

In primary Shouldice repairs the incidence is small; the Shouldice clinic reports a 1% incidence in 28 760 repairs,[356] while Wantz reports a 0.36% incidence in 2240 Shouldice operations.[964] In the Stockton-on-Tees series one case occurred in 858 (0.1%) primary operations.[244] In operations for recurrent hernias, the incidence is as high as 5%.[450] Extensive dissection of the fundus of large scrotal indirect hernias predisposes to this complication, suggesting that dissection which disturbs the pudendal/scrotal anastomosis at the external ring is important in pathogenesis.[963]

The extensive dissection required to repair a recurrent hernia using an anterior approach hazards the testicular vessels with a much higher incidence of testicular ischaemia – up to 5% in some series. This is a very powerful argument for employing the extraperitoneal (preperitoneal) approach, which does not entail risk to the scrotal/pudendal anastomosis when operating on recurrent groin hernias.

In all complete or scrotal indirect hernias care should be exercised in dissecting the distal sac. Indeed, it is not necessary to remove all the sac; it is adequate to identify the neck of the sac, divide it and close the proximal peritoneum leaving the distal sac unclosed *in situ*. No complications of the sac are consequent on this manoeuvre. This is the procedure of choice in the circumstances.

The spermatic cord can be divided at the deep ring, or within the canal, without hazard if the extra-aponeurotic cord and scrotal contents are undisturbed. Heifetz divided the cord electively in 112 primary hernioplasties. There were no untoward sequelae in one-third of his cases; two-thirds developed ischaemic orchitis and of these only half subsequently progressed to atrophy. Testicular necrosis occurred in only one patient.[414]

Ischaemic orchitis is generally held to be surgeon-dependent (i.e. a failure of technique), the surgeon being blamed for damaging the cord, closing the external ring too tightly or snugging the deep ring too narrowly around the vas, the veins and the testicular artery.[309, 968] You cannot make the deep ring too tight because the superolateral boundary of the deep ring is soft and pliant; the ring is in reality a 'U' shaped sling, not a rigid band as a wedding ring. The superficial ring cannot be incriminated because in anterior hernioplasty it is not tightened; the external oblique is merely re-assembled.[968] The rich collateral circulation of the testes indicates that too tight a closure of the internal ring is not the correct hypothesis and histological examination of the testis reveals that anaemic infarction is not the pathology, i.e. necrosis does not take place. Constriction of the deep veins at the level of the deep ring does not produce testicular venous congestion unless the collateral venous circulation has been interrupted, either at the time of surgery or by previous scrotal operation. Nevertheless, reconstruction of the internal ring by adequate closure is essential to reduce the incidence of indirect recurrences. The cause of ischaemic orchitis is now generally attributed to surgical trauma to the testicular veins, which may amount to little more than merely stretching during operation. The pathogenesis can be explained entirely on the basis of testicular vein thrombosis. Thus, extensive dissection of the cord is not recommended. In the Stockton-on-Tees experience of the Shouldice operation, the complication was not encountered from 1970 to 1982 (718 primary operations) and was experienced for the first time in 1985 in an elderly male with a scrotal indirect hernia; thus in primary repairs it occurred once in 858 operations. Koontz reports a similar experience: 'Atrophy of the testicle sometimes follows a simple primary operation for inguinal hernia repair in which neither the collateral nor the primary circulation has been molested as far as the surgeon is aware. The same surgeon may operate on two entirely similar hernias in exactly the same way, in different patients, and atrophy of the testicle will occur in one and not the other.'[513] The almost chance incidence and unpredictability of this condition is a further argument against simultaneous bilateral primary inguinal hernia repair in a young man.

Halsted observed that skeletonizing the cord led to an unacceptable incidence of pampiniform plexus thrombosis and testicular atrophy. Perhaps this observation, with subsequent studies attributing testicular ischaemia to extensive dissection of scrotal sacs or recurrent hernias, gives us a clue to the origin of this unfortunate complication. Wantz hypothesises that the most important aetiologic factor is trauma to the pampiniform veins, leading to progressive thrombosis of the venous drainage and hence true infarction (L. *infarcire*, to stuff) of the testicle and its appendages. This thesis fits the clinical course of the syndrome, with the slow onset of pain and swelling at first in the cord and then in the testicle, followed by gradual resolution and atrophy. Nontraumatic and meticulous dissection of the inguinal canal and cord, non-disturbance of the cord or removal of extensive lipomas within the cord, avoidance of dissection of the cord or scrotal contents distal to the pubic tubercle and leaving the distal sac in indirect hernias *in situ* are technical details that minimize the risk of this complication. Anomalies of testicular blood supply are bound to occur and these may lead to sporadic cases following the most perfect and experienced surgery. In repairing the deep ring during sutured repairs due care must be given to placing the peritoneal stump deep to the suture line and then carefully reconstructing the deep ring around the medial side of the cord so that the venous drainage is not impeded.

If the complication occurs an expectant policy is advised; analgesics and a scrotal support enable the condition to settle. Antibiotics have no role in this abacterial inflammation. Anticoagulants have a theoretical but untested place on the therapeutic menu. Re-exploration is very unlikely to achieve any benefit. Chronic pain is not a feature of the condition.

The effect of testicular atrophy on fertility was studied by Yavetz and colleagues.[999] Among 8500 patients attending a fertility clinic during the period 1979–1990, 565 men (6.65%) reported an incident of inguinal hernioplasty, with or without subsequent atrophy of the testes. Additional pathology was present in 41 men and these were excluded from the study, as were 96 who had undergone bilateral hernia repair. Of the remaining 428 patients, 49 (11.4%) were found to have atrophy of one testis. Semen quality (sperm concentration, motility and morphology) of these patients was markedly reduced in comparison to that of fertile men. Thus, in cases where hernioplasty was followed by atrophy of the testes, the sperm characteristics and Sertoli cell function were damaged, although there were no changes in luteinizing hormone or testosterone levels. These results indicate the serious consequences for fertility in young men previously having hernia repair, which resulted in testicular atrophy.

INJURY TO THE VAS DEFERENS

The vas deferens should only rarely be damaged during primary hernia repair in adults. It should never be injured in children (see page 119). In recurrent hernias the vas, like the vessels, may be traumatized, particularly if an anterior approach is used to repair a multiply recurrent hernia. Vas transection should immediately be repaired using a magnifying loop or microscope to achieve adequate end-to-end apposition with a row of interrupted circumferential suture of very fine Prolene.

Matsuda and colleagues studied 724 patients attending a male infertility clinic.[622] Unilateral obstruction of the vas deferens occurred in 12 of 45 patients (27%) who were subfertile and gave a history of inguinal hernia repair during childhood. The diagnosis was made by palpation of the scrotal contents as a suitable non-invasive method. Moreover, half of the 12 patients had dysfunction of the contralateral testes and successful vasovasotomy was possible only in five, with pregnancy later occurring in only two cases. This series points to the disastrous long-term consequences of damage to the vas occurring after childhood hernia repair.

HYDROCELE

Postoperative hydrocele complicates Shouldice repair of an inguinal hernia in approximately 1% of cases. The hydrocele is lax and resolves spontaneously. Obney, from the Shouldice clinic, analyses their experience of postoperative hydrocele and observes that the greatest incidence of hydrocele at the clinic occurred in 1948, a year in which a now abandoned policy of extensive stripping of the fat out of the spermatic cord was used.[711] History repeating itself! Halsted made this observation 50 years earlier.

Provided the cord is not maltreated, hydrocele is very infrequent. Postoperative hydrocele usually requires no treatment. If it is troublesome, a once-off sterile aspiration allows it to resolve.

Hydrocele as a complication of a distal retained hernial sac, left deliberately to avoid distal dissection (see page 150), also occurs. Again, these hydroceles resolve as the cord lymphatics regain their function postoperatively. Surgical interference with these hydroceles can hazard the blood supply of the testicle – a hazard that leaving the distal sac *in situ* is intended to avoid. Slitting the anterior wall of the distally retained sac for a short distance without traumatizing any cord structures may alleviate this problem.

GENITAL OEDEMA

Oedema of the penis and scrotum is a common sequel to groin hernia repair in men. It generally settles spontaneously within 72 h of operation. After preperitoneal mesh placement for bilateral recurrent or giant hernias, more extensive oedema of the pubic area, penis and scrotum is common. Although sometimes this appears horrific to the patient, it always settles spontaneously. Reassurance and a scrotal support is all that is required.

IMPOTENCE

Men frequently complain of impotence in the immediate aftermath of a hernia repair. No organic cause for this can be identified, and firm counselling usually resolves the problem. Patients can be assured that hernia repair does not compromise sexual efficiency.

Special complications

NERVE INJURY

The iliohypogastric (L1), ilio-inguinal (L1) and genitofemoral (L1 and L2) nerves are liable to trauma during inguinal hernioplasty. Virtually all patients have some numbness in an area inferior and medial to the incision after operation. The ilio-inguinal and iliohypogastric nerves penetrate the internal oblique laterally and then run deep to the external oblique aponeurosis 2 or 3 cm cephalad to the superficial inguinal ring. The iliohypogastric nerve supplies the skin of the lower abdomen. The ilio-inguinal nerve penetrates the internal oblique near the anterior part of the iliac crest, then it enters the inguinal canal to run deep to the cord and emerge from the superficial inguinal ring. It provides cutaneous sensation to the root of the penis, the side of the scrotum and a variable area of the upper medial thigh. The size of the ilio-inguinal nerve is in inverse proportion to that of the iliohypogastric nerve. The iliohypogastric and ilio-inguinal nerves are purely sensory.

The genitofemoral nerve is a mixed nerve, the genital branch giving a motor supply to the cremaster and the femoral branch a sensory supply to the upper more medial part of the skin of the femoral triangle. The genital branch enters the inguinal canal through the deep ring. In addition to the motor supply to the cremaster, the nerve carries sensation from a variable area of the scrotum and base of the penis. The femoral branch passes behind the inguinal ligament and enters the femoral sheath lateral to the femoral artery. It then pierces the anterior femoral sheath and fascia lata to supply the skin of the upper medial thigh.[1010]

There is considerable overlap between the sensory areas supplied by each of these nerves.

The ilio-inguinal nerve is most at risk when the external oblique is first opened to isolate the spermatic cord. The iliohypogastric nerve lying above the canal is vulnerable during dissection and particularly vulnerable if a relaxing incision is needed in the anterior rectus sheath.

Attitudes to these nerves during hernioplasty vary. Division of any one causes little if any permanent disturbance because of the degree of overlap of their sensory functions. The motor function of the genitofemoral nerve is effectively abolished by dissection and division of the cremaster, with loss of its suspensory function and the cremaster reflex in the inguinal canal during the Shouldice operation. Because fenestration, and not excision, of the cremaster muscle is all that is required for the mesh tension-free hernioplasty, it is to be expected that complications arising from damage or division of the genito-femoral nerve will not occur with such frequency after this operation. If damage has occurred, an area of numbness is almost always complained of; this invariably settles in months. An attempt should be made to protect the function of the ilio-inguinal and iliohypogastric nerves, but if these nerves are damaged or stretched they should be cleanly divided and ligated to prevent regenerative penetration of adjacent mesodermal scar tissue and neuroma formation. Neuroma formation can cause persistent postoperative pain and require ablation by phenol injection or operation.

When the extraperitoneal approach with extensive mesh reinforcement is being employed for recurrent herniation, it is important to identify and avoid the femoral nerve. Injury to this nerve or a suture snagging it will result in paresis of the extensors of the thigh. The femoral nerve should not be at risk during primary anterior hernioplasty when the fascia transversalis is reconstructed medial to the deep ring. However, sutures through the fascia transversalis lateral to the deep ring and emergent cord are very dangerous; they are prone to catch the nerve and should never be used. They are unnecessary anyway, the object of anterior repair being to restore the normal shutter mechanism of the deep ring medial to the cord. Sutures on the lateral side only destroy this shutter mechanism. The deep ring should always be reconstructed from the medial side under direct vision.

In the extraperitoneal repair of recurrent hernia with polypropylene mesh, there is often much scar tissue to be transversed and dissected. The femoral nerve lies on the psoas muscle lateral to the femoral sheath. It is covered by dense fascia and can scarcely be at risk of injury by dissection. However, laterally placed sutures to fix the prosthesis may catch it if care is not taken.

Chronic residual neuralgia can be the end result of nerve damage.[968] The consequences of such damage are accompanied by a range of vegetative, and potentially medicolegal, manifestations. Two types of pain can be attributed to nerve damage:

1. Nociceptive pain due to proliferation of nerve fibres outside the neurolemma can result in a burning pain. In specialist centres with appropriate expertise this condition can be treated by genitofemoral or ilio-inguinal neurectomy.[490] Kennedy and colleagues treated 23 patients over a nine-year period, who had been symptomatic for an average of 3.3 years and had previously undergone 3.1 operations before referral. Of the patients, 15 underwent L1 to L2 paraspinus nerve block and 13 had pain relief; three patients had persistent neuralgia associated with significant orchialgia. This series supports the concept of early referral for neurectomy in selected cases.
2. Deafferentation resulting in delayed-type hyperaesthesia. Selective nerve-block is often successful in alleviating this problem.

Wantz, in giving advice as to the avoidance of chronic residual neuralgia, advises the intentional division of the sensory nerves which may be necessary in up to 25% of inguinal hernioplasties.[968]

PERSISTENT POSTOPERATIVE PAIN

Persistent pain at or adjacent to the pubic tubercle and nearby bone is sometimes a complaint after successful hernioplasty. Periostitis of the pubis, adductor strain, nerve entrapment, strain of the origin of abdominal muscles, the rectus, pectineus or conjoint tendon are all mentioned. The differential diagnosis between each of these entities is almost impossible. Deep sutures through the periosteum of the pubic tubercle can lead to periostitis; it was a complication frequently reported when biological derived sutures, silk, catgut and tendon, were employed in hernioplasty. There are no reports of this periostitis with modern polymer suture materials. Periosteal suture should be avoided and is unnecessary anyway.

If pain at the pubic tubercle persists and if there is local bone tenderness, a radiograph of the bone should be advised to exclude osteitis. If no bone pathology is identified, injection with local anaesthetic and corticosteroids invariably alleviates the symptoms.

FEMORAL VEIN COMPRESSION

Compression of the femoral vein can occur if sutures or a prosthesis are placed too far laterally in repair of a femoral hernia or in a Cooper's ligament type repair of an inguinal hernia. Oedema of the lower limb and pulmonary embolus could be in the presenting signs of femoral vein compression.[124] The diagnosis can be confirmed by phlebography or venous Duplex scanning.[704] Systemic anticoagulation and reoperation should be undertaken immediately.[303] There is a real risk of major pulmonary embolism occurring in these circumstances.

The femoral vein is also at risk of being snagged by a suture during repair of the fascia transversalis to the iliopubic tract/anterior femoral sheath during both inguinal and femoral hernia repair. If sutures are placed too deeply or carelessly the vein will be injured and blood will well up and fill the space deep to the repair. Removal of the suture and firm pressure usually stems the venous leak.

URINARY RETENTION

Urinary retention is reported by up to 30% of male patients in the immediate aftermath of a groin hernia repair operation. Usually, simple methods such as mobilization and the upright posture or standing by a running-water tap resolve the problem. However, if retention persists a once-only catheterization is advised before the bladder becomes too distended.

Caution is advised in older men with bladder neck obstruction. If there is a history to suggest prostatism, this should be evaluated and treated before hernioplasty. Cramer and colleagues reported on the outcome in 44 patients who had symptomatic prostatic obstruction that required either transuretheral or open prostatic resection within 12 months of hernia repair.[203] Twenty-seven of these patients had prostatectomy prior to hernia repair, 16 had hernia repair prior to prostatectomy, and one had simultaneous prostatectomy and hernia repair. No urinary tract infections occurred after hernia surgery when prostatectomy was performed first. However, in five of 16 patients urinary tract infection occurred after hernia surgery when prostatectomy was delayed. This incidence of urinary tract infection (31%) correlated with the need for, and duration of, bladder catheterization as a result of prostatic obstruction. Cramer thus recommended that, in cases of inguinal hernia and symptomatic prostatic obstruction, prostatectomy should be performed first to reduce the incidence of urinary tract infection consequent upon catheterization with no additional risk related to the hernia. This is an important recommendation because inguinal hernia is found in 25% of prostatectomy patients and 11–30% of inguinal hernia patients develop prostatic symptoms. Both inguinal hernia and prostatic enlargement are common conditions, occurring in 3% and 50% of men over the age of 65 respectively.

Early mobilization prevents urinary retention. General anaesthesia, increasing age, and moderate volumes of perioperative fluid administration increase the incidence of postoperative urinary retention.[741] In a retrospective study of 295 patients, Petros and colleagues found the incidence to be 19% in patients having general anaesthesia versus 8% in those undergoing spinal anaesthesia, 14% in patients under the age of 53 versus 27% in those over the age of 53, and 16% in those having less than 1200 ml of perioperative fluid administration versus 25% in those receiving more than this amount. By avoiding general anaesthesia altogether, Finlay and colleagues virtually eliminated urinary retention in a series of 880 patients after adopting spinal anaesthesia.[302] The Shouldice clinic reports that catheterization is required less than once in 1000 postoperative patients.[449]

OSTEITIS PUBIS

Osteitis pubis is a rare complication of hernioplasty. The condition is well known as a complication of a urological and gynaecological procedures and is a condition recognized in athletes.[475, 550] The pathogenesis is unclear but is probably related to periosteal trauma which seems to be the initiating event. The inflammatory process generated then leads to pelvic pain, which can radiate from the pubic area to the adductor region and over the ischial tuberosities. This is disabling and results in a waddling gate, intermittent fever and sometimes anorexia or weight loss.

Radiological appearances include widening of the symphysis pubis, loss of definition of the adjacent cortical surfaces followed by periosteal new bone formation and finally sclerosis of bone and bony fusion of the symphysis. Rarely the condition is associated with osteomyelitis in which case the remedy is antibiotic treatment rather than anti-inflammatory medication. However, the distinction is difficult and relies on bone biopsy. Unless there are good grounds for suspecting infection the condition should be treated as inflammatory.

Osteitis pubis as a complication of open herniorrhaphy is extremely rare, with only a few cases reported in the literature.[405] Although the condition is self-limiting, conservative measures with physical rest and anti-inflammatory drugs may take several months to resolve the condition.

Laparoscopic herniorrhaphy has also been reported to result in the complication of osteitis pubis both secondary to mesh infection and as a *prima facie* inflammatory pathology.[591] The relative frequency of this complication occurring as a result of the open or laparoscopic procedure is unknown.[591]

General complications

VISCERAL INJURY

A distinction should be made between visceral injury to structures forming the wall of sliding hernia and injury to the contents of a hernial sac.

The bladder medially in direct inguinal and in femoral hernias, the sigmoid colon or caecum and appendix laterally in indirect hernias and the ureter in the inferior wall of both direct and indirect hernias are at risk during dissection. Bladder diverticula can complicate the medial side of direct hernia sac walls or prolapse into the sac.

The bladder is a frequent component of indirect hernias in infants and great care must be taken to avoid injury to it. If the bladder is inadvertently opened, it should be closed with two layers of fine absorbable sutures; bladder catheterization with a thin catheter (10 f.g.) is then maintained for seven days to allow healing to take place. Ureteric injuries are similarly managed by inserting a pigtail catheter from renal pelvis to bladder and carefully suturing the damaged ureter with fine absorbable sutures. The pigtail catheter can be removed endoscopically after seven days. In adults, the best advice to avoid bladder injury (which is rare) is to refrain from seeking a peritoneal sac in the broad-based direct bulge hernia. Just put the inverted direct hernia behind the fascia transversalis repair; it is not necessary to excise direct sacs. If a direct

sac must be opened because of a narrow neck or adherent contents, commence the incision laterally on the side wall of the sac away from the bladder. An important landmark is the obliterated umbilical artery lying in the extraperitoneal fat of the medial umbilical fold. It is invariably identifiable and lies lateral to the bladder wall which may be indistinct in the areolar tissue.

In femoral hernia in adults, the bladder is often in the medial wall of the sac, which is frequently fibrous and thickened from repeated irritation where it abuts on the margin of the lacunar ligament. The same approach to a femoral hernial sac from the lateral side and the same advice about visceral injuries pertains.

In infants and children, the hernia is indirect; the sac may have the bladder in the medial wall and in the female the fallopian tube may slide into the lateral wall and the ovary into the sac proper. All indirect sacs in children should be opened before they are excised and ligated. Their contents and their walls warrant careful examination.

Caecum and sigmoid colon form a portion of the wall of right and left indirect sliding hernias, respectively. The bowel in these sacs may be injured by entering it directly or by dissection damage to its blood supply. Great care must be taken with a sliding hernia; it is quite unnecessary to 'invent' a sac in these cases. Any redundant peritoneal sac, well clear of the bowel, should be removed and the peritoneum closed. The bowel is then reduced and the repair made anteriorly. The extraperitoneal mesocolic wall does not need dissection.

Penetrating injuries to the large bowel should be immediately closed; whether they should then be exteriorized or a proximal diverting stoma performed requires fine judgement. Caution and prudence suggest that an injury to unprepared loaded colon is best exteriorized.

Visceral contents of hernial sacs include omentum, small and large intestine, stomach, ureters and internal genitalia. All indirect sacs or incompletely reducible direct sacs should be opened and their contents inspected. Enteric and vascular injured viscera can all too easily be returned to the peritoneal cavity. If this happens, confused signs of peritoneal irritation will appear postoperatively, diagnosis will be late and management delayed. When there is a possibility of devitalized or perforated gut it is better to perform immediately laparotomy rather than await events.

INCIDENTAL APPENDICECTOMY

Appendicectomy at right inguinal hernioplasty is not recommended. Although there is one trial which suggests that appendicectomy with antibiotic cover can be safely accomplished, the case for prophylactic appendicectomy, which is what it is, is not proved in the UK experience.

Pollack and Nyhus advise differently. They note that 2200 patients die annually of appendicitis in the USA and one in three patients older than 70 years may require appendicectomy. They, and Condon, therefore advise incidental appendicectomy.[191, 750] Eiseman and colleagues concur in this view that appendicectomy should be performed as an adjunct to hernioplasty if (a) there is no complicating disease to contraindicate prolongation of the operating time, and (b) the entire appendix can be visualized from base to tip and appendicectomy and invagination of the base can be accomplished without enlargement of the hernial aperture or sac.[278]

Ludbrook and Spears (1965), using New Zealand data, refute these arguments; they estimate the risk of appendicitis at birth as one in five. This risk falls and is at its lowest in the 50–70 years age group, the age group of most adult inguinal hernia repairs. The risk of appendicitis is greatest in the 15–19 years age group.

Based on these data, a logical policy recommended by the authors is to remove the appendix if it easily presents during herniotomy in childhood up to adolescence. In these circumstances no non-absorbable repair of the inguinal canal is being made; hence the risk of ongoing groin infection and sinus formation, which is ever present when full-scale hernioplasty is made, is not a consideration.[582] For all these reasons, incidental appendicectomy is not performed during inguinal hernioplasty in adults.

In order to avoid the risk of sepsis and because appendicitis is not frequent in the elderly, incidental appendicectomy is not recommended during inguinal hernioplasty in adults.

PNEUMOPERITONEUM, AIR EMBOLISM AND THE LE VEEN SHUNT

At laparotomy air enters the peritoneal cavity, remains in the peritoneum for 10–12 days and is maximally demonstrated at X-ray some 48 h after the laparotomy. A similar phenomenon occurs after major abdominal hernia repair. The amount of air entering the peritoneal cavity after straightforward inguinal or femoral hernia repair is very small, so small that there is often no air demonstrated on the most careful X-ray examination after these operations.[377] There are two consequences of these observations. First, if a considerable pneumoperitoneum is detected after a groin hernia repair the clinician should suspect major pathology – a perforated colon if there has been dissection of a sliding hernia or a perforated peptic ulcer if there is epigastric pain. Secondly, small quantities of air do enter the peritoneal cavity whenever it is opened and this may lead to air embolism if a peritoneovenous shunt has been inserted previously.

A peritoneojugular Le Veen shunt is often inserted in cirrhotic patients with intractable ascites.[541] Due to the raised intra-abdominal pressure caused by the ascites, there is an increased incidence of inguinal and umbilical hernia in these patients. These hernias cause discomfort and pain. Although the patient's general medical status may be poor, surgical repair is advisable because the hernias can incarcerate and strangulate. Air embolism via the peritoneojugular shunt is a hazard of hernioplasty in these patients. To avoid an embolism at surgery and in the postoperative period, the shunt should be clamped with a small bulldog clamp below the clavicle before operation. The venous side of the shunt should be injected with heparin solution to prevent blockage by blood clot, and ascitic fluid should be aspirated from the peritoneal side to ensure patency. The infraclavicular incision should then be closed, leaving the bulldog clamp *in situ*.[370]

At operation, special care is needed when the sac is explored – the catheter tip may be in the sac. After the hernioplasty is completed, the abdomen should be X-rayed daily and the bulldog clamp removed once all the air has been absorbed from the peritoneal cavity. Normally, 7–14 days elapse before the peritoneal cavity becomes air- free on X-ray. The bulldog clamp must never be removed until pneumoperitoneum has been excluded.

CHEST INFECTION

It is traditionally taught in the UK that the risk of chest infection is greater during the inclement British winter. This traditional wisdom is used as an excuse for not undertaking elective hernia repair in wintertime. In the past this may have been a wise policy.

In a review of all the complications in 19 550 adult (18 285 male and 1265 female) patients undergoing elective inguinal hernia repair in the Northern Region in 1984, there was no evidence to suggest seasonal variations in chest infection rates, in infective (wound complications) and non-infective (DVT, pulmonary embolus) rates. Indeed, the duration of stay did not show any seasonal variation either, indicating no adverse consequences of the cold Northern winter. There were no in-hospital deaths in the sample (Table 24.4).[244]

DEEP VEIN THROMBOSIS AND PULMONARY EMBOLISM

With elective hernioplasty and immediate ambulation, deep vein thrombosis and pulmonary embolism is a rare phenomenon. In 10 years of experience in Stockton (1970–80) there was one case of pulmonary embolism; this occurred in a 27-year-old man who had undergone a day-case hernia repair 10 days previously. Treatment by systemic anticoagulation resolved the problem. On the basis of this experience we estimate the incidence of pulmonary embolism to be less than 1 in 1500 elective inguinal hernioplasties.

Table 24.4 Complications of elective inguinal hernioplasty in 19 550 adult males, Northern Region, UK, 12 months in 1984[244]

Month	Average duration of stay (days)	Infective complications (%)	Non-infective complications (%)	Total complications (%)	Patients staying in hospital >7 days (%)	Patients staying in hospital >10 days (%)
January	8.3	1.0	0.6	1.6	45.2	15.8
February	7.2	1.2	0.2	1.4	49.0	16.7
March	6.9	0.5	0.5	1.0	45.0	14.3
April	6.7	0.9	0.4	1.3	43.9	14.4
May	6.8	0.6	0.3	0.9	45.7	14.4
June	6.9	0.8	0.4	1.1	45.2	14.1
July	6.9	0.8	0.5	1.3	45.0	14.2
August	6.6	0.8	0.6	1.4	44.7	13.0
September	6.6	0.9	0.2	1.1	43.9	13.8
October	6.7	0.6	0.7	1.3	46.6	13.4
November	6.6	0.4	0.4	0.8	44.4	15.1
December	6.3	0.5	0.3	0.8	38.5	11.9

(1) Infective complications include wound infections and chest infections. Non-infective complications include deep vein thrombosis and pulmonary embolism.
(2) A similar study of 1265 adult females shows no significant differences.

Mortality from elective hernia repair

The mortality rate for elective hernia repair must be carefully separated from the mortality rate for emergency hernia repair. Emergency hernia repair for incarceration and strangulation carries a substantial mortality, especially in the older age groups.

Iles, in 1969, compared the mortality rate for elective inguinal hernioplasty in public hospitals in North America with the results from the Shouldice clinic: in public hospitals the death rate was 4.1 per 1000 compared with the Shouldice clinic rate of 0.5 per 1000.[450] Many factors may account for this great difference in the perioperative death rate between the American public hospitals and the Shouldice clinic: early ambulation and local anaesthesia, different patient selection, and the fact that all the Shouldice patients are motivated to seek the best medical care for their hernioplasty. In 1974, Ponka reported a perioperative death rate of 0.5% in a series of 200 patients over 70 years old undergoing elective hernia repair.[754] Rutledge (1980) reports one operative death in 758 Cooper's ligament repairs – a 65-year-old man suffering a fatal myocardial infarction.[813] In a two-year period, 1986–1987, Gilbert repaired 175 hernias in patients over the age of 65 years,[340] 58% of the patients were ASA grade 3, having severe systemic disease which limited activity but was not incapacitating, and most of this comprised vascular disease. The majority of patients (124) underwent local anaesthesia or epidural anaesthesia (34). Strict protocols were adhered to with preoperative control of systemic medical conditions, careful choice of anaesthesia, and the avoidance of perioperative complications. There were no deaths, even though 19 patients presented as an emergency with an incarcerated hernia. In a study of hospital costs and morbidity in

octogenarians undergoing surgery, Gardner and Palaski confirmed that death was a result of complications of the primary disease rather than the general surgical condition such as hernia.[327]

In contrast, there is a considerable mortality related to strangulated inguinal hernias. The Confidential Enquiry into Perioperative Deaths in the UK estimate the death rate for adults with strangulated groin hernias to be 7.0%.[128] More recently, the report of the National Confidential Enquiry into Perioperative Deaths 1991/1992 studied the year 1990 for the management of strangulated hernia.[148] During that year 210 English residents died as a result of complications of inguinal hernias, and a further 120 died following complications of femoral hernia. Several recommendations were made as a result of this report. Firstly, the experience of the anaesthetist

Table 24.5 Outcome after operation for strangulated inguinal and femoral hernias: Northern Region, UK, 1973–1982[244]*

Age	Outcome		Total	Death rate
	Discharged alive	Dead		
<60	870	9	879	0.010
60–64	216	6	222	0.027
65–69	331	15	346	0.043
70–74	408	28	436	0.064
75–79	449	39	488	0.080
80–84	387	48	435	0.110
85+	400	47	447	0.105
Total	3061	192	3253	0.059

* The test statistic $\chi^2 = 85.087$ is highly significant ($P < 0.001$ on 6 d.f.). The conclusion is that there is a highly significant association between outcome and age.

Table 24.6 Outcome after operation for strangulated inguinal and femoral hernias – effect of age: Northern Region, UK, 1973–1982[244]*

Age	Outcome		Total
	Discharged alive	Dead	
<60	870	9	879
85+	400	47	447
Total	1270	56	1326

*The test statistic $\chi^2 = 65.98$ is highly significant ($P < 0.001$ on 1 d.f.). The conclusion is that there is a significantly higher proportion of deaths in the older group than in the younger group.

and surgeon attending the patient should be matched to the ASA grade of the patient, i.e. elderly frail patients should be attended by consultants. Secondly, patients must be prepared adequately for surgery by adequate and timely resuscitation. Thirdly, prompt access to emergency operating theatres must be available, and high-dependency units should be available for intensive care and postoperative management of these frequently unstable patients. Finally, some patients may be too ill for surgery and a more humane approach to their care should be considered. This should be a consultant's decision

We have reviewed the death rates for strangulated inguinal and femoral hernia in the Northern Region for the 10 years 1973–82 inclusive. These show an overall death rate of 5.9%, with a highly significant increase in the older age patients (Tables 24.5 and 24.6). Comparison of reported series in the past 25 years reveals the improvement in outcome (Table 24.7).

Table 24.7 Complications of groin hernioplasty

	Rydell (1963)[820]	Dodd (1964)[253]	Gaston (1970)[330]	Palumbo and Sharp (1971)[721]	Ponka and Brush (1974)[754]	Berliner (1984)[92]	Glasgow (1984)[356]	Devlin et al. (1986)[248]		Alexander (1986)[10]
No. operations in series	961	624	621	3572	200	2259	10 353	718	7367	150 000
Wound problems:										
Haematoma and ecchymosis	0.7%	—	15.1%	—	3.5%	—	—	—	0.2%	—
Infection	1.3%	1.4% from 1929–50; none from 1950–64	0.3%	—	3.5%	1.6% prior to 1975; 0.1% since 1975	—	0.3%	0.2%	0.5%
Sinus formation	—	3	—	—	—	0.13%	—	0.6%*	—	—
Scrotal complications:										
Oedema	2.6%	—	1.1%	—	1.5%	0.8%	—	—	—	—
Hydrocele	0.5%	2	0	—	—	1	—	—	—	—
Oedema and testicular atrophy	1.8%	—	1.7%	—	—	0.3%	—	0.1%	—	0.001%
Oedema and scrotal infection	—	—	0.16%	—	—	—	—	—	—	—
Urinary retention	1.0%	—	0.48%	—	10%	1	—	0	0.04%	—
Osteitis pubis	—	1	0	—	—	—	—	0	—	—
Missed hernia	—	—	—	—	—	—	—	0	—	—
Recurrence	—	—	—	1%	2%	1.1%	1.1%	0.8%	—	—
Myocardial infarction	0.2%	—	0.16%	1 case	—	—	—	0	—	12 cases
Deep vein thrombosis	1.4%	—	0.32%	—	15%	—	—	—	—	—
Pulmonary embolus	—	4	0.16%	—	—	—	—	1 case	—	—
Chest infection	—	—	0	—	—	—	—	—	—	—
Deaths (28 day mortality)	0.3%	4	0	0.05%	—	1	—	0	—	14 cases
		All these patients were aged over 50 yr		One interesting death in a 42-year-old man from peritonitis following a perforation of the ascending colon		All operations using a fascia transversalis (Shouldice) repair			Operations at Shouldice clinic in 1984	First 150 000 cases at Shouldice clinic

* Sinuses occurred with braided polyester sutures only.

BIOGRAPHICAL NOTES

Edoardo Bassini, MD (1844–1924)
Italian Senator; Professor of Surgical Pathology and subsequently of Clinical Surgery, University of Padua.

Bassini had a lifelong interest in applied anatomy. He advanced herniology in four important ways: (a) he ligated the peritoneal sac flush with the peritoneum; (b) he reconstructed the posterior wall of the inguinal canal, especially the fascia transversalis from the deep ring to the pubic tubercle, taking in the lateral margin of the rectus sheath medially; (c) he used non-absorbable (silk) sutures; (d) he performed adequate audit and follow-up of his patients – itself a major clinical advance.

Bassini and his Italian pupils were quite explicit about his technique both in text and in diagram. Anyone seeking to check the anatomic details can refer to Catterina's English monograph.[153]

Bassini's reputation has suffered immensely at the hands of many English (and Irish) surgeons who have inadequately performed his operation and blamed him for their failure to read his work and follow his instructions. He appreciated the importance of the fascia transversalis and used non-absorbable sutures. Colleagues who neglect the fascia transversalis and use catgut should understand that they are not performing Bassini's operation.

Jean-Annet Bogros (1786–1825)

Bogros was born in Messiex Auvergne, France, on 14 June 1786. He studied in Paris with Dupuytren and Bechard. In 1817 he was appointed Assistant in Anatomy. He obtained his MD in 1823.

The doctoral thesis that established his name challenged and improved the technique of ligation of the epigastric and iliac vessels which had been put forward by Abernethy and Astley-Cooper. His thesis *Essai Sur L'Anatomie Chirurgicale De La Region Iliaque* was published in 1823.

Bogros' untimely death in 1825, probably of pulmonary tuberculosis, at the age of 39, deprived us of a fine pragmatic French surgeon.

William Bradley Coley, MD, Hon FRCS (1851–1936)
Surgeon-in-Chief, New York Hospital for Ruptured and Crippled.

Much of Coley's surgical enterprise was to the management of bone sarcomas. By 1911 he was able to report successful management of 65 cases of inoperable sarcoma in which the tumour regressed after treatment. He used a mixed toxin (Coley's fluid), derived from erysipelas and *Bacillus prodigiosus*, and later combined with this X-ray therapy.

Coley contributed to inguinal hernia surgery, reporting and following up techniques and patients. Unfortunately he introduced suturing of the fascia transversalis and musculature lateral to the deep ring, 'Coley's stitch'. This negated the sling/shutter mechanism of the deep ring and was inevitably followed by recurrence.[183]

Abraham Colles, MD, FRCSI (1733–1843)
Professor of Anatomy, Physiology and Surgery to the Royal College of Surgeons in Ireland and, subsequently, twice President of that College; Surgeon to Dr Steeven's Hospital, Dublin.

Colles was educated at Trinity College, Dublin, and Edinburgh University. In 1797 he left Edinburgh to work as assistant to Astley Cooper (q.v.) at Guy's Hospital, London. He assisted Cooper in the dissections necessary for Cooper's monumental work on hernias.[189, 190]

There are many Colles eopnyms – the fascia, the fracture, the law, the ligament and the space. We are concerned with the triangular ligament of Colles, known in modern nomenclature as the reflected part of the inguinal ligament: from the crest of the pubis, anteriorly to the insertion of the internal oblique and transversalis tendons, passing immediately behind the external abdominal tendon until it reaches the lines alba in which it terminates.[184]

Astley Paston Cooper, Kt, FRCS, FRS (1768–1841)
Lecturer in Anatomy, Surgeons' Hall; Surgeon, Guy's Hospital; twice Hunterian Professor and twice President of the Royal College of Surgeons of England.

In 1793, on the same day that Marie Antoinette was guillotined in Paris, Cooper was appointed Lecturer in Anatomy at Surgeons' Hall. This post entailed public dissections of recently executed criminals in the Old Bailey yard. Cooper performed well, was an entertaining lecturer and drew great crowds and much applause.

In 1800 Cooper, now aged 32, was appointed to the staff at Guy's. In 1804 he published the first volume of his greatest work on hernias.[189] He was assisted in the research and dissections for this by Abraham Colles (q.v.) who had come to London to study with him.

Francis Sydney Alfred Doran, MD, FRCS (1910–1996)
Consultant Surgeon, Worcester Hospital.

Educated at Cambridge and Manchester Royal Infirmary, Doran served in Burma during World War II. After the war he returned to Manchester where he was appointed Surgical Chief Assistant. He applied both anatomic and mathematical skills to the investigation of hernia repair techniques. His advocacy of randomized trials in surgery in the 1950s and 1960s brought a deluge of criticism from a conservative profession who intuitively knew, from Baconian empiricism, what was correct! Nevertheless he succeeded, sorted out the morass of spurious hernia statistics and, not content, went on to develop day-case surgery.

Eric Leslie Farquharson, MD FRCS Edin., FRCS Eng. (1905–1970)
Surgeon, Royal Infirmary, Edinburgh

Eric Leslie Farquharson was educated at Edinburgh Academy and qualified in medicine from Edinburgh University in 1928. He was house surgeon at Edinburgh Royal Infirmary and held further junior appointments at Kirkcaldy and Leicester Royal Infirmary before returning to Edinburgh Royal Infirmary as surgical tutor. He obtained the FRCS Edin. in 1931 and MD in 1932. He then had a spell of postgraduate study in Paris, Vienna and Heidelberg. Just before World War II he was appointed temporary assistant surgeon to Edinburgh Royal Infirmary. After war service in East Africa, Ceylon and India he returned to Edinburgh Royal Infirmary as assistant surgeon and subsequently as full surgeon. He obtained the FRCS Eng. after the war. He was an examiner for this FRCS and then served on the council of both the English and the Edinburgh Royal Colleges of Surgeons. He is most renowned for his textbook of operative surgery which first appeared in 1954 but which arose from his teaching of surgical anatomy. Many of the drawings were done by himself. His interest in hernia surgery with local anaesthesia arose from his experience of local anaesthesia for major abdominal surgery in Paris and his interest in early ambulation of hernia patients in the army in East Africa in 1940.

Alexander Hugh Ferguson (1853–1912)
Professor of Surgery, College of Physicians and Surgeons, Chicago.

Ferguson was born in Ontario and qualified from the University of Toronto. He studied in London, Edinburgh and Berlin and then set up in surgical practice in Winnipeg in 1882. In 1894 Ferguson moved to Chicago and became a professor of surgery in the College of Physicians and Surgeons there.

He was the first to abandon and openly speak out against the transposition of the cord advocated by Halsted.

Henri Rene Fruchaud (1894–1960)
Professor of Clinical Surgery, Angers, Anjou, France.

Fruchaud 'was a tiger who could work for hours on end'. During World War I Fruchaud studied medicine in Paris and served as a corporal stretcher bearer and then as a *sous-aide-major*, an assistant doctor at the front. After finishing his surgical training in 1924 he went on a world surgical tour of Germany (Berlin, Heidelberg and Hamburg), Austria (Vienna), England, Switzerland, Italy and Belgium. He was appointed Professor of Surgery in 1937, his inaugural lecture 'Praise of Surgical Spirit' says all about him. He did not allow himself to be buried in the armistice of June 1940 so he joined DeGaulle in London and became chief surgeon of the 'Forces Francaises Libres'. He served with elan during the war, in London, in Syria and in Italy.

His written output covered five topics, surgical oncology and radiation therapy, the surgery of pulmonary tuberculosis, abdominal surgery, war surgery and hernias. His 1956 books *L'Anatomie Chirurgical de la Region l'Aine* and *Le Traitement Chirurgical des Hernies de l'Aine* were very important works on the anatomy and development of groin hernias. Fruchaud concept of the groin funnel, the abdomino–crural–fascial funnel, through the myopectineal orifice drew together all the anatomy of the groin into one concept of repair.

William Edward Gallie, MD (Toronto), FRCS, FRCS (Canada), Hon FRCSE, FACS (1882–1959)
Professor of Surgery, Toronto; Hunterian Professor, Royal College of Surgeons of England; President of the American College of Surgeons.

Gallie qualified from the University of Toronto in 1903 and was only 39 when he was appointed Surgeon-in-Chief to Toronto Children's Hospital. Eight years later he was appointed Professor of Surgery in the University of Toronto. He developed the first co-ordinated surgical training scheme in Canada and in 1941 was elected President of the American College of Surgeons. Because of the war he held office for six strenuous years.

Although he remained a general surgeon, his principal

interests were in bone and joint surgery and particularly in fascial healing. From 1921 to 1937 he published extensively on fascial grafts. With a colleague, Le Mesurier, he published his work on 'Living sutures in the treatment of Hernia' in the *Canadian Medical Journal*.[618] This description of the use of fascial strips on grafts in hernia repair was very influential and was championed in Britain by Keynes.

Frank Glassow, MD, FRCS, FRCS (Canada) (1917–)
Contemporary. Surgeon, Shouldice Hospital, Toronto, Canada; Hunterian Professor, Royal College of Surgeons of England.

Glassow was educated at Cambridge University and Newcastle upon Tyne. During World War II he served with the 15th Scottish Infantry Division at the Normandy landings and afterwards in Northern Europe. After the war he joined the staff of Newcastle Royal Victoria Infirmary. He emigrated to Canada in 1952 and joined the staff of the Shouldice Hospital.

A prolific author and lecturer, he has done much to increase awareness of the beneficial results of good surgery for all types of hernias.

Terence Percy Norman Jenkins, FRCS (1913–)
Contemporary. Surgeon to Guildford Hospitals.

Jenkins was educated at University College, London, and at University College Hospital. He served in the RAMC during World War II. Jenkins' contribution to the understanding of fascial healing was gleaned from 27 years' experience of NHS hospital practice. He initially closed the abdomen with catgut, with inevitable dehiscence. Then he used nylon, again with dehiscence, and this led him to seek a mechanical cause. Hence we now have 'Jenkins' rule', concerning the ratio of suture length to wound length.

Arthur Keith, Kt, FRS, DSc, MD, FRCS (1866–1955)
Curator of the Hunterian Museum, Royal College of Surgeons of England.

Keith was born and received his initial education in Aberdeen. After qualifying, he first entered general practice in Mansfield. Then, seeking adventure, he went to Siam as medical officer to a gold mine. His work in Siam on the anatomy of Catarrhina monkeys brought him a Gold Medal.

After Siam he proceeded to University College, London, and thence to Leipzig for postgraduate experience. When he returned to England he launched his scientific career as anatomy demonstrator at the London

Hospital. He was greatly interested in comparative anatomy, anthropology and embryology, subjects then fashionable and developing rapidly. In 1908 he was appointed Curator of the Hunterian Museum at the Royal College of Surgeons and remained in the post for 25 years. In May 1941 the college was bombed, but Keith recovered the remains of the museum and built it up again after the war.

Geoffrey Langton Keynes, Kt, MA, FRCS, FRCP, FRCOG (1887–1982)
Surgeon, London Truss Society; Surgeon, St Bartholomew's Hospital; Hunterian Professor, Royal College of Surgeons of England.

The younger brother of the economist John Maynard Keynes, he became a scholar at Cambridge, where he took first-class honours, after which he read medicine at St Bartholomew's Hospital. During World War I he served in France and was mentioned in dispatches. His appointment as Surgeon to the City of London Truss Society gave him a unique insight into working men and their problems with ruptures. He understood trusses and their disadvantages.

Almost as a second life Keynes was a scholar, bibliophile, artist and literateur. He wrote biographies of John Donne, John Evelyn, Bishop Berkeley and William Blake and designed stage settings for Job. At the age of 90 he published his autobiography *The Gates of Memory*.

Irving Lichtenstein (1920–)
Surgeon, Cedars-Sinai Hospital, Los Angeles

Lichtenstein received his medical training at Hahneman Medical School. He is a Fellow of the American College of Surgeons. He founded the Lichtenstein Hernia Institute in Los Angeles in 1952 while a surgeon at the Cedars-Sinai Medical Center. His monograph in 1970 introduced four concepts: (1) hernia surgery can be performed as an outpatient procedure; (2) it is best performed by an experienced surgeon; (3) a 'tensionless' mesh procedure has enormous advantages; (4) local anaesthesia also has advantages. Early ambulation and return to unrestricted activity and labour is encouraged and brings economic advantages.

Lichtenstein is an important and influential iconoclast.

Charles Barrett Lockwood, FRCS (1856–1914)
Surgeon, St Bartholomew's Hospital; Hunterian Professor and Vice-President, Royal College of Surgeons of England.

Lockwood was born in Stockton-on-Tees and attended Stockton Grammar School. After school he was apprenticed to a firm of surgeons in Stockton. In 1874 he entered St Bartholomew's Hospital where he spent the remainder of his career, eventually retiring as a full surgeon in 1912. In 1914 he pricked his finger when operating for gangrenous appendicitis and died five weeks later from septicaemia.

William James Lytle, MB, FRCS (1896–1986)
Surgeon, Sheffield Royal Infirmary.

Lytle was born in Maghera, County Londonderry, and educated at Campbell College and Queen's University, Belfast. During World War I he served in the Royal Navy. He was Consultant Surgeon, then Assistant Professor, then Postgraduate Dean in Sheffield.

His work on the anatomy of the fascia transversalis and, in particular, his fine colour film showing the action of the internal inguinal ring are very important contributions.

Charles Bidwell McVay, PhD, MD, FACS (1911–1987)
Professor of Surgery, University of South Dakota; Chief of Surgery, Yankton Clinic, Yankton, South Dakota; Regent American College of Surgeons.

McVay was born in Yankton, South Dakota, and initially educated there. He went to medical school in North Western University, Chicago, and was a resident at the University of Michigan School of Medicine. He served in the US Army in Europe in World War II.

McVay became Clinical Professor of Surgery and also Professor of Anatomy in the University of South Dakota. He was a Fellow of the American College of Surgeons.

His contributions to the anatomy of the abdominal wall and herniology are numerous. Perhaps his most important contribution is his groin anatomy, based on the dissection of 500 body halves.

Rodney Honor Maingot, FRCS (1893–1982)
Surgeon, Royal Waterloo Hospital and Royal Free Hospital, London.

Maingot was born in Trinidad of British parents and educated at Ushaw College, Durham. He studied medicine at St Bartholomew's in London and qualified with the conjoint diploma in 1916. He then joined the RAMC, serving in Egypt and Palestine, and was twice mentioned in dispatches. He returned to Bart's after the war and took the FRCS in 1920. He was appointed Consulting Surgeon to the Royal Waterloo Hospital and Southend General Hospital. In 1945 he joined the staff of the Royal Free Hospital.

Maingot was a deft and meticulous surgeon whose

major interest was in the abdomen. A prodigious writer and editor, his Abdominal Operations was first published in 1931 with himself as sole author. This classic textbook is still in print, but is now a multi-author colossus. Sequential reading of the editions will give a well-referenced and accurate summary of the development of each aspect of hernia surgery over the years.

Henry Orlando Marcy, MD, AM, LLD (1837–1924)
Surgeon, Cambridge, Massachusetts; served in the Union Army 1861-65; President of the American Medical Association.

A graduate of Harvard, Marcy studied in Europe where he became a convert to Lister's doctrine of antisepsis and the use of carbolized catgut ligatures. He was the first surgeon to reconstruct the internal ring for inguinal hernia. 'In 1871 I first published two cases in which I closed the (internal) ring with interrupted sutures of carbolized catgut, followed by permanent cure.'

Marcy described his operation to the International Medical Congress in London in 1881 and Bassini (q.v.) was in the audience. Bassini got the message and hurried home to Padua to put it to the test – to reconstruct the fascia transversalis and the deep ring.

Marcy's life was not only concerned with hernias; he was responsible for many civil engineering projects, including reclaiming the land to build the Massachusetts Institute of Technology and renovating the Charles River Basin in his native Cambridge, Massachusetts.

Austin Joseph Marsden, ChM, FRCS (1919–)
Contemporary. Consultant Surgeon, Liverpool and Ormskirk Hospitals; Research Associate, Liverpool University.

Educated at Liverpool University, Marsden's contribution was to the follow-up and assessment of inguinal hernia results in the Liverpool hospitals during 1951–57. He has had a long-standing interest in inguinal hernia and has personally operated on, and followed up, over 3000 cases. His study of recurrent hernia using a 'lace' technique, a relaxed loose nylon darn with meticulous technique, is a paradigm of observational and operative clinical surgery.

William James Mayo, MD (1861–1939)
Surgeon, Rochester, Minnesota.

The brothers William and Charles Mayo, with their father, William Worall Mayo, were the triumvirate which founded the Medical and Surgical Clinic,

Rochester, Minnesota. William W. Mayo was born in Eccles, Lancashire, and studied medicine at Owen's College, Manchester. He emigrated to the USA and practised as a pioneer in Rochester. His sons, William James (born 1861) and Charles Horace (born 1865), qualified in medicine and devoted themselves to medicine, research and teaching. The Mayo Clinic was founded in 1894. They invested all their savings and energies in the enterprise, drawing a small salary only for themselves. When the surgery in the clinic was divided up, Charles inclined to head and neck and prostatectomy and William to abdominal surgery. The brothers worked together all their lives and shared a common pocket notebook into which they wrote their share of day-to-day experiences and observations.

Lloyd Milton Nyhus, BA, MD, FACS (1923–)
Contemporary. Surgeon, Head of the Department of Surgery, University of Illinois College of Medicine; Surgeon-in-Chief, University of Illinois Hospital, Chicago.

Nyhus is a contributor to the surgical literature on reflux oesophagitis and the stomach and duodenum, as well as on the subject of hernia. His book Hernia is the most comprehensive contemporary text. Nyhus is an important advocate of the preperitoneal approach to the groin. Nyhus has long been an advocate of individualizing operations for inguinal hernia; his classification system underpinning this concept is an important contribution to groin hernia surgery.

William Heneage Ogilvie, KBE, MCh, MD, FRCS (1894–1971)
Surgeon, Guy's Hospital, London; Hunterian Professor and Vice President of the Royal College of Surgeons of England.

Ogilvie was a powerful surgical character, imbued with a spirit of heterodoxy. He was a deft operator and skilled medical journalist. His views on hernia management were given full scope in World War II, during which he was Consulting Surgeon to the Mediterranean forces, with the rank of Major-General. His post-war book Hernia was the standard work of its day.

Always outspoken, honest and combative, in 1949 while visiting the USA he caused consternation when he announced that he liked working in the British National Health Service.

Raymond Charles Read, MD, PhD, FRCS, FACS (1921–)
Contemporary. Surgeon-in-Chief, Veterans Administration Medical Center, and Professor of Surgery, Little Rock, Arkansas.

Read was born in Beckenham, Kent. He was a Scholar at Cambridge, where he took his tripos Part II in Anatomy and became interested in hernia. He was a Rockefeller Student at the University of Minnesota, where he received his surgical training.

His studies of the causation of hernia, in particular his contributions on collagen failure, have led to the concept of 'metastatic emphysema'.

Edward Earle Shouldice, MD (1890–1965)
Lecturer in Anatomy, University of Toronto.

Shouldice was born in Ontario, Canada and graduated in medicine from the University of Toronto in 1916. He then served in the Canadian Forces in World War I. After the war he set up in private practice in Toronto and was appointed Lecturer in Anatomy in the University of Toronto.

He became interested in hernia surgery during World War II when treating recruits for military service. After the war he opened a small private hospital for the surgical treatment of hernias, with the emphasis on local anaesthesia and early ambulation.

Since 1969 the hospital has moved to a large modern facility on the outskirts of Toronto. It has five operating theatres and several operating teams; 7000 hernia repairs are performed there annually.

Cecil Pembrey Greay Wakeley, Bart., KBE, CB, DSc, FRCS (1882–1979)
Consultant Surgeon, King's College Hospital; Surgeon Rear Admiral, Royal Navy, President, Royal College of Surgeons of England.

Wakeley served in the Royal Navy in both world wars. During World War I he treated large numbers of burned men after the Battle of Jutland. He initiated treatment by exposure and early skin grafting and produced convincing evidence of the detrimental effects of the picric acid treatment, then in vogue as a first aid measure. During World War II he served as Rear Admiral in charge of surgical services at the Royal Naval Hospital, Haslar.

An enthusiastic anatomist, he was, for 50 years, an anatomy teacher at King's College in the Strand. He was Consultant Surgeon at King's College Hospital from 1922 until his retirement in 1957. As Vice-President and then President of the Royal College of Surgeons of England he was the guiding hand behind the rebuilding of the Lincoln's Inn Fields premises after the war. He was Editor of the Annals for 20 years and Editorial Secretary of the British Journal of Surgery for 30 years! A prolific and enthusiastic surgical journalist, he contributed many articles on hernia, his most typical – combining anatomy with clinical observation and operative technique – being his classic on obturator hernia.

Leo M Zimmerman, MD, FACS
Contemporary. Professor of Surgery, Chicago Medical School.

Zimmerman was an associate of Anson and McVay (q.v.) and was chiefly noted for his anatomic display of the leaves of the semilunar line and the anatomy of Spigelian hernias.

REFERENCES AND
FURTHER READING

1   Abrams BL, Alisikafi FH, Waterman NG. Colostomy: a new look at morbidity and mortality. *Annals of Surgery* 1979; **45**: 462.

2   Abramson JH, Gofin J, Hoppe, Makler A. The epidemiology of inguinal hernia. A survey in western Jerusalem. *Journal of Epidemiology and Community Health* 1978; **32**: 59–67.

3   Ackerman LV Tumours of the retroperitoneum mesentery and peritoneum. In *Atlas of Tumour Pathology*. Washington DC: Armed Forces Institute of Pathology, 1954; 134–135.

4   Adams HD, Smith DC. Obturator hernia. *Journal of the American Medical Association* 1948; 948–950.

5   Adamson RJW. A case of bilateral hernia through Petit's triangle with two associated abnormalities. *British Journal of Surgery* 1958; **46**: 88–89.

6   Adler MW. Randomized controlled trial of early discharge for inguinal hernia and varicose veins. *Annals of the Royal College of Surgeons of England* 1977; **59**: 251–254.

7   Aird I. The association of inguinal hernia with traumatic perforation of the intestine. *British Journal of Surgery* 1935; **24**: 529–533.

8   Aird I. *Companion in Surgical Studies*, 2nd edn. Edinburgh: Churchill Livingstone, 1957

9   Akman PC. A study of 500 incisional hernias. *Journal of the International College of Surgeons* 1962; **37**: 125–142.

10 Alexander MAJ. How to select suitable procedures for out-patient surgery: the Shouldice Hospital experience. *American College of Surgeons Bulletin* 1986; **71**: 9–11.

11 Allegra SR, Broderick PA. Desmoid fibroblastoma. Intracytoplasmic collagen synthesis in a peculiar fibroblastic tumour: light and ultrastructural study of a case. *Human Pathology* 1973; **4**: 419–429.

12 Allen PIM, Zager M, Goldman M. Elective repair of groin hernias in the elderly. *British Journal of Surgery* 1987; **74**: 987.

13 Allen RP, Condon VR. Transitory extraperitoneal hernia of the bladder in infants (bladder ears). *Radiology* 1961; **77**: 979–983.

14 Alsarrage SAM, Godbole CSM. A randomized trial to compare local with general anaesthesia for inguinal hernia repair. *Journal of the Kuwait Medical Association* 1990; **24**: 31–34.

15 Altman B. Interstitial presenting as Spigelian hernia. *British Journal of Surgery* 1960; **48**: 60–62.

16 American Society of Anaesthesiologists. *Classification of Physical Status*, 1985.

17 Amid PK, Shulman AG, Lichtenstein IL. Selecting synthetic mesh for the repair of groin hernia. *Postgraduate Medical Journal* 1992; **4**: 150–155.

18 Amid PK, Shulman AG, Lichtenstein IL. Critical suturing of the tension free hernioplasty. *American Journal of Surgery* 1993; **165**: 369–372.

19 Amid PK, Shulman AG, Lichtenstein IL. Local anaesthesia for inguinal hernia repair: step-by-step procedure. *Annals of Surgery* 1994; **220**: 735–737.

20 Amid PK, Shulman AG, Lichtenstein IL. Biomaterials and abdominal wall hernia surgery. In *Inguinal Hernia; Advances or Controversies?* Eds ME Arregui, RF Nagan. Oxford and New York: Radcliffe Medical Press, 1994; 107–114.

21 Anderson GR. Obturator hernia. *Liverpool Medico-Chirurgical Journal* 1900; **20**: 271–275.

22 Andren-Sandberg A, Ihse I. False hernias through parametric defects. *Acta Chirurgica Scandinavica* 1981; **147**: 381–384.

23 Andrews WE, Topuzlu C, Mackay AG. Special indications for preperitoneal hernioplasty. *Archives of Surgery* 1968; **96**: 25–26.

24 Andrews WE. Imbrication of lap joint method: a plastic operation for hernia. *Chicago Medical Recorder* 1895; **9**: 67–77.

25 Andrews NJ. Presentation and outcome of strangulated external hernia in a district general hospital. *British Journal of Surgery* 1981; **68**: 329–332.

26 Angelini GD, Butchart EG, Armistead SH, Breckenridge IM. Comparative study of leg wound skin closure in coronary artery bypass graft operations. *Thorax* 1984; **39**: 942–945.

27 Annandale T. Reducible oblique and direct inguinal and femoral hernia. *Edinburgh Medical Journal* 1876; **21**: 1087–1091.

28 Anson BJ, Morgan EH, McVay CB. Surgical anatomy of the inguinal region based upon a study of 500 body halves. *Surgery, Gynecology and Obstetrics* 1960; **III**: 707–725.

29 Arbman G. Strangulated obturator hernia: a simple method for closure. *Acta Chirurgica Scandinavica* 1984; **150**: 337–339.

30 Archampong EQ. Preoperative diagnosis of strangulated obturator hernia. *Postgraduate Medical Journal* 1968; **44**: 140–143.

31 Archampong EQ. Strangulated obturator hernia with acute gangrenous appendicitis. *British Medical Journal* 1969; **1**: 230.

32 Armitage EN, Howat JM, Long FW. A day surgery programme for children incorporating anaesthetic outpatient clinic. *Lancet* 1975; **ii**: 21–23.

33 Armstrong DN, Kingsnorth AN. Local anaesthesia in inguinal herniorrhaphy: influence of dextran and saline solutions on duration of action of bupivacaine. *Annals of the Royal College of Surgeons of England* 1986; **68**: 207–208.

34 Arnaud JP, Eloy R, Weill-Bousson M, Grenier JF, Adloff M. Resistance et tolerance biologique de 6 prostheses 'inertes' utilisees dans la reparation de la paroi abdominale. *Journal de Chirurgie, Paris* 1977; **113**: 85–100.

35 Arnbjornsson E. A neuromuscular basis for the development of right inguinal hernia after appendectomy. *American Journal of Surgery* 1982; **143**: 367–369.

36 Arnbjornsson E. Development of right inguinal hernia after appendectomy. *American Journal of Surgery* 1982; **143**: 174–175.

37 Arregui ME. A laparoscopic perspective of the anatomy of the peritoneum, preperitoneal fascia, trasversalis fascia and structures in the space of Bogros. *Postgraduate General Surgery* 1995; **6**: 30–36.

38 Artandi C. A revolution in sutures. *Surgery, Gynecology and Obstetrics* 1980; **150**: 235–236.

39 Ashby EC. Chronic obscure groin pain is commonly caused by enthesopathy: 'tennis elbow' of the groin. *British Journal of Surgery* 1994; **81**: 1632–1634.

40 Ashley GT. Hernia in East Africa – an anatomical analvsis of 700 cases. *East African Medical Journal* 1954; **31**: 315–319.

41 Askar O. Surgical anatomy of the aponeurotic expansions of the anterior abdominal wall. *Annals of the Royal College of Surgeons of England* 1977; **59**: 313–321.

42 Askar O. A new concept of the aetiology and surgical repair of para-umbilical and epigastric hernias. *Annals of the Royal College of Surgeons of England* 1978; **60**: 42–48.

43 Askar OM. Aponeurotic hernias. Recent observations upon para-umbilical and epigastric hernias. *Surgical Clinics of North America* 1984; **64**: 315–354.

44 Asmussen T, Jensen FU. A follow-up study of recurrence after inguinal hernia repair. *Surgery, Gynecology and Obstetrics* 1983; **156**: 198–200.

45 Association of Anaesthetists of Great Britain and Ireland. *Recommendations for standards of monitoring during anaesthesia and recovery. Revised edition 1994*. London: AAGBI, 1994.

46 Astudillo R, Merrell R, Sanchez J, Olmedo S. Ventral herniorrhaphy aided by pneumoperitoneum. *Archives of Surgery* 1986; **121**: 935–936.

47 Attah M, Jibril JA, Kalayi GD, Nmadu PT. Congenital sciatic hernia *Journal of Pediatric Surgery* 1992; **27**: 1603–1604.

48 Atwell JD. Inguinal hernia and the testicular feminization syndrome in infancy and childhood. *British Journal of Surgery* 1962; **49**: 367–371.

49 Atwell JD. Inguinal hernia in female infants and children. *British Journal of Surgery* 1962; **50**: 294–297.

50 Atwell JD, Burn JMS, Dewar AK, Freeman NV. Paediatric day case surgery. *Lancet* 1973; **ii**: 895–897.

51 Ausobsky JR, Evans M, Pollock AV. Does mass closure of midline laparotomies stand the test of time? A random controlled clinical trial. *Annals of the Royal College of Surgeons of England* 1985; **67**: 159–161.

52 Babcock WW. The range of usefulness of commercial stainless steel cloths in general and special forms of surgical practice. *Annals of Western Medicine and Surgery* 1952; **6**: 15–23.

53 Badoe EA. Acute intestinal obstruction in Korie Bu Teaching Hospital, Accra: 1965–1969. *Ghana Medical Journal* 1970; **9**: 283–287.

54 Badoe EA. External hernia in Accra-some epidemiological aspects. *African Journal of Medical Science* 1973; **4**: 51–58.

55 Badruddoja M, Bush IM, Angres G, Ansari SA, Schwartz MP, Sullivan KP. The role of herniography in undiagnosed groin pain. In *Inguinal Hernia: Advances or Controversies?* Eds ME Arregui, RF Nagan. Oxford: Radcliffe Medical Press, 1994; 323–331

56 Bailey D. Spigelian hernia. *British Journal of Surgery* 1957; **44**: 502–506.

57 Bailey J. The economics of day surgery. In *Guidelines for Day Case Surgery*. London: Royal College of Surgeons of England, 1992.

58 Baillie RC. Incarceration of a Meckel's inguinal hernia in an infant. *British Journal of Surgery* 1959; **46**: 459–461.

59 Bain IM, Bishop HM. Spontaneous rupture of an infantile umbilical hernia. *British Journal of Surgery* 1995; **82**: 35.

60 Bakwin H. Indirect inguinal hernia in twins. *Journal of Pediatric Surgery* 1971; **6**: 165–168.

61 Ball L. The repair of inguinal hernia and the use of filigrees. *British Journal of Surgery* 1958; **45**: 562–564.

62 Barker AK., Smiddy FG. Mass reduction of inguinal hernia. *British Journal of Surgery* 1970; **57**: 264–266.

63   Barkun JS, Wexler MJ, Hinchley EJ, Thibeault D, Meakins JL. Laparoscopic versus open inguinal herniorrhaphy: preliminary results of a randomized controlled trial. *Surgery* 1995; **118**: 703–710.

64   Barnes JP. Inguinal hernia repair with routine use of Marlex mesh. *Surgery, Gynecology and Obstetrics* 1987; **165**: 33–37.

65   Baron HC. Umbilical hernia secondary to cirrhosis of the liver. Complications of surgical correction. *New England Journal of Medicine* 1960; **263**: 824.

66   Barron J. Pectineus fascia for femoral hernia repair. Quoted by Ponka JL, Brush BE, Problems of femoral hernia. *Archives of Surgery* 1971; **102**: 417–423.

67   Barst HH. Pneumoperitoneum as an aid in the surgical treatment of giant hernia. *British Journal of Surgery* 1972; **59**: 360–364.

68   Bartlett W. An improved filigree for the repair of large defects in the abdominal wall. *Annals of Surgery* 1903; **38**: 47.

69   Barwell NJ. Recurrence and early activity after groin hernia repair. *Lancet* 1981; **2**: 985.

70   Barwell NJ. Personal letter, 1984.

71   Baskerville PA, Jarrett PE. Day case inguinal hernia repair under local anaesthesia. *Annals of the Royal College of Surgeons of England* 1983; **65**: 224–225.

72   Bassini E. Nuova technica per la cura radicale dell'ernia. *Atti del Associazione Medica Italiano Congresso* 1887; **2**: 179–182.

73   Bassini E. Nuova technica per la cura dell'ernia inguinali. *Societa Italiana di Chirurgica* 1887; **4**: 379–382.

74   Bassini E. Ueber die Behandlung des Leistenbruches. *Archiv fur Klinische Chirurgie* 1890; **40**: 429–476.

75   Bassini E. Neue operations – Methode zur Radicalbehandlung der Schenkelhernia. *Archiv fur Klinische Chirurgie* 1894; **47**: 1–25.

76   Battle WH. A clinical lecture on femoral hernia. *Lancet* 1901; **i**: 302–305.

77   Baumer CD. Groin hernia. *British Journal of Surgery* 1971; **58**: 667–669.

78   Bayley AC. The clinical and operative diagnosis of Maydl's hernia: a report of five cases. *British Journal of Surgery* 1970; **5**: 687–690.

79   Beacon J, Hoile RW, Ellis H. A trial of suction drainage in inguinal hernia repair. *British Journal of Surgery* 1980; **67**: 554–555.

80   Beattie WM. Distinguishing direct and indirect inguinal hernias. *British Medical Journal* 1980; **1**: 1321.

81   Beets GL, Van Geldere D, Baeten CGMI, Go PMNYH. Long-term results of giant prosthetic reinforcement of the visceral sac for complex recurrent inguinal hernia. *British Journal of Surgery* 1996; **83**: 203–206.

82   Behnia R, Hashemi F, Stryker SJ, Ujicki GT, Policka SM. A comparison of general versus local anaesthesia during inguinal herniorrhaphy *Surgery, Gynecology and Obstetrics* 1992; **174**: 277–280.

83   Belcher DW, Nyame DK, Wurapa FJ. The prevalence of inguinal hernia in adult Ghanaian males. *Tropical and Geographical Medicine* 1978; **30**: 39–43.

84   Belham GJ, Emery RJ, Cheslyn-Curtis S, Ralphs DNL. Early discharge despite post-operative pyrexia after inguinal herniorrhaphy in unselected patients. *British Journal of Surgery* 1985; **72**: 973–975.

85   Bellis CJ. Immediate return to unrestricted work after inguinal herniorrhaphy. Personal experiences with 27,267 cases, local anaesthesia, and mesh. *International Surgery* 1992; **77**: 167–169.

86   Bendavid R. The space of Bogros and the deep inguinal circulation. *Surgery, Gynecology and Obstetrics* 1992; **174**: 355–358.

87   Bendavid R. *Prostheses and abdominal wall hernias*. Austin: Landes Biomedical, 1994.

88   Bennett C. Appendiceal pus in a hernia sac simulating strangulated inguinal hernia. *British Medical Journal* 1919; **2**: 75.

89   Berger P. La hernie inguino-interstitielle et son traitment par la cure radicale. *Revue de Chirurgie, Paris* 1902; **25**: 1.

90   Bergstein JM, Condon RE. Obturator hernia: Current diagnosis and treatment. *Surgery* 1996; **119**: 133–136.

91   Berliner SD. Inguinal hernia: a handicapping condition? *Journal of the American Medical Association* 1983; **249**: 727.

92   Berliner SD. An approach to groin hernia. *Surgical Clinics of North America* 1984; **64**: 197–213.

93   Berliner SD. When is surgery necessary for a groin hernia? *Postgraduate Medicine* 1990; **87**: 149–152.

94   Berliner SD. Clinical experience with an inlay expanded polytetrafluoroethylene soft tissue patch as an adjunct in inguinal hernia repair. *Surgery, Gynecology and Obstetrics* 1993; **176**: 323–326.

95   Berliner S, Burson L, Kate P, Wise L. An anterior transversalis fascia repair for adult inguinal hernia. *American Journal of Surgery* 1978; **135**: 633–636.

96   Bhatti IH. A case of strangulated inguinal hernia in a 37 day old infant. *British Journal of Surgery* 1963; **5**: 452–453.

97   Billroth T. *Clinical Surgery. Extracts from reports of surgical practice between the years 1860–1876. Translated from the original by C.T. Dent.* London: New Sydenham Society, 1891.

98   Binns JH, Cross RM. Hernia uteri inguinalis in a male. *British Journal of Surgery* 1967; **54**: 571–575.

99 Birnbaum W, Ferrier P. Complications of abdominal colostomy *American Journal of Surgery* 1952; **83**: 64–67.

100 Black S. Sciatic hernia. In *Hernia*, 4th edn. Eds LM Nyhus, RE Condon. Philadelphia: Lippincott, 1995.

101 Blau JS, Keating TM, Stockinger FS. Radiologic diagnosis of inguinal hernia in children. *Surgery, Gynecology and Obstetrics* 1973; **136**: 401–405.

102 Blodgett JB, Beattie, EJ. The effect of early postoperative rising on the recurrence rate of hernia. *Surgery, Gynecology and Obstetrics* 1947; **84**: 716–718.

103 Bloodgood JC. The transplantation of the rectus muscle in certain cases of inguinal hernia in which the conjoined tendon is obliterated. *Bulletin of the Johns Hopkins Hospital* 1898; **9**: 96–100.

104 Bloodgood JC. Operations on 459 cases of hernia in the Johns Hopkins Hospital from June 1889 – January 1899. *Johns Hopkins Hospital Reports* 1899; **7**: 223–563.

105 Bloodgood JC. The transplantation of the rectus muscle or its sheath for the cure of inguinal hernia when the conjoined tendon is obliterated. The transplantation of the sartorius muscle for the cure of recurrent hernia when Poupart's ligament has been destroyed. *Annals of Surgery* 1919; **70**: 81–88.

106 Blumberg NA. Infantile umbilical hernia. *Surgery, Gynecology and Obstetrics* 1980; **150**: 187–192.

107 Bock JE, Sobye JV. Frequency of contralateral inguinal hernia in children. *Acta Chirurgica Scandinavica* 1970; **136**: 707–709.

108 Bohde YG. Condition of the testicle after division of cord in treatment of hernia. *British Medical Journal* 1959; **1**: 1507–1510.

109 Boley SJ, Kleinhams S. A place for the Cheatle/Henry approach in paediatric surgery? *Journal of Pediatric Surgery* 1966; **1**: 394–397.

110 Bourke JB. Strangulated femoral hernia in a female child of three years and nine months. *British Journal of Surgery* 1968; **55**: 880–881.

111 Bourke JB, Lear PA, Taylor M. Effect of early return to work after elective repair of inguinal hernia: clinical and financial consequences at one and three years. *Lancet* 1981; **2**: 623–625.

112 Bower H. A safety net cast over new surgery. *Hospital Doctor* 1996; 16 May.

113 Boyce DE, Shandall AA, Crosby DL. Aspects of hernia surgery in Wales. *Annals of the Royal College of Surgeons of England* 1995; **77**: 198–201.

114 Brandt WE. Unusual complications of hernia repairs: large symptomatic granulomas. *American Journal of Surgery* 1956; **92**: 640–643.

115 Brennan SS, Leaper DJ. The effect of antiseptics on the healing wound: a study using the rabbit ear chamber. *British Journal of Surgery* 1985; **72**: 780–782.

116 Brenner A. Zur radical operation der Leistenhernien. *Zentralblatt fur Chirurgie* 1898; **25**: 1017–1023.

117 Brenner J. Mesh materials in hernia repair. In *Inguinal Hernia Repair*. Eds Schumpelick V, Wantz GE. Basel: Karger, 1995.

118 Brenner J, Sordillo PP, Magill GB. An unusual presentation of malignant mesothelioma. The incidental finding of tumour in the hernia sac during hernioplasty. *Journal of Surgical Oncology* 1981; **18**: 159–161.

119 Brereton RJ. Hernia repair in children. *Lancet* 1980; **i**: 156.

120 Bridger P, Rees M. What a difference a day makes. *Health Service Journal* 1995; **20 April**: 22–23.

121 Bristol JB, Bolton RA. The results of Ramstedt's operation in a district general hospital. *British Journal of Surgery* 1981; **68**: 590–592

122 Britton BJ, Morris PJ. Local anaesthetic hernia repair. An analysis of recurrence. *Surgical Clinics of North America* 1984; **64**: 245–256.

123 Bronsther B, Abrams MW, Elboim C. Inguinal hernias in childhood – a study of 1,000 cases and a review of the literature. *Journal of the American Medical Women's Association* 1972; **27**: 522–535.

124 Brown RE, Kinateder RJ, Rosenburg N. Ipsilateral thrombophlebitis and pulmonary embolism after Cooper's ligament herniorrhaphy. *Surgery* 1980; **87**: 230–232.

125 Browse NL. Distinguishing direct and indirect inguinal hernias. *British Medical Journal* 1980; **1**: 1270.

126 Browse NL, Hurst P. Repair of long, large midline incisional hernias using reflected flaps of anterior rectus sheath reinforced with Marlex mesh. *American Journal of Surgery* 1979; **138**: 738–739.

127 Bryant AL. Spigelian hernias. *American Journal of Surgery* 1947; **73**: 396–397.

128 Buck N, Devlin HB, Lunn JN. *The Report of a Confidential Enquiry into Perioperative Deaths*. London: Nuffield Provincial Hospital Trust and the King Edward's Hospital Fund for London, 1987.

129 Bucknall TE, Ellis H. Abdominal wound closure. A comparison of monofilament nylon and polyglycolic acid. *Surgery* 1981; **89**: 672–677.

130 Bucknall TE, Cox PJ, Ellis H. Burst abdomen and incisional hernia: a prospective study of 1129 major laparotomies. *British Medical Journal* 1982; **284**: 931–933.

131 Bull WT. Notes on cases of hernia which have relapsed after various operations for radical cure. *New York Medical Journal* 1891; **53**: 615–617.

132 Bulman JFH. The use of floss nylon in the repair of inguinal hernia. *British Journal of Surgery* 1963; **50**: 636–640.

133 Burdick CG, Higginbotham NL. Division of the spermatic cord as an aid in operating on selected types of inguinal hernia. *Annals of Surgery* 1935; **102**: 863–874.

134 Burdick CG, Gillespie DHM, Higinbotham NL. Fascial suture operations for hernia. *Annals of Surgery* 1937; **106**: 333–345.

135 Burgess P, Matthew VV, Devlin HB. A review of terminal colostomy complications following abdominoperineal resection for carcinoma. *British Journal of Surgery* 1984; **71**: 1004.

136 Burn JMB. Responsible use of resources: day surgery. *British Medical Journal* 1983; **286**: 492–493.

137 Burns FJ. Complications of colostomy. *Diseases of the Colon and Rectum* 1970; **13**: 448–450.

138 Byers JM, Steinberg JB, Postier RG. Repair of parastomal hernias using polypropylene mesh. *Archives of Surgery* 1992; **127**: 1246–1247.

139 Calcagno D, Wantz GE. Suture tension and the Shouldice repair. *Lancet* 1985; **ii**: 1446

140 Caldironi MW, Romano M, Bozza F, Pluchinotta AM, Pelizzo MR, Toniato A, Ranzato R. Progressive pneumoperitoneum in the management of giant incisional hernias: a study of 41 patients. *British Journal of Surgery* 1990; **77**: 306–308.

141 Caldwell KPS. Femoral hernia: the collar stud operation. *Journal of the International College of Surgeons* 1959; **32**: 618–620.

142 Callisen H. Herniorum rarioram bigna acta societas medicae hafniae. *Haanniae* 1777; **2**: 321.

143 Callum KG, Doig RL, Kinmonth JB. The results of the nylon darn repair for inguinal hernia. *Archives of Surgery* 1974; **108**: 25–27.

144 Calne RY. Repair of bilateral hernia: a technique using Merselene mesh behind the rectus abdominis. *British Journal of Surgery* 1967; **54**: 917–920.

145 Cameron AEP. Accuracy of clinical diagnosis of direct and indirect inguinal hernia. *British Journal of Surgery* 1994; **81**: 250.

146 Campbell HE. The incidence of malignant growth in the undescended testicle: A reply and re-evaluation. *Journal of Urology* 1959; **81**: 663–668.

147 Campbell RC, Dudley HAF. Hospital stay of patients undergoing minor surgical procedures. *Lancet* 1964; **2**: 403–405.

148 Campling EA, Devlin HB, Hoyle RW, Lunn JN. *The report of a National Confidential Enquiry into Perioperative Deaths 1991/1992*. London,1993.

149 Cannon DJ, Read RC. Metastatic emphysema. A mechanism for acquiring inguinal herniation. *Annals of Surgery* 1981; **194**: 270–276.

150 Cannon DJ, Casteel L, Read RC. Abdominal aortic aneurysm, Leriche's syndrome, inguinal herniation and smoking. *Archives of Surgery* 1984; **119**: 387–389.

151 Cannon SR, Ralphs DNL, Bolton JP, Wood JJ, Allan A. Early discharge following hernia repair in unselected patients. *British Journal of Surgery* 1982; **69**: 112–113.

152 Capozzi JA, Berkenfeld JA, Cherry JK. Repair of an inguinal hernia in the adult with prolene mesh. *Surgery, Gynecology and Obstetrics* 1988; **167**: 124–128.

153 Carbonell JF, Sanchez JLA, Peris RT, Ivorra JC, Delbano MJP, Sanchez C, Araez JIG, Greus PC. Risk factors associated with inguinal hernias: a case control study. *European Journal of Surgery* 1993; **159**: 481–486.

154 Carey LC. Acute appendicitis occurring in hernias: a report of 10 cases. *Surgery* 1967; **61**: 236–238.

155 Carnett JB. lnguinal hernia of the caecum. *Annals of Surgery* 1909; **49**: 491–515.

156 Carriquiry LA, Pineyro A. Pre-operative diagnosis of non strangulated obturator hernia, the contribution of herniography. *British Journal of Surgery* 1988; **75**: 785.

157 Castelein RM, Saunter AJM. Lumbar hernia in an iliac bone graft defect. *Acta Orthopaedica Scandinavica* 1985; **56**: 273–274.

158 Castleden WM. Meckel's diverticulum in an umbilical hernia. *British Journal of Surgery* 1970; **57**: 932–934.

159 Catterina A. *Bassini's Operation*. London: Lewis, 1934.

160 Catterina A. *L'operatione di Bassini der la cura radicale dell'ernia inguinale*. Bolognia, Italia: L. Capelli, 1932

161 Celestin LR. The indirect inguinal hernia. *British Journal of Surgery* 1964; **51**: 423–429.

162 Celsus AC. *Of Medicine*. Translated by James Grieve, London 1756.

163 Cevese P, D'Amico D, Biasiato R *et al*. Peristomal hernia following end colostomy: a conservative approach. *Italian Journal of Surgical Science* 1984; **14**: 207–209.

164 Chamary VL. Femoral hernia: intestinal obstruction is an unrecognized source of morbidity and mortality. *British Journal of Surgery* 1993; **80**: 230–232.

165 Champault G, Benoit J, Lauroy J, Rizk P. Hernies de l'aine de l'adulte. Chirugie Laparoscopique vs operation de Shouldice. Etude randomise controlee 181 patients. Resultats preliminaires. *Annales de Chirurgie (Paris)* 1994, **48**: 1003–1008.

166 Chan MK, Baillod RA, Tanner RA *et al*. Abdominal hernias in patients receiving continuous

ambulatory peritoneal dialysis. *British Medical Journal* 1981; **283**: 826.

167 Chang FC, Farha GJ. Inguinal herniorrhaphy under local anaesthesia. *Archives of Surgery* 1977; **112**: 1069–1071.

168 Chapman B, Snell AM, Rowntree L. Decompensated portal cirrhosis: report of one hundred and twelve cases. *New England Journal of Medicine* 1931; **97**: 237.

169 Charlton JE. Monitoring and supplemental oxygen during endoscopy. *British Medical Journal* 1995; **310**: 886–887.

170 Chatterjee SK. Spontaneous rupture of umbilical hernia with evisceration of small intestine. *Journal of the Indian Medical Association* 1972; **59**: 287.

171 Cheatle GL. An operation for radical cure of inguinal and femoral hernia. *British Medical Journal* 1920; **2**: 68–69.

172 Cheatle GL. An operation for inguinal hernia. *British Medical Journal* 1921; **2**: 1025–1026.

173 Cheek CM, Williams MH, Farndon JR. Trusses in the management of hernia today. *British Journal of Surgery* 1995; **82**: 1611–1613.

174 Cheek C, Black NA, Devlin HB, Kingsnorth AN, Taylor RS, Watkins D. Systematic review on groin hernia surgery. *Annals of the Royal College of Surgeons of England* (1998); **80** (Suppl.).

175 Cheselden W. *The Anatomy of the Human Body*, 12th Edn. London: Livingston, Dodsley, Cadell, Baldwin and Lowndes, 1784.

176 Chevrel JP (Ed.) *Chirurgie des parois de l'abdomen*. Berlin: Springer-Verlag, 1985.

177 Chilvers C, Pike MC, Foreman D, Fogelman K, Wadsworth MEJ. Apparent doubling of frequency of undescended testis in England and Wales 1962–1981. *Lancet* 1984; **ii**: 330–332.

178 Chung-Kuao Chou, Liu GC, Chen LT, Jaw TS. The use of M.R.I. in bowel obstruction. *Abdominal Imaging* 1993; **18**: 131–135.

179 Clain A. Traumatic hernia. *British Journal of Surgery* 1964; **51**: 549–550.

180 Clear JJ. Ten year statistical study of inguinal hernias. A comparison of the rate of recurrence following repair by the Halsted I and other operations. *Archives of Surgery, Chicago* 1951; **62**: 70–78.

181 Cleland J, Mackay JY, Young RB. The relations of the aponeurosis of the transversalis and internal oblique muscles to the deep epigastric artery and the inguinal canal. *Memoirs and Memoranda in Anatomy* 1889; **1**: 142.

182 Cloquet J. Recherches anatomiques sur les hernies de l'abdomen. Theses, Paris, 1817, 133: 129.

183 Cloud DT, Reed WA, Ford JL, Linkner LN, Trump DS, Dorman GW. The 'Surgicenter': a fresh concept in outpatient pediatric surgery. *Journal of Paediatric Surgery* 1972; **7**: 206.

184 Coe RC. Changing methods best way to cut costs. *American Medical News* 1981; **24**: 5.

185 Coetzee T, Phillips WR. Torsion of a myomatous uterus incarcerated in an umbilical hernia. *British Journal of Surgery* 1960; **48**: 342–344.

186 Cole GJ. Strangulated hernia in Ibadan. *Transactions of the Royal Society of Tropical Medicine and Hygiene* 1964; **58**: 441–447.

187 Cole P. The filigree operation for inguinal hernia. *British Journal of Surgery* 1942; **29**: 168–181.

188 Coley WB. The operative treatment of hernia with a report of 200 cases. *Annals of Surgery* 1895; **21**: 389–437.

189 Colles AA. *Treatise on Surgical Anatomy*. Dublin: Gilbert and Hodges, 1811.

190 Condon RE. Surgical anatomy of the transversus abdominis and transversalis fascia. *Annals of Surgery* 1971; **173**: 1–5.

191 Condon RE. In *Hernia*, 4th ed. Eds LM Nyhus, RE Condon. Philadelphia: Lippincott, 1989

192 Condon RE, Nyhus LM. Complications of groin hernia and of hernia repair. *Surgical Clinics of North America* 1971; **51**: 1325–1336.

193 Cooper A. *The Anatomy and Surgical Treatment of Inguinal and Congenital Hernia I*. London: T. Cox, 1804.

194 Cooper A. *The Anatomy and Surgical Treatment of Hernia II*. London: Longman, Hurst, Rees and Orme, 1807.

195 Cooper A. *Lectures on the Principles and Practice of Surgery III*. London: Simpkin and Marshall, 1827.

196 Cooper JL, Nicholls AJ, Simms IM. Genital oedema in patients treated by continuous ambulatory peritoneal dialysis: an unusual presentation of inguinal hernia. *British Medical Journal* 1983; **286**: 1923–1924.

197 Cope Z. *The Early Diagnosis of the Acute Abdomen*, 4th ed. London; Oxford University Press, 1972.

198 Copeman WSC, Ackerman WL. Fibrositis of the back. *Quarterly Journal of Medicine* 1944; **13**: 37–40.

199 Corbitt JD. Laparoscopic herniorraphy. *Surgical Laparoscopy and Endoscopy* 1991; **1**: 23–25.

200 Coulter A, McPherson K. Socioeconomic variations in the use of common surgical operations. *British Medical Journal* 1985; **291**: 183–187.

201 Cox KR. Bilateral pre-vascular femoral hernia. *Australian and New Zealand Journal of Surgery* 1962; **31**: 318–321.

202 Craig RDP. Strangulated obturator hernia. *British Journal of Surgery* 1962; **49**: 426–428.

203 Cramer SO, Malangoni MA, Schulte WJ, Condon RE. Inguinal hernia repair before and after prostatic resection. *Surgery* 1983; **94**: 627–630.

204 Criado FJ. A simplified method of umbilical

herniorrhaphy. *Surgery, Gynecology and Obstetrics* 1981; **153**: 904–905.

205 Cronin K, Ellis H. Pus collections in hernial sacs. *British Journal of Surgery* 1959; **46**: 364–367.

206 Crump ED. Umbilical hernia. 1. Occurrence of the infantile type in Negro infants and children. *Journal of Pediatrics* 1952; **40**: 214–223.

207 Cubillo E. Obturator hernia diagnosed by computed tomography *American Journal of Roentgenology* 1983; **140**: 735–736.

208 Cuschieri A. *Minimal Access Surgery: Implications for the NHS.* Edinburgh: HMSO, 1994.

209 Cuschieri A, Dubois F, Mouiel J *et al.* The European experience with laparoscopic cholecystectomy. *American Journal of Surgery* 1991; **161**: 385–387.

210 Cushing H. The employment of local anaesthetics in the radical cure of certain cases of hernia with a note on the nervous anatomy of the inguinal region. *Annals of Surgery* 1900; **31**: 1.

211 Cuthbertson AM, Collins JP. Strangulated para-ileostomy hernia *Australian and New Zealand Journal of Surgery* 1977; **47**: 86–87.

212 Czeizel A, Gardonyi J. A family study of congenital inguinal hernia. *American Journal of Medical Genetics* 1979; **4**: 247–254.

213 Czerny V. Studien zur Radikalbehandlung der Hernien. *Wiener Medizinische Wochenschrift* 1877; **27**: 497–500.

214 Daniel WJ, Aarons BJ, Hamilton NT, Duffy DB. Paravesical granuloma presenting as a late complication of herniorrhaphy. *Australian and New Zealand Journal of Surgery* 1973; **43**: 38.

215 Daniell SJ. Strangulated small bowel hernia within a prolapsed colostomy stoma. *Journal of the Royal Society of Medicine* 1981; **74**: 687–688.

216 Datta P, Zaidi A, Devlin HB. Short stay surgery for inguinal hernia. *Lancet* 1980; **ii**: 99–100.

217 Daum R, Meinel A. Die operative behandlung der kindlichen leistenhernie analyse von 3, III fallen. *Chirurgica* 1972; **43**: 49–54.

218 Davey WW. *Companion to Surgery in the Tropics.* Edinburgh and London: Livingstone, 1968.

219 Davey WW, Strange SL. The stomach as a content of inguinal and femoral hernias. *British Journal of Surgery* 1954; **41**: 651–658.

220 Davidson BR, Bailey JS. Incisional herniae following median sternotomy incisions – their incidence and aetiology. *British Journal of Surgery* 1986; **73**: 995–997.

221 Davies M, Najmaldin A, Burge DM. Irreducible inguinal hernia in children below two years of age. *British Journal of Surgery* 1990; **77**: 1291–1292.

222 Davies N, Thomas MG, McIlroy B, Kingsnorth AN. Early results with the Lichtenstein tension-free hernia repair. *British Journal of Surgery* 1994; **81**: 1478–1479.

223 Davies JOF, Barr A. Survey of hospital treatment of uncomplicated herniorrhaphy. *British Journal of Surgery* 1965; **52**: 569–573.

224 Davis PR. The causation of herniae by weight lifting. *Lancet* 1969; **ii**: 155–157.

225 De Boar A. Inguinal hernia in infants and children. *Surgery* 1957; **75**: 920–927.

226 De Chauliac, G. *La Grande Chirurgie composée en 1363. Revue avec des notes, une introduction sur le moyenage. Sur la vie et les oeuvres de Guy de Chauliac par E. Nicaise.* Paris: Felix Alcan, 1890.

227 De Garengeot RJC. *Traite des operations de chirurgie,* 2nd ed. Paris: Huart, 1731; pp. 369–371.

228 De Gimbernat A. *Nuevo metodo de operar en la hernia crural.* Madrid: Ibarra, 1793.

229 De Giuli M, Festa V, Denoye GC, Morino M. Large post-operative umbilical hernia following laparoscopic cholecystectomy: a case report. *Surgical Endoscopy* 1994; **8**: 904–905.

230 De Grood PMRM, Harbers JBM, Van Egmond J, Crul JF. Anaesthesia for laparoscopy – a comparison of five techniques including propofol, etomidate, thiopentone and isoflurane. *Anaesthesia* 1987; **42**: 815– 823.

231 De Ruiter P, Bijnen AB. Successful local repair of paracolostomy hernia with a newly developed prosthetic device. *International Journal of Colorectal Disease* 1992; **7**: 132–134.

232 Deitch EA, Engel JM. Spigelian hernia. *Archives of Surgery* 1980; **115**: 93.

233 Deitch EA, Engel JM. Ultrasonic diagnosis of surgical disease of the anterior abdominal wall. *Surgery, Gynecology and Obstetrics* 1980; **151**: 484–486.

234 Department of Health. Press release 94/251, 1994.

235 Department of Health. Press release 95/82, 1995.

236 Department of Health and Social Security. *Hospital Plan.* London: HMSO, 1964.

237 Deshpande PV. Testicular gangrene in infancy due to incarcerated inguinal hernia. *British Journal of Surgery* 1964; **51**: 237–238.

238 Detmar DE, Buchannan-Davidson DJ. Ambulatory surgery. *Surgical Clinics of North America* 1982; **62**: 685–704.

239 Deva AK, Quinn MJ, Nettle WJS. The difficult problem of a groin lump in a morbidly obese patient. *Australian and New Zealand Journal of Surgery* 1993; **63**: 664–665.

240 Devlin HB. Hernia. In *Recent Advances in Surgery II.* Ed. RCG Russell. Edinburgh: Churchill Livingstone, 1982.

241 Devlin HB. Time for the economist and the surgeon to rub shoulders. *Health and Social Services Journal* 1980; **Jan. 11**.

242 Devlin HB. The economics of day case surgery. In *Guidelines for Day Case Surgery.* London: Royal College of Surgeons of England, 1985.

243 Devlin HB. *Stoma Care Today.* Medicine (Oxford), 1985.

244 Devlin HB. *Management of abdominal hernias.* London: Butterworth,1988.

245 Devlin HB. *History of Surgical Procedures. Sonderdruck aus Hygeine in Chirurgischen Alltag.* Berlin: De Gruyter 1993.

246 Devlin HB, Nicholson S. Hernias of the abdominal wall and pelvis: Incisional hernias and parastomal herniation. In *Operative Surgery and Management*, 3rd ed. Eds Keen G, Farndon J. Oxford: Butterworth Heinemann, 1994.

247 Devlin HB, Russell IT, Muller D, Sahay AK, Tiwari PN. Short stay surgery for inguinal hernia. *Lancet* 1977; **i**: 847–849.

248 Devlin HB, Gillen PHA, Waxman BP, Macnay RA. Short stay surgery for inguinal hernia: experience of the Shouldice operation 1970–1982. *British Journal of Surgery* 1986; **73**: 123–124.

249 Deysine M, Grimson RC, Soroff HS. Inguinal herniorrhaphy: reduced morbidity by service standardization. *Archives of Surgery* 1991; **126**: 628–630.

250 Deysine M, Soroff HS. Must we specialize herniorrhaphy for better results? *American Journal of Surgery* 1990; **160**: 239–241.

251 Dierking GW, Dahl JB, Kanstrup J, Dahl A, Kehlet H. Effect of pre- vs postoperative inguinal field block on postoperative pain after hernoirrhaphy. *British Journal of Anaesthesia* 1992; **68**: 344–348.

252 Dillon E, Renwick M. The antenatal diagnosis and management of abdominal wall defects: the Northern Regional experience. *Clinical Radiology* 1995; **50**: 855–859.

253 Dodd EH Inguinal herniae in older persons. *British Journal of Surgery* 1964; **51**: 833–836.

254 Doeven JJ. Results of treatment of incisional hernias with extractable prostheses. *Archivum Chirurgicum Neerlandicum* 1975; **27**: 245–255.

255 Doherty VC, O'Donovan TR, Hill GJ. *Current status of ambulatory surgery in the United States in Out-patient surgery*, 3rd ed. Philadelphia: Hill George J Saunders, 1988.

256 Doig CM . Appendicitis in umbilical hernial sac. *British Medical Journal* 1970; **2**: 113–114.

257 Donaldson DR, Hegarty JH, Brennan TC, Guillou RJ, Finan RJ, Hall TJ. The lateral paramedian incision – experience with 850 cases. *British Journal of Surgery* 1982; **69**: 630–632.

258 Doolin W. Inflamed appendix in a hernial sac. *British Medical Journal* 1919; **2**: 239.

259 Doran FSA. Nylon darn repairs of herniae. *Lancet* 1958; **i**: 637.

260 Doran FSA, White M, Drury M. The scope and safety of short stay surgery in the treatment of groin herniae and varicose veins. *British Journal of Surgery* 1972; **59**: 333–339.

261 Doran FSA. Three methods of repairing the deep abdominal ring in men with primary indirect inguinal herniae. *British Journal of Surgery* 1962; **49**: 642–649.

262 Doran FSA. A clinical trial to determine whether a Lytle's repair of a primary indirect inguinal hernia needs the addition of a rectus flap. *British Journal of Surgery* 1972; **59**: 339–345.

263 Doran FSA, Lonsdale WN. A simple experimental method of evaluation for the Bassini and allied types of herniorrhaphy. *British Journal of Surgery* 1949; **36**: 339–345.

264 Doran FSA, Gibbins RE, Whitehead R. A report on 313 inguinal herniae repaired with nylon nets. *British Journal of Surgery* 1961; **48**: 430–434.

265 Douglas DM. Repair of large herniae with tantalum gauze. An experimental study. *Lancet* 1948; **i**: 936–939.

266 Douglas DM. The healing of aponeurotic incisions. *British Journal of Surgery* 1952; **40**: 79–82.

267 Douglas DM, Forrester JC, Ogilvie RR. Physical characteristics of collagen in the later stages of wound healing. *British Journal of Surgery* 1969; **56**: 219–222.

268 Douglas L. The parastomal hernia. *Surgical Clinics of North America* 1984; **64**: 407–415.

269 Downs SH, Black NA, Devlin HB, Royston CMS, Russell RCG. Systematic review of the effectiveness and safety of laparoscopic cholecystectomy. *Annals of the Royal College of Surgeons of England* 1996; **78**: part II.

270 Ducharmé JC, Bertrand R, Chacar R. Is it possible to diagnose inguinal hernia by X-ray? *Journal of the Canadian Association of Radiologists* 1967; **18**: 448.

271 Dutta CR, Katzarski M. The anatomical basis for the inguinal hernia in Ghana. *Ghana Medical Journal* 1969; **8**: 185–186.

272 Duvie SO. Femoral hernia in Ilesa, Nigeria. *West African Journal of Medicine* 1988; **8**: 246–250.

273 Eames NWA, Deans GT, Lawson JT, Irwin ST. Heriography for occult hernia and groin pain. *British Journal of Surgery* 1994; **81**: 1529–1530.

274 Eaton AC. A controlled trial to evaluate and compare sutureless skin closure technique (op-site skin closure) with conventional skin suturing and clipping in surgery. *British Journal of Surgery* 1980; **67**: 857–860.

275 Editorial. Surgical innovation under scrutiny. *Lancet* 1993; **342**: 187–188.

276 Edwards H. Discussion on hernia. *Proceedings of the Royal Society of Medicine* 1943; **36**: 186–189.

277 Edwards H. Inguinal hernia. *British Journal of Surgery* 1943; **31**: 172–185.

278 Eiseman B, Robinson RM, Brown JH. Simultaneous appendectomy and herniorrhaphy

without prophylactic antibiotic therapy. *Surgery* 1962; **51**: 578–582.

279 Ekberg O, Lasson A, Kesek P, Van Westen D. Ipsilateral multiple groin hernias. *Surgery* 1995; **115**: 557–562.

280 Ekwueme O. Strangulated external hernia associated with generalised peritonitis. *British Journal of Surgery* (1973), 60, 929–933

281 Elechi EN. External abdominal wall hernias: experiences with elective and emergency repairs in Nigeria. *British Journal of Surgery* 1987; **74**: 834–835.

282 Ellis H. *Famous Operations*. Pennsylvania: Harwell Publishing Media, 1984.

283 Ellis H, Gajraj H, George CD. Incisional hernias, when do they occur? *British Journal of Surgery* 1983; **70**: 290–321.

284 Engeset J, Youngson GG. Ambulatory peritoneal dialysis and hernial complications. *Surgical Clinics of North America* 1984; **64**: 385–392.

285 Esposito TJ, Fedorak I. Traumatic lumbar hernia. Case report & review of the literature. *Journal of Trauma* 1994; **37**: 123–126.

286 Evans AG. The comparative incidence of umbilical hernias in colored and white infants. *Journal of the National Medical Association* 1941; **33**: 158.

287 Evans PAS. Health survey in 300 African males. *Central African Medical Journal* 1961; **7**: 55–61.

288 Evans RG, Robinson GC. Surgical day care: measurements of the economic pay off. *Canadian Medical Association Journal* 1980; **123**: 873–881.

289 Faille RJ. Low back pain and lumbar fat herniation. *The American Surgeon* 1978; **44**: 359–361.

290 Fakim A, Walker MA, Byrne DJ, Forrester JC. Recurrent strangulated obturator hernia *Annales Chirurgiae et Gynaecologiae* 1991; **80**: 317–320.

291 Fallis LS. Direct inguinal herniation. *Annals of Surgery* 1938; **107**: 572.

292 Farquharson EL. Early ambulation with special reference to herniorrhaphy as an out-patient procedure. *Lancet* 1955; **ii**: 517–519.

293 Fawcett AN, Rooney PS. Inguinal canal lipoma. *British Journal of Surgery* 1997; **84**; 1169–1170.

294 Fear RE. Laparoscopic: a valuable aid in gynecologic diagnosis. *Obstetrics and Gynecology* 1968; **31**: 297–304.

295 Ferguson AH. On the radical cure of inguinal and femoral hernias by operation. *Annals of Surgery* 1895; **21**: 547–564.

296 Ferguson AH. Oblique inguinal hernia. Typic operation for its radical cure. *Journal of the American Medical Association* 1899; **33**: 6–14.

297 Ferguson AH. *The technic of modern operation for hernia*. Chicago: Cleveland Press, 1907

298 Ferzli GS, Massad A, Albed P. Extraperitoneal Endoscopic inguinal hernia repair. *Journal of Laparoendoscopic Surgery* 1992; **2**: 281–285.

299 Ficarra BJ. Hernia: masquerader of surgical disorders. *Surgical Clinics of North America* 1971; **51**: 1401–1414.

300 Fines G. *Les toiles metalliques dans le traitement des recidives der hernies et des eventrations*. Toulouse: RI (imprimerie), 1972.

301 Fingerhut A, Hay JM. Seventh annual meeting of the French Association for Surgical Research (A.R.C.), and first French-German joint meeting with the permanent working party on clinical studies (C.A.S.) of the German Surgical Society, 27th March, 1993 in Paris, France: Shouldice or not Shouldice? Late results in a controlled trial in 1,593 patients. *Theoretical Surgery* 1993; **8**: 163–167.

302 Finley RK, Miller SF, Jones LM. Elimination of urinary retention following inguinal herniorrhaphy. *American Surgeon* 1991; **57**: 486–489.

303 Fitzgerald, P Mehigan IE. A complication resulting from the use of a rigid inlay in repair of an inguinal hernia. *British Journal of Surgery* 1959; **46**: 422.

304 Fitzgibbons RJ Jr, Salerno GM, Filipl CJ, Hunter WJ, Watson P. Laparoscopic intraperitoneal onlay mesh technique for the repair of an indirect inguinal hernia. *Annals of Surgery* 1994; **219**: 144–156.

305 Fitzgibbons RJ, Camps J, Cornet DA *et al*. Laparoscopic inguinal herniorrhaphy. Results of a multicenter trial. *Annals of Surgery* 1995; **221**: 3–13.

306 Flanagan LJR, Bascom JV. Herniorrhaphies performed upon out-patients under local anaesthesia. *Surgery, Gynecology and Obstetrics* 1981; **153**: 557–560.

307 Flanagan LJR, Bascom JV. Repair of groin hernia: out-patient approach with local anaesthesia. *Surgical Clinics of North America* 1984; **64**: 257–268.

308 Flich J, Alfonso JL, Delgrado F, Prado MJ, Cortina P. Inguinal hernias and certain risk factors *European Journal of Epidemiology* 1992; **8**: 277–282.

309 Fong Y, Wantz GE. Prevention of ischaemic orchitis during inguinal hernioplasty. *Surgery, Gynecology and Obstetrics* 1992; **174**: 399–402.

310 Fonkalsrud EW, De Lorimier AA, Clatworthy HW. Femoral and direct inguinal hernias in infants and children. *Journal of the American Medical Association* 1965; **192**: 597.

311 Ford JL, Reed WA. The Surgicentre: An innovation in the delivery and cost of medical care. *Arizona Medicine* 1969; **26**: 801–804.

312 Forrest I. Current concepts in soft connective tissue wound healing. *British Journal of Surgery* 1983; **70**: 133–140.

313 Forrest J. Repair of massive inguinal hernia with pneumoperitoneum and without mesh replacement. *Archives of Surgery* 1979; **114**: 1087–1088.

314 Franco P. Traite des hernies contenant une ample declaration de toutes leurs especes et autres excellentes parites de la chirurgie, assauoir de la pierre, des cataractes des yeux, et autres maladies, desquelles comme la cure est perilluese, aussi est elle de' peu d'hommes bien exercee. Lyon: Thibauld Payan, 1561.

315 Frankau C. Strangulated hernia: a review of 1,487 cases. *British Journal of Surgery* 1931; **19**: 176–191.

316 Friedman DW, Boyd CD, Norton P, Greco RS, Boyarsky AH, Mackenzie JW, Deak SB. Increases in Type III collagen gene expression and protein expression in patients with inguinal hernias. *Annals of Surgery* 1993; **218**: 754–760.

317 Fruchaud H. *Le traitement chirurgicale des hernies de l'aine chez l'adulte*. Paris: G. Doin, 1956.

318 Fruchaud H. *L'Anatomie Chirurgicale de l'Aine*. Paris: C Doin & Co, 1956.

319 Fruchaud H. *Anatomie chirurgicale des hernies de l'aine*. Paris: G. Doin, 1956.

320 Fry ENS. Hypoglycaemia in children undergoing operations. *British Medical Journal* 1976; **2**: 639.

321 Fung A. Inguinal herniotomy in young infants. *British Journal of Surgery* 1992; **79**: 1071.

322 Gallegos NC, Dawson J, Jarvis M, Hobsley M. Risk of strangulation in groin hernias. *British Journal of Surgery* 1991; **78**: 1171–1173.

323 Gallie WE, Le Mesurier AB. Living sutures in the treatment of hernia. *Canadian Medical Association Journal* 1923; **13**: 468–480.

324 Gallie WE, Le Mesurier AB. The transplantation of the fibrous tissues in the repair of anatomical defects. *British Journal of Surgery* 1924; **12**: 289–320.

325 Ganesaratnam M. Maydl's hernia: report of a series of seven cases and review of the literature. *British Journal of Surgery* 1985; **72**: 737–738.

326 Gans SL. Sliding inguinal hernia in female infants. *Archives of Surgery* 1959; **79**: 109.

327 Gardner B, Palasti S. A comparison of hospital costs and morbidity between octogenerians and other patients undergoing general surgical operations. *Surgery, Gynecology and Obstetrics* 1990; **171**: 299–304.

328 Garland EA. Femoral appendicitis. *Journal of the Indiana State Medical Association* 1955; **48**: 1292–1296.

329 Gaster, J. *Hernia: One day repair*. Darien, Connecticut: Hafner, 1970.

330 Gaston EA Inguinal herniorrhaphy. *Archives of Surgery* 1970; **101**: 472–474.

331 Gaunt ME, Tan SG, Dias J. Strangulated obturator hernia masquerading as pain from a total hip replacement. *Journal of Bone and Joint Surgery* 1992; **74b**: 782–783.

332 Gaur DD. Venous distension in strangulated femoral hernia. *Lancet* 1967; **i**: 816.

333 Geis WP, Saletta JD. Lumbar Hernia. In *Hernia*, 3rd ed. Eds LM Nyhus, RE Condon. Philadelphia: Lippincott, 1989.

334 George CD, Ellis H. The results of incisional hernia repair: a twelve year review. *Annals of the Royal College of Surgeons of England* 1986; **68**: 185–187.

335 Ger R. The management of certain abdominal herniae by intra-abdominal closure of the neck of the sac. *Annals of the Royal College of Surgeons of England* 1982; **64**: 342–344.

336 Ger R, Monroe K, Duvivier R, Mishrick A. Management of indirect hernias by laparoscopic closure of the neck of the sac. *American Journal of Surgery* 1990; **159**: 371–373.

337 Ghahremani GG, Michael AS. Sciatic hernia with incarcerated ileum – C.T. and radiographic diagnosis. *Gastro-intestinal Radiology* 1991; **16**: 120–122.

338 Gibson C. Post-operative intestinal obstruction. *Annals of Surgery* 1916; **63**: 442–451.

339 Gibson CL. Operation for cure of large ventral hernia. *Annals of Surgery* 1920; **72**: 214–217.

340 Gilbert AI. Hernia repair in the aged and infirmed. *Journal of the Florida Medical Association* 1988; **75**: 742–744.

341 Gilbert AI. An anatomic and functional classification for the diagnosis and treatment of inguinal hernia. *American Journal of Surgery* 1989; **157**: 331–333.

342 Gilbert AI. Inguinal hernia repair: biomaterials and sutureless repair. *Perspectives in General Surgery* 1991; **2**: 113–119.

343 Gilbert AI. Sutureless repair of inguinal hernia. *American Journal of Surgery* 1992; **163**: 331–335.

344 Gilbert M, Clatworthy HW. Bilateral operations for inguinal hernia and hydrocele in infancy and childhood. *American Journal of Surgery* 1959; **97**: 255–259.

345 Gilbert AI, Felton LL. Infection in inguinal hernia repair considering biomaterials and antibiotics. *Surgery, Gynecology and Obstetrics* 1993; **177**: 126–130.

346 Gilsdorf JR, Friedman RH, Shapiro P. Electromyographic evaluation of the inguinal region in patients with hernia of the groin. *Surgery, Gynecology and Obstetrics* 1988; **167**: 466–468.

347 Glassow F. Inguinal hernia in the female. *Surgery, Gynecology and Obstetrics* 1963; **116**: 701–704.

348 Glassow F. Is post-operative wound infection following simple inguinal herniorrhaphy a predisposing cause of recurrent hernia? *Canadian Medical Association Journal* 1964; **91**: 870–871.

349 Glassow F. Femoral hernia: review of 1,143 consecutive repairs. *Annals of Surgery* 1966; **163**: 227–232.

350 Glassow F. Recurrent inguinal and femoral hernia. *British Medical Journal* 1970; **1**: 215–219.

351 Glassow F. Femoral hernia following inguinal herniorrhaphy. *Canadian Journal of Surgery* 1970; **13**: 27–30.

352 Glassow F. Femoral hernia in men. *American Journal of Surgery* 1971; **121**: 637–640.

353 Glassow F. The surgical repair of inguinal and femoral hernias. *Canadian Medical Association Journal* 1973; **108**: 308–313.

354 Glassow F. Short stay surgery (Shouldice technique) for repair of inguinal hernia. *Annals of the Royal College of Surgeons of England* 1976; **58**: 133–139.

355 Glassow F. Inguinal hernia repair: a comparison of the Shouldice and Cooper ligament repair of the posterior inguinal wall. *American Journal of Surgery* 1976; **131**: 306–311.

356 Glassow F. Inguinal hernia repair using local anaesthesia. *Annals of the Royal College of Surgeons of England* 1984; **66**: 382–387.

357 Glassow, F. Ambulatory hernia repair (a discussion with M. Ravitch and G. Wantz). *Contemporary Surgery* 1984; **24**: 107–130.

358 Goligher JC. *Surgery of the Anus, Rectum and Colon*, 4th ed. London: Bailliere Tindall, 1980.

359 Goligher JC, Irvin TT, Johnston D, De Dombal, FT, Hill GL, Horrocks JC. A controlled clinical trial of three methods of closure of laparotomy wounds. *British Journal of Surgery* 1975; **62**: 823–827.

360 Gong ,Y, Shao C, Sun Q *et al*. Genetic study of indirect inguinal hernia. *Journal of Medical Genetics* 1994; **31**: 187–192.

361 Gough AS. A report on the use of nylon tape in the repair of inguinal hernia. *British Journal of Surgery* 1963; **50**: 932–934.

362 Gray HT. Lesions of the isolated appendix vermiformis in the hernial sac. *British Medical Journal* 1910; **2**: 1142–1145.

363 Gray SW, Skandalakis JE, Soria RE, Rowe JS. Strangulated obturator hernia. *Surgery* 1974; **75**: 20–27.

364 Green EW. Colostomies and their complications. *Surgery, Gynecology and Obstetrics* 1966; **122**: 1230–1232.

365 Griffith CA. Inguinal hernia: an anatomic surgical correlation. *Surgical Clinics of North America* 1959; **39**: 531–556.

366 Griffiths JC, Toomey WF. Large bowel obstruction due to a herniated carcinoma of sigmoid colon, *British Journal of Surgery* 1964; **51**: 715–717

367 Griffiths M, Water WE, Acheson ED. Variation in hospital stay after inguinal herniorrhaphy. *British Medical Journal* 1979; **1**: 787–789.

368 Grosfield JL. Current Concepts in Inguinal Hernia in Infants and Children. *World Journal of Surgery* 1989; **13**: 506–515.

369 Grosfield JL. Groin hernia in infants and children. In *Hernia*. Eds LM Nyhus, RE Condon. Philadelphia: Lippincott, 1994.

370 Grosfield JL, Cooney DR. Inguinal hernia after ventriculo-peritoneal shunt for hydrocephalus. *Journal of Pediatric Surgery* 1974; **9**: 311–315.

371 Gross RE. Inguinal hernia. In *Surgery of Infancy and Childhood*. Philadelphia: Saunders, 1955; pp. 107–120.

372 Grotzinger U. Ambulante Herniechirurgie. *Therapeutische Umschau* 1992; **49**: 478–481.

373 Gue, S. Development of right inguinal hernia following appendicectomy. *British Journal of Surgery* 1972; **59**: 352–353.

374 Gui D, Giangiuliani G, Veneziani A, Giorgi G, Sganga G. Inguinal hernia repair in patients with peritoneo-venous shunt: risk of an embolism. *British Journal of Surgery* 1986; **73**: 122.

375 Guillou PJ, Hall TJ, Donaldson DR, Broughton AC, Brennan TG. Vertical abdominal incisions – a choice. *British Journal of Surgery* 1980; **67**: 395–399.

376 Gullmo A. Herniography. *World Journal of Surgery* 1989; **13**: 560–568.

377 Gullmo A, Broome A, Smedberg S. Herniography. *Surgical Clinics of North America* 1984; **64**: 229–246.

378 Gumrich H. Klinik und Behandlungsergebisse der epigastrichen Hernie. *Bruns Beitrage zur Klinischen Chirurgie* 1972; **219**: 256–262.

379 Guttman FM, Bertrand R, Ducharme JC. Herniography and the paediatric contralateral inguinal hernia. *Surgery, Gynecology and Obstetrics* 1972; **135**: 551–555.

380 Hackney RG. The sports hernia: a cause of chronic groin pain. *British Journal of Sports Medicine* 1993; **27**: 58–62.

381 Hahn-Pedersen J, Lund L, Hansen-Hojhus J, Bojsen-Moller F. Evaluation of direct and indirect inguinal hernia by computed tomography. *British Journal of Surgery* 1994; **81**: 569–572.

382 Haidenthaller J. Die Radicaloperationen der Hernien in der Klinik des Hofraths Professor Dr. Billroth, 1877–1889. *Archiv fur Klinische Chirurgie* 1890; **40**: 493–555.

383 Halsall AK, Benson EA Pneumoperitoneum following hernia repair. *British Journal of Surgery* 1978; **65**: 416.

384 Halsted WS. The radical cure of hernia. *Bulletin of the Johns Hopkins Hospital* 1889; i: 12–13.

385 Halsted WS. The operative treatment of hernia. *American Journal of Medical Science* 1895; **110**: 13–17.

386 Halsted WS. An additional note on the operation for inguinal hernia. In *Surgical Papers by William Stuart Halsted, Vol 1*. Baltimore: Johns Hopkins Press, 1924; pp. 306–308.

387 Halverson K, McVay CH. Inguinal and femoral hernioplasty: a 22 year study of the author's methods. *Archives of Surgery* 1970; **101**: 127–135.

388 Hamer DB, Duthie HL Pneumoperitoneum in the management of abdominal incisional hernia. *British Journal of Surgery* 1972; **59**: 372–375.

389 Hamer-Hodges DW, Scott NB. Replacement of an abdominal wall defect using expanding PTFE sheet (Gortex). *Journal of the Royal College of Surgeons of Edinburgh* 1985; **30**: 65–67.

390 Hamilton JF. The repair of large or difficult hernias with mattressed outlay grafts of fascia lata: a 21 year experience. *Annals of Surgery* 1968; **167**: 85–90.

391 Hamilton, R.W. Spontaneous rupture of an incisional hernia. *British Journal of Surgery* 1966; **53**: 477–479.

392 Hamlin JA, Kahn AM. Herniography in symptomatic patients following inguinal hernia repair. *Western Journal of Medicine* 1995; **162**: 28–31.

393 Hancock BD. Strangulated hernia in Uganda and Manchester. *Journal of the Royal College of Surgeons of Edinburgh* 1975; **20**: 134–137.

394 Handley WS. A method for the radical cure of inguinal hernia (darn and stay-lace method). *Practitioner* 1918; **100**: 466–471.

395 Hanley JA, Hanna BKB. Obturator hernia: A report of three cases with strangulation occurring twice in two patients. *Journal of the Irish Medical Association* 1970; **63**: 396–398.

396 Hannington-Kiff JG. Absent thigh adductor reflex in obturator hernia. *Lancet* 1980; i: 180.

397 Hardie RM. Day Surgery Assessment Nurse. *Journal of One-Day Surgery* 1993; **2**: 19–20.

398 Harding KG, Mudge M, Leinster SJ, Hughes LE. Late development of incisional hernia: an unrecognised problem. *British Medical Journal* 1983; **286**: 519–520.

399 Harding-Jones D, Robson P. Rupture of an infantile umbilical hernia. *British Medical Journal* 1965; **1**: 498.

400 Hardy JC, Costin JR. Femoral hernias: a ten year review. *Journal of the American Osteopathic Association* 1969; **68**: 696–704.

401 Harper RC, Cacia A, Sin C. Inguinal hernia: a common problem of premature infants weighing 1000 gm or less at birth. *Pediatrics* 1975; **56**: 112.

402 Harrison CA, Morris S, Harvey JS. Effect of ilioinguinal and iliohypogastric nerve block and wound infiltration with 0.5% bupivacaine on postoperative pain after hernia repair. *British Journal of Anaesthesia* 1994; **72**: 691–693.

403 Harrison LA, Keesling CA, Martin NL, Lee KR, Wetzel LH. Abdominal wall hernias: Review of herniography and correlation with cross-sectional imaging. *Radiographics* 1995; **15**: 315–332.

404 Harshaw DH, Gardner B, Vives A, Sundaram KN. The effect of technical factors upon complications from abdomino-perineal resections. *Surgery, Gynecology and Obstetrics* 1974; **139**: 756–760.

405 Harth M, Bourne RB. Osteitis pubis: an unusual complication of herniorrhaphy. *Canadian Journal of Surgery* 1981; **24**: 407–409.

406 Hartley RC. Spontaneous rupture of incisional herniae. *British Journal of Surgery* 1962; **49**: 617–618.

407 Harvald B. Genetic epidemiology of Greenland. *Clinical Genetics* 1989; 36: 364–367.

408 Harvey MH, Johnston MJS, Fossard DP. Inguinal herniotomy in children: a five year survey. *British Journal of Surgery* 1985; 72: 485–487.

409 Hass BE, Schrager RE. Small bowel obstruction due to Richter's hernia after laparoscopic procedures. *Journal of Laparoendoscopic Surgery* 1993; 3: 421–423.

410 Haydorm WH, Velanovich V. A five year U.S. Army experience with 36,250 abdominal hernia repairs. *American Surgeon* 1990; 56: 596.

411 Healy TEJ, Un EN. General anaesthesia for day stay surgery. In *Clinical Anaesthesiology; Anaesthesia for Day Case Surgery*. Ed. TEJ Healy, 1990; pp. 667–677.

412 Heasman, M A and Carstairs V In-patient management: variations in some aspects of practice in Scotland. *British Medical Journal* 1971; 1: 495–498.

413 Heifetz CJ. Resection of the spermatic cord in selected inguinal hernias: twenty years experience. *Archives of Surgery* 1971; 102: 36.

414 Heifetz CJ, Bilson ZT, Gaus WW. Observations on the disappearance of umbilical hernias in infancy and childhood. *Surgery, Gynecology and Obstetrics* 1963; 120: 469–473.

415 Heister L. *A General System of Surgery in Three Parts* (translated into English from the Latin). London: Innys, Davis, Clark, Manby and Whiston, 1743.

416 Heithold DL, Ramshaw BJ. Tucker JG *et al*. 500 total extraperitoneal approach (TEPA) laparoscopic herniorrhaphies – a single institution review. *Surgical Endoscopy* 1996; 10: 572.

417 Helwig H. von. Uber sogennante Spontonrupturen von Hernien. *Schweizerische Medizinische Wochenschrift* 1958; 27: 662–666.

418 Henry AK. Operation for femoral hernia by a midline extraperitoneal approach: with a preliminary note on the use of this route for reducible inguinal hernia. *Lancet* 1936; i: 531–533.

419 Herlock DJ, Smith S. Complications resulting from a patent processus vaginalis in two patients on

continuous ambulatory peritoneal dialysis. *British Journal of Surgery* 1984; **71**: 477.

420 Herman RE. Abdominal wound closure using a new polypropylene monofilament suture. *Surgery, Gynecology and Obstetrics* 1974; **138**: 84–86.

421 Hermann JB, Kavhouwa S, Kelley RJ, Burns WA. Fibrosarcoma of the thigh associated with a prosthetic vascular graft. *New England Journal of Medicine* 1971; **284**: 91.

422 Herrman NIB. Tensile strength and knot security of surgical suture materials. *The American Surgeon* 1971; **37**: 209–217.

423 Hertzeld G. Hernia in infancy. *American Journal of Surgery* 1938; **39**: 422–428.

424 Hesselbach FK. *Neueste Anatomisch-Pathologische Untersuchungen uber den Ursprung und das Fortschreiten der Leisten und Schenkelbruche.* Warzburg: Baumgartner, 1814.

425 Hesselink VJ, Luijendijk RW, de Wilt JHW, Heide R. An evaluation of risk factors in incisional hernia recurrence. *Surgery, Gynecology and Obstetrics* 1993; **176**: 228–234.

426 Heydorn WH, Velanovich V. A five year U.S. Army experience with 36,250 abdominal hernia repairs. *American Surgeon* 1990; **56**: 596–600.

427 Hiller N, Alberton Y, Shapira Y, Hadas-Halpern I. Richter's hernia strangulated in a Spigelian hernia: ultrasonic diagnosis. *Journal of Clinical Ultrasound* 1994; **22**: 503–505.

428 Hilton J. Case of Obturator Hernia with symptoms of intestinal obstruction within the abdomen, to relieve which the abdomen was opened. *Lancet* 1848; **2**: 103.

429 Hoffman HC, Traverso ALV. Preperitoneal prosthetic herniorrhaphy: one surgeon's successful technique. *Archives of Surgery* 1993; **128**: 964–970.

430 Hoguet JB. Direct inguinal hernia. *Annals of Surgery* 1920; **72**: 671–674.

431 Hoguet JP. Right inguinal hernia following appendectomy. *Annals of Surgery* 1911; **54**: 673–676.

432 Holder LE, Schneider HJ. Spigelian hernias: anatomy and roentgenographic manifestation. *Radiologic Diagnosis* 1974; **112**: 309–313.

433 Homans J. *Three Hundred and Eighty-four Laparotomies for Various Diseases.* Boston: Nathan Sawyer, 1887.

434 Horgan K, Hughes LE. Para-ileostomy hernia: failure of a local repair technique. *British Journal of Surgery* 1986; **73**: 439–440.

435 Horner CH *et al.* Cited in Van Mameren H, Go PMNYH. Anatomy and Variations of the Internal Inguinal Region. In *Inguinal Hernia Repair.* Eds V Schumpelick, GE Wantz. Basel: Karger 1994.

436 Horton MC, Florence MG. Simplified preperi-

toneal Marlex hernia repair. *American Journal of Surgery* 1993; **165**: 595–599.

437 Horwich M. Hernia repair using nylon tricot implant. *British Journal of Surgery* 1958; **45**: 320–322.

438 Howes EL. The strength of wounds sutured with catgut and silk. *Surgery, Gynecology and Obstetrics* 1933; **57**: 309.

439 Howes EL. Effects of suture material on the tensile strength of wound repair. *Annals of Surgery* 1933; **98**: 153–155.

440 Hsu C-H, Wang C-C, Jeng L-BB, Chen M-F. Obturator hernia: a report of eight cases. *American Surgeon* 1993; **59**: 709– 711.

441 Hughson W. The persistent or preformed sac in relation to oblique inguinal hernia. *Surgery, Gynecology and Obstetrics* 1925; **41**: 610–614.

442 Hulten L, Kewenter J, Kock NG. Komplicationen der Ileostomie und Colostomie und ihre Behandlung. *Chirurg* 1976; **47**: 20.

443 Hunt DM. Primary defect in copper transport underlies mottled mutant in mouse. *Nature* 1974; **249**: 852–854.

444 Hunter J. Palmer's edition of Hunter's works, published 1837, London, vol. iv, p. 1

445 Hunter RR. Anatomical repair of midline incisional hernia. *British Journal of Surgery* 1971; **58**: 888–891.

446 Hurst JW. Measuring the benefits and costs of medical care – the contribution of health status measurement. *Health Trends* 1984; **16**: 16–19.

447 Iason AH. *Hernia.* Philadelphia: Blakiston, 1941.

448 Ijiri R, Kanamaru H, Yokoyama H, Shirakawa M, Hashimoto H, Yoshino G. Obturator hernia: The usefulness of computed tomography in diagnosis. *Surgery* 1996; **119**: 137–140.

449 Iles JDH. Specialisation in elective herniorrhaphy. *Lancet* 1965; **i**: 751–755.

450 Iles JDH Mortality from elective hernia repair. *Journal of Abdominal Surgery* 1969; **May**: 87–95.

451 Immordino PA. Femoral hernia in infancy and childhood. *Journal of Pediatric Surgery* 1972; **7**: 40.

452 Ingall JRF. Femoral hernia in childhood. *British Journal of Surgery* 1964; **51**: 438–440.

453 Ingimarsson O, Spak I. Inguinal and femoral hernias: long-term results in a community hospital. *Acta Chirurgica Scandinavica* 1983; **149**: 291–287.

454 Irvin TT, Koffman CG, Duthie HL. Layer closure of laparotomy wounds with absorbable and non-absorbable suture materials. *British Journal of Surgery* 1976; **63**: 793–796.

455 Isaac RE. Inguinal hernia and the ilio-pectineal line. *British Journal of Surgery* 1961; **49**: 204–208.

456 Israelsson L. Wound complications in the midline laparotomy incisions: the importance of suture

technique. Thesis. The department of surgery, Lund University, Malmo, Sweden, 1995.

457 Israelsson L, Jonsson T. Suture length to wound length ratio in the healing of midline laparotomy incisions. *British Journal of Surgery* 1993; **80**: 1284–1286.

458 Ivanov NT, Losanoff JE, Kjossev KT. Recurrent Sciatic Hernia treated by prosthetic mesh, reinforcement of the pelvic floor. *British Journal of Surgery* 1994; **81**: 447.

459 Jackson DJ, Mocklen LH. Umbilical hernia: a retrospective study. *California Medicine* 1970; 113.

460 Jacoby HI, Brodie DA. *Laparoscopic Herniorrhaphy*. American Medical Association, 1996.

461 James PM Jr. The problem of hernia in infants and adolescents. *Surgical Clinics of North America* 1971; **51**: 1361–1370.

462 James T. Umbilical hernia in Xhosa infants and children. *Journal of the Royal Society of Medicine* 1982; **75**: 537–541.

463 Jan SE, Wu CW, Lui WY. Shouldice inguinal hernioplasty. *Chinese Medical Journal* 1992; **50**: 26–28.

464 Jarrett MED. Personal communication.

465 Jelliffe D. The racial incidence of umbilical hernias. *Journal of Tropical Hygiene and Medicine* 1954; **57**: 270–272.

466 Jenkins TPN. The burst abdominal wound: a mechanical approach. *British Journal of Surgery* 1976; **63**: 873–876.

467 Jenkins TPN. Incisional hernia repair: a mechanical approach. *British Journal of Surgery* 1980; **67**: 335–336.

468 Jenner RE. Strangulated obturator hernia. *Annals of the Royal College of Surgeons of England* 1975; **56**: 266–269.

469 Johnson CD. Appendicitis in external herniae. *Annals of the Royal College of Surgeons of England* 1982; **64**: 283.

470 Johnson-Nurse C, Jenkins DHR. The use of flexible carbon fibre in the repair of experimental large abdominal incisional hernias. *British Journal of Surgery* 1980; **67**: 135–137.

471 Jones DJ. Braided versus monofilament sutures in inguinal hernia. *British Journal of Surgery* 1986; **73**: 414.

472 Jones PF, Towns FM. An abdominal extraperitoneal approach for the incarcerated inguinal hernia of infancy. *British Journal of Surgery* 1983; **70**: 719–720.

473 Jones TCL. Partial enterocele: strangulated. *Lancet* 1904; **i**: 1280.

474 Judd ES. The prevention and treatment of ventral hernia. *Surgery, Gynecology and Obstetrics* 1912; **14**: 175–182.

475 Julsrud ME. Osteitis pubis. *Journal of the American Pediatric Medical Association* 1986; **76**: 562–565.

476 Kahnan OR. Accidents of hernia operations. *New York State Medical Journal* 1913; 13: 200.

477 Kalsbeek HL. Experience with the use of teflon mesh in the repair of incisional hernias. *Archivum Chirurgicum Neerlandicum* 1974; **26**: 71–75.

478 Kapadia CR. Ligatures and suture materials. In *Rob and Smith's Operative Surgery, vol. 1*. Eds HAF Dudley, WJ Poirees. London: Butterworths, 1983; pp. 119–123.

479 Kaplan GW. Iatrogenic cryptorchism resulting from hernia repair. *Surgery, Gynecology and Obstetrics* 1976; **142**: 671–672.

480 Kaplan SA, Snyder WH Jr, Little S. Inguinal hernia in females and the testicular feminization syndrome. *American Journal of Diseases of Children* 1969; **117**: 243–251.

481 Kapur BML, Shah DK. Strangulated obturator presenting as subcutaneous emphysema of the thigh. *Canadian Journal of Surgery* 1969; **12**: 233–235.

482 Karatassas A, Morris RG, Walsh D, Hung P, Slavotinek AH. Evaluation of the safety of inguinal hernia repair in the elderly using lignocaine infiltration anaesthesia. *Australian and New Zealand Journal of Surgery* 1993; **63**: 266–269.

483 Kark AE, Kurzer M, Waters KJ. Tension-free mesh hernia repair: review of 1,098 cases using local anaesthesia in a day unit. *Annals of the Royal College of Surgeons of England* 1995; 77: 299–304.

484 Kasson MA, Munoz E, Laughlin A, Margolis IB, Wise L. Value of routine pathology in herniorrhaphy performed upon adults. *Surgery, Gynecology and Obstetrics* 1986; 163: 518–522.

485 Kastrissios H, Triggs EJ, Sinclair F, Moran P, Smithers. Plasma concentrations of bupivacaine after wound infiltration of an 0.5% solution after inguinal herniorrhaphy; a preliminary study. *European Journal of Clinical Pharmacology* 1993; **44**: 555–557.

486 Kavey NB, Altshuler KZ. Sleep in herniorrhaphy patients. *American Journal of Surgery* 1979; **138**: 682–687.

487 Keith A. On the origin and nature of hernia. *British Journal of Surgery* 1924; **11**: 455–475.

488 Kemp DA (ed.) *Kemp and Kemp: The Quantum of Damages*. Revised edn, vol. 1. London: Sweet and Maxwell, 1975.

489 Kennedy CM, Matyas JA. Use of expanded polytetrafluoroethylene in the repair of the difficult hernia. *American Journal of Surgery* 1994; **168**: 304–306.

490 Kennedy EM, Harms BA, Starling JB. Absence of maladaptive neuronal plasticity after genito-femoral–ilioinguinal neurectomy. *Surgery* 1994; **116**: 665–671.

491 Keynes G. The modern treatment of hernia. *British Medical Journal* 1927; 173–179.

492 Keynes WM, Withycombe J. Hudson's operation for femoral hernia. In *Hernia*. eds LM Nyhus, HN Hawkins. London; Pitman Medical, 1984.

493 Kiely EM, Spitz L Layered versus mass closure of abdominal wounds in infants and children. *British Journal of Surgery* 1985; **72**: 739–740.

494 Kieswetter WB, Oh KS. Unilateral inguinal hernias in children. *Archives of Surgery* 1980; **115**: 1443–1445.

495 Kieswetter WB, Parenzan L. When should inguinal hernia in the infant be treated bilaterally? *Journal of the American Medical Association* 1959; **171**: 287–290.

496 King LR. Optimal treatment of children with undescended testicles. *Journal of Urology* 1984; **131**: 734–735.

497 Kingsnorth AN, Britton BJ, Morris PJ. Recurrent inguinal hernia after local anaesthetic repair. *British Journal of Surgery* 1981; **68**: 273–275.

498 Kingsnorth AN, Gray MR, Nott DM. Prospective, randomized trial comparing the Shouldice technique and plication darn for inguinal hernia. *British Journal of Surgery* 1992; **79**: 1068–1070.

499 Kingsnorth AN, Wijesinha SS, Grixti CJ. Evaluation of dextran with local anaethesia for short stay inguinal herniorrhaphy. *Annals of the Royal College of Surgeons of England* 1979; **61**: 456–458.

500 Kirk RM. The incidence of burst abdomen: comparison of layered opening and closing with straight through one layered closure. *Proceedings of the Royal Society of Medicine* 1973; **66**: 1092.

501 Kirk RM. Intra-abdominal replacement of testis as an aid to the repair of difficult and recurrent inguinal hernias. *British Journal of Surgery* 1974; **61**: 540.

502 Kirk RM. Which inguinal hernia repair? *British Medical Journal* 1983; **287**: 4–5.

503 Kirschner M. Die praktischen ergebnisse der freien Fascien-Transplantation. *Archiv fur Klinische Chirurgie* 1910; **92**: 889–912.

504 Klinkosch JT. *Programma Quo Divisionem Herniarum, Novumque Herniae Ventralis Specium Proponit*. Rotterdam: Beman, 1764.

505 Knapp RW, Mullen JT. Clinical evaluation of the use of local anaesthesia for the repair of inguinal hernia. *American Surgeon* 1976; **42**: 908–910.

506 Knox AJS, Caldwell KPS. New method of femoral hernia repair using a silastic stud. *British Medical Journal* 1971; **1**: 604–605.

507 Knox G. The incidence of inguinal hernia in Newcastle children. *Archives of Diseases in Childhood* 1959; **34**: 482–484.

508 Kocher T. *Chirurgische operationslehre*. Jena: Verlag von Gustav Fischer, 1907.

509 Kodner IJ. Colostomy and ileostomy. *Ciba Clinical Symposia* 1978; **30**: 2–36.

510 Komura JI, Yano H, Uchida M, Shima I. Paediatric spigelian hernia: reports of three cases. *Surgery Today* 1994; **24**: 1081–1084.

511 Koontz AR. Preliminary report on the use of tantalum mesh in the repair of ventral hernias. *Annals of Surgery* 1948; **127**: 1079–1085.

512 Koontz AR. *Hernia*. New York; Appleton-Century-Crofts, 1963.

513 Koontz AR. Atrophy of the testicle as a surgical risk. *Surgery, Gynecology and Obstetrics* 1965; **120**: 511–513.

514 Koslowski JM, Beal JM. Obturator hernia: an elusive diagnosis. *Archives of Surgery* 1977; **112**: 1001–1002.

515 Kretschmer HL. Lumbar hernia of the kidney. *Journal of Urology* 1851; **65**: 944–948.

516 Kreymer M. Inguinal hernien bei centralafrikanern. *Munchenener Medizinische Wochenschrift* 1968; **110**: 1750–1755.

517 Kronberg O, Kramhohft J, Backer O, Sprechler M. Late complications following operations for cancer of the rectum and anus. *Diseases of the Colon and Rectum* 1974; **17**: 750.

518 Krug F, Herold A, Wenk H, Bruch HP Nabenhernien nach laparoskopischen eingriffen. *Der Chirurgie* 1995; **66**: 419–423.

519 Krukowski ZH, Matheson NA Button-hole incisional hernia: a late complication of wound closure with continuous non-absorbable sutures (case report). *British Journal of Surgery* 1987; **74**: 824–825.

520 Kux M, Fuchsjager N, Feichter A. Lichtenstein patch versus Shouldice – Technik bei primaren Leistenhernien mit hoher rezidivge fahrdung. *Der Chirurgie* 1994; **65**: 59–62.

521 Kux M, Fuchsjager N, Schemper M. Shouldice is superior to Bassini inguinal herniorrhaphy. *American Journal of Surgery* 1994; **168**: 15–18.

522 Kwong KH, Ong GB. Obturator hernia. *British Journal of Surgery* 1966; **53**: 23–25.

523 Lamb JP, Vitale T, Kaminski DL. Comparative evaluation of synthetic meshes used for abdominal wall replacement. *Surgery* 1983; **93**: 643–648.

524 Langenbuch. Quoted in Ponka (1980) (Ref. 753).

525 LaRoque GP. The permanent cure of inguinal and femoral hernia. A modification of the standard operative procedures. *Surgery, Gynecology and Obstetrics* 1919; **29**: 507–511.

526 Larson GM, Harrower HW. Plastic mesh repair of incisional hernia. *American Journal of Surgery* 1978; **135**: 559–563.

527 Larson GM, Vandertoll DJ. Approaches to repair of ventral hernia and full thickness loss of the

abdominal wall. *Surgical Clinics of North America* 1984; **64**: 335–350.

528 Larson GM, Vitale GC, Casey J *et al.* Multipractice analysis of laparoscopic cholecystectomy in 1,983 patients. *American Journal of Surgery* 1991; **163**: 221–226.

529 Lassaletta L, Fonkalsrud EW, Tover JA, Dudgeon D, Asch MJ. The management of umbilical hernias in infancy and childhood. *Journal of Pediatric Surgery* 1975; **10**: 405–409.

530 Laugier S. Note sur une nouvelle espece de hernie de l'abdomen a travers le ligament de Gimbernat. *Archives Generales de Medecine, Paris* 1833; **2**: 27–37.

531 Laurell CB, Ericksson S. The electrophoretic alpha-l-globulin pattern of serum alpha-l-antitrypsin deficiency. *Scandinavian Journal of Clinical and Laboratory Investigation* 1963; **15**: 132–140.

532 Law NA. A comparison of polypropylene mesh, expanded polytetrafluoroethylene patch and polyglycolic acid mesh for the repair of experimental abdominal wall defects. *Acta Chirurgica Scandinavica* 1990; **156**: 759–762.

533 Law NW, Trapnell JE. Does a truss benefit a patient with inguinal hernia? *British Medical Journal* 1992; **304**: 1092.

534 Lawrence K, McWhinne D, Goodwin A *et al.* Randomised controlled trial of laparoscopic versus open repair of inguinal hernia: Early results. *British Medical Journal* 1995; **311**: 981–985.

535 Lawrence, K, McWhinnie D, Goodwin A *et al.* An economic evaluation of laparoscopic vs open inguinal hernia repair. *Journal of Public Health Medicine* 1996, **18**: 41–48.

536 Lawrenz K, Hollman, Carachi R, Cacciagnerra S. Ultrasound assessment of the contralateral groin in infants with unilateral inguinal hernia. *Clinical Radiology* 1994; **49**: 546–548.

537 Lawrie P. A survey of the absorbability of commercial surgical catgut. *British Journal of Surgery* 1959; **46**: 634–637.

538 Lawrie P, Angus G-E, Reese AJM. The absorption of surgical catgut. *British Journal of Surgery* 1959; **46**: 638–642.

539 Lawrie P, Angus G-E, Reese, AJM. The absorption of surgical catgut: II The influence of size. *British Journal of Surgery* 1960; **47**: 551–555.

540 Le Dran HF. *The Operations in Surgery.* London; Dodsley and Lay, 1781; 59–60.

541 Le Veen H, Christondias G. Peritoneo-venous shunting for ascites. *Annals of Surgery* 1974; **180**: 580–591.

542 Leaper DJ. Laparotomy closure. *British Journal of Hospital Medicine* 1985; **33**: 317–322.

543 Leaper DJ, Pollock AV, Evans M. Abdominal wound closure: a trial of nylon, polyglycolic acid and steel sutures. *British Journal of Surgery* 1977; **64**: 603–606.

544 Leaper DJ, Allan A, May RE, Corfield AP, Kennedy RH. Abdominal wound closure: a controlled trial of polyamide (nylon) and polydioxanone suture (PDS). *Annals of the Royal College of Surgeons of England* 1985; **67**: 273–275.

545 Leech P, Waddell G, Main RG. The incidence of right inguinal hernia following appendicectomy. *British Journal of Surgery* 1972; **59**: 623.

546 Lees W. Carcinoma of colon in inguinal hernial sacs. *British Journal of Surgery* 1966; **53**: 473–474.

547 Legorreta AP, Silber JH, Constantino GN *et al.* Increased cholecystectomy rate after the introduction of laparoscopic cholecystectomy. *Journal of the American Medical Association* 1993; **270**: 1429–1432.

548 Lehnert B, Wadouh F. High coincidence of inguinal hernias and abdominal aortic aneurysms. *Annals of Vascular Surgery* 1992; **6**: 134–137.

549 Lejars F. Neoplasmes herniares et peri-herniares. *Gazette des Hopitaux Civils et Militaires* 1889; **62**: 801–811.

550 Lentz SM. Osteitis pubis: a review. *Obstetrics and Gynecology Survey* 1995; **50**: 310–315.

551 Leonetti JP, Aranha GV, Wilkinson WA, Stanley M, Greenlee HB. Umbilical herniorrhaphy in cirrhotic patients. *Archives of Surgery* 1984; **119**: 442–445.

552 Lerwick E. Studies of the efficacy and safety of polydioxanone monofilament absorbable suture. *Surgery, Gynecology and Obstetrics* 1983; **156**: 51–55.

553 Leslie MD, Slater ND, Smallwood CI. Small bowel fistula from a Littre's hernia. *British Journal of Surgery* 1983; **70**: 244.

554 Lestor R, Bourke JR. Strangulated femoral hernia containing appendices. *Journal of the Royal College of Surgeons of Edinburgh* 1979; **24**: 102–103.

555 Levack JH. En masse reduction of strangulated hernia. *British Journal of Surgery* 1963; **50**: 582–585.

556 Levene CL, Ockleford CD, Harber CL. Scurvy: a comparison between ultrastructural and biochemical changes observed in cultured fibroblasts and the collagen they synthesize. *Virchows Archiv pt B, Cell Pathology* 1977; **23**: 325–338.

557 Lewis RT. Knitted polypropylene (Marlex) mesh in the repair of incisional hernias. *Canadian Journal of Surgery* 1984; **27**: 155–157.

558 Liakakos T, Karanikas I, Panagiotidis H, Dendrinos S. Use of Marlex mesh in the repair of recurrent incisional hernia. *British Journal of Surgery* 1994; **81**: 248–249.

559 Lichtenstein IL. *Hernia Repair Without Disability.* St Louis: C.V. Mosby, 1970.

560 Lichtenstein IL. *Hernia Repair Without Disability*, 2nd ed. St Louis/Tokyo: Ishiyaku Euromerica, 1986.

561 Lichtenstein IL. Herniorrhaphy – a personal experience with 6,321 cases. *American Journal of Surgery* 1987; **153**: 553–559.

562 Lichtenstein IL, Shore JM. Simplified repair of femoral and recurrent inguinal hernias by a 'plug' technique. *American Journal of Surgery* 1974; **128**: 439–444.

563 Lichtenstein IL, Shore JM. Exploding the myths of hernia repair. *American Journal of Surgery* 1976; **132**: 307–315.

564 Lichtenstein IL, Shulman AG, Amid PK, Montilier MM. The tension-free hernioplasty. *American Journal of Surgery* 1989; **157**: 188–193.

565 Lickley HLA, Trusler GH. Femoral hernia in children. *Journal of Pediatric Surgery* 1966; **1**: 338.

566 Liem MS, Van Steensel CJ, Boelhouwer RU *et al.* The learning curve for totally extraperitoneal laparoscopic inguinal hernia repair. *American Journal of Surgery* 1996; **171**: 281–285.

567 Liem MSL, Van der Graaf Y, Van Steensel CJ *et al.* Comparison of conventional anterior surgery and laparoscopic surgery for inguinal hernia repair. *New England Journal of Medicine* 1997; **336**: 1541–1547.

568 Lifschutz H, Juler GL. The inguinal darn. *Archives of Surgery* 1986; **121**: 717–719.

569 Lillemoe, KD, Yeo CJ, Talamini MA, Wang BH, Pitt HA, Gadacz TR. Selective cholangiography: current role in laparoscopic cholecystectomy. *Annals of Surgery* 1992; **215**: 669–76.

570 Lister, J. Note on the preparation of catgut for surgical purposes. *British Medical Journal* 1908; **1**: 125–126.

571 Littré, A. Observation sur une nouvelle espece de hernie. *Histoire de l'Academie des Sciences (1700), Paris mem.*, 300–310.

572 Lobe TE, Schropp KP. Inguinal hernias in pediatrics: initial experience with laparoscopic inguinal exploration of the asymptomatic contralateral side. *Journal of Laparo-endoscopic Surgery* 1992; **2**: 135–141.

573 Lockwood CB The radical cure of femoral and inguinal hernia. *Lancet* 1893; **2**: 1297–1302.

574 Lockwood CB. *The Radical Cure of Hernia, Hydrocele and Varicocele*. Edinburgh and London: Young, 1898.

575 Loder R. A local anaesthetic solution with longer action. *Lancet* 1960; **2**: 346–347.

576 Loh A, Rajkumar JS, South LM. Anatomical repair of large incisional hernias. *Annals of the Royal College of Surgeons of England* 1992; **74**: 100–105.

577 Londono-Schimmer EE, Leong APK, Phillips RKS. Life Table analysis of complications following colostomy. *Diseases of the Colon and Rectum* 1994; **37**: 916–920.

578 Losanoff J, Kjossev KT. Sciatic Hernia. *Acta Chirurgica Belgica* 1995; **95**: 269–270.

579 Lotheissen G. Zur Radikaloperation den Schenkelhernien. *Centralblatt fur Chirurgie* 1898; **21**: 548–549.

580 Lubbers EJC, Devlin HB. The complications of a permanent ileostomy. Poster: 8th World Congress of Collegium Internationale Chirurgiae Digestivae, Amsterdam, 11–14 September, 1984.

581 Lucus-Championniere J. *Chirurgie operatoire: Cure radicale des hernies; avec une etude statistique de deux cents soixante-quinze operations et cinquante figures intercalees dans le texte*. Paris: Rueff, 1892.

582 Ludbrook J, Spears GFS. The risk of developing appendicitis. *British Journal of Surgery* 1965; **52**: 856–858.

583 Lynch TH, Waymont B, Beacock CJ, Wallace DMA. Paravesical suture granuloma: a problem following herniorrhaphy. *Journal of Urology* 1992; **147**: 460–462.

584 Lynn HB, Johnson WW. Inguinal herniorrhaphy in children: a critical analysis of 1,000 cases. *Archives of Surgery* 1961; **83**: 573.

585 Lytle W.J. Internal inguinal ring. *British Journal of Surgery* 1945; **32**: 441–446.

586 Lytle W J Femoral hernia. *Annals of the Royal College of Surgeons of England* 1957; **21**: 244–262.

587 Lytle WJ. The deep inguinal ring, development, function and repair. *British Journal of Surgery* 1970; **57**: 531–536.

588 Mabogunje OA, Grundy DJ, Lawrie JH. Orchidectomy in a rural African population. *Transactions of the Royal Society of Tropical Medicine and Hygiene* 1980; **74**: 749–751.

589 MacArthur DC, Greive DC, Thompson JD, Greig JD, Nixon SJ. Herniography for groin pain of uncertain origin. *British Journal of Surgery* 1997; **84**: 684–685.

590 MacEwen W. On the radical cure of oblique inguinal hernia by internal abdominal peritoneal pad and the restoration of the valved form of the inguinal canal. *Annals of Surgery* 1886; **4**: 89–119.

591 MacFadyen BV, Arregui ME, Corbitt JD. Complications of laparoscopic herniorrhaphy. *Surgical Endoscopy* 1993; **7**: 155–8.

592 Mack NK. The incidence of umbilical hernia in Africans. *East African Medical Journal* 1945; **22**: 369.

593 Maclennan A. The radical cure of inguinal hernia in children. *British Journal of Surgery* 1921–22; **9**: 445–449.

594 Macleod C. The treatment of indirect inguinal hernia: a critical review of a small personal series. *Lancet* 1955; **2**: 106–110.

595 Madden JL, Hakim S, Agorogiannis AB. The anatomy and repair of inguinal hernias. *Surgical Clinics of North America* 1971; 1269–1292.

596 Maddern GJ, Rudkin G, Bessell JR, Devitt P, Ponte L. A comparison of laparoscopic and open hernia repair as a day surgical procedure. *Surgical Endoscopy* 1994; **8**: 1404–1408.

597 Magnus R. Late bowel obstruction due to kinking of the damaged loop following reduction of a strangulated hernia. *British Journal of Surgery* 1965; **52**: 121–122.

598 Maguire J, Young D. Repair of epigastric incisional hernia. *British Journal of Surgery* 1976; **63**: 125–127.

599 Maingot R. The floss silk lattice posterior repair for direct inguinal hernia. *British Medical Journal* 1941; **1**: 777–778.

600 Maingot R. A further report on the 'keel' operation for large diffuse incisional hernias. *The Medical Press* 1958; **240**: 989–993.

601 Maingot R. Operations for sliding herniae and large herniae. *British Journal of Clinical Practice* 1961; **15**: 993.

602 Maingot R. *Abdominal Operations*, 4th ed. New York: Appleton-Century-Crofts, 1961; p. 939.

603 Maingot R. The choice of operation for femoral hernia with special reference to McVay's technique. *British Journal of Clinical Practice* 1968; **22**: 323–329.

604 Mair GB. Preliminary report on the use of whole skin grafts as a substitute for fascial sutures in the treatment of herniae. *British Journal of Surgery* 1945; **32**: 381–385.

605 Mair GB. Analysis of a series of 454 inguinal hernias with special references to morbidity and recurrence after the whole skin graft method. *British Journal of Surgery* 1946; **34**: 42.

606 Malycha P, Lovell G. Inguinal surgery in athletes with chronic groin pain: The 'sportsman's hernia'. *Australian and New Zealand Journal of Surgery* 1992; **62**: 123–125.

607 Manninen MJ, Lavonius M, Perhoniemi VJ. Results of incisional hernia repair. A retrospective study of 172 unselected hernioplasties. *European Journal of Surgery* 1991; **157**: 29–31.

608 Marcy HO. A new use of carbolized catgut ligatures. *Boston Medical Surgical Journal* 1871; **85**: 315–316.

609 Marcy HO. The cure of hernia. *Journal of the American Medical Association* 1887; **8**: 589–592.

610 Marcy HO. Note on mortality after operation for large incarcerated hernia. *Annals of Surgery* 1900; **31**: 65–74.

611 Margoles JS, Braun RA. Pre-peritoneal versus classical hernioplasty. *American Journal of Surgery* 1971; **121**: 641–643.

612 Margotta R. *An illustrated history of medicine*. Ed. L. Lewis. English translation. Middlesex: Hamlyn, 1968.

613 Marks CG, Ritchie J. The complications of synchronous combined excision for adenocarcinoma of the rectum at St Mark's Hospital. *British Journal of Surgery* 1975; **62**: 901–905.

614 Marsden AJ. Inguinal hernia: a three year review of one thousand cases. *British Journal of Surgery* 1958; **46**: 234–243.

615 Marsden AJ. Inguinal hernia: a three year review of two thousand cases. *British Journal of Surgery* 1962; **49**: 384–394.

616 Marsden AJ. The results of inguinal hernia repairs: a problem of assessment. *Lancet* 1959; **i**: 461–462.

617 Marshall FF, Leadbetter WF, Dretler SP. Ileal conduit parastomal hernias. *Journal of Urology* 1975; **113**: 40–42.

618 Martin MC, Welch TP. Obturator hernia. *British Journal of Surgery* 1974; **61**: 547–548.

619 Martin RE, Max CC. Primary inguinal hernia repair with prosthetic mesh. *Hospimedica* 1984; **1**.

620 Mason ML, Allen HS. The rate of healing of tendons: an experimental study of tensile strength. *Annals of Surgery* 1941; **113**: 424.

621 Matapurkar BG, Gupta AK, Agarwal AK. A new technique of 'Marlex-peritoneal sandwich' in the repair of large incisional hernias. *World Journal of Surgery* 1991; **15**: 768–770.

622 Matsuda T, Horii Y, Yoshida O. Unilateral obstruction of the vas deferens caused by childhood inguinal herniorrhaphy in male infertility patients. *Fertility and Sterility* 1992; **58**: 609–613.

623 Mattson H. Use of rectus sheath and superior pubic ligament in direct and recurrent inguinal hernia. *Surgery* 1946; **19**: 498–503.

624 Maydl C. Ueber retrograde Incarceration der Tuba und des Processus Vermiformis in Leisten und Schenkelhernien. *Wiener Klinische Rundschau* 1895; **9**: 17–18 and 33–35.

625 Mayer AD, Ausobsky JR, Evans M, Pollock AV. Compression suture of the aboominal wall: a controlled trial in 302 major laparotomies. *British Journal of Surgery* 1981; **68**: 632–634.

626 Mayo WJ. An operation for the radical cure of umbilical hernia. *Annals of Surgery* 1901; **31**: 276–280.

627 Mayo WJ. Further experience with the vertical overlapping operation for the radical cure of umbilical hernia. *Journal of the American Medical Association* 1903; **41**: 225–228.

628 McArthur LL. Autoplastic suture in hernia and other diastases. *Journal of the American Medical Association* 1901; **37**: 1162–1165.

629 McCarthy MC, Lemmon GW. Traumatic lumbar hernia: a seat belt injury. *Journal of Trauma,*

Injury, Infection and Critical Care 1996; **40**: 121–122.

630 McCarthy MP. Obturator hernia of the urinary bladder. *Urology* 1976; **7**: 312–314.

631 McCleane G, Mackle E, Stirling I. The addition of triamcinalone acetonide to bupivacaine has no effect on the quality of analgesia produced by ilioinguinal nerve block. *Anaesthesia* 1994; **49**: 819–820.

632 McDowell E. Quoted in Scharchner, A. *Ephraim McDowell: Father of Ovariotomy and Father of Abdominal Surgery*. Philadelphia: Lippincott, 1921.

633 McEntee GP, O'Carroll A, Mooney B, Egan TJ, Delaney PV. Timing of strangulation in adult hernias. *British Journal of Surgery* 1989; **76**: 725–726.

634 McEvedy PG. Femoral hernia. *Annals of the Royal College of Surgeons of England* 1950; **7**: 484–496.

635 McGavin L. The double filigree operation for the radical cure of inguinal hernia. *British Medical Journal* 1909; **2**: 357–363.

636 McKernan JB, Laws HL. Laparoscopic repair of inguinal hemias using a totally extraperitoneal prosthetic approach. *Surgical Endoscopy* 1993; **7**: 26–28.

637 McLean AB. Spontaneous rupture of an umbilical hernia in an infant. *British Journal of Surgery* 1950; **37**: 239.

638 McNealy RW, Glassman JA. Experience with Vitallium plates in the repair of hernias. *Surgery* 1950; **27**: 753.

639 McPherson K, Coulter A, Stratton I. Increasing use of private practice by patients in Oxford requiring common elective surgical operations. *British Medical Journal* 1985; **291**: 797–799.

640 McVay CB. The anatomy of the relaxing incision in inguinal hernioplasty. *Quarterly Bulletin of North West University Medical School* 1962; **36**: 245–252.

641 McVay CB. The normal and pathologic anatomy of the transversus abdominis muscle in inguinal and femoral hernia. *Surgical Clinics of North America* 1971; **51**: 1251–1261.

642 McVay CB. The anatomic basis for inguinal and femoral hernioplasty. *Surgery, Gynecology and Obstetrics* 1974; **139**: 931–945.

643 McVay CB, Anson BJ. Inguinal and femoral hernioplasty. *Surgery, Gynecology and Obstetrics* 1949; **88**: 473–485.

644 McVay CB, Chapp JD. Inguinal and femoral hernioplasty. *Annals of Surgery* 1958; **148**: 499–512.

645 Meckel JF. Ueber die divertikel am Darmkanal. *Archiv fur die Physiologie* 1809; **9**: 421.

646 Melick DW. Nylon suture. *Annals of Surgery* 1942; **115**: 475–476.

647 Melone JH, Schwartz MZ, Tyson KRT, Marr CC, Greenholz SK, Taub JE, Hough VJ. Outpatient inguinal herniorrhaphy in Premature Infants: is it safe? *Journal of Pediatric Surgery* 1992; **27**: 203–208.

648 Menardi G, Saur H. Hodengangran als Komplikation der Inkarzeration der Sauglinshernie. *Z. Kinderchir.* 1975; **16**: 421–425.

649 Merrett ND, Waterworth MW, Green MF. Repair of giant inguinoscrotal inguinal hernia using Marlex mesh and scrotal skin flaps. *Australian and New Zealand Journal of Surgery* 1994; **64**: 380–383.

650 Mikkelsen WP, Berne CJ. Femoral hernioplasty: suprapubic extraperitoneal (Cheatle–Henry) approach. *Surgery* 1954; **35**: 743–748.

651 Milamed DR, Hedley-White J. Contributions of the surgical sciences to a reduction of the mortality rate in the United States for the period 1968 to 1988. *Annals of Surgery* 1994; **219**: 94–102.

652 Millat B, Fingerhut A, Gignoux M, Hay JM, The French Associations for Surgical Research. Factors associated with early discharge after inguinal hernia repair in 500 consecutive unselected patients. *British Journal of Surgery* 1993; **80**: 1158–1160.

653 Miller AR, Van Heerden JA, Naessens JM, O'Brien PC. Simultaneous bilateral inguinal hernia repair: a case against conventional wisdom. *Annals of Surgery* 1991; **213**: 272–276.

654 Milligan ETC. The inguinal route for radical cure of obturator hernia. *British Medical Journal* 1919; **2**: 134–135.

655 Millikan, KW, Deziel DJ. The management of hernia: considerations in cost-effectiveness. *Surgical Clinics of North America* 1996; **76**: 105–116.

656 Mitchell-Heggs F. Tantulum gauze: a 10 year survey. *British Journal of Surgery* 1963; **50**: 907–923.

657 Molloy RG, Moran KT, Waldron RP, Brady MP, Kirwan WO. Massive incisional hernia: abdominal wall replacement with Marlex mesh. *British Journal of Surgery* 1991; **78**: 242–244.

658 Moloney GE, Gill WG, Barclay RC. Operations for hernia – technique of nylon darn. *Lancet* 1948; **2**: 45–48.

659 Moloney GE. Treatment of inguinal hernia. *Lancet* 1960; **1**: 333.

660 Monasch S. *Breuken in het Gebied Van de Lies*. Rotterdam: N.V. Universitaire, 1964.

661 Montagu AMF. A case of familial inheritance of oblique inguinal hernia. *Journal of Heredity* 1942; **33**: 355–356.

662 Moore CA. Hypertrophic fibrosis of the gut causing chronic obstruction: a sequel to a strangulated hernia. *British Journal of Surgery* 1913; **1**: 361–365.

663 Moore CR, Oslund R. Experiments on sheep testis, cryptochidism, vasectomy and scrotal insulation. *American Journal of Physiology* 1924; **67**: 595–607.

664 Moreno IG. Chronic eventuation and large hernias. *Surgery* 1947; **22**: 945–953.

665 Morgan M, Paul E, Devlin HB. Lengths of stay for three common surgical procedures: variations between districts. *British Journal of Surgery* 1987; **74**: 884–889.

666 Morris D, Ward AWM, Handyside AJ. Early discharge after hernia repair. *Lancet* 1968; **1**: 681–685.

667 Morris GE, Jarrett PEM. Recurrence rates following local anaesthetic day case inguinal hernia repair by junior surgeons in a DGH. *Annals of the Royal College of Surgeons of England* 1987; **69**: 97–99.

668 Morris JM. The syndrome of testicular feminization in male pseudohermaphrodites. *American Journal of Obstetrics and Gynecology* 1953; **65**: 1192–1211.

669 Morris T, Tracey J. Ligocaine: its effects on wound healing. *British Journal of Surgery* 1977; **64**: 902–903.

670 Morrison AS. Cryptorchidism, hernia and cancer of the testis. *Journal of the National Cancer Institute* 1976; **56**: 731–733.

671 Morris-Stiff G, Coles G, Moore R, Jurewicz, Lord R. Abdominal wall hernia in autosomal dominant polycystic kidney disease. *British Journal of Surgery* 1997; **84**: 615–617.

672 Morton NS, Raine PAM. *Paediatric Day Case Surgery*. Oxford: Oxford University Press, 1995.

673 Moschowitz AV. Femoral hernia: a new operation for radical cure. *New York Journal of Medicine* 1907; 396–400.

674 Moschowitz AV. The rational treatment of sliding hernia. *American Journal of Surgery* 1966; **112**: 52.

675 Moss CM, Levine R, Messenger N, Dardik I. Sliding colonic Maydl's hernia: report of a case. *Diseases of the Colon and Rectum* 1976; **19**: 636–638.

676 Moure P, Martin R. Le role du ligament du foie dans les hernies epigastrique et ombilicales douloureuses. *Bulletin et Memoires de la Societe Nationale de Chirurgie* 59: 1011–1017.

677 Moynihan BGA. *Retroperitoneal Hernia*. London: Baillière Tindall, 1899 (revised 1906, London and New York: Wm. Wood).

678 Moynihan BGA. The ritual of a surgical operation. *British Journal of Surgery* 1920; **8**: 27–35.

679 Mozingo DW, Walters MJ, Otchy DP, Rosenthal D. Properitoneal synthetic mesh repair of recurrent inguinal hernias. *Surgery, Gynecology and Obstetrics* 1992; **174**: 33–35.

680 Mudge M, Hughes LE. Incisional hernia and post-thrombotic syndrome – an observed association. *Annals of the Royal College of Surgeons of England* 1984; **66**: 351–352.

681 Mudge M, Hughes LE. Incisional hernia: a ten year prospective study of incidence and attitudes. *British Journal of Surgery* 1985; **72**: 70–71.

682 Mudge M, Harding KG, Hughes LE Incisional hernia. *British Journal of Surgery* 1986; **73**: 82.

683 Murdoch RWG. Testicular strangulation from incarcerated inguinal hernia in infants. *Journal of the Royal College of Surgeons of Edinburgh* 1979; **24**: 97–101.

684 Murphy JL, Freeman JB, Dionne PG. Comparison of Marlex and Gore-Tex to repair abdominal wall defects in rats. *Canadian Journal of Surgery* 1989; **32**: 244–247.

685 Musgrove JE, McReady FJ. The Henry approach to femoral hernia. *Surgery* 1949; **26**: 608–611.

686 Myers B, Rightor M, Donovan W. Inguinal hernia repair: an experimental model in the rat to evaluate technical factors. *Archives of Surgery* 1981; **116**: 463–465.

687 Myers RN, Shearburn EW. The problem of recurrent inguinal hernia. *Surgical Clinics of North America* 1973; **53**: 555–558.

688 Mynors JM. A large lumbar hernia. *British Journal of Surgery* 1955; **42**: 554–555.

689 Nagahama T, Nakashima A, Ashikawa T, Sugano N, Kawamura T, Ootawa S, Sato Y, Endo M. Obturator hernia diagnosed by herniography. In *Inguinal Hernia: Advances or Controversies?* Eds ME Arregui, RF Nagan. Oxford: Radcliffe Medical Press, 1994; 333–341.

690 Narath A Ueber eine Eigenartige Form von Hernia Cruralis (prevascularis) in Anschlusse an die unblutige Behandlung angeborener Huftgelenskverrenkung. *Archiv fur Klinische Chirurgie* 1899; **59**: 396–424.

691 National Centre For Health Statistics. *Health Interview responses compared with medical records. Health Statistics from the US. National Health Survey Series D*. Washington DC: US Dept of Health, Education and Welfare, 1961.

692 *National Confidential Enquiry into Perioperative Deaths*. London, 1995.

693 Nayak RN. Malignant mucocele of the appendix in a femoral hernia. *Post-Graduate Medical Journal* 1974; **50**: 24, 249.

694 Naylor J. Combination of Spigelian and Richter's hernias: a case report. *The American Surgeon* 1978; **44**: 750–752.

695 Neuhauser D. Elective inguinal herniorrhaphy versus truss in the elderly. In *Costs, Risks and Benefits of Surgery*. Eds JP Bunker, BA Barnes, F Mosteller. New York: Oxford University Press, 1977; pp. 223–229.

696 Neutra RR. See Neuhauser (1977) (ref. 695).

697 Ng Lung Kit HK, Collins REC. Leiomyoma of the broad ligament in an obturator hernia presenting as a lump in the groin. *Journal of the Royal Society of Medicine* 1986; 79: 174–175.

698 Nichol JH. The surgery of infancy. *British Medical Journal* 1909; 2: 753–754.

699 Nicholl JP, Beeby NR, Williams BT. Comparison of the activity of short stay independent hospitals in England and Wales, 1981 and 1986. *British Medical Journal* 1989; 298: 239–242.

700 Nicholls JC. Necessity into choice: an appraisal of inguinal herniorrhaphy under local anaesthesia. *Annals of the Royal College of Surgeons of England* 1977; 59: 124–127.

701 Nicholson S, Keane TE, Devlin HB. Femoral hernia: an avoidable sense of surgical mortality. *British Journal of Surgery* 1990; 77: 307–308.

702 Nielsen DF, Bulow S. The incidence of male hermaphroditism in girls with inguinal hernia. *Surgery, Gynecology and Obstetrics* 1976; 142: 875–876.

703 Nilsson F, Anderberg B, Bragmark M, Eriksson T, Fordell R, Happaniemi S, Heuman R, Kald A, Stubberod A, Svensson P. Hernia surgery in a defined population: improvements possible in outcome and cost-effectiveness. *Ambulatory Surgery* 1993; 1: 150–153.

704 Normington EY, Franklin DP, Brotman SI. Constriction of the femoral vein after McVay inguinal hernia repair. *Surgery* 1992; 111: 343–347.

705 Nussbaum A. Ein einfaches hifsmittet beis der reposition der sanglinge. *Munchen Medizinische Wochenschrift* 1913; 60: 1434.

706 Nyhus LM, Donohue PE. Groin hernia repair: past, present and future. *Problems in General Surgery* 1995; 12: 7–11.

707 Nyhus LM, Condon RE, Harkins HN. Clinical experiences with pre-peritoneal hernial repair for all types of hernia of the groin. *American Journal of Surgery* 1960; 100: 234–244.

708 Nyhus LM, Harkins HN. *Hernia.* London: Pitman Medical/Philadelphia; Lippincott, 1965. Also *ibid.*, 2nd ed (Ed. RE Condon) Philadelphia: Lippincott, 1978.

709 Nyhus LM, Pollak R, Bombeck T, Donahue PE. The preperitoneal approach and prosthetic buttress repair for recurrent hernia: the evolution of a technique. *Annals of Surgery* 1988; 208: 733–737.

710 O'Donoghue PD. Strangulation of an ulcerated incisional hernia. *British Journal of Surgery* 1955; 43: 329–330.

711 Obney N. Hydroceles of the testicle complicating inguinal hernias. *Journal of the Canadian Medical Association* 1956; 75: 733–736.

712 Obney N. An analysis of 192 consecutive cases of incisional hernia. *Journal of the Canadian Medical Association* 1957; 77: 463–469.

713 Ogilvie H. *Hernia.* London: Edward Arnold, 1959.

714 Onukak EE, Grundy DJ, Lawrie JH. Hernia In Northern Nigeria. *Journal of the Royal College of Surgeons of Edinburgh* 1983; 28: 147–150.

715 Orchard C. Comparing healthcare outcomes. *British Medical Journal* 1994; 308: 1496–1499.

716 Orr KB. Perforated appendix in an inguinal hernial sac: Amyand's hernia. *Medical Journal of Australia* 1993; 159: 762–763.

717 Ortiz H, Sara MJ, Armedariz M, de Miguel M, Marti J, Chocarro C. Does the frequency of para-colostomy hernias depend on the position of the colostomy in the abdominal wall? *International Journal of Colorectal Disease* 1994; 9: 65–67.

718 Page CM, Edwards H, Lloyd Williamson JCF, Parker GE, Badenoch AW, Wright AD, Heritage K. Discussion on hernia. *Proceedings of the Royal Society of Medicine* 1942; 36: 185–189.

719 Pailler JL, Baranger B, Darrieu H, Schill H, Neveux Y. Clinical analysis of expanded PTFE in the teatment of recurrent and complex groin hernias. *Postgraduate Medical Journal* 1992; 4: 168–170.

720 Palmer BV. Incarcerated inguinal hernia in children. *Annals of the Royal College of Surgeons of England* 1978; 60: 121–124.

721 Palumbo LT, Sharp WS. Primary inguinal hernioplasty in the adult. *Surgical Clinics of North America* 1971; 51: 1293–1308.

722 Palumbo LT, Sharpe WS, Shirley WG, Benetti, AF. Primary direct inguinal hernioplasty: sixteen years study of 686 operations. *American Journal of Surgery* 1964; 108: 815–819.

723 Panos RG, Beck DE, Maresh JF, Harford FJ. Preliminary results of a prospective randomized study of Cooper's ligament versus Shouldice herniorrhaphy technique. *Surgery, Gynecology and Obstetrics* 1992; 175: 315–319.

724 Paterson-Brown S, Dudley HAF. Knotting in continuous mass closure of the abdomen. *British Journal of Surgery* 1986; 73: 676–680.

725 Paul A, Troidl H, Williams JI, Rixen D, Langen R and the Cologne Hernia Study Group. Randomized trial of modified Bassini versus Shouldice inguinal hernia repair. *British Journal of Surgery* 1994; 81: 1531–1534.

726 Payne JH, Grininger LM, lzawa MT, Podoll EF, Lindahl PJ, Balfour J. Laparoscopic or open inguinal herniorrhaphy? A randomised prospective trial. *Archives of Surgery* 1994; 129: 973–981.

727 Peacock EE. Here we are: behind again! *American Journal of Surgery*

728 Peacock EE, Madden JW. Studies on the biology and treatment of recurrent inguinal hernia: 11. Morphological changes. *Annals of Surgery* 1974; 179: 567–571.

729 Pearl RK, Prasad ML, Orsay CP, Abcarian H, Tan AB, Melzl MT. Early local complications from

intestinal stomas. *Archives of Surgery* 1985; **120:** 1145.

730   Pearl RK, Prasad ML, Orsay CP, Abcarian H, Tan AB. A survey of technical considerations in the construction of intestinal stomas. *Annals of Surgery* 1988; **51:** 462–465.

731   Pearse HE. Strangulated hernia reduced en masse. *Surgery, Gynecology and Obstetrics* 1931; **53:** 822–828.

732   Pedersen VM, Jensen BS, Hansen B. Skin closure in abdominal incisions: continuous nylon suture versus Steristrip tape suture. *Acta Chirurgica Scandinavica* 1981; **147:** 619–622.

733   Peevy KJ, Speed FA, Hoff CJ. Epidemiology of inguinal hernia in pre-term neonates. *Paediatrics* 1986; **77:** 246–247.

734   Pelosa OA, Wilkinson LH. The chain stitch knot. *Surgery, Gynecology and Obstetrics* 1974; **139:** 599–600.

735   Pemberton J, De J, Curry FS. The symptomatology of epigastric hernia: analysis of 296 cases. *Minnesota Medicine* 1936; **19:** 109–112.

736   Pender BWT. Recurrent obstruction of an obturator hernia. *British Medical Journal* 1950; **2:** 1038.

737   Percival WL. Ureter within a sliding inguinal hernia. *Canadian Journal of Surgery* 1983; **26:** 283–286.

738   Pergament E, Himler A, Shah P. Testicular feminisation and inguinal hernia. *Lancet* 1973; **2:** 740–741.

739   Perlman JA, Hoover HC, Safer PK. Femoral hernia with strangulated Meckel's diverticulum (Littré's hernia). *American Journal of Surgery* 1980; **139:** 286–289.

740   Pescovitz MO. Umbilical hernia repair in patients with cirrhosis. No evidence for increased evidence of variceal bleeding. *Annals of Surgery* 1984; 199–325.

741   Petros JG, Rimm EB, Robillard RJ, Argy O. Factors influencing postoperative urinary retention in patients undergoing elective inguinal herniorrhaphy. *American Journal of Surgery* 1991; **161:** 421–423.

742   Philip PJ. Afferent limb internal strangulation in obstructed inguinal hernia. *British Journal of Surgery* 1967; **54:** 96–99.

743   Phillips EH, Arregui M, Carroll BJ *et al.* Incidence of complications following laparoscopic hernioplasty. *Surgical Endoscopy* 1995; **9:** 16–21.

744   Phillips P, Pringle W, Evans C, Keighley M Analysis of hospital based stomatherapy service. *Annals of the Royal College of Surgeons of England* 1985; **67:** 37–40.

745   Pickford IR, Brennan SS, Evans M, Pollock AV. Two methods of skin closure in abdominal operations: a controlled clinical trial. *British Journal of Surgery* 1983; **70:** 226–228.

746   Piper JV. A comparison between whole thickness skin graft and Bassini methods of repair of inguinal hernia. *British Journal of Surgery* 1969; **56:** 345–348.

747   Pitkin RM. Abdominal hysterectomy in obese women. *Surgery, Gynecology and Obstetrics* 1976; **142:** 532–536.

748   Plaus WJ. Laparoscopic trocar site hernias. *Journal of Laparoendoscopic Surgery* 1993; **3:** 393–397.

749   Pless TK, Pless JE. Giant ventral hernias and their repair: a 10 year follow up study. *Scandinavian Journal of Plastic Reconstruction and Hand Surgery* 1993; **27:** 311–315.

750   Pollack R, Nyhus LM. Complications of groin hernia repair. *Surgical Clinics of North America* 1983; **63:** 1363–1371.

751   Pollack HM, Popky GL, Blumberg ML. Hernias of the ureter: an anatomic roentgenographic study. *Radiology* 1975; **117:** 275.

752   Ponka JL. *Hernias of the Abdominal Wall.* Philadelphia: WB Saunders, 1980.

753   Ponka JL, Brush BE. Problems of femoral hernia. *Archives of Surgery* 1971; **102:** 417–423.

754   Ponka JL, Brush BE. Experiences with the repair of groin hernia in 200 patients aged 70 or older. *Journal of the American Geriatrics Society* 1974; **22:** 18–24.

755   Ponka JL, Sapala JA. Bupivacaine as a local anaesthetic for hernia repair. *Henry Ford Hospital Medical Journal* 1976; **24:** 31.

756   Pories WJ. Personal communication, 1983.

757   Pott P. *Treatise on Ruptures.* London: Hitch and Hawes, 1757.

758   Powell J. All on our own: away from the district hospital. *Journal of One-Day Surgery* 1995; **2:** 11.

759   Powell RW. Intra-operative diagnostic pneumoperitoneum in pediatric patients with unilateral inguinal hernias: the Goldstein test. *Journal of Pediatric Surgery* 1985; 20: 418.

760   Power DA, Edward N, Catto GDR, Muirhead N, Macleod A, Engeset J. Richter's hernia: an unrecognised complication of chronic ambulatory peritoneal dyalysis. *British Medical Journal* 1981; **283:** 528.

761   Powers JH. Early ambulation: its influence on postoperative complications and return to work following hernioplasty in a rural population. *Annals of the New York Academy of Sciences* 1954; 524–535.

762   Prian GW, Sawyer RB, Sawyer KC. Repair of peristomal colostomy hernias. *American Journal of Surgery* 1975; **130:** 694–696.

763   Puri P, Guiney EJ, O'Donnell B. Inguinal hernia in infants: the fate of the testis following incarceration. *Journal of Pediatric Surgery* 1984; **19:** 44–46.

764 Pye JK, Wijewardane PA, Crumplin MKH. Skin discolouration following inguinal hernia repair. *British Journal of Surgery* 1987; **74**: 1171–1173.

765 Quill DS, Devlin HB, Plant JA, Denham KR, McNay RA, Morris D. Surgical operations rates: a twelve year experience in Stockton-on-Tees. *Annals of the Royal College of Surgeons of England* 1983; **65**: 248–253.

766 Quillinan RH. Repair of recurrent inguinal hernia. *American Journal of Surgery* 1969; **118**: 593.

767 Qvist G. Saddlebag hernia. *British Journal of Surgery* 1977; **64**: 442–444.

768 Radhakrishnan J. Umbilical Hernia. In *Hernia*, 4th ed. Eds LM Nyhus, RE Condon. Philadelphia: JB Lippincott, 1994.

769 Rains AJH. Contribution to the principles of the surgery of inguinal hernia. *British Journal of Surgery* 1951; **39**: 211.

770 Ralphs DNL, Cannon SR, Bolton JB. Skin closure of inguinal herniorrhaphy wounds in short stay patients. *British Journal of Surgery* 1982; **69**: 341–342.

771 Ramayya GR. Volvulus of an ileal conduit in an inguinal hernia. *British Journal of Surgery* 1984; **71**: 637.

772 Ravitch MM. Ventral hernia. *Surgical Clinics of North America* 1971; **51**: 1341–1346.

773 Ray IA, Doddi N, Regula D, Williams JA, Melveger A. Polydioxanone (PDS) a novel monofilament synthetic absorbable suture. *Surgery, Gynecology and Obstetrics* 1981; **153**: 497–507.

774 Read RC. Attenuation of the rectus sheath in inguinal herniation. *American Journal of Surgery* 1970; **120**: 610–614.

775 Read RC. Bilaterality and the prosthetic repair of large recurrent inguinal hernias. *American Journal of Surgery* 1979; **138**: 788–793.

776 Read RC. Marcy's priority in the development of inguinal herniorraphy. *Surgery* 1980; **88**: 682–685.

777 Read RC. Can relaxing rectus sheath incision predispose to recurrent direct inguinal hernia? *Archives of Surgery* 1981; **116**: 1493.

778 Read RC. The development of inguinal herniorrhaphy. *Surgical Clinics of North America* 1984; **64**: 185–196.

779 Read RC. The centenary of Bassini's contribution to inguinal herniorrhaphy. *American Journal of Surgery* 1987; **153**: 324–326.

780 Read RC. Cooper's Posterior lamina of transversalis fascia. *Surgery, Gynecology and Obstetrics* 1992; **174**: 426–434.

781 Read RC, White HJ. Inguinal herniation 1777–1977. *American Journal of Surgery* 1978; **136**: 651–654.

782 Reid I, Devlin HB. Testicular atrophy as a consequence of inguinal hernia repair. *British Journal of Surgery* 1994; **81**: 91–93.

783 Reinhard W. Surgical treatment of infantile hernia. *Archiv fur Klinische Chirurgie* 1939; **195**: 678–681.

784 Reinhoff WF Jr. The use of the rectus fascia for closure of the lower or critical angle of the wound in the repair of inguinal hernia. *Surgery* 1940; **8**: 326–339.

785 Richter A. *Abhandlung von den Bruchen*. Gottingen; I.C. Dietrich, 1785.

786 Rider MA, Baker DM, Locker A, Fawcett AN. Return to work after inguinal hernia repair. *British Journal of Surgery* 1993; **80**: 745–746.

787 Ries E. Some radical changes in the after treatment of celiotomy cases. *Journal of the American Medical Association* 1899; **33**: 454–459.

788 Rignault DP. Properitoneal prosthetic inguinal hernioplasty through a Pfannenstiel approach. *Surgery, Gynecology and Obstetrics* 1986; **163**: 465–468.

789 Robertson GSM, Hayes IG, Burton PR. How long do patients convalesce after inguinal hernioplasty? Current principles and practice. *Annals of the Royal College of Surgeons of England* 1993; **75**: 30–33.

790 Robin AP. Epigastric Hernia. In *Hernia*, 4th ed. Eds LM Nyhus, RE Condon. Philadelphia: Lippincott, 1995.

791 Rockwell E. Out-patient repair of inguinal hernia. *American Journal of Surgery* 1982; **143**: 559–560.

792 Rosai J. *Ackerman's Surgical Pathology*, 6th ed, vol. 2. St. Louis: Mosby, 1981.

793 Rosai J, Dehner LP. Nodular mesothelial hyperplasia in hernia sacs. A benign reactive condition simulating a neoplastic process. *Cancer* 1975; **35**: 165–175.

794 Rose E, Santull TV. Sliding appendiceal inguinal hernia. *Surgery, Gynecology and Obstetrics* 1978; **146**: 626–627.

795 Roslyn JJ, Stable BE, Rangeneath C. Cancer in inguinal and femoral hernias. *The American Surgeon* 1980; **46**: 358–362.

796 Ross APJ. Incidence of inguinal hernia recurrence: effect of time off work after repair. *Annals of the Royal College of Surgeons of England* 1975; **57**: 326–328.

797 Rowe MI, Copelson LW, Clatworthy HW. The patent processus vaginalis and the inguinal hernia. *Journal of Pediatric Surgery* 1969; **4**: 102–107.

798 Royal College of General Practitioners, OPCS. 1981–82. *Morbidity Statistics from General Practice. Third National Study*. London: HMSO, 1986.

799 Royal College of Surgeons of England. *Guidelines for Day Case Surgery*, 1985.

800 Royal College of Surgeons of England. *Guidelines for Day Case Surgery*, 1992.

801 Royal College of Surgeons of England. *Clinical Guidelines for the management of groin hernias in adults.* London, 1993.

802 Royal College of General Practitioners: Royal College of Surgeons of England. Clinical Guidelines for the Management of Groin Hernia in Adults. London: RCGP, 1997.

803 Rubin M, Schoetz DJ, Matthews JB. Para-stomal hernia: is the stoma relocation superior to fascial repair. *Archives of Surgery* 1994; **129**: 413–419.

804 Ruckley, C V Day Care and short stay surgery for hernia. *British Journal of Surgery* 1978; **65**: 1–4.

805 Ruckley CV, Cuthbertson C, Fenwick N, Prescott RJ, Garraway WM. Day care after operations for hernia or varicose veins: a controlled trial. *British Journal of Surgery* 1978; **65**: 456–459.

806 Ruge, 1908. Cited in Rauber's Lehrbuch der Anatomie des Menschen, Kopsch FR Abt 5; Nervensystem: 388, 1920.

807 Russell IT, Devlin HB, Fell M, Glass NJ, Newell DJ. Day case surgery for hernias and haemorrhoids. *Lancet* 1977; **1**: 844–847.

808 Russell H. The saccular theory of hernia and the radical operation. *Lancet* 1906; **3**: 1197–1203.

809 Rutkow I. A selective history of groin herniorrhaphy in the 20th century. *Surgical Clinics North America* 1993; **73**: 395–411.

810 Rutkow I. *Surgery, An Illustrated History.* St Louis: Mosby, 1993.

811 Rutkow IM, Robbins AW. Demographic, classificatory, and socio-economic aspects of hernia repair in the United States. *Surgical Clinics of North America* 1993; **73**: 413–426.

812 Rutkow IM, Robbins AW. Open mesh plug hernioplasty. *Problems in General Surgery* 1995; **12**: 121–127.

813 Rutledge RH. Cooper's ligament repair for adult groin hernias. *Surgery* 1980; **87**: 601–610.

814 Rutledge RH. Technique for all groin hernias in adults. *Surgery* 1988; **103**: 1–10.

815 Rutledge RH. Theodor Billroth: A century later. *Surgery* 1995; **118**: 36–43.

816 Rutten P, Ledecq M, Hoebeke Y, Roeland A, van den Oever R, Croes I. Hernie inguinal primaire: hernioplastie ambulatoire selon Lichtenstein: premiers resultats cliniques et implications economiques etude des 130 premiers cas operes. *Acta Chirurgica Belgica* 1992; **92**: 168–171.

817 Ryan EA. An analysis of 313 consecutive cases of indirect sliding inguinal hernias. *Surgery, Gynecology and Obstetrics* 1956; **102**: 45–58.

818 Ryan EA. Hernias related to pelvic fractures. *Surgery, Gynecology and Obstetrics* 1971; **133**: 440–446.

819 Ryan WJ. Hernia of the vermiform appendix. *Annals of Surgery* 1937; **105**: 135.

820 Rydell WB. Inguinal and femoral hernias. *Archives of Surgery* 1963; **87**: 493–499.

821 Saha SP, Rao N, Stephenson SE Jr. Complications of colostomy. *Diseases of the Colon and Rectum* 1973; **16**: 515–516.

822 Salcedo-Wasicek CM, Thirlby RC. Postoperative course after inguinal herniorrhaphy: a case-controlled comparison of patients receiving worker's compensation vs patients with commercial insurance. *Archives of Surgery* 1995; **130**: 29–32.

823 Salter RB. Innominate osteotomy in the treatment of dislocation and subluxation of the hip. *Journal of Bone and Joint Surgery* 1961; **43-B**: 518–539.

824 Sames CP. The use of the vas deferens in inguinal herniorrhaphy. *British Journal of Surgery* 1975; **62**: 495–496.

825 Sandblom P. The tensile strength of healing wounds. *Acta Chirurgica Scandinavica* 1944; suppl. 89–90: 1.

826 Santora TA, Roslyn JJ. Incisional hernia. *Surgical Clinics of North America* 1993; **73**: 557–570.

827 Savatguchi S, Matsunaga E, Honna T. A genetic study on indirect inguinal hernia. *Japanese Journal of Human Genetics* 1975; **20**: 187–195.

828 Scarpa A. Sull'ernia, memorie anatomico-chirurgiche. Pavia Galleazzi, 1819.

829 Schapp HM, Van De Pavoordt HDWM, Bast TJ. The preperitoneal approach in the repair of recurrent inguinal hernias. *Surgery, Gynecology and Obstetrics* 1992; **174**: 460–464.

830 Schilling JA. Advances in knowledge related to wounding, repair and healing: 1885–1984. *Annals of Surgery* 1985; **201**: 268–277.

831 Schofield TL. Polyvinyl alcohol sponge: an inert plastic for use as a prosthesis in the repair of large hernias. *British Journal of Surgery* 1955; **42**: 618–621.

832 Schultz L, Graber J, Pietraffita *et al.* Laser laparoscopic herniorraphy: A clinical trial. Preliminary results. *Journal of Laparoendoscopic Surgery* 1991; **1**: 41–45.

833 Schumpelick V, Ault G. The Aachen Classification of Inguinal Hernia. *Problems in General Surgery* 1995; **12**: 57–58.

834 Schumpelick V, Wantz GE, Eds. *Inguinal Hernia Repair.* Basel: Karger, 1995.

835 Schumpelick V, Treutner KH, Arit G. Inguinal hernia repair in adults. *Lancet* 1994; **344**: 375–379.

836 Schurgers ML, Boelaert JRO, Daneels RF, Robbens EJ, Vandelanotte MM. Genital oedema in patients treated by continuous ambulatory peritoneal dialysis: an unusual presentation of inguinal hernia. *British Medical Journal* 1983; **388**: 358–359.

837 Scorer CG, Farrington GH. *Congenital Deformities of the Testis and Epididymis.* London: Butterworths, 1971.

838 Scottish Health Service. *Scottish in-patient statistics 1974*. Edinburgh: Common Services Agency, Information Services Division, 1974.

839 Scotte M, Majerus B, Sibert L, Teniere P. Incarceration vesicale dans une hernie de spiegel. *Journal de Chirurgie (Paris)* 1991; **128**: 74–75.

840 Sculpher M. Phase II Medical Laser Technology Assessment. HERG Research Report No. 15, Brunel University 1993.

841 See WA, Cooper CS, Fisher RJ. Predictors of laparoscopic complications after formal training in laparoscopic surgery. *Journal of the American Medical Association* 1993; **270**: 289–2692.

842 Semmence A, Kynch J. Hernia repair and time off work in Oxford. *Journal of the Royal College of General Practitioners* 1980; **30**: 90–96.

843 Senapati, A. Spontaneous dehiscence of an incisional hernia. *British Journal of Surgery* 1982; **69**: 313.

844 Serpell JW, Jarrett PEM, Johnson CD. A prospective study of bilateral inguinal hernia repair. *Annals of the Royal College of Surgeons of England* 1990; **72**: 299–303.

845 Shaw A, Santulli TV. Management of sliding hernias of the urinary bladder in infants. *Surgery, Gynecology and Obstetrics* 1967; **124**: 1315–1316.

846 Shearburn EW, Myers RN. Shouldice repair for inguinal hernia. *Surgery* 1969; **66**: 450–459.

847 Sheehan V. Spigelian hernia. *Journal of the Irish Medical Association* 1951; **29**: 87–91.

848 Sheen A, Puri P. Inguinal hernia in the newborn: A 15 year review. *Pediatric Surgery International* 1988; **3**: 156–157.

849 Shepherd JA. Acute appendicitis. A historical survey. *Lancet* 1954; **ii**: 299–302.

850 Shouldice EE. Obesity and ventral hernia repair. *Modern Medicine of Canada* 1953; **August**: 89.

851 Shouldice EE. The treatment of hernia. *Ontario Medical Review* 1953; 1–14.

852 Shouldice EE, Glassow F, Black N. Sinus formation following infected herniorrhaphy incisions. *Journal of the Canadian Medical Association* 1961; **84**: 576–579.

853 Shrock P. The processus vaginalis and gubernaculum. Their raison d'etre redefined. *Surgical Clinics of North America* 1971; **51**: 1263–1268.

854 Shulman A, Amid P. Which Lichtenstein method? *Archives of Surgery* 1994; **129**: 561.

855 Shulman AG, Amid PK, Lichtenstein lL. The 'plug' repair of 1402 recurrent inguinal hernias: 20-year experience. *Archives of Surgery* 1990; **125**: 265–267.

856 Shulman AG, Amid PK, Lichtenstein IL. The safety of mesh repair for primary inguinal hernias: results of 3019 operations from five diverse surgical sources. *American Surgeon* 1992; **58**: 255–257.

857 Shulman AG, Amid PK, Lichtenstein IL. Patch or plug for groin hernia – which? *American Journal of Surgery* 1994; **167**: 331–336.

858 Shulman AG, Amid PK, Lichtenstein IL. Returning to work after herniorrhaphy. *British Medical Journal* 1994; **309**: 216–217.

859 Shuttleworth KED, Davies WH. Treatment of inguinal herniae. *Lancet* 1960; **1**: 126–127.

860 Simpson JG, Gunnlangsson GH, Dawson B, Lynn HB. Further experience with bilateral operations for inguinal hernia in infants and children. *Annals of Surgery* 1969; **169**: 450.

861 Simpson PI, Hughes DR, Long DH. Prolonged local analgesia for inguinal herniorrhaphy with bupivacaine and dextran. *Annals of the Royal College of Surgeons of England* 1982; **64**: 243–246.

862 Sinha SN, De Costa AE. Obturator hernia. *Australian and New Zealand Surgery* 1983; **53**: 349–351.

863 Sjodahl R, Anderberg B, Bolin T. Parastomal hernia in relation to the site of the abdominal wall stoma. *British Journal of Surgery* 1988; **75**: 339–341.

864 Skandalakis JE, Gray SW, Burns WB, Sangmalee U, Sorg JL. Internal and External Supra-vesical hernia. *American Surgeon* 1976; **42**: 142.

865 Skandalakis JE, Colborn GL and Skandalakis LJ. The embryology of the inguino-femoral area: an overview. *Hernia* 1997; **1**: 45–54.

866 Skandalakis LJ, Gadacz TR, Mansberger AR, Mitchell WE, Colborn GL, Skandalakis IE. *Modern Hernia Repair*. New York: Parthenon Publishing, 1996.

867 Skandalakis PN, Skandalakis LJ, Gray SW, Skandalakis JE. Supra-vesical hernia. In *Hernia*, 4th ed. Eds LM Nyhus, RE Condon. Philadelphia: Lippincott, 1995.

868 Skidmore FD. Umbilical hernia in child swimmers. *British Medical Journal* 1979; **2**: 494.

869 Smedberg SGG. Herniography. In *Hernia*, 4th ed. Eds LM Nyhus, RE Condon. Philadelphia: Lippincott, 1995.

870 Smedberg S, Broome A, Elmer O, Gullmo A. Herniography in the diagnosis of obscure groin pain *Acta Chirurgica Scandinavica* 1985; **151**: 663–667.

871 Smedberg SGG, Broome AEA, Gullmo A, Roos H. Herniography in athletes with groin pain. *American Journal of Surgery* 1985; **149**: 378–382.

872 Smith I. Irreducible inguinal herniae in children. *British Journal of Surgery* 1954; **42**: 271–274.

873 Smith MP, Sparkes RS. Familial inguinal hernia. *Surgery* 1965; **57**: 807–812.

874 Smith RS. The use of prosthetic materials in the repair of hernias. *Surgical Clinics of North America* 1971; **51**: 1387–1399.

875 Snyder WH. *Paediatric Surgery*, vol I. Chicago: Year Book, 1962; p. 573.

876 Somell A, Ljungdahl L, Spangen L. Thigh neuralgia as a symptom of obturator hernia. *Acta Chirurgica Scandinavica* 1976; **142:** 457–459.

877 Soper NJ, Brunt LM, Kerbl K. Laparoscopic general surgery. *New England Journal of Medicine* 1994; **330:** 409–419.

878 Spangen L. Spigelian hernia. *Acta Chirurgica Scandinavica Suplementum* 1976; **462:** 1–47.

879 Spangen L. Spigelian hernia. *Surgical Clinics of North America* 1984; **64:** 351–366.

880 Spangen L. Spigelian hernia. *World Journal of Surgery* 1989; **13:** 573–580.

881 Spangen L, Andersson R, Ohlsson L. Nonpalpable inguinal hernia in women. In *Hernia*, 3rd ed. Eds LM Nyhus, RE Condon, 1989.

882 Sparkman RJ. Bilateral exploration of inguinal hernias in juvenile patients. *Surgery* 1962; **51:** 393–402.

883 Sparnon AL, Kiely EM, Spitz L. Incarcerated inguinal hernia in infants. *British Medical Journal* 1986; **293:** 376–377.

884 Spaw AT, Reddick EJ, Olsen DO. Laparoscopic laser cholecystectomy: a comparison with mini-lap cholecystectomy. *Surgical Endoscopy* 1991; **1:** 2–7.

885 Spiegel A. *Opera Quae Extant Omnia*. Amsterdam: John Bloew, 1645.

886 Spittal MJ, Hunter SJ. A comparison of bupivacaine instillation and inguinal field block for control of pain after herniorrhaphy. *Annals of the Royal College of Surgeons of England* 1992; **74:** 85–88.

887 Stanton E, Mac D. Post-operative ventral hernia. *New York Journal of Medicine* 1916; **16:** 511–515.

888 Steele C. On operations for the radical cure of hernia. *British Medical Journal* 1874; **2:** 584.

889 Stephens FC, Dudley HAF. An out-patient organisation for out-patient surgery. *Lancet* 1961; **1:** 1042–1045.

890 Stephenson BM, Phillips RKS. Para-stomal hernia: local resiting and mesh repair. *British Journal of Surgery* 1995; **82:** 1395–1396.

891 Sternhill B, Schwartz S. Effect of hypaque on mouse peritoneum. *Radiology* 1960; **75:** 81–84.

892 Stirk DI. Strangulated inguino-femoral hernia with descent of the testis through the femoral canal. *British Journal of Surgery* 1955; **43:** 331–332.

893 Stock FE. Faecal fistula and bilateral strangulated hernia in an infant. *British Medical Journal* 1951; **1:** 171.

894 Stoker DL, Wellwood JM. Return to work after inguinal hernia surgery. *British Journal of Surgery* 1993; **80:** 1354–1355.

895 Stoker DL, Spiegelhalter DJ, Singh R, Wellwood JM. Laparoscopic versus open inguinal hernia repair: Randomised prospective trial. *Lancet* 1994; **343:** 1243–1245.

896 Stoppa R, Warlaumont CR, Verhaeghe PJ, Odimba BKFE, Henry X. Comment, pourquoi, quand utiliser les prostheses de tulle de Dacron pour traiter les hernies et les eventrations. *Chirurgie* 1982; **108:** 570–575.

897 Stoppa RE, Rives JL, Warlaumont CR, Palot JP, Verhaeghe PJ, Delattre JF. The use of Dacron in the repair of hernias of the groin. *Surgical Clinics of North America* 1984; **64:** 269–285.

898 Stoppa RF, Warlaumont CR. The preperitoneal approach and prosthetic repair of groin hernia. In *Hernia*, 3rd ed. Eds LM Nyhus, RE Condon. New York: Lippincott, 1989.

899 Stotter AT, Kapadia CR, Dudley HAF. Sutures in surgery. In *Recent Advances in Surgery*. Ed. RCG Russell. London: Churchill Livingstone, 1986.

900 Strange SL. Spontaneous rupture of an umbilical hernia in an infant. *Postgraduate Medical Journal* 1956; **32:** 39.

901 Stromayr. Practica Copiosa – Lindau 1559. Cited by Rutkow IM. *Surgery, An Illustrated History.* Mosby: St Louis, 1993

902 Stuckej AL, Lutjko GD, Tivarovskij VI. Hernias of the spigeli line. *Tsitologiia* 1973; **15:** 10–13.

903 Sturdy DE. Incarcerated inguinal hernia in infancy with testicular gangrene. *British Journal of Surgery* 1960; **48:** 210–211.

904 Szell K. Local anaesthesia and inginal hernia repair: a cautionary tale. *Annals of the Royal College of Surgeons of England* 1994; **76:** 139–140.

905 Tagart REB. The suturing of abdominal incisions. A comparison of monofilament nylon and catgut. *British Journal of Surgery* 1967; **54:** 952–957.

906 Tait L A discussion on treatment of hernia by median abdominal section. *British Medical Journal* 1891; **2:** 685–691.

907 Tam PKH, Lister J. Femoral hernia in children. *Archives of Surgery* 1984; **119:** 1161–1164.

908 Tanner NC. A slide operation for inguinal and femoral hernia. *British Journal of Surgery* 1942; **29:** 285–289.

909 Taube M, Porter RJ, Lord PH. A Combination Of Subcuticular Suture And Sterile Micropore Tape Compared With Conventional Interrupted Sutures For Skin Closure. *Annals of the Royal College of Surgeons of England* 1983; **65:** 164–166.

910 Taylor EW, Dewar EP. Early return to work after repair of a unilateral inguinal hernia. *British Journal of Surgery* 1983; **70:** 599–600.

911 Tchupetlowsky S, Losanoff J, Kjossev K. Bilateral obturator hernia: a new technique and a new prosthetic material for repair- case report and review of the literature. *Surgery* 1995; **117:** 109–112.

912 Teasdale D, McCrum A, Williams NB, Horton RE. A randomized controlled trial to compare local with general anaesthesia for short stay inguinal hernia repair. *Annals of the Royal College of Surgeons of England* 1982; **64**: 238–242.

913 The Southern Surgeon's Club. A prospective analysis of 1518 laparoscopic cholecystectomies. *New England Journal of Medicine* 1991; **324**: 1073–1078.

914 Thieme ET. Recurrent inguinal hernia. *Archives of Surgery* 1971; **103**: 238–242.

915 Thomas D. Strangulated femoral hernia. *Medical Journal of Australia* 1967; **1**: 258–260.

916 Thomas JM. Groin strain versus occult hernia: uncomfortable alternatives or incompatible rivals? *Lancet* 1995; **345**: 1552–1553.

917 Thomas WEG, Vowles KDL, Williamson RCN. Appendicitis in external herniae. *Annals of the Royal College of Surgeons of England* 1982; **64**: 121–122.

918 Thomeret G, Dubost C, Pillo, P. L'utilisation de la toile d'acier inoxydable dans la cure des eventerations et des hernies. *Academie de Chirurgie* 1960; **86**: 500–507.

919 Thompson W. Radical cure of inguinal hernia with a plastic insert. *Lancet* 1948; **2**: 182–183.

920 Thorndike A, Ferguson CF. Incarcerated inguinal hernia in infancy and childhood. *American Journal of Surgery* 1938; **39**: 429–437.

921 Throckmorton TC. Repair of obturator hernia with a tantalum gauze implant. *Surgery* 1950; **27**: 888–892.

922 Throckmorton TD. Tantalum gauze in the repair of hernias complicated by tissue deficiency. *Surgery* 1948; **23**: 32–46.

923 Tilson MD, Davis G. Deficiences of copper and a compound with iron exchange characteristics of pyridinoline in skin from patients with abdominal aortic aneurysms. *Surgery* 1983; **94**: 134–141.

924 Tingwald GR, Cooperman M. Inguinal and femoral hernia repair in geriatric patients. *Surgery, Gynecology and Obstetrics* 1982; **154**: 704–706.

925 Todd IP. *Intestinal Stomas*. London: Heinemann, 1978.

926 Ton JG. Tijdelijke prothesen bij het sluiten van geinfecteerde littekenbreuken. *Nederlands Tijdschrift voor Geneeskunde* 1967; **112**: 972.

927 Tong HWC, Kupczyk-Joeris D, Rotzscher VM, Schumpelick V. Chronic inguinal pain following Shouldice repair of primary inguinal hernias. *Contemporary Surgery* 1990; **37**: 24–30.

928 Tran VK, Putz T, Rohde H. A randomized controlled trial for inguinal hernia repair to compare the Shouldice and the Bassini–Kirschner opration. *International Surgery* 1992; **77**: 235–237.

929 Treves F. Richter's hernia or partial enterocele. *Medico-Chirurgical Transactions, London* 1887; **52**: 149–167.

930 Trimbos. Factors relating to the volume of surgical knots. *International Journal of Gynecology and Obstetrics* 1989; **30**: 355–359.

931 Troung SN, Pfingsten F, Dreuw B, Schumpelick V. Value of ultrasound in the diagnosis of undetermined findings in the abdominal wall and inguinal region. In *Inguinal Hernia*. Eds V Schumpelick, GE Wantz. Basel: Karger, 1995; pp. 29–41.

932 Tsutsui S, Kitamura M, Shirabe K, Yoshizawa S, Yoshida M. Radiographic diagnosis of obturator hernia. *British Journal of Surgery* 1994; **81**: 1371–1372.

933 Turnbull RB, Weakley FI. *Atlas of Intestinal Stomas*. St Louis: Mosby, 1967.

934 Turnock RR. Preperitoneal approach to irreducible inguinal hernia in infants. *British Journal of Surgery* 1994; **81**: 251.

935 Ulbak S, Ornsholt J. Para-inguinal hernia: an atypical spigelian variant. *Acta Chirurgica Scandinavica* 1983; **149**: 335–336.

936 Underhill BML. Strangulated femoral hernia in an infant boy aged five weeks. *British Journal of Surgery* 1954; **42**: 332–333.

937 Usher FC. Hernia repair with Marlex mesh. *Archives of Surgery* 1962; **84**: 73–76.

938 Usher FC. New technique for repairing incisional hernias with Marlex mesh. *American Journal of Surgery* 1979; **138**: 740–741.

939 Usher FC. The repair of incisional and inguinal hernias. *Surgery, Gynecology and Obstetrics* 1970; **131**: 525–530.

940 Usher FC. Further observations on the use of Marlex mesh. A new technique for the repair of inguinal hernias. *American Surgeon* 1959; **25**: 792–795.

941 Usher FC. Technique for repairing inguinal hernias with Marlex mesh. *American Journal of Surgery* 1982; **143**: 382–384.

942 Usher FC, Allen JE, Crosthwait RW, Cogan JE. Polypropylene monofilament. A new biologically inert suture for closing contaminated wounds. *Journal of the American Medical Association* 1962; **179**: 180.

943 Validire J, Imbaud P, Dutet D, Duron JJ. Large abdominal incisional hernias: repair by fascial approximation reinforced with a stainless steel mesh. *British Journal of Surgery* 1986; **73**: 8–10.

944 Van Den Berg JC, Strijk SP. Groin hernia: role of herniography. *Radiology* 1992; **184**: 191–194.,

945 Van Der Lei B, Bleichrodt RP, Simmermocher RKJ, Van Schilfgaarde R. Expanded polytetrafluoroethylene patch for the repair of large abdominal wall defects. *British Journal of Surgery* 1989; **76**: 803–805.

946 Van Mameren H, Go PMNYH. Anatomy and variations of the internal inguinal region. In *Inguinal Hernia Repair* Eds Schumpelick V, Wantz GE. Basel: Karger, 1995.

947 Van Meurs DPP. Strangulation of the ovary and fallopian tube in an obturator hernia. *British Journal of Surgery* 1945; **32**: 539–540.

948 Van Winkle W. The tensile strength of wounds and factors that influence it. *Surgery, Gynecology and Obstetrics* 1969; **129**: 819–842.

949 Van Winkle WJR, Hastings JC. Considerations in the choice of suture materials for various tissues. *Surgery, Gynecology and Obstetrics* 1972; **135**: 113–126.

950 Van Winkle W, Hastings JC, Barker E, Hines D, Nichols W. Effect of suture materials on healing wounds. *Surgery, Gynecology and Obstetrics* 1975; **140**: 7–12.

951 Verges J, Jaupitre A. Cure de hernie inguinale par plaque metallique avec adenomectomie prostatique en seul temps:a propos de 7 cas. *Annals Urologie* 1973; **7**: 55–57.

952 Vohr BR, Rosenfield AG, Oh W. Umbilical hernia in low birthweight infants (less than 1,500 gm). *Journal of Pediatrics* 1977; **90**: 807–808.

953 Vowles KDJ. Intestinal complications of strangulated hernia. *British Journal of Surgery* 1959; **47**: 189–192.

954 Waddington RT. Femoral hernia: a recent appraisal. *British Journal of Surgery* 1971; **58**: 920–922.

955 Wagh PV, Leverich AP, Sun CN, White JH, Read RC. Direct inguinal herniation in man: a disease of collagen. *Journal of Surgical Research* 1974; **17**: 425–433.

956 Wagman ID, Barnhart GR, Sugerman HJ. Recurrent midline hernial repair. *Surgery, Gynecology and Obstetrics* 1985; **161**: 181–182.

957 Wakeley CPG. Obturator hernia: its aetiology, incidence and treatment with two personal operative cases. *British Journal of Surgery* 1939; **26**: 515–525.

958 Wakeley CPG. Treatment of certain types of external herniae. *Lancet* 1940; **1**: 822–826.

959 Wakeley C, Childs P. Spigelian hernia: hernia through the linea semilunaris. *Lancet* 1951; **1**: 1290–1291.

960 Walters GAB. A retropubic operation for femoral herniae. *British Journal of Surgery* 1965; **52**: 678–682.

961 Walton JM, Bass JA. Spigelian hernia in infants: reports of two cases. *Canadian Journal of Surgery* 1995; **38**: 95–96.

962 Wantz GE. Suture tension in Shouldice's hernioplasty. *Archives of Surgery* 1981; **116**: 1238–1239.

963 Wantz GE. Testicular atrophy as a risk of inguinal hernioplasty. *Surgery, Gynecology and Obstetrics* 1982; **154**: 570–571.

964 Wantz GE. Complications of inguinal hernia repair. *Surgical Clinics of North America* 1984; **64**: 287–298.

965 Wantz GE. The operation of Bassini as described by Attilio Catterina. *Surgery, Gynecology and Obstetrics* 1989; **168**: 67–80.

966 Wantz GE. Giant prosthetic replacement of the visceral sac. *Surgery, Gynecology and Obstetrics* 1989; **169**: 408–417.

967 Wantz GE. *Atlas of Hernia Surgery.* Raven Press, 1991.

968 Wantz GE. Testicular atrophy and chronic residual neuralgia as risks of inguinal hernioplasty. *Surgical Clinics of North America* 1993; **73**: 571–581.

969 Wara P, Sorensen K, Berg V. Proximal fecal diversion: Review of ten years experience. *Diseases of the Colon and Rectum* 1981; **24**: 114–119.

970 Watkins KM. Appendix abscess in a femoral hernia sac. *Post-Graduate Medical Journal* 1981; **57**: 306–307.

971 Watkins RM, Leach RD, Ellis H. Bilateral obturator herniae and associated femoral hernia. *Post-Graduate Medical Journal* 1981; **57**: 466.

972 Watson LF. *Hernia: Anatomy, Etiology, Symptoms, Diagnosis, Differential Diagnosis, Prognosis, and the Operative and Injection Treatment*, 2nd edn. London: Harry Kimpton, 1938.

973 Webster TR, Tracy TF. Groin hernias and hydroceles. In *Paediatric Surgery* 2nd ed. Eds Ashcraft KW, Holder TM. Philadelphia: WB Saunders, 1993; 562–570.

974 Wechsler R, Kurtz AB, Needleman L. Pictorial essay: cross-sectional imaging of abdominal wall hernias. *American Journal of Roentgenology* 1989; **153**: 517–521.

975 Weimer BR. Congenital inheritance of inguinal hernia. *Journal of Heredity* 1949; **40**: 219–220.

976 Wells CA. Hernia – incisional and umbilical. *Annals of the Royal College of Surgeons of England* 1956; **19**: 316–318.

977 Welsh DRJ. Sliding inguinal hernias. *Journal of Abdominal Surgery* 1964; **6**.

978 Welsh DRJ. The Shouldice Inguinal Repair. *Problems in General Surgery* 1995; **12**: 93–100.

979 Welsh DR, Alexander MA. The Shouldice Repair. *Surgical Clinics of North America* 1993; **73**: 451.

980 West LS. Two pedigrees showing inherited predisposition to hernia. *Journal of Heredity* 1936; **27**: 449–455.

981 Wheatley RG, Samaan AK. Postoperative pain relief. *British Journal of Surgery* 1995; **82**: 292–295.

982 Wheeler MH. Femoral hernia: analysis of the results of surgical treatment. *Proceedings of the Royal Society of Medicine* 1975; **68**: 177–178.

983 Whipple AO. The use of silk in the repair of clean wounds. *Annals of Surgery* 1933; **98**: 662–671.

984 White HJ, Sun CN, Read RC. Inguinal hernia: a true collagen disease. *Laboratory Investigations* 1977; **36**: 359.

985 Wijesinha SS. Inguinal hernia-the local experience. *Sri Lanka Journal of Surgery* 1991; **7**: 7–9.

986 Williams DI. Urology in childhood. In *Encyclopaedia of Urology*. New York, 1974.

987 Williams BT, Nicholl JP, Thomas KJ, Knowlenden J. Differences in duration of stay for surgery in the N.H.S. and private hospitals in England and Wales. *British Medical Journal* 1985; **290**: 978–980.

988 Williams JG, Etherington R, Hayward MWJ, Hughes LE. Para-ileostomy hernia: a clinical and radiological study. *British Journal of Surgery* 77: 1355–1357.

989 Williams M, Frankel S, Nanchalal K, Coast J, Donovan J. *Hernia Repair: Epidemiologically Based Needs Assessment*. Health Care Evaluation Unit, University of Bristol Print Services, 1992.

990 Winslet MC, Obeid ML, Kumar V. On-table pneumoperitoneum in the management of complicated incisional hernias. *Annals of the Royal College of Surgeons of England* 1993; **75**: 186–188.

991 Witherington R. Cryptorchism and approaches to its surgical management. *Surgical Clinics of North America* 1984; **64**: 367–384.

992 Wobbes T. Chrassords-Koops H, Oldhoff J. Relationship between testicular tumours, undescended testicles and inguinal hernias. *Journal of Surgical Oncology* 1980; **14**; 45–51.

993 Wolfe BM, Gardiner BN, Leary BF, Frey CF. Endoscopic cholecystecomy: an analysis of complications. *Archives of Surgery* 1991; **126**: 1192–1198.

994 Wolfler A. Zur radikaloperation des Freien Leistenbruches In *Beitr. Chir.* (Festchr. Geuidmet Theodor Billroth). Stuttgart: Hoffman, 1892; pp. 552–603.

995 Wolstenholme JT. Use of commercial Dacron fabric in the repair of inguinal hernias and abdominal wall defects. *Archives of Surgery* l956; **73**: 1004–1008.

996 Woods GE. Some observations on umbilical hernias in infants. *Archives of Disease in Childhood* 1953; **28**: 450–462.

997 Wright D, Baxter JN, O'Dwyer PJ. Effect of extraperitoneal insufflation on intraoperative blood gas and haemodynamic changes. *Surgical Endoscopy* 1995; **9**: 1169–1172.

998 Wright DM, Kennedy A, Baxter JN *et al.* Early outcome after open versus extraperitoneal endoscopic tension-free hernioplasty: A randomised clinical trial. *Surgery* 1996; **119**: 552–557.

999 Yavetz H, Harash B, Yogev L, Hamomnai ZT, Paz G. Fertility of men following inguinal hernia repair. *Andrologia* 1991; **23**: 443–446.

1000 Yeates WK. Pain in the scrotum *British Journal of Hospital Medicine* 1985; **133**: 101–104.

1001 Yip AWC, Ah Chong AK, Lam KH. Obturator hernia: A continuing diagnostic challenge. *Surgery* 1993; **113**: 266–269.

1002 Yordanov YS, Stoyanov SK. The incidence of hernia on the Island of Pemba. *East African Medical Journal* 1969; **46**: 687–691.

1003 Young D. Repair of epigastric incisional hernia. *British Journal of Surgery* 1961; **48**: 514–516.

1004 Zaman K, Taylor JD, Fossard DP. Femoral hernia in children. *Annals of the Royal College of Surgeons of England* 1985; **67**: 249–250.

1005 Zimmerman LM, Anson BJ. *Anatomy and Surgery of Hernia*, 2nd edn. Baltimore: Williams and Wilkins, 1967; pp. 216–227.

1006 Zimmerman LM, Anson BJ, Morgan EH, McVay CB. Ventral hernia due to normal banding of the abdominal muscles. *Surgery, Gynecology and Obstetrics* 1944; **78**: 535–540.

1007 Zimmerman LM, Laufman H. Sliding hernia. *Surgery, Gynecology and Obstetrics* 1942; **75**: 76–78.

1008 Zinanovic S. The anatomical basis for the high frequency of inguinal and femoral hernia in Uganda. *East African Medical Journal* 1968; **45**: 41–46.

1009 Zuckerkandl M. Hernia inflammata in Folge Typhilitis des Wormfortsatzes in einem Leistebruche. *Wiener Klinische Wodzenschrift* 1891; **4**: 305.

1010 Storling JR, Harms BA. The diagnosis and treatment of genito-femoral and ilio-inguinal neuralgia. *World Journal of Surgery* 1989; **13**: 586–591.

INDEX